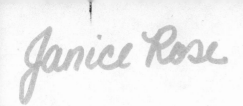

Women and Health
in America

WOMEN AND HEALTH IN AMERICA

Historical Readings

Edited by
JUDITH WALZER LEAVITT

The University of Wisconsin Press

Published 1984

The University of Wisconsin Press
114 North Murray Street
Madison, Wisconsin 53715

The University of Wisconsin Press, Ltd.
1 Gower Street
London WC1E 6HA, England

First printing

Printed in the United States of America

For LC CIP information see the colophon

ISBN 0-299-09640-8 cloth
ISBN 0-299-09644-0 paper

For
Lewis
T.L.

CONTENTS

Women and Health
in America

WOMEN AND HEALTH IN AMERICA:
AN OVERVIEW

During the past fifteen years a quiet revolution has taken place within the field of history, reflecting the activity of the women's movement and the sociopolitical context of our times as well as the growing sophistication of the discipline. The articles collected in this volume represent the best such scholarship in one area, women and health, and illustrate how the new studies can alter and enhance our understanding of life in the past. This recent scholarship emerged from three separate, but related, movements: the new social history, the new medical history, and modern feminism.

Social history developed in the 1920s and 1930s under the aegis of scholars like Arthur Schlesinger and Charles and Mary Beard, and it was characterized by an interest in the experiences of nonelites.[1] The new social history, a product of the 1960s, matured when scholars applied a more analytical approach to writing history, questioning why and how things happened the way they did and following new methodologies learned from the social sciences. Historians writing the new history sought to understand the relationship between people and society by analyzing the role of economic interests, power inequalities, cultural diversity, and sex differences and by applying quantitative tests to determine the validity and reliability of their observations. The study of women, one group among others forgotten under the more traditional history, burgeoned within social history.[2]

Historians of medicine adopted many techniques and perspectives from both the old and the new social history. Two scholars in particular, Richard Harrison Shryock and John B. Blake, early brought the topic of women in medicine under the new analysis. In a pivotal 1950 article, Shryock bridged the gap between the earlier narrative approach and the new methodologies. Writing on the subject of women physicians, Shryock analyzed the

social factors that influenced women's medical careers and celebrated women's achievements within the context of their struggles against discrimination. Blake, who had been a fellow at the Johns Hopkins Institute for the History of Medicine with Shryock, followed suit with another path-breaking article on women in medicine published in 1965.[3] Thus both social history and medical history had by the 1960s recognized the significance of studying the history of women and health from the new perspectives.[4]

The earliest "corrective" scholarship emanating from the influence of the feminist movement made its points with a political emphasis. Believing that historians had virtually ignored the study of women, scholars also identified a male conspiracy in the past against women. Two pamphlets by Barbara Ehrenreich and Deirdre English, *Witches, Midwives and Nurses* and *Complaints and Disorders: The Sexual Politics of Sickness* (1973), argued that male medicine had played a particularly onerous role in the oppression of women both as patients and within the health professions. These essays have been enormously influential, because the authors dared to be explicit in their accusations and because the omissions they pointed to were so flagrant. But the polemical nature of the conspiracy argument could not stand the test of time in a historical climate in which scholars have so successfully emphasized the interconnected nature of multiple factors in historical development. Women's historians, like Regina Markell Morantz, whose influential essay appears on pp. 239–45, were quick to criticize the early characterizations. Emphasizing the complexity of historical change and providing examples of women's unique cultural development, scholars are establishing that specific male influence was only one factor molding the shape of women's lives. Despite the limitations of the arguments about women as victims and men as oppressors, these interpretations have pointed to new directions and asked new questions that historians cannot now ignore.

Leading the response toward a more complex analysis, incorporating new social and medical history perspectives and methodologies, on the one hand, with a feminist understanding, on the other, were Charles Rosenberg and Carroll Smith-Rosenberg. (See pp. 12–27.) Writing together and separately in a series of articles, they successfully put to rest the impression that feminist history had to be polemical.[5] In the hands of such scholars, gender analysis, which focused on the cultural implications of gender dualisms and analyzed how the subordinate status of "other" in American society influenced women's lives, broadened our understanding of the past rather than narrowed it and made a major contribution to new conceptualizations. In addition to increasing the analytic component of historical scholarship, the change of emphasis altered the ways historians used their material. Whereas menstruation could have been a topic of interest to earlier medical historians seeking to understand the evolution of medical thinking, historians writing from the new perspectives analyzed medical theory of the menstrual cycle to shed light on the larger question of women's social and political subordination. Thus historians no longer accept the job as chroniclers of medicine's greatness, but increasingly use their scholarship to analyze critically directions in American history, to explain the forces that have influenced women's lives, and to uncover the motivations and interests that have produced change.

Perhaps the best way to understand the impact of the new historical writing is to compare it directly with what preceded it. During the 1940s historians showed some interest in the subject area of women and health. Scholars at that time concentrated on famous people and medical advances. Articles with titles like "Louisiana's Contributions to Obstetrics and Gynecology" (1948), "Grace Revere Osler: Her Influence on Men of Medicine" (1949), and "The First Woman Dentist, Lucy Hobbs Taylor, D.D.S. (1833–1910)" (1951) indicate the typical range of topics.[6] The early articles could be characterized as encompassing the "great lady" approach and the "great men conquering women's diseases" approach, both parallel to medicohistorical scholarship in general during the middle years

of the twentieth century. Historians struggled to identify significant people and to record major contributions of the past, and they saw as their job the documentation of the march of medical progress. Where women fit into this model, as when they were pioneers like Elizabeth Blackwell or wives of famous doctors like Grace Osler, they became relevant subjects for historical writing. Similarly, the male doctors who conquered women's health problems were likely targets of study. Historians today, as the articles in this book testify, have moved beyond this celebratory stage to more comprehensive analyses of the meaning of women's experiences.

Using a sample of four journals, the graph illustrates that both periods of interest in the history of women and health correspond to times of increased participation and visibility of women in American society.[7] Although men wrote most of the articles published during the 1940s, they were probably influenced by the cultural and patriotic value of women's World War II participation in areas previously dominated by men. Similarly, the second wave of American feminism since the late 1960s revitalized interest in women's history. This time, women themselves are writing many of the historical articles and are helping move scholarship in women's health history in new directions.

The articles in this collection, with two exceptions, were published since 1973, and they all represent the new trends.[8] The volume organizes the representative articles into two parts. The first half provides twenty articles on the health of women and examines the menstrual cycle, sexuality, birth control, childbirth, and women's diseases and treatments. The second half offers fifteen articles on women in the health occupations, including midwives, health reformers, physicians, and nurses. Most of the articles have been previously published; five appear here for the first time.

Both sections of this book address women's physical and mental capacities and analyze how perceptions of them have changed over time. Theory about what could be expected from women in large part determined how society and the medical profession defined and reacted to women's health problems. In the first half of the nineteenth century doctors learned that women's bodies were regulated by the uterus—the organ that Philadelphia physician Charles Meigs called the "disturb-

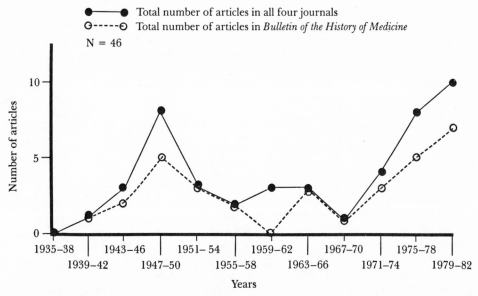

●————● Total number of articles in all four journals
◒-----◒ Total number of articles in *Bulletin of the History of Medicine*

N = 46

Number of articles on women and health in America appearing in *Bulletin of the History of Medicine, Journal of the History of Medicine and Allied Sciences, Journal of American History,* and *Journal of Social History* from 1935–1982.

ing radiator" of women's constitution—and their diagnoses frequently reverted solely to finding fault with the reproductive system.[9] As a result, when women tried to move into jobs outside the traditional domestic ones in the nineteenth century, they found the way blocked by the biological argument that their reproductive systems governed their lives and limited their capacity for other activity. The argument of women's limited physical and mental capacity and the centrality of reproduction for understanding women's bodies thus defined medical treatments and views of women's health and sickness and sustained traditional roles for women in the culture at large. As compelling as the "anatomy is destiny" conception was, however, biology's influence over women's lives was rarely total. Although most women did bear children, they were not perpetually confined by their bodies. American women participated widely in nondomestic and nonreproductive activity, providing factory and farm labor for America's burgeoning economy, creating active service organizations, and, as illustrated in this book, entering the professions in substantial numbers. Women's lives were influenced by their reproductive capacities, but physiology alone did not define womanhood.[10]

The two sections of this volume also address the question of women's control over their bodies and how this issue influenced women's health and women's participation in the health occupations. As today, women in the past wanted control over their bodies, and they went to extreme lengths at various times to get it. They actively sought birth control measures against the wishes of their husbands or religious advisers; they aborted, putting their lives in jeopardy with knitting needles and toxic substances; they used potentially dangerous drugs to alleviate their painful and out-of-control childbirths; and they did these things both as individuals and as members of organizations formed to increase women's power over their lives. How much control women wanted and what form it took varied from group to group and over time, but the issue was relevant to women's lives in the past as it remains today.

The essays in both sections of this volume examine women's questions in relation to medical history and medical questions in relation to women's history. The interrelationships between these two subfields of American history, both of which have independent existences and large bodies of literature, are significant. One without the other would produce lopsided perceptions of women's lives and health in the past. For example, women's medical education cannot be understood outside of the context of nineteenth-century women's lives and changing values. Medicine was one field among others that attracted women, and the attraction originated in women's traditional experiences. Similarly, the sexuality section of this book unites medical views about the relationship between sexual activity and health with the significant literature now available on sexual expression within women's sphere. Women's social and emotional network is central to understanding how women coped with their health problems together, but this female bonding itself can be understood only within an examination of women's physical lives and the forces that produced a female domestic culture. Women's history and medical history are thus inextricably connected; together they have the ability to open new windows on the past.

The field of the history of women and health as illustrated by the articles in this book is evolving. Much remains to be accomplished. While socioeconomic class, race, and ethnicity have been the focus of the new social history's analysis of the past, these factors have so far in the women-and-health historiography lagged behind historians' attempts to introduce the variable of gender. Today, though, historians of women and health recognize that gender is only one of many factors that need to be combined in a complex and multifaceted analysis of the process of historical experience and change. The biggest gap in this volume is the one created by the fact that historical study using the lens of race and class has not yet produced a significant body of literature on women and health.[11] My hopes are that a future edition of this reader would be able to add examples of this promising and unfulfilled area, so that the health of black, minority, and poor women can be addressed to correct what is here a too-strong emphasis on the health experiences of white, middle-class women. So too would the next edition benefit from the addition of more articles like the one here by Darlene Clark Hine (see pp. 497–506) on the unique struggles of black and minority women in the health professions. Similarly, the particular health problems of aging women need to be analyzed within the historical context, as do explorations of generational gaps among women in the health professions.[12] It is only by a thorough analysis of the experiences of all women that we can begin to understand the particular role played by gender and how this one variable interacted with others to shape the course of American history.

Some of the conclusions reached in this volume are still controversial, while others are by now widely accepted; some methodologies used in the articles will cause debate, others will not. The diversity, I think, reflects the struggles of a new field to find its métier and the excitement of new investigations and new investigators. Regardless of perspective, the scholars studying the history of women and health share a commitment to the inherent value of women's experiences. Whether historians approach the subject of women and health from a feminist perspective or because they found some interesting documents about women in the family attic, their contributions are valuable. The most useful criterion in sifting worthy from unworthy should be the author's ability to listen to the evidence within its contemporary framework. We must be faithful to the historical record, so that our generation and our children's generation can learn to use the past to improve the future.

I hope readers will like the diversity in this volume and will be able to find here represented writing that has personal as well as historical meaning. I also hope that this volume will illustrate that the new history with its analytical emphasis still knows how to tell a good story.

I want to thank the students in my course "Women and Health in American History" who have helped mold my conceptualization of the field. My colleagues in the History of Medicine Department and in the Women's Studies Program at the University of Wisconsin are enormously supportive of my teaching and research in the area of women and health. I especially want to thank Rima D. Apple, Ruth Bleier, Susan Friedman, Marjorie Klein, Diane Kravetz, Lewis Leavitt, Barbara Melosh, Ronald L. Numbers, and Mariamne Whatley for their suggestions, challenges, and help over the years. To the authors whose essays are included in this volume and the historians whose good work in the field could not be included because of space considerations, I owe a special debt. I have learned so much from them all, and their work has enriched my life both personally and professionally.

NOTES

1   Arthur M. Schlesinger, *New Viewpoints in American History* (1922) and Charles A. Beard and Mary R. Beard, *The Rise of American Civilization* (4 vols., 1927–1942). See also Schlesinger's edited 13-volume series *A History of American Life* published between 1926 and 1948 (with Dixon Ryan Fox).

2   See for example Samuel P. Hays, "A systematic social history," in *American History: Retrospect and Prospect*, ed. George Athan Billias and Gerald N. Grob (New York: Free Press, 1971).

3   Richard Harrison Shryock, "Women in American medicine," *Journal of the American Medical Women's Association*, 1950, *5:* 371–79; John B. Blake,"Women and medicine in ante-bellum America," *Bulletin of the History of Medicine*, 1965, *39:* 99–123.

4   For a history of medical history see Ronald L. Numbers, "The history of American medicine: a field in ferment," *Reviews in American History*, 1982, *10:* 243–63. See also Susan Reverby and David Rosner, "Beyond 'the great doctors,'" in their *Health Care in America: Essays in Social History* (Philadelphia: Temple University Press, 1979), 3–16.

5   In addition to "The female animal: medical and biological views of woman and her role in 19th-century America," reprinted in this volume, see Charles E. Rosenberg, "Sexuality, class and role in 19th-century America," *American Quarterly*, 1973, *25:* 131–53, and Carroll Smith-Rosenberg, "From puberty to menopause: the cycle of femininity in nineteenth-century America," *Clio's Consciousness Raised: New Perspectives on the History of Women*, ed. Mary Hartman and Lois V. Banner (New York: Harper Colophon Books, 1974), 23–37, and her "The hysterical women: sex roles and role conflict in 19th-century America," *Social Research*, 1972, *39:* 652–78.

6   Thomas Benton Sellers, "Louisiana's contributions to obstetrics and gynecology," *Bulletin of the History of Medicine*, 1948, *22:* 196–207; John F. Fulton, "Grace Revere Osler: her influence on men of medicine," ibid., 1949, *23:* 341–51; and Ralph W. Edwards, "The first woman dentist, Lucy Hobbs Taylor, D.D.S. (1833–1910)," ibid., 1951, *25:* 277–83.

7   I would like to thank Kathy Holtgraver for her help in collecting articles from the four journals, the *Bulletin of the History of Medicine* (1932–1982), *Journal of the History of Medicine and Allied Sciences* (1946–1982), *Journal of American History* (formerly *Mississippi Valley Historical Review*), 1913–1982, and the newer *Journal of Social History* (1967–1982). The *Bulletin of the History of Medicine* published three-quarters of the articles; other journals, such as the *Journal of Interdisciplinary History, American Quarterly, Signs*, and the *Journal of the American Medical Women's Association*, occasionally published articles in the field, but were not systematically reviewed here.

8   Readers should consult the bibliography, pp. 509–14, for a selected listing of articles and books in the field.

9   Charles Meigs, *Woman: Her Diseases and Remedies: A Series of Letters to His Class*, 3d ed. (Philadelphia: Blanchard and Lea, 1854).

10 Edward Shorter's *A History of Women's Bodies* (New York: Basic Books, 1982) argues that anatomy has been destiny for women in Western Europe and America. Shorter credits twentieth-century medical advances with freeing women from the physical sufferings that enslaved them earlier and permitting, among other things, the emergence of feminism.

11 Some scholars have addressed questions of race, ethnicity, and class. See Linda Gordon, *Woman's Body, Woman's Right: A Social History of Birth Control in America* (New York: Viking Books, 1976); Rima D. Apple, "Lillie Rosa Minoka-Hill (1876–1952)," *Women and Health*, 1979, *4:* 329–31; Edward Shorter and Phillips Cutright, "The effects of health on the completed fertility of nonwhite and white U.S. women born between 1867 and 1935," *Journal of Social History*, 1979, *13:* 191–217.

12 See, for example, Virginia G. Drachman, "Female solidarity and professional success: the dilemma of women doctors in late-nineteenth century America," *Journal of Social History* 15 (Summer 1982): 607–19.

PART I

THE HEALTH OF WOMEN

MENSTRUAL CYCLE

To many members of the medical profession in the nineteenth century, the reproductive life cycle, beginning with puberty and the onset of the menstrual cycle and ending with menopause and the years "beyond the reach of sexual storms," defined the productive boundaries of women's lives. The centrality of reproductive capability was almost overwhelming; it was, also, based on more than simple biological theory. The two articles in this section investigate the social context in which the theory of reproductive control thrived and posit some connections between the expanding directions of women's lives and medical reactions.

How women themselves reacted to their monthly menstrual periods and how these periodic episodes shaped women's activities and perceptions of themselves remain shrouded in the veils of modesty and privacy. Historical investigation has revealed women's strong opinion against Edward H. Clarke's theory that women could not simultaneously experience puberty and gain an education. But historians know far less about how women coped with their periods each month and how the lack of disposable sanitary napkins may have limited women's activity. How, for example, did Elizabeth Blackwell manage her menstrual periods when she attended an all-male medical school in 1848 and 1849, where her presence was required for long hours each day and where it must have been difficult to arrange for privacy and impossible to consult with another woman? We know of course, that she found a solution; but the personal costs involved in her pioneer triumph remain speculation. Similarly, how did women farm or factory workers contend with their long hours away from home? Not until after the post–World War I years, when nurses returning from the battlefields showed industry and women that the surplus bandages had a domestic use, did women have an easy way to collect and dispose of the monthly discharges. How did the difficulty of menstrual management affect women's lives in the past?

Whether or not women believed that their reproductive abilities controlled their life choices and set limits on their activities, the recurring insistence of the menstrual cycle influenced women's lives. The questions raised when historians begin to address the meaning of the menstrual cycle are interesting; answers to them should reveal the quality of life in the past in a new light. But because of the silence surrounding menstruation, historians will have to be inventive to uncover the missing data. Combinations of oral histories, histories of sanitary napkin companies, examinations of guides for girls, and study of women's personal diaries and letters will be needed to understand this important and pervasive dimension of women's lives.

1

The Female Animal: Medical and Biological Views of Woman and Her Role in Nineteenth-Century America

CARROLL SMITH-ROSENBERG AND CHARLES ROSENBERG

Since at least the time of Hippocrates and Aristotle, the roles assigned women have attracted an elaborate body of medical and biological justification. This was especially true in the nineteenth century as the intellectual and emotional centrality of science increased steadily. Would-be scientific arguments were used in the rationalization and legitimization of almost every aspect of Victorian life, and with particular vehemence in those areas in which social change implied stress in existing social arrangements.

This essay is an attempt to outline some of the shapes assumed by the nineteenth-century debate over the ultimate bases for women's domestic and childbearing role.[1] In form it resembles an exercise in the history of ideas; in intent it represents a hybrid with social and psychological history. Biological and medical views serve as a sampling device suggesting and illuminating patterns of social continuity, change, and tension.

The relationships between social change and social stress are dismayingly complex and recalcitrant to both psychological theorists and to the historian's normal modes of analysis. In an attempt to gain insight into these relationships the authors have chosen an analytic approach based on the study of normative descriptions of the female role at a time of widespread social change; not surprisingly emotion-laden attempts to reassert and redefine this role constitute one response to the stress induced by such social change.

CARROLL SMITH-ROSENBERG is Professor of History, University of Pennsylvania, Philadelphia, Pennsylvania.
CHARLES E. ROSENBERG is Professor of History, University of Pennsylvania, Philadelphia, Pennsylvania.
Reprinted with permission from *Journal of American History*, 60 (Sept., 1973), 332–356.

This approach was selected for a variety of reasons. Role definitions exist on a level of prescription beyond their embodiment in the individuality and behavior of particular historical persons. They exist rather as a formally agreed upon set of characteristics understood by and acceptable to a significant proportion of the population. As formally agreed upon social values they are, moreover, retrievable from historical materials and thus subject to analysis. Such social role definitions, however, have a more than platonic reality; for they exist as parameters with which and against which individuals must either conform or define their deviance. When inappropriate to social, psychological, or biological reality such definitions can themselves engender anxiety, conflict, and demands for change.

During the nineteenth century, economic and social forces at work within Western Europe and the United States began to compromise traditional social roles. Some women at least began to question—and a few to challenge overtly—their constricted place in society. Naturally enough, men hopeful of preserving existing social relationships, and in some cases threatened themselves both as individuals and as members of particular social groups, employed medical and biological arguments to rationalize traditional sex roles as rooted inevitably and irreversibly in the prescriptions of anatomy and physiology. This essay examines the ideological attack mounted by prestigious and traditionally minded men against two of the ways in which women expressed their dissatisfaction and desire for change: women's demands for improved educational opportunities and their decision to resort to birth control and abortion. That much of this often emotionally charged debate was oblique and couched in would-be scientific and medical language and metaphor makes it even more significant; for few spokesmen could explicitly and consciously confront those changes which impinged upon the bases of their particular emotional adjustment.

The Victorian woman's ideal social characteristics—nurturance, intuitive morality, domesticity, passivity, and affection—were all assumed to have a deeply rooted biological basis. These medical and scientific arguments formed an ideological system rigid in its support of tradition, yet infinitely flexible in the particular mechanisms which could be made to explain and legitimate woman's role.

Woman, nineteenth-century medical orthodoxy insisted, was starkly different from the male of the species. Physically, she was frailer, her skull smaller, her muscles more delicate. Even more striking was the difference between the nervous system of the two sexes. The female nervous system was finer, "more irritable," prone to overstimulation and resulting exhaustion. "The female sex," as one physician explained in 1827,

> is far more sensitive and susceptible than the male, and extremely liable to those distressing affections which for want of some better term, have been denominated nervous, and which consist chiefly in painful affections of the head, heart, side, and indeed, of almost every part of the system.[2]

"The nerves themselves," another physician concurred a generation later, "are smaller, and of a more delicate structure. They are endowed with greater sensibility, and, of course, are liable to more frequent and stronger impressions from external agents on mental influences."[3] Few if any questioned the assumption that in males the intellectual propensities of the brain dominated, while the female's nervous system and emotions prevailed over her conscious and rational faculties. Thus it was only natural, indeed inevitable, that women should be expected and permitted to display more affect than men; it was inherent in their very being.

Physicians saw woman as the product and prisoner of her reproductive system. It was the ineluctable basis of her social role and behavioral characteristics, the cause of her most common ailments; woman's uterus and ovaries controlled her body and behavior from puberty through menopause. The male reproductive system, male physi-

cians assured, exerted no parallel degree of control over man's body. Charles D. Meigs, a prominent Philadelphia gynecologist, stated with assurance in 1847 that a woman is "a moral, a sexual, a germiferous, gestative and parturient creature."[4] It was, another physician explained in 1870, "as if the Almighty, in creating the female sex, had taken the uterus and built up a woman around it."[5] A wise deity had designed woman as keeper of the hearth, as breeder and rearer of children.

Medical wisdom easily supplied hypothetical mechanisms to explain the interconnection between the female's organs of generation and the functioning of her other organs. The uterus, it was assumed, was connected to the central nervous system; shocks to the nervous system might alter the reproductive cycle—might even mark the gestating fetus—while changes in the reproductive cycle shaped emotional states. This intimate and hypothetical link between ovaries, uterus, and nervous system was the logical basis for the "reflex irritation" model of disease causation so popular in middle- and late-nineteenth century medical texts and monographs on psychiatry and gynecology. Any imbalance, exhaustion, infection, or other disorders of the reproductive organs could cause pathological reactions in parts of the body seemingly remote.[6] Doctors connected not only the paralyses and headaches of the hysteric to uterine disease but also ailments in virtually every part of the body. "These diseases," one physician explained, "will be found, on due investigation, to be in reality, no disease at all, but merely the sympathetic reaction or the symptoms of one disease, namely, a disease of the womb."[7]

Yet despite the commonsensical view that such ailments resulted from childbearing, physicians often contended that far greater difficulties could be expected in childless women. Motherhood was woman's normal destiny, and those females who thwarted the promise immanent in their body's design must expect to suffer. The maiden lady, many physicians argued, was fated to a greater incidence of both physical and emotional disease than her married sisters and to a shorter life span.[8] Her nervous system was placed under constant pressure, and her unfulfilled reproductive organs—especially at menopause—were prone to cancer and other degenerative ills.

Woman was thus peculiarly the creature of her

internal organs, of tidal forces she could not consciously control. Ovulation, the physical and emotional changes of pregnancy, even sexual desire itself were determined by internal physiological processes beyond the control or even the awareness of her conscious volition.[9] All women were prisoners of the cyclical aspects of their bodies, of the great reproductive cycle bounded by puberty and menopause, and by the shorter but recurrent cycles of childbearing and menstruation. All shaped her personality, her social role, her intellectual abilities and limitations; all presented as well possibly "critical" moments in her development, possible turning points in the establishment—or deterioration—of future physical and mental health. As the president of the American Gynecological Society stated in 1900: "Many a young life is battered and forever crippled in the breakers of puberty; if it crosses these unharmed and is not dashed to pieces on the rock of childbirth, it may still ground on the ever-recurring shallows of menstruation, and lastly, upon the final bar of the menopause ere protection is found in the unruffled waters of the harbor beyond the reach of sexual storms."[10]

Woman's physiology and anatomy, physicians habitually argued, oriented her toward an "inner" view of herself and her worldly sphere. (Logically enough, nineteenth-century views of heredity often assumed that the father was responsible for a child's external musculature and skeletal development, the mother for the internal viscera, the father for analytical abilities, the mother for emotions and piety.)[11] Their secret internal organs, women were told, determined their behavior; their concerns lay inevitably within the home.[12] In a passage strikingly reminiscent of some mid-twentieth-century writings, a physician in 1869 depicted an idealized female world, rooted in the female reproductive system, sharply limited socially and intellectually, yet offering women covert and manipulative modes of exercising power:

> Mentally, socially, spiritually, she is more interior than man. She herself is an interior part of man, and her love and life are always something interior and incomprehensible to him. . . . Woman is to deal with domestic affections and uses, not with philosophies and sciences. . . . She is priest, not king. The house, the chamber, the closet, are the centres

of her social life and power, as surely as the sun is the centre of the solar system. . . . Another proof of the interiority of woman, is the wonderful secretiveness and power of dissimulation which she possesses. . . . Woman's secrecy is not cunning; her dissimulation is not fraud. They are intuitions or spiritual perceptions, full of tact and wisdom, leading her to conceal or reveal, to speak or be silent, to do or not to do, exactly at the right time and in the right place.[13]

The image granted women in these hypothetical designs was remarkably consistent with the social role traditionally allotted them. The instincts connected with ovulation made her by nature gentle, affectionate, and nurturant. Weaker in body, confined by menstruation and pregnancy, she was both physically and economically dependent upon the stronger, more forceful male, whom she necessarily looked up to with admiration and devotion.

Such stylized formulae embodied, however, a characteristic yet entirely functional ambiguity. The Victorian woman was more spiritual than man, yet less intellectual, closer to the divine, yet prisoner of her most animal characteristics, more moral than man, yet less in control of her very morality. While the sentimental poets placed woman among the angels and doctors praised the transcendent calling of her reproductive system, social taboos made woman ashamed of menstruation, embarrassed and withdrawn during pregnancy, self-conscious and purposeless during and after menopause. Her body, which so inexorably defined her personality and limited her role, appeared to woman often degrading and confining.[14] The very romantic rhetoric which tended to suffocate nineteenth-century discussions of femininity only underlined with irony the distance between behavioral reality and the forms of conventional ideology.

The nature of the formalistic scheme implied as well a relationship between the fulfilling of its true calling and ultimate social health. A woman who lived "unphysiologically"—and she could do so by reading or studying in excess, by wearing improper clothing, by long hours of factory work, or by a sedentary, luxurious life—could produce only weak and degenerate offspring. Until the twentieth century, it was almost universally assumed that acquired characteristics in the form of damage from disease and improper life-styles in parents would be transmitted through heredity; a nervous and debilitated mother could have only nervous, dyspeptic, and undersized children.[15] Thus appropriate female behavior was sanctioned not only by traditional injunctions against individual sin in the form of inappropriate and thus unnatural modes of life but also by the higher duty of protecting the transcendent good of social health, which could be maintained only through the continued production of healthy children. Such arguments were to be invoked with increasing frequency as the nineteenth century progressed.

In mid-nineteenth-century America it was apparent that women—or at least some of them—were growing dissatisfied with traditional roles. American society in mid-nineteenth century was committed—at least formally—to egalitarian democracy and evangelical piety. It was thus a society which presumably valued individualism, social and economic mobility, and free will. At the same time it was a society experiencing rapid economic growth, one in which an increasing number of families could think of themselves as middle class and could seek a life-style appropriate to that station. At least some middle-class women, freed economically from the day-to-day struggle for subsistence, found in these values a motivation and rationale for expanding their roles into areas outside the home. In the Jacksonian crusades for piety, for temperance, for abolition, and in pioneering efforts to aid the urban poor, women played a prominent role, a role clearly outside the confines of the home. Women began as well to demand improved educational opportunities—even admission to colleges and medical schools. A far greater number began, though more covertly, to see family limitation as a necessity if they would preserve health, status, economic security and individual autonomy.

Only a handful of nineteenth-century American women made a commitment to overt feminism and to the insecurity and hostility such a commitment implied. But humanitarian reform, education, and birth control were all issues which presented themselves as real alternatives to every respectable churchgoing American woman.[16] Contemporary medical and biological arguments identified, reflected, and helped to eliminate two of these threats to traditional role definitions: demands by women for higher education and family limitation.

Since the beginnings of the nineteenth-century, American physicians and social commentators generally had feared that American women were physically inferior to their English and Continental sisters. The young women of the urban middle and upper classes seemed in particular less vigorous, more nervous than either their own grandmothers or European contemporaries. Concern among physicians, educators, and publicists over the physical deterioration of American womanhood grew steadily during the nineteenth century and reached a high point in its last third.

Many physicians were convinced that education was a major factor in bringing about this deterioration, especially education during puberty and adolescence. It was during these years that the female reproductive system matured, and it was this process of maturation that determined the quality of the children which American women would ultimately bear. During puberty, orthodox medical doctrine insisted, a girl's vital energies must be devoted to development of the reproductive organs. Physicians saw the body as a closed system possessing only a limited amount of vital force; energy expended in one area was necessarily removed from another. The girl who curtailed brain work during puberty could devote her body's full energy to the optimum development of its reproductive capacities. A young woman, however, who consumed her vital force in intellectual activities was necessarily diverting these energies from the achievement of true womanhood. She would become weak and nervous, perhaps sterile, or more commonly, and in a sense more dangerously for society, capable of bearing only sickly and neurotic children—children able to produce only feebler and more degenerate versions of themselves.[17] The brain and ovary could not develop at the same time. Society, midcentury physicians warned, must protect the higher good of racial health by avoiding situations in which adolescent girls taxed their intellectual faculties in academic competition. "Why," as one physician pointedly asked, "spoil a good mother by making an ordinary grammarian?"[18]

Yet where did America's daughters spend these years of puberty and adolescence, doctors asked, especially the daughters of the nation's most virtuous and successful middle-class families? They spent these years in schools; they sat for long hours each day bending over desks, reading thick books, competing with boys for honors. Their health and that of their future children would be inevitably marked by the consequences of such unnatural modes of life.[19] If such evils resulted from secondary education, even more dramatically unwholesome was the influence of higher education upon the health of those few women intrepid enough to undertake it. Yet their numbers increased steadily, especially after a few women's colleges were established in the East and state universities in the Midwest and Pacific Coast began cautiously to accept coeducation. Women could now, critics agonized, spend the entire period between the beginning of menstruation and the maturation of their ovarian systems in nerve-draining study. Their adolescence, as one doctor pointed out, contrasted sadly with those experienced by healthier, more fruitful forebears: "Our great-grandmothers got their schooling during the winter months and let their brains lie fallow for the rest of the year. They knew less about Euclid and the classics than they did about housekeeping and housework. But they made good wives and mothers, and bore and nursed sturdy sons and buxom daughters and plenty of them at that."[20]

Constant competition among themselves and with the physically stronger males disarranged the coed's nervous system, leaving her anxious, prey to hysteria and neurasthenia. One gynecologist complained as late as 1901:

> the nervous force, so necessary at puberty for the establishment of the menstrual function, is wasted on what may be compared as trifles to perfect health, for what use are they without health? The poor sufferer only adds another to the great army of neurasthenia and sexual incompetents, which furnish neurologists and gynecologists with so much of their material . . . bright eyes have been dulled by the brain-fag and sweet temper transformed into irritability, crossness and hysteria, while the womanhood of the land is deteriorating physically.
>
> She may be highly cultured and accomplished and shine in society, but her future husband will discover too late that he has married a large outfit of headaches, backaches and spine aches, instead of a woman fitted to take up the duties of life.[21]

Such speculations exerted a strong influence upon educators, even those connected with institutions which admitted women. The state universities, for example, often prescribed a lighter course load for females or refused to permit women admission to regular degree programs. "Every physiologist is well aware," the Regents of the University of Wisconsin explained in 1877, "that at stated times, nature makes a great demand upon the energies of early womanhood and that at these times great caution must be exercised lest injury be done. . . . Education is greatly to be desired," the Regents concluded:

> but it is better that the future matrons of the state should be without a University training than that it should be produced at the fearful expense of ruined health; better that the future mothers of the state should be robust, hearty, healthy women, than that, by over study, they entail upon their descendants the germs of disease.[22]

This fear for succeeding generations born of educated women was widespread. "We want to have body as well as mind," one commentator noted, "otherwise the degeneration of the race is inevitable."[23] Such transcendent responsibilities made the individual woman's personal ambitions seem trivial indeed.

One of the remedies suggested by both educators and physicians lay in tempering the intensely intellectualistic quality of American education with a restorative emphasis on physical education. Significantly, health reformers' demands for women's physical education were ordinarily justified not in terms of freeing the middle-class woman from traditional restrictions on bodily movement, but rather as upgrading her ultimate maternal capacities. Several would-be physiological reformers called indeed for active participation in housecleaning as an ideal mode of physical culture for the servant-coddled American girl. Bed making, clothes scrubbing, sweeping, and scouring provided a varied and highly appropriate regimen.[24]

Late-nineteenth-century women physicians, as might have been expected, failed ordinarily to share the alarm of their male colleagues when contemplating the dangers of coeducation. No one, a female physician commented sardonically, worked harder or in unhealthier conditions than the washerwoman; yet, would-be saviors of American womanhood did not inveigh against this abuse—washing, after all, was appropriate work for women. Women doctors often did agree with the general observation that their sisters were too frequently weak and unhealthy; however, they blamed not education or social activism but artificialities of dress and slavery to fashion, aspects of the middle-class woman's life-style which they found particularly demeaning. "The fact is that girls and women can bear study," Alice Stockham explained, "but they cannot bear compressed viscera, tortured stomachs and displaced uterus," the results of fashionable clothing and an equally fashionable sedentary life. Another woman physician, Sarah Stevenson, wrote in a similar vein: "'How do I look?' is the everlasting story from the beginning to the end of woman's life. Looks, not books, are the murderers of American women."[25]

Even more significant than this controversy over woman's education was a parallel debate focusing on the questions of birth control and abortion. These issues affected not a small percentage of middle- and upper-middle-class women, but all men and women. It is one of the great and still largely unstudied realities of nineteenth-century social history. Every married woman was immediately affected by the realities of childbearing and child rearing. Though birth control and abortion had been practiced, discussed—and reprobated—for centuries, the mid-nineteenth century saw a dramatic increase in concern among spokesmen for the ministry and medical profession.[26]

Particularly alarming was the casualness, doctors charged, with which seemingly respectable wives and mothers contemplated and undertook abortions, and how routinely they practiced birth control. One prominent New York gynecologist complained in 1874 that well-dressed women walked into his consultation room and asked for abortions as casually as they would for a cut of beefsteak at their butcher.[27] In 1857, the American Medical Association nominated a special committee to report on the problem; then appointed another in the 1870s; between these dates and especially in the late 1860s, medical societies throughout the country passed resolutions attacking the prevalence of abortion and birth control and condemning physicians who performed and condoned such illicit practices. Nevertheless, abortions could in the 1870s

be obtained in Boston and New York for as little as ten dollars, while abortifacients could be purchased more cheaply or through the mail. Even the smallest villages and rural areas provided a market for the abortionist's services; women often aborted any pregnancy which occurred in the first few years of marriage. The Michigan Board of Health estimated in 1898 that one-third of all the state's pregnancies ended in abortion. From 70 to 80 percent of these were secured, the board contended, by prosperous and otherwise respectable married women who could not offer even the unmarried mother's "excuse of shame."[28] By the 1880s, English medical moralists could refer to birth control as the "American sin" and warn against England's women following in the path of America's faithless wives.[29]

So general a phenomenon demands explanation. The only serious attempts to explain the prevalence of birth control in this period have emphasized the economic motivations of those practicing it—the need in an increasingly urban, industrial, and bureaucratized society to limit numbers of children so as to provide security, education, and inheritance for those already brought into the world. As the nineteenth century progressed, it has been argued, definitions of appropriate middle-class life-styles dictated a more and more expansive pattern of consumption, a pattern—especially in an era of recurring economic instability—particularly threatening to those large numbers of Americans only precariously members of the secure economic classes. The need to limit offspring was a necessity if family status was to be maintained.[30]

Other aspects of nineteenth-century birth control have received much less historical attention. One of these needs only to be mentioned for it poses no interpretative complexities; this was the frequency with which childbirth meant for women pain and often lingering incapacity. Death from childbirth, torn cervixes, fistulae, prolapsed uteri were widespread "female complaints" in a period when gynecological practice was still relatively primitive and pregnancy every few years common indeed. John Humphrey Noyes, perhaps the best-known advocate of family planning in nineteenth-century America, explained poignantly why he and his wife had decided to practice birth control in the 1840s:

The [decision] was occasioned and even forced upon me by very sorrowful experiences. In the course of six years my wife went through the agonies of five births. Four of them were premature. Only one child lived. . . . After our last disappointment, I pledged my word to my wife that I would never again expose her to such fruitless suffering.[31]

The Noyeses' experience was duplicated in many homes. Young women were simply terrified of having children.[32]

Such fears, of course, were not peculiar to nineteenth-century America. The dangers of disability and death consequent upon childbirth extended back to the beginning of time, as did the anxiety and depression so frequently associated with pregnancy. What might be suggested, however, was that economic and technological changes in society added new parameters to the age-old experience. Family limitation for economic and social reasons now appeared more desirable to a growing number of husbands; it was, perhaps, also, more technically feasible. Consequently married women could begin to consider, probably for the first time, alternative life-styles to that of multiple pregnancies extending over a third of their lives. Women could begin to view the pain and bodily injury which resulted from such pregnancies not simply as a condition to be borne with fatalism and passivity, but as a situation that could be avoided. It is quite probable, therefore, that, in this new social context, increased anxiety and depression would result once a woman, in part at least voluntarily, became pregnant. Certainly, it could be argued, such fears must have altered women's attitudes toward sexual relations generally. Indeed the decision to practice birth control must necessarily have held more than economic and status implications for the family; it must have become an element in the fabric of every marriage's particular psychosexual reality.[33]

A third and even more ambiguous aspect of the birth control controversy in nineteenth-century America relates to the way in which attitudes toward contraception and abortion reflected role conflict within the family. Again and again, from the 1840s on, defenders of family planning—including individuals as varied and idealistic as Noyes

and Stockham, on the one hand, and assorted quack doctors and peddlers of abortifacients, on the other—justified their activities not in economic terms, but under the rubric of providing women with liberty and autonomy. Woman, they argued with remarkable unanimity, must control her own body; without this she was a slave not only to the sexual impulses of her husband but also to endless childbearing and rearing. "Woman's equality in all the relations of life," a New York physician wrote in 1866, "implies her absolute supremacy in the sexual relation. . . . it is her absolute and indefeasible right to determine when she will and when she will not be exposed to pregnancy." "God and Nature," another physician urged, "have given to the female the complete control of her own person, so far as sexual congress and reproduction are concerned."[34] The assumption of all these writers was clear and unqualified: women, if free to do so, would choose to have sexual relations less frequently, and to have far fewer pregnancies.

Implied in these arguments as well were differences as to the nature and function of sexual intercourse. Was its principal and exclusively justifiable function, as conservative physicians and clergymen argued, the procreation of children, or could it be justified as an act of love, of tenderness between individuals? Noyes argued that the sexual organs had a social, amative function, separable from their reproductive function. Sex was justifiable as an essential and irreplaceable form of human affection; no man could demand this act unless it was freely given.[35] Nor could it be freely given in many cases unless effective modes of birth control were available to assuage the woman's anxieties. A man's wife was not his chattel, to be violated at will, and forced—ultimately—to bear unwanted and thus almost certainly unhealthy children.

Significantly, defenders of women's right to limit childbearing employed many of the same arguments used by conservatives to attack women's activities outside the home; all those baleful hereditary consequences threatened by overeducation were seen by birth control advocates as resulting from the bearing of children by women unwilling and unfit for the task, their vital energies depleted by excessive childbearing. A child, they argued, carried to term by a woman who desired only its death could not develop normally; such children proved inevitably a source of physical and emotional degeneracy. Were women relieved from such accustomed pressures, they could produce fewer but better offspring.[36]

Many concerned mid-nineteenth-century physicians, clergymen, and journalists failed to accept such arguments. They emphasized instead the unnatural and thus necessarily deleterious character of any and all methods of birth control and abortion. Even coitus interruptus, obviously the most common mode of birth control in this period, was attacked routinely as a source of mental illness, nervous tension, and even cancer. This was easily demonstrated. Sex, like all aspects of human bodily activity, involved an exchange of nervous energy; without the discharge of such accumulated energies in the male orgasm and the soothing presence of the male semen "bathing the female reproductive organs," the female partner could never, the reassuring logic ran, find true fulfillment. The nervous force accumulated and concentrated in sexual excitement would build up dangerous levels of undischarged energy, leading ultimately to a progressive decay in the unfortunate woman's physical and mental health. Physicians warned repeatedly that condoms and diaphragms—when the latter became available after midcentury—could cause an even more startlingly varied assortment of ills. In addition to the mechanical irritation they promoted, artificial methods of birth control increased the lustful impulse in both partners, leading inevitably to sexual excess. The resultant nervous exhaustion induced gynecological lesions, and then through "reflex irritation" caused such ills as loss of memory, insanity, heart disease, and even "the most repulsive nymphomania."[37]

Conservative physicians similarly denounced the widespread practice of inserting sponges impregnated with supposedly spermicidal chemicals into the vagina immediately before or after intercourse. Such practices, they warned, guaranteed pelvic injury, perhaps sterility. Even if a woman seemed in good health despite a history of practicing birth control, a Delaware physician explained in 1873 that "as soon as this vigor commences to decline . . . about the fortieth year, the disease [cancer] grows as the energies fail—the cancerous fangs penetrating deeper and deeper until, after excruciating suffering, the writhing victim is yielded up to its terrible embrace."[38] Most importantly, this argument followed, habitual attempts at contra-

ception meant—even if successful—a mother permanently injured and unable to bear healthy children. If unsuccessful, the children resulting from such unnatural matings would be inevitably weakened. And if such grave ills resulted from the practice of birth control, the physical consequences of abortion were even more dramatic and immediate.[39]

Physicians often felt little hesitation in expressing what seems to the historian a suspiciously disproportionate resentment toward such unnatural females. Unnatural was of course the operational word; for woman's presumed maternal instinct made her primarily responsible for decisions in regard to childbearing.[40] So frequent was this habitual accusation that some medical authors had to caution against placing the entire weight of blame for birth control and abortion upon the woman; men, they reminded, played an important role in most such decisions.[41] In 1871, for example, the American Medical Association Committee on Criminal Abortion described women who patronized abortionists in terms which conjured up fantasies of violence and punishment:

> She becomes unmindful of the course marked out for her by Providence, she overlooks the duties imposed on her by the marriage contract. She yields to the pleasures—but shrinks from the pains and responsibilities of maternity; and, destitute of all delicacy and refinement, resigns herself, body and soul, into the hands of unscrupulous and wicked men. Let not the husband of such a wife flatter himself that he possesses her affection. Nor can she in turn ever merit even the respect of a virtuous husband. She sinks into old age like a withered tree, stripped of its foliage; with the stain of blood upon her soul, she dies without the hand of affection to smooth her pillow.[42]

The frequency with which attacks on family limitation in mid-nineteenth-century America were accompanied by polemics against expanded roles for the middle-class woman indicates with unmistakable clarity something of one of the motives structuring such jeremiads. Family limitation necessarily added a significant variable within conjugal relationships generally; its successful practice implied potential access for women to new roles and a new autonomy.

Nowhere is this hostility toward women and the desire to inculcate guilt over women's desire to avoid pregnancy more strikingly illustrated than in the warnings of "race suicide" so increasingly fashionable in the late nineteenth century. A woman's willingness and capacity to bear children was a duty she owed not only to God and husband but to her "race" as well.[43] In the second half of the nineteenth century, articulate Americans forced to evaluate and come to emotional terms with social change became, like many of their European contemporaries, attracted to a world view which saw racial identity and racial conflict as fundamental. And within these categories, birthrates became all-important indices to national vigor and thus social health.

In 1860 and again in 1870, Massachusetts census returns began to indicate that the foreign born had a considerably higher birthrate than that of native Americans. Indeed, the more affluent and educated a family, the fewer children it seemed to produce. Such statistics indicated that native Americans in the Bay State were not even reproducing themselves. The social consequences seemed ominous indeed.

The Irish, though barely one-quarter of the Massachusetts population, produced more than half of the state's children. "It is perfectly clear," a Boston clergyman contended in 1884, "that without a radical change in the religious ideas, education, habits, and customs of the natives, the present population and their descendants will not rule that state a single generation."[44] A few years earlier a well-known New England physician, pointing to America's still largely unsettled western territories, had asked: "Shall they be filled by our own children or by those of aliens? This is a question that our own women must answer; upon their loins depends the future destiny of the nation." Native-born American women had failed themselves as individuals and society as mothers of the Anglo-Saxon race. If matters continued for another half-century in the same manner, "the wives who are to be mothers in our republic must be drawn from trans-Atlantic homes. The Sons of the New World will have to re-act, on a magnificent scale, the old story of unwived Rome and the Sabines."[45]

Such arguments have received a goodly amount of historical attention, especially as they figured in the late nineteenth and early twentieth centuries as part of the contemporary rationale for immigration restriction.[46] Historians have interpreted the race suicide argument in several fashions. As an incident in a general Western acceptance of racism, it has been seen as product of a growing alienation of the older middle and upper classes in the face of industrialization, urbanization, and bureaucratization of society. More specifically, some American historians have seen these race suicide arguments as rooted in the fears and insecurities of a traditionally dominant middle class as it perceived new and threatening social realities.

Whether or not historians care to accept some version of this interpretation—and certainly such motivational elements seem to be suggested in the rhetorical formulae employed by many of those bemoaning the failure of American Protestants to reproduce in adequate numbers—it ignores another element crucial to the logical and emotional fabric of those arguments. This is the explicit charge of female sexual failure. To a significant extent, contemporaries saw the problem as in large measure woman's responsibility; it was America's potential mothers, not its fathers, who were primarily responsible for the impending social cataclysm. Race suicide seemed a problem in social gynecology.

Though fathers played a necessary role in procreation, medical opinion emphasized that it was the mother's constitution and reproductive capacity which most directly shaped her offspring's physical, mental, and emotional attributes. And any unhealthy mode of life—anything in short which seemed undesirable to contemporary medical moralists, including both education and birth control—might result in a woman's becoming sterile or capable of bearing only stunted offspring. Men, it was conceded, were subject to vices even more debilitating, but the effects of male sin and imprudence were, physicians felt, "to a greater extent confined to adult life; and consequently do not, to the same extent, impair the vitality of our race or threaten its physical destruction." Women's violation of physiological laws implied disaster to "the unborn of both sexes."[47]

Though such social critics tended to agree that woman was at fault, they expressed some difference of opinion as to the nature of her guilt. A few felt that lower birthrates could be attributed simply to the conscious and culpable decision of American women to curtail family size. Other physicians and social commentators, while admitting that many women felt little desire for children, saw the roots of the problem in somewhat different—and perhaps even more apocalyptic—terms. It was not, they feared, simply the conscious practice of family limitation which resulted in small families; rather the increasingly unnatural life-style of the "modern American woman" had undermined her reproductive capacities so that even when she would, she could not bear adequate numbers of healthy children. Only if American women returned to the simpler life-styles of the eighteenth and early nineteenth centuries could the race hope to regain its former vitality; women must from childhood see their role as that of robust and self-sacrificing mothers. If not, their own degeneration and that of the race were inevitable.

Why the persistence and intensity of this masculine hostility, of its recurring echoes of conflict, rancor, and moral outrage? There are at least several possible, though by no means exclusive, explanations. One centers on the hostility implied and engendered by the sexual deprivation—especially for the male—implicit in many of the modes of birth control employed at this time. One might, for example, speculate—as Oscar Handlin did some years ago—that such repressed middle-class sexual energies were channeled into a xenophobic hostility toward the immigrant and the black and projected into fantasies incorporating the enviable and fully expressed sexuality of these alien groups.[48] A similar model could be applied to men's attitudes toward women as well; social, economic, and sexual tensions which beset late-nineteenth-century American men might well have caused them to express their anxieties and frustrations in terms of hostility toward the middle-class female.[49]

Such interpretations are, however, as treacherous as they are inviting. Obviously, the would-be scientific formulations outlined here mirror something of postbellum social and psychic reality. Certainly some middle-class men in the late nineteenth century had personality needs—sexual inadequacies or problems of status identification—which made traditional definitions of gender roles functional to them. The hostility, even the violent imagery expressed toward women who chose to limit the number of children they bore indicates a sig-

nificant personal and emotional involvement on the part of the male author. Some women, moreover, obviously used the mechanisms of birth control and, not infrequently, sexual rejection as role-sanctioned building blocks in the fashioning of their particular adjustment. Their real and psychic gains were numerous: surcease from fear and pain, greater leisure, a socially acceptable way of expressing hostility, and a means of maintaining some autonomy and privacy in a life which society demanded be devoted wholeheartedly to the care and nurturance of husband and children. Beyond such statements, however, matters become quite conjectural. At this moment in the development of both historical methodology and psychological theory great caution must be exercised in the development of such hypotheses—especially since the historians of gender and sexual behavior have at their disposal data which from a psychodynamic point of view are at best fragmentary and suggestive.[50]

What the nineteenth-century social historian can hope to study with a greater degree of certainty, however, is the way in which social change both caused and reflected tensions surrounding formal definitions of gender roles. Obviously, individuals as individuals at all times and in all cultures have experienced varying degrees of difficulty in assimilating the prescription of expected role behavior. When such discontinuities begin to affect comparatively large numbers and become sufficiently overt as to evoke a marked ideological response one can then speak with assurance of having located fundamental cultural tension.[51]

Students of nineteenth-century American and Western European society have long been aware of the desire of a growing number of women for a choice among roles different from the traditional one of mother and housekeeper. It was a theme of Henry James, Henrik Ibsen, and a host of other, perhaps more representative if less talented, writers. Women's demands ranged from that of equal pay for equal work and equal education for equal intelligence to more covert demands for abortion, birth control information, and sexual autonomy within the marriage relationship. Their demands paralleled and were in large part dependent upon fundamental social and economic developments. Technological innovation and economic growth, changed patterns of income distribution, population concentrations, demographic changes in terms of life expectancy and fertility all affected woman's behavior and needs. Fewer women married; many were numbered among the urban poor. Such women had to become self-supporting and at the same time deal with the changed self-image that self-support necessitated. Those women who married generally did so later, had fewer children, and lived far beyond the birth of their youngest child. At the same time ideological developments began to encourage both men and women to aspire to increased independence and self-fulfillment. All these factors interacted to create new ambitions and new options for American women. In a universe of varying personalities and changing economic realities, it was inevitable that some women at least would—overtly or covertly—be attracted by such options and that a goodly number of men would find such choices unacceptable. Certainly for the women who did so the normative role of home-bound nurturant and passive woman was no longer appropriate or functional, but became a source of conflict and anxiety.

It was inevitable as well that many men, similarly faced with a rapidly changing society, would seek in domestic peace and constancy a sense of the continuity and security so difficult to find elsewhere in their society. They would—at the very least—expect their wives, their daughters, and their family relationships generally to remain unaltered. When their female dependents seemed ill disposed to do so, such men responded with a harshness sanctioned increasingly by the new gods of science.

NOTES

1   For historical studies of women's role and ideological responses to it in nineteenth-century America, see William L. O'Neill, *Everyone Was Brave: The Rise and Fall of Feminism in America* (Chicago, 1969); William Wasserstrom, *Heiress of All the Ages: Sex and Sentiment in the Victorian Tradition* (Minneapolis, 1959); Eleanor Flexner, *Century of Struggle: The Woman's Rights Movement in the United States* (New York, 1968); Aileen S. Kraditor, *The Ideas of the Woman Suffrage Movement, 1890–1920* (New York, 1965). For studies emphasizing the interaction between social change and sex role conflict, see Carroll Smith-Rosenberg, "Beauty, the Beast and the militant woman: a case study in sex roles and social stress in Jacksonian America," *American Quarterly* (Oct. 1971):562–84; Carroll Smith-Rosenberg, "The hysterical woman: sex roles and role conflict in 19th-century America," *Social Research* 39 (Winter 1972): 652–78. The problem of sexuality in the English-speaking world has been a particular subject of historical concern. Among the more important, if diverse, attempts to deal with this problem are Peter T. Cominos, "Late-Victorian sexual respectability and the social system," *International Review of Social History,* 1963, *8:* 18–48, 216–50; Stephen Nissenbaum, "Careful love: Sylvester Graham and the emergence of Victorian sexual theory in America, 1830–1840," Ph.D. diss., University of Wisconsin, 1968; Graham J. Barker-Benfield, "The Horrors of the Half Known Life: Aspects of the Exploitation of Women by Men," Ph.D. diss., University of California, Los Angeles, 1968; Nathan G. Hale, Jr., *Freud and the Americans: The Beginnings of Psychoanalysis in the United States, 1876–1917* (New York, 1971), 24–

46; David M. Kennedy, *Birth Control in America: The Career of Margaret Sanger* (New Haven, 1970), 36–71; Steven Marcus, *The Other Victorians: A Study of Sexuality and Pornography in Mid-Nineteenth-Century England* (New York, 1966). See also Charles E. Rosenberg, "Sexuality, class and role in 19th-Century America," *American Quarterly,* 25 (May 1973): 131–54.

2   Marshall Hall, *Commentaries on Some of the More Important of the Diseases of Females,* in three parts (London, 1827), 2. Although this discussion centers on the nineteenth century, it must be understood that these formulations had a far longer pedigree.

3   Stephen Tracy, *The Mother and Her Offspring* (New York, 1860), xv; William Goodell, *Lessons in Gynecology* (Philadelphia, 1879), 332; William B. Carpenter, *Principles of Human Physiology: With Their Chief Applications to Pathology, Hygiène, and Forensic Medicine,* 4th ed. (Philadelphia, 1850), 727. In mid-nineteenth century many of these traditional views of woman's peculiar physiological characteristics were restated in terms of the currently fashionable phrenology. For example, see Thomas L. Nichols, *Woman, in All Ages and Nations: A Complete and Authentic History of the Manners and Customs, Character and Condition of the Female Sex in Civilized and Savage Countries, from the Earliest Ages to the Present Time* (New York, ca. 1849), xi.

4   Charles D. Meigs, *Lecture on Some of the Distinctive Characteristics of the Female, Delivered before the Class of the Jefferson Medical College, January 5, 1847* (Philadelphia, 1847), 5.

5   M. L. Holbrook, *Parturition without Pain: A Code of Directions for Escaping from the Primal Curse* (New York,

1882), 14–15. See also Edward H. Dixon, *Woman, and her Diseases, from the Cradle to the Grave: Adapted Exclusively to Her Instruction in the Physiology of Her System, and All the Diseases of Her Critical Periods* (New York, 1846), 17; M. K. Hard, *Woman's Medical Guide: Being a Complete Review of the Peculiarities of the Female Constitution and the Derangement to Which It Is Subject, with a Description of Simple Yet Certain Means for Their Cure* (Mt. Vernon, Ohio, 1848), 11.

6 In the hypothetical pathologies of these generations, the blood was often made to serve the same function as that of the nerves; it could cause general ills to have local manifestations and effect systemic changes based on local lesions. By midcentury, moreover, physicians had come to understand that only the blood supply connected the gestating mother to her child.

7 M. E. Dirix, *Woman's Complete Guide to Health* (New York, 1869), 24. So fashionable were such models in the late nineteenth century that America's leading gynecologist in the opening years of the present century despaired of trying to dispel such exaggerated notions from his patients' minds. "It is difficult," he explained, "even for a healthy girl to rid her mind of constant impending evil from the uterus and ovaries, so prevalent is the idea that woman's ills are mainly 'reflexes' from the pelvic organs." Gynecological therapy was the treatment of choice for a myriad of symptoms. Howard A. Kelly, *Medical Gynecology* (New York, 1908), 73.

8 [Dr. Porter], *Book of Men, Women, and Babies: The Laws of God Applied to Obtaining, Rearing, and Developing the Natural, Healthful, and Beautiful in Humanity* (New York, 1855), 56; Tracy, *Mother and Offspring*, xxiii; H. S. Pomeroy, *The Ethics of Marriage* (New York, 1888), 78.

9 On the involuntary quality of female sexuality, see Alexander J. C. Skene, *Education and Culture as Related to the Health and Diseases of Women* (Detroit, 1889), 22.

10 George Engelmann, *The American Girl of To-Day: Modern Education and Functional Health* (Washington, 1900), 9–10.

11 Alexander Harvey, "On the relative influence of the male and female parents, in the reproduction of the animal species," *Monthly Journal of Medical Science* 19 (Aug. 1854): 108–18; M. A. Pallen, "Heritage, or hereditary transmission," *St. Louis Medical and Surgical Journal* 14 (Nov. 1856): 495. William Warren Potter, *How Should Girls be Educated? A Public Health Problem for Mothers, Educators, and Physicians* (Philadelphia, 1891), 9.

12 As one clerical analyst explained, "All the spare force of nature is concerned in this interior nutritive system, unfitting and disinclining the woman for strenuous muscular and mental enterprise, while providing for the shelter and nourishment of offspring throughout protracted periods of embryo and infancy." William C. Conant, "Sex in nature and society," *Baptist Quarterly* 4 (April 1870): 183.

13 William H. Holcombe, *The Sexes Here and Hereafter* (Philadelphia, 1869), 201–2. William Holcombe was a Swedenborgian, and these contrasting views of the masculine and feminine also reflect New Church doctrines.

14 In regard to pregnancy many middle-class women "sought to hide their imagined shame as long as possible," by tightening corsets and then remaining indoors, shunning even the best of friends—certainly never discussing the impending event. Henry B. Hemenway, *Healthful Womanhood and Childhood: Plain Talks to Non-Professional Readers* (Evanston, Ill., 1894); Elizabeth Evans, *The Abuse of Maternity* (Philadelphia, 1875), 28–29.

15 For a brief summary of late-nineteenth-century assumptions in regard to human genetics, see Charles E. Rosenberg, "Factors in the development of genetics in the United States: some suggestions," *Journal of the History of Medicine*, 22 (Jan. 1967): 31–33.

16 Since both male and female were ordinarily involved in decisions to practice birth control, the cases are not strictly analogous. Both, however, illustrate areas of social conflict organized about stress on traditional role characteristics. This discussion emphasizes only those aspects of the birth control debate which placed responsibility on the woman. Commentators did indeed differ in such emphases; in regard to abortion, however, writers of every religious and ideological persuasion agreed in seeing the matter as woman's responsibility.

17 "The results," as Edward H. Clarke put it in his widely discussed polemic on the subject, "are monstrous brains and puny bodies; abnormally active cerebration, and abnormally weak digestion; flowing thought and constipated bowels; lofty aspirations and neuralgic sensations." Edward H. Clarke, *Sex in Education; or, A Fair Chance for Girls* (Boston, 1873), 41. Thomas A. Emmett, in his widely used textbook of gynecology, warned in 1879 that girls of the better classes should spend the year before and two years after puberty at rest. "Each menstrual period should be passed in the recumbent position until her system becomes accustomed to the new order of life." Thomas Addis Emmett, *The Principles and Practice of Gynecology* (Philadelphia, 1879), 21.

18 T. S. Clouston, *Female Education from a Medical Point of View* (Edinburgh, 1882), 20; Potter, *How Should Girls Be Educated?* 9.

19 The baleful hereditary effects of woman's second-

ary education served as a frequent sanction against this unnatural activity. Lawrence Irwell, "The competition of the sexes and its results," *American Medico-Surgical Bulletin* 10 (Sept. 19, 1896): 319–20. All the doyens of American gynecology in the late nineteenth century—Emmett, J. Marion Sims, T. Gaillard Thomas, Charles D. Meigs, William Goodell, and Mitchell—shared the conviction that higher education and excessive development of the nervous system might interfere with woman's proper performance of her maternal functions.

20 William Goodell, *Lessons in Gynecology* (Philadelphia, 1879), 353.

21 William Edgar Darnall, "The pubescent schoolgirl," *American Gynecological and Obstetrical Journal* 18 (June 1901): 490.

22 Board of Regents, University of Wisconsin, *Annual Report, for the Year Ending, September 30, 1877* (Madison, 1877), 45.

23 Clouston, *Female Education,* 19.

24 James E. Reeves, *The Physical and Moral Causes of Bad Health in American Women* (Wheeling, W.Va., 1875), 28; John Ellis, *Deterioration of the Puritan Stock and Its Causes* (New York, 1884), 7; George Everett, *Health Fragments; or, Steps toward a True Life: Embracing Health, Digestion, Disease, and the Science of the Reproductive Organs* (New York, 1874), 37; Nathan Allen, "The law of human increase; or, population based on physiology and psychology," *Quarterly Journal of Psychological Medicine* 2 (April 1868): 231; Nathan Allen, "The New England family," *New Englander* (March 1882): 9–10; Pye Henry Chavasse, *Advice to a Wife on the Management of Her Own Health, And on the Treatment of Some of the Complaints Incidental to Pregnancy, Labour and Suckling with an Introductory Chapter Especially Addressed to a Young Wife* (New York, 1886), 73–75.

25 Sarah H. Stevenson, *The Physiology of Woman, Embracing Girlhood, Maternity and Mature Age,* 2d ed. (Chicago, 1881), 68, 77; Alice Stockham, *Tokology: A Book for Every Woman,* rev. ed. (Chicago, 1887), 257. Sarah H. Stevenson noted acidly that "the unerring instincts of woman have been an eloquent theme for those who do not know what they are talking about." Stevenson, *Physiology of Woman,* 79. The dress reform movement held, of course, far more significant implications than one would gather from the usually whimsical attitude with which it is normally approached; clothes were very much a part of woman's role. Health reformers, often critical as well of the medical establishment whose arguments we have—essentially—been describing, were often sympathetic to women's claims that not too much, but too little, mental stimulation was the cause of their ills, especially psychological ones. M. L. Hol-

brook, *Hygiene of the Brain and Nerves and the Cure of Nervousness* (New York, 1878), 63–64, 122–23; James C. Jackson, *American Womanhood: Its Peculiarities and Necessities* (Dansville, N.Y., 1870), 127–31.

26 For documentation of the progressive drop in the white American birthrate during the nineteenth century, and some possible reasons for this phenomenon, see Yashukichi Yasuba, *Birth Rates of the White Population in the United States, 1800–1860: An Economic Study* (Baltimore, 1862); J. Potter, "American population in the early national period," in *Proceedings of Section V of the Fourth Congress of the International Economic History Association,* Paul Deprez, ed. (Winnipeg, Canada, 1970), 55–69. For a more general background to this trend, see A. M. Carr-Saunders, *World Population: Past Growth and Present Trends* (London, 1936).

27 A. K. Gardner, *Conjugal Sins against the Laws of Life and Health (New York, 1874), 131.* H. R. Storer of Boston was probably the most prominent and widely read critic of such "conjugal sins." Abortion had in particular been discussed and attacked since early in the century, though it was not until the postbellum years that it became a widespread concern of moral reformers. Alexander Draper, *Observations on Abortion, With an Account of the Means both Medicinal and Mechanical, Employed to Produce that Effect . . .* (Philadelphia, 1839); Hugh L. Hodge, *On Criminal Abortion: A Lecture* (Philadelphia, 1854). Advocates of birth control routinely used the dangers and prevalence of abortion as one argument justifying their cause.

28 *Report of the Suffolk District Medical Society on Criminal Abortion and Ordered Printed . . . May 9, [1857]* (Boston, 1857), 2. The report was almost certainly written by Storer. The Michigan report is summarized in William D. Haggard, *Abortion: Accidental, Essential, Criminal,* Address before the Nashville Academy of Medicine, Aug. 4, 1898 (Nashville, Tenn., 1898), 10. For samples of contemporary descriptions of prevalence, cheapness, and other aspects of abortion and birth control in the period, see Ely Van de Warker, *The Detection of Criminal Abortion, and a Study of Foeticidal Drugs* (Boston, 1872); Evans, *Abuse of Maternity;* Horatio R. Storer, *Why Not? A Book for Every Woman,* 2d ed. (Boston, 1868); N. F. Cook, *Satan in Society: By a Physician* (Cincinnati, 1876); Discussion, *Transactions of the Homeopathic Medical Society of New York,* 1866, *4:* 9–10; H. R. Storer and F. F. Heard, *Criminal Abortion* (Boston, 1868); H. C. Ghent, "Criminal abortion, or foeticide," *Transactions of the Texas State Medical Association at the Annual Session, 1888–89* (1888–89), 119–46; Hugh Hodge, *Foeticide, or Criminal Abortion: A Lecture Introductory to the Course on Obstetrics, and Diseases of*

Women and Children, University of Pennsylvania (Philadelphia, 1869), 3–10. Much of the medical discussion centered on the need to convince women that the traditional view that abortion was no crime if performed before quickening was false and immoral and to pass and enforce laws and medical society proscriptions against abortionists.

29 Compare the warning of Pomeroy, *Ethics of Marriage*, v, 56, with the editorial "A conviction for criminal abortion," *Boston Medical and Surgical Journal* 106 (Jan. 5, 1882): 18–19. It is significant that discussions of birth control in the United States always emphasized the role and motivations of middle-class women and men; in England, following the canon of the traditional Malthusian debate, the working class and its needs played a far more prominent role. Not until late in the century did American birth control advocates tend to concern themselves with the needs and welfare of the working population. It is significant as well that English birth control advocates often used the prevalence of infanticide as an argument for birth control; in America this was rarely discussed. And one doubts if the actual incidence of infanticide was substantially greater in London than New York.

30 For a guide to literature on birth control in nineteenth-century America, see Norman Himes, *Medical History of Contraception* (Baltimore, 1936). See also J. A. Banks, *Prosperity and Parenthood: A Study of Family Planning among the Victorian Middle Classes* (London, 1954), and J. A. Banks and Olive Banks, *Feminism and Family Planning in Victorian England* (Liverpool, 1964); Margaret Hewitt, *Wives and Mothers in Victorian Industry* (London, ca. 1958). For the twentieth century, see David M. Kennedy, *Birth Control in America.*

31 John Humphrey Noyes, *Male Continence* (Oneida, N.Y., 1872), 10–11.

32 It is not surprising that the design for a protodiaphragm patented as early as 1846 should have been called "The Wife's Protector." J. B. Beers, "Instrument to prevent conception, patented Aug. 28th, 1846," design and drawings (Historical Collections, Library of the College of Physicians of Philadelphia).

33 In some marriages, for example, even if the male had consciously chosen, indeed urged, the practice of birth control, he was effectively deprived of a dimension of sexual pleasure and of the numerous children which served as tangible and traditional symbols of masculinity as well as the control over his wife which the existence of such children implied. In some marriages, however, birth control might well have brought greater sexual fulfillment because it reduced the anxiety of the female part-

ner. Throughout the nineteenth century withdrawal was almost certainly the most common form of birth control. One author described it as "a practice so universal that it may well be termed a national vice, so common that it is unblushingly acknowledged by its perpetrators, for the commission of which the husband is even eulogized by his wife." [Cook], *Satan in Society*, 152. One English advocate of birth control was candid enough to argue that "the real objection underlying the opposition, though it is not openly expressed, is the idea of the deprivation of pleasure supposed to be involved." Austin Holyyoake, *Large or Small Families* (London, 1892), 11.

34 R. T. Trall, *Sexual Physiology: A Scientific and Popular Exposition of the Fundamental Problems in Sociology* (New York, 1866), xi, 202. As women awoke to a realization of their own "individuality," as a birth control advocate explained it in the 1880s, they would rebel against such "enforced maternity." E. B. Foote, Jr., *The Radical Remedy in Social Science; or, Borning Better Babies* (New York, 1886), 132. See also Stevenson, *Physiology of Women*, 91; T. L. Nichols, *Esoteric Anthropology* (New York, 1824). E. H. Heywood, *Cupid's Yokes; or, the Binding Force of Conjugal Life* (Princeton, Mass., 1877); Stockham, *Tokology*, 250; Alice Stockham, *Karezza: Ethics of Marriage* (Chicago, 1896); E. B. Foote, *Medical Commonsense Applied to the Causes, Prevention and Cure of Chronic Diseases and Unhappiness in Marriage* (New York, 1864), 365; J. Soule, *Science of Reproduction and Reproductive Control: The Necessity of Some Abstaining from Having Children; the Duty of All to Limit Their Families According to Their Circumstances Demonstrated; Effects of Continence Effects of Self-Pollution—Abusive Practices; Seminal Secretion—Its Connection with Life; with All the Different Modes of Preventing Conception, and the Philosophy of Each* (n.p., 1856), 37; L. B. Chandler, *The Divineness of Marriage* (New York, 1872). To radical feminist Tennie C. Claflin, man's right to impose his sexual desires upon woman was the issue underlying all opposition to woman suffrage and the expansion of woman's role. Tennie C. Claflin, *Constitutional Equality: A Right of Woman; or A Consideration of the Various Relations Which She Sustains as a Necessary Part of the Body of Society and Humanity; with Her Duties to Herself—together with a Review of the Constitution of the United States, Showing That the Right to Vote Is Guaranteed to All Citizens; Also a Review of the Rights of Children* (New York, 1871), 63. Particularly striking are the letters from women desiring birth control information. Margaret Sanger, *Motherhood in Bondage* (New York, 1928); E. B. Foote, Jr., *Radical Remedy*, 114–20; Henry C. Wright, *The Unwelcome Child; or The Crime of an Undesigned and Un-*

desired Maternity (Boston, 1858). This distinction between economic, "physical," and role consideration is, quite obviously, justifiable only for the sake of analysis; these considerations must have coexisted within each family in particular configuration.

35 Noyes, *Male Continence,* 16; Frederick Hollick, *The Marriage Guide; or, Natural History of Generation; A Private Instructor for Married Persons and Those about to Marry, Both Male and Female* (New York, ca. 1860), 348; Trall, *Sexual Physiology,* 205–6.

36 Indeed, in these post-Darwinian years it was possible for at least one health reformer to argue that smaller families were a sign of that higher nervous evolution which accompanied civilization. [M. L. Holbrook], *Marriage and Parentage* (New York, 1882). For the eugenic virtues of fewer but better children, see E. R. Shepherd, *For Girls: A Special Physiology: Being a Supplement to the Study of General Physiology,* 20th ed. (Chicago, 1887), 213; M. L. Griffith, *Ante-Natal Infanticide* (n.p. [1889]), 8.

37 See Louis François Etienne Bergeret, *The Preventive Obstacle; or, Conjugal Onanism,* trans. P. de Marmon, (New York, 1870); C. H. F. Routh, *Moral and Physical Evils Likely to Follow If Practices Intended to Act as Checks to Population Be Not Strongly Discouraged and Condemned* 2d ed. (London, 1879), 13; Goodell, *Lessons in Gynecology,* 371, 374; Thomas Hersey, *The Midwife's Practical Directory; or, Woman's Confidential Friend: Comprising, Extensive Remarks on the Various Casualties and Forms of Diseases Preceeding, Attending and Following the Period of Gestation, with Appendix,* 2d ed. (Baltimore, 1836), 80; William H. Walling, *Sexology* (Philadelpia, 1902), 79.

38 J. R. Black, *The Ten Laws of Health; or, How Disease is Produced and Can Be Prevented* (Philadelphia, 1873), 251. See also C. A. Greene, *Build Well: The Basis of Individual Home, and National Elevation, Plain Truths Relating to the Obligations of Marriage and Parentage* (Boston, ca. 1885), 99; E. P. LeProhon, *Voluntary Abortion; or Fashionable Prostitution, with Some Remarks upon the Operation of Craniotomy* (Portland, Me., 1867), 15; M. Solis-Cohen, *Girl, Wife, and Mother* (Philadelphia, 1911), 213.

39 There is an instructive analogy between these ponderously mechanistic sanctions against birth control and abortion and the psychodynamic arguments against abortion used so frequently in the twentieth century; both served precisely the same social function. In both cases, the assumption of woman's childbearing destiny provided the logical basis against which a denial of this calling produced sickness, in the nineteenth century through physiological, and ultimately, pathological processes—in the twentieth century through guilt and psychological but again, ultimately, pathological processes.

40 A. K. Gardner, for example, confessed sympathy for the seduced and abandoned patron of the abortionist, "but for the married shirk, who disregards her divinely-ordained duty, we have nothing but contempt." Gardner, *Conjugal Sins,* 112. See also E. Frank Howe, *Sermon on Ante-Natal Infanticide Delivered at the Congregational Church in Terre Haute, on Sunday Morning, March 28, 1869* (Terre Haute, Ind., 1869); J. H. Tilden, *Cursed before Birth* (Denver, ca. 1895); J. M. Toner, *Maternal Instinct, or Love* (Baltimore, 1864), 91.

41 It must be emphasized that this is but one theme in a complex debate surrounding the issue of birth control and sexuality. A group of more evangelically oriented health reformers tended to emphasize instead the responsibility of the "overgrown, abnormally developed and wrongly directed amativeness of the man" and to see the woman as victim. John Cowan, Henry C. Wright, and Dio Lewis were widely read exemplars of this point of view. This group shared a number of assumptions and presumably psychological needs, and represents a somewhat distinct interpretive task. John Cowan, *The Science of a New Life* (New York, 1874), 275.

42 W. L. Atlee and D. A. O'Donnell, "Report of the Committee on Criminal Abortion," *Transactions of the American Medical Association,* 1871, *22:* 241.

43 The most tireless advocate of these views was Nathan Allen, a Lowell, Massachusetts, physician and health reformer. Nathan Allen, "The law of human increase; or, population based on physiology and psychology," *Quarterly Journal Psychological Medicine* 2 (April 1868): 209–66; Nathan Allen, *Changes in New England Population, Read at the Meeting of the American Social Science Association, Saratoga, September 6, 1877* (Lowell, Mass., 1877); Nathan Allen, "The physiological laws of human increase," *Transactions of the American Medical Association,* 1870, *21:* 381–407; Nathan Allen, "Physical degeneracy," *Journal of Psychological Medicine* 4 (Oct. 1870): 725–64; Nathan Allen, "The normal standard of woman for propagation," *American Journal of Obstetrics* 9 (April 1876): 1–39.

44 Ellis, *Deterioration of Puritan Stock,* 3; Storer, *Why Not?* 85.

45 Clarke, *Sex in Education,* 63. For similar warnings, see Henry Gibbons, *On Feticide* (San Francisco, 1878), 4; Charles Buckingham, *The Proper Treatment of Children, Medical or Medicinal* (Boston, 1873), 15; Edward Jenks, "The education of girls from a medical stand-point," *Transaction of the Michigan State Medical Society,* 1889, *13:* 52–62; Paul Paquin, *The Supreme Passions of Man* (Battle Creek, Mich., 1891), 76.

46 These arguments, first formulated in the 1860s, had

become clichés in medical and reformist circles by the 1880s. See Barbara Miller Solomon, *Ancestors and Immigrants: A Changing New England Tradition* (Cambridge, Mass., 1956); John Higham, *Strangers in the Land: Patterns of American Nativism, 1860–1925* (New Brunswick, N.J., 1955). Such arguments exhibited a growing consciousness of class as well as of ethnic sensitivity; it was the better-educated and more sensitive members of society, anti-Malthusians began to argue, who would curtail their progeny, while the uneducated and coarse would hardly change their habits. H. S. Pomeroy, *Is Man Too Prolific? The So-Called Malthusian Idea* (London, 1891), 57–58.

47　Ellis, *Deterioration of Puritan Stock*, 10.

48　Oscar Handlin, *Race and Nationality in American Life*, 5th ed. (Boston, 1957), 139–66.

49　One might postulate a more traditionally psychodynamic explanatory model, one which would see the arguments described as a male defense against their own consciousness of sexual inadequacy or ambivalence or of their own unconscious fears of female sexual powers. These emphases are quite distinct. The first—though it also assumes the reality of individual psychic mechanisms such as repression and projection—is tied very much to the circumstances of a particular generation, to social location, and to social perception. The second kind of explanation is more general, time-free, and based on a presumably ever-recurring male fear of female sexuality and its challenge to the capacity of particular individuals to act and live an appropriately male role. For the literature on this problem, see Wolfgang Lederer, *The Fear of Women* (New York, 1968).

50　At this time, moreover, most psychiatric clinicians and theoreticians would agree that no model exists to extend the insights gained from individual psychodynamics to the behavior of larger social groups such as national populations or social classes.

51　Most societies provide alternative roles to accommodate the needs of personality variants—as, for example, the shaman role in certain Siberian tribes or the accepted man-woman homosexual of certain American Indian tribes. In the nineteenth-century English-speaking world such roles as that of the religious enthusiast and the chronic female invalid or hysteric may well have provided such modalities. But a period of peculiarly rapid or widespread social change can make such available role alternatives inadequate mechanisms of adjustment for many individuals. Others in the same society may respond to the same pressures of change by demanding an undeviating acceptance of traditional role prescriptions and refusing to accept the legitimacy of such cultural variants. The role of the hysterical woman in late-nineteenth-century America suggests many of the problems inherent in creating such alternative social roles. While offering both an escape from the everyday duties of wife and mother, and an opportunity for the display of covert hostility and aggression, this role inflicted great bodily (though nonorganic) pain, provided no really new role or interest, and perpetuated—even increased—the patient's dependence on traditional role characteristics, especially that of passivity. The reaction of society, as suggested by the writings of most male physicians, can be described as at best an unstable compromise between patronizing tolerance and violent anger. See Carroll Smith-Rosenberg, "The hysterical woman: sex roles and role conflict in 19th-century America," 652–78. For useful discussions of hysteria and neurasthenia, see Ilza Veith, *Hysteria: The History of a Disease* (Chicago, 1965); Henri F. Ellenberger, *The Discovery of the Unconscious: The History and Evolution of Dynamic Psychiatry* (New York, 1970); Charles E. Rosenberg, "The place of George M. Beard in nineteenth-century psychiatry," *Bulletin of the History of Medicine* 36 (May–June 1962): 245–59; John S. Haller, Jr., "Neurasthenia: the medical profession and the 'New Woman' of late nineteenth-century," *New York State Journal of Medicine* 71 (Feb. 15, 1971): 473–82. Esther Fischer-Homberger has recently argued that these diagnostic categories masked an endemic male-female conflict: "Hysterie und Mysogynie—ein Aspekt der Hysteriegeschichte," *Gesnerus*, 1969, *26:* 117–27.

2

Women, Menstruation, and Nineteenth-Century Medicine

VERN BULLOUGH AND MARTHA VOGHT

One of the recurrent themes in medical history is the reluctance of physicians to accept new scientific findings. This may well be due to the innate conservatism of medical practitioners and their unwillingness to use patients as guinea pigs for treatment about which they are unsure. Sometimes, too, the reluctance comes because new findings demonstrate that previous practices might have been harmful to the patient; this turn of events is difficult to accept. Often, however, the reluctance is not attributable to any medical reason but results when new findings upset the emotional attachments, some would say political prejudices, that most physicians hold and which have little to do with medicine itself. This paper is concerned with this kind of opposition.

When the belief structure of the physician is threatened, even in fields outside of medicine, he often uses his medical expertise to justify his prejudices and in the process strikes back with value-laden responses which have nothing to do with scientific medicine. Unfortunately, since he is assumed to speak with authority, his response, perhaps as he intended, has influence far beyond that of ordinary men. One of the best examples of this is the controversy over the physical disabilities of women which took place in the last part of the nineteenth century as women began to demand more education and greater political equality and to challenge many of the male stereotypes about woman's place. Since medical practitioners were

almost all men, and many of them were hostile to any change in the status quo in male-female relationships, they inevitably entered the struggle with arguments which not only appear today as ludicrous, but even in the period they were writing were not based upon any scientific findings and in fact went contrary to those findings. This is particularly true in their understanding of the consequences of menstruation.

During the last part of the nineteenth century American physicians toyed with several theories of menstruation. In general they were aware of the theories of John Power of London who postulated that ovulation and menstruation were connected. American medical journals also made an attempt to keep their readers current on the English researchs which tended to support his theories.[1] At the same time, however, many physicians seriously discussed various folk theories about menstruation, retaining with little change in content ideas which appear in the Hippocratic corpus or in Aristotle. Many still held that it was the effect of the moon upon women that caused them to menstruate; others held that the fetus was formed from the menstrual flow. The popular underground pseudonymous marriage manual *Aristotle's Masterpiece* held that menstruation was due to the casting out of the excess blood which would have nourished the embryo if pregnancy had occurred.[2] Even as late as the 1890s when the first experimental work leading to the understanding of human hormones was taking place, American physicians were still discussing the question of whether the ovaries triggered menstruation, whether the uterus was an independent organ and performed the menstrual function without external aid, or whether the fallopian tubes were responsible for the monthly flow.[3] A few, however, perhaps influenced by the Victo-

VERN L. BULLOUGH is Dean of the Faculty of Natural and Social Sciences, State University of New York College, Buffalo, New York.
MARTHA L. VOGHT is a free-lance writer of educational materials in Bishop, California.
Reprinted with permission from *Bulletin of the History of Medicine* 47 (1973): 66–82.

rian disgust at the sexual and reproductive processes, considered menstruation a pathological condition. These physicians believed that in Paradise humans had reproduced asexually and it was only when man had fallen that perfection had been replaced by the evil of sex. An article in the *American Journal of Obstetrics* in 1875, for example, argued that menstruation was pathological, proof of the inactivity and threatened atrophy of the uterus. As evidence of its unnaturalness the author claimed that conception was most likely when intercourse occurred during the monthly flow, but intercourse at such times was dangerous and forbidden because the menstrual blood was the source of male gonorrhea. Since menstruation therefore stood in the way of fruitful coitus it obviously had not been ordained by nature.[4]

In 1861 E. F. W. Pflüger demonstrated that menstruation did not take place in women whose ovaries had been removed, a finding which reinforced the ovarian theory but did not end the debate since Pflüger himself in 1863 hypothesized that there was a mechanical stimulus of nerves by the growing follicle which was responsible for congestion and menstrual bleeding. This led him to believe that menstruation and ovulation occurred simultaneously.[5] It was not until the twentieth century and a better understanding of the hormonal process that the timing of ovulation was fully understood. In the meantime, many American physicians accepted Pflüger's theory that nervous stimulation triggered menstruation, and it was this belief which led large numbers of physicians to express opposition to any emancipation of women.

This paper is not the place to discuss the movement for female emancipation, but even a brief synopsis must point out that women were much more assertive of their rights in the last part of the nineteenth century than earlier. Though traditionally women in the United States had received some sort of primary education, if only to learn to read the Bible, they had been denied entrance to any of the grammar schools or colleges. In 1783, for example, twelve-year-old Lucinda Foote was examined for admission to Yale and found capable of giving the "true meaning of passages in the *Aeneid* of Virgil, the *Select Orations* of Cicero and the Greek *Testament*." She was, however, declared unqualified to enter the college because of her sex.[6] Physicians

of the time were generally more inclined to favor female education than oppose it. Perhaps the best example is Benjamin Rush. He urged female education on the grounds that it would allow women to better fulfill their familial responsibilities, be less prone to superstition, have talent in managing their family's affairs, and be better teachers for their sons. Rush also pointed out to his fellow males who might be somewhat hesitant to accept his ideas that the ignorant were the most difficult to govern and an educated wife could, by virtue of her education, be more easily shown the wisdom of her husband's orders and decisions.[7] It was only later that a significant portion of the medical community appear in opposition to female education.

During the first part of the nineteenth century the female academies and seminaries began to multiply, and in the 1830s full-fledged colleges were proposed for women and Oberlin College opened its doors to both sexes.[8] Soon medical schools also found themselves under attack for failure to admit women, and a few women such as Elizabeth Blackwell managed to receive medical training. Most women, however, turned to nursing as an alternative to challenging the male bastion of medicine,[9] but it is perhaps no accident that medical opposition to feminine emancipation began to increase as the physician himself felt threatened by the few women attempting to enter medical school. About 1870 several medical writers began proclaiming that education for women was a disastrous error since girls between twelve and twenty could not stand the strain of higher education, in large part because of the physiological strains which puberty and ovulation put upon them.

Among the first theorists of menstrual disability, by far the most influential was Edward H. Clarke, a professor of materia medica at Harvard and a fellow of the American Academy of Arts and Sciences. In 1873 he wrote that though women undoubtedly have the right to do anything of which they are physically capable, one of the things they could not do and still retain their good health was to be educated on the pattern and model of men. He held that while the male developed steadily and gradually from birth to manhood, the female, at puberty, had a sudden and unique period of growth when the development of the reproductive system took place.[10] If this did not take place at puberty, it would never occur, and since the system can never do "two things well at the same time," the female between twelve and twenty must concentrate on developing her reproductive system. To digest one's dinner, he held it was necessary to temper exercise and brain work; likewise, during the growth of the female reproductive system, brain work must be avoided. The overuse of the central nervous system would overload the switchboard, so to speak, and signals from the developing organs of reproduction would be ignored in favor of those coming from the overactive brain. Even after puberty females were not to exercise their minds without restriction because of their monthly cycle. The menstrual period was vital, Clarke held, and any mental activity during the "catamenial week" would interfere with ovulation and menstruation,[11] the necessary physiological processes of being female.

He then proceeded to demonstrate, at least to his own satisfaction, that higher education left a great number of its female adherents in poor health for life. He was alarmed that the increase in the number of young women being educated would so deplete the population that within fifty years "the wives who are to be mothers in our republic must be drawn from trans-Atlantic homes."[12] For proof of his assertion he offered as evidence the cases of young women he had as patients whose ill health he ascribed to hard study. One had entered a female seminary at fifteen in good health but after a year of application to her studies and following the routine of the school, which included standing to recite, she was pale and tired "every fourth week." A summer's rest restored her but by the end of the second year she was not only pale but suffering from an "uncontrollable twitching of a rhythmical sort" in the muscles of her face. On the advice of the family physician she was taken for a year of travel in Europe and returned cured. Unfortunately she then returned to school where she studied without regard to her menstrual periods and, though she graduated at nineteen as valedictorian, she was an invalid and it took two years in Europe for her to recover. Her illness, according to Dr. Clarke's diagnosis, resulted from making her body do two things at once. He reported the case of another young woman, a student at Vassar, who began to have fainting spells and suffer painful and sparse menses. Inevitably she graduated at nineteen as an invalid, suffering from constant headaches. Dr. Clarke believed this was because

she suffered from the arrested development of her reproductive system due to her education. As evidence he claimed she not only had menstrual troubles but was rather flat chested. Another young college woman came to him with a history of diminishing menstrual flow, constant headaches, mental depression, acne, and rough skin. Eventually Dr. Clarke committed her to an asylum.[13] It was also of some concern to Dr. Clarke that young women of the lower classes were expected, during puberty, to take jobs in domestic service or in factories. In his practice he had seen evidences of ill health among such women which he blamed upon their work. Yet, he concluded that labor in factory at a loom was far less damaging than study to a woman, because it worked the body, not the brain. It was primarily brain work which destroyed feminine capabilities.[14]

Women who concentrated upon education rather than the development of their reproductive system also underwent mental changes, according to Clarke. Not possessing the physical attributes of a man, they also tended to lose the "maternal instincts" of a woman to become coarse and forceful. By educating women, said Dr. Clarke, we were creating a class of sexless humans analogous to eunuchs. To solve this alarming problem, he recommended strict separation of the sexes during education, particularly after elementary school. He urged that female schools provide periodic rest periods for students during their menstrual periods. The young women would also have shorter study periods since they were by nature weak and less able to cope with long hours.

> A girl cannot spend more than four, or, in occasional instances, five hours of force daily upon her studies, and leave sufficient margin for the general physical growth that she must make. . . . If she puts as much force into her brain education as a boy, the brain or the special apparatus (i.e., the reproductive system) will suffer.[15]

He held up as models some reports on German education, showing that menstrual rest for female students was practiced.[16]

Though there was immediate unfavorable reaction to Clarke's thesis, it still became widely accepted. His critics pointed out, for example, that Clarke had done no scientific study on the matter, that he generalized from a few clinical cases in his own practice, and that his description of periodic rests in European education were totally untrue. One critic commented that "Dr. Clarke has thrown out to a popular audience a hypothesis of his own, which has no place in physiological or medical science. . . . His whole reasoning is singularly unsound."[17] There was some suspicion that Clarke's argument was designed to end speculation at Harvard about admitting female students.[18] Nevertheless, the popularity of his message is indicated by the fact that within thirteen years, *Sex in Education* went through seventeen editions.

Those physicians who followed Clarke tended to exaggerate his position and to ascribe far more harm to the education of women than even he had dared. T. S. Clouston, a physician of Edinburgh, Scotland, wrote a lengthy series for the *Popular Science Monthly* to demonstrate to the public the dangers of the education of females. He pointed out that it was medically accepted that the "female organism is far more delicate than that of men; . . . it is not fitted for the regular grind that the man can keep up." Overstimulation of the female brain causes stunted growth, nervousness, headaches and neuralgias, difficult childbirth, hysteria, inflammation of the brain, and insanity. The female character is likewise altered by education; the educated woman becomes cultured, but "is unsympathetic; learned, but not self denying." Clouston admitted the weak point of his argument, "that it is not founded on any basis of collated statistical facts," based only upon observations of physicians of their own patients. Nonetheless, he expressed the hope that research to gather the facts would be carried on in the future.[19]

This, in fact, began to happen but the results were not what Clouston anticipated. The Massachusetts Labor Bureau made the first report on the health of American college women based upon statistical evidence and not the "haphazard estimate of physicians and college instructors."[20] The results indicated that of 705 college women, 78 percent were in good or excellent health, 5 percent were classed as in fair health, and 17 percent were in poor health. When these women had started college, 20 percent were in poor health. The report concluded that there were no marked differences in health between college women and the national average.[21] John Dewey, in his analysis of

the report, decided that worry over personal matters was more harmful to health than overstudy.[22]

In spite of the publicity given the study, there was little change in attitudes among those who believed women and education made a dangerous mixture. In the same year that it appeared, Henry Maudsley wrote in *Sex in Mind and in Education* that the concurrence of puberty and higher education meant that mental development was accomplished at the expense of physical. While acknowledging that there were no facts to provide an answer to the question—what are the effects of coeducation?—he nonetheless answered the question by citing Clarke and declaring that girls educated in the traditional ways were losing "their strength and health." The imperfect development of the reproductive system interfered with the development of the feminine character, leaving the educated woman without a sufficiently feminine frame of mind. The education of women must be designed to prepare them for their proper sphere.

> It will have to be considered whether women can scorn delights and live laborious days of intellectual exercise and production, without injury to their functions as the conceivers, mothers, and nurses of children. For, it would be an ill thing, if it should so happen that we got the advantage of a quantity of female intellectual work at the price of a puny, enfeebled, and sickly race.[23]

Clarke and most of his imitators subscribed to the Pflüger theory of menstruation, but it was not a necessary preliminary to the belief in the physical disability of women. John Goodman, a Louisville physician, believed that the ovular theory of menstruation was untenable. Instead menstruation was "presided over by a law of monthly periodicity," a "menstrual wave" which affected the entire female being and from whose dictates women could not escape.[24] This theory, although in conflict with that of Pflüger, was appropriated to the cause of those who opposed female education. A good example is George J. Engelmann who, in his presidential address before the American Gynecological Society in 1900, expressed the opinion that female schools should heed the "instability and susceptibility of the girl during the functional waves which permeate her entire being," and provide rest during the menstrual periods. At the same time he said that menstruation was controlled by "physical conditions and nerve influences," and that the first menses were accelerated by mental stimulation. His observations contradicted those of Clarke, since while Clarke found educated women ceasing menstruation, Engelmann found that mental work increased the frequency of menstrual flow.[25] Nevertheless he would agree with Clarke that women could not endure the rigors of higher education.

J. H. Kellogg, whose *Plain Facts for Old and Young* was responsible for inculcating vast numbers of Americans with the idea that masturbation led to insanity, added also to the public misinformation about menstruation. Part of Kellogg's success was due to the fact that he appeared to be so scientific:

> There has been a great amount of speculation concerning the cause and nature of the menstrual process. No entirely satisfactory conclusions have been reached, however, except that it is usually accompanied by the maturation and expulsion from the ovary of an ovum, which is termed ovulation. But menstruation may occur without ovulation, and vice versa.[26]

He then stated that the first occurrence of menstruation is a very critical period in the life of a female, that each recurrence renders her specially susceptible to morbid influences and liable to serious derangements, and that she must carefully watch out during these periods.

> There is no doubt that many young women have permanently injured their constitutions while at school by excessive mental taxation during the catamenial period, to which they were prompted by ambition to excel, or were compelled by the "cramming" system too generally pursued in our schools, and particularly in young ladies' seminaries.

He adds, however, that a moderate amount of study would not be injurious, and he had no doubt that a large share of the injury which has been attributed to overstudy during the catamenia was caused by improper dress, exposure to cold, keeping late hours, and improper diet. Kellogg also wondered about women workers and felt that female workers should be protected during their periods. He felt it was wrong that women in order to keep their situations were required to be on hand daily and

allowed no opportunity for rest at the menstrual period.

> In many cases, too, they are compelled to remain upon their feet all day behind a counter, or at a work table, even at periods when a recumbent position is actually demanded by nature. There should be less delicacy in relation to this subject on the part of young women, and more consideration on the part of employers.[27]

As the movement for female emancipation grew, the physicians who discussed the frailties of the female did so with increasing emotional fervor. The president of the Oregon State Medical Society, F. W. Van Dyke, in 1905, claimed that hard study killed sexual desire in women, took away their beauty, and brought on hysteria, neurasthenia, dyspepsia, astigmatism, and dysmenorrhea. Educated women, he added, could not bear children with ease because study arrested the development of the pelvis at the same time it increased the size of the child's brain, and therefore its head. The result was extensive suffering in childbirth by educated women. Van Dyke concluded by declaring that the women who were remembered in history were faithful wives and good mothers such as Penelope, Cornelia, St. Elizabeth; and these would still be remembered when "the name of the last graduate of the woman's college shall have faded from the recollection of men forever."[28]

Dr. Ralph W. Parsons in the *New York Medical Journal* in 1907 cited many of the above authorities to show that the results of higher education for women could lead only to ill health. He claimed college women suffered from digestive disorders as well as nervous and mental diseases.

> The nervous system has been developed at the expense of other bodily organs and structures. The delicate organism and sensitive and highly developed nervous system of our girls was never intended by the Creator to undergo the stress and strain of the modern system of higher education, and the baneful results are becoming more and more apparent as the years go by.[29]

He offered as proof the fact that in 1902, 42 percent of the women admitted to New York insane asylums were well educated, while only 16 percent of the men admitted had gone beyond grade school. He concluded that women "who have undergone the strain of the modern system of education, are much more liable to become victims of insanity than men of the same class."

One of the mental diseases to which college women were prone was the modification of feminine traits of mind. These women developed distaste for the duties of home life, were egotistical, assumed independence of speech and manner, and were not attentive to the advice of their parents. Educated women neglected to cultivate refined speech, had loud voices, laughed with gusto, and sometimes even used slang and profanity. "They do not exhibit," said Dr. Parsons, "the modesty of demeanor which we have been taught to believe is one of the most admirable traits of the feminine character." Colleges encouraged unwomanly behavior. At one school girls publicly appeared on stage in knee breeches, and in the performance used such words as "devilish" and "damned." Such women as these would never be able to fulfill their female functions, for not only was their reproductive apparatus stunted by education, but no man would ever love them. This was because men had deep sentiment for women with "feminine traits of character with which God intended they should be endowed."

Parson's solution went far beyond anything proposed in the nineteenth century by medical men. Girls, he decided, should not learn Latin, Greek, civics, political economy, or higher math, for these subjects could be of no use to them in their proper sphere. They should have shorter school hours than boys, and spend most of their time in home economics classes.[30]

All of these twentieth-century physicians had available to them a careful study on the health of college and noncollege women, printed in the *Publications* of the American Statistical Association, 1900–1901. This study, carried out during the 1890s, compared college women, not to the "average" woman of the census, as past projects had done, but to a control group of noncollege women composed of their own relatives and friends of their own social class. The study found that though college women married two years later than noncollege women there was a growing tendency to marry later among both groups. Noncollege women had "a slightly larger number of children," but college

women had more children per years of married life. There were no differences in problems of pregnancy and mortality of children. The health of the children was roughly equal; although among college-educated mothers the researchers felt they detected slightly fewer delicate children and slightly more robust children. The study found no significant difference between the health of the two groups of women before or after college age. Seventy-five percent of the college women had been employed before marriage, while only 34 percent of the noncollege women had had outside employment. The college women chose different kinds of husbands than the control group. Seventy-five percent of them married college men, while their noneducated cousins married a college-educated husband in only half the cases. Sixty-five percent of college women married professional men, while only 37 percent of the noncollege women had husbands in the professions.[31]

The physicians who persisted in accepting the theories of Clarke et al. simply ignored such studies. G. Stanley Hall who, though one of the outstanding psychologists of the early twentieth century, strongly believed that woman's place was in the home, simply dismissed the statistical studies as inaccurate. Instead, he felt, physicians who treated overeducated women were more likely to see the true circumstances. Inevitably Hall's classic *Adolescence* repeated all the fears and superstitions concerning female education. For example, he connected menstruation to mental exercise. As proof he offered the fact that American girls had their first menses at an average of 14 years of age, while European girls were, on the average, 15.5 years of age before menstruation started. This precocity of American girls was "due chiefly to mentality and nerve stimulation," in other words, education. "Education," theorized Hall, "in a temperate or subartic zone is more productive of precocity than in the south, and if general nervous stimulus is the cause, the same schooling is more dangerous in the city than in the country."[32] Hall was heavily influenced by Clarke's concept of rest during the menstrual periods, and suggested that the female, rather than observing the weekly Sabbath, should have rest periods of four successive days per month. These days would be devoted to leisure and religion, since during menstruation the female was inclined "to a natural piety and sense of dependence," which accounted for the fact that women were more religious than men.[33] Women were by nature intuitive, Hall claimed, not mental. By being "bookish" woman lapsed into male manners and fashions, declined from "her orbit," and obscured her "original divinity."[34]

He believed with Goodman that the ruling factor of female life was periodicity. For most of her life a women had no alternative but to give way to its dictates, and for this reason special schools should be established for girls. Under no circumstances should coeducation exist, for putting adolescents in the intimacy of the classroom destroyed "the bloom and delicacy" of the girls. Female schools should be in the country, with plenty of places for exercise and privacy. All students should observe the "monthly Sabbath" during their menstrual periods, during which time

> the paradise of stated rest should be revisited, idleness be actively cultivated; reverie, in which the soul, which needs these seasons of withdrawal for its own development, expatiates over the whole life of the race, should be provided for and encouraged in every legitimate way, for in rest the whole momentum of heredity is felt in ways most favorable to full and complete development. Then woman should realize that *to be* is greater than *to do;* should step reverently aside from her daily routine and let Lord Nature work.[35]

Such opinions as this were unlikely, in 1905, to go unchallenged by the feminists. Martha Carey Thomas, president of Bryn Mawr College, attacked this lyrical report on periodicity as "sickening sentimentality" and "pseudo-scientific." She held that the seventh and seventeenth chapters of Hall's work were more degrading to womanhood than anything written since Michelet's *La Femme.* She recalled her student days, when she was "terror-struck lest I, and every other woman with me, were doomed to live as pathological invalids in a universe merciless to woman as a sex." Now "we know" that it is not "we," but the "man who believes such things about us, who is himself pathological, blinded by neurotic mists of sex, unable to see that women form one-half of the kindly race of normal, healthy human creatures in the world."[36]

Serious research also questioned the point of view Hall represented. One such study hypothesized that if the menstrual cycle had such influence on women, it ought to show up on tests comparing motor and mental abilities of both men and women. When the results were analyzed it was found that none of the efficiency curves correlated with the menstrual cycles and that the males in the tests had varying efficiencies similar to the females rather than being stable and unvarying as had been thought. In fact, the curves produced by the two sexes were indistinguishable when the notations of the menstrual periods were removed. How, asked the researcher Leta Stetter Hollingworth, was such a striking disparity from what had been the accepted scientific position to be accounted for. Two possible explanations were offered. First the scientific and medically accepted facts were not facts at all but traditions carried on by mystic and romantic writers that "woman is a mysterious being, half hysteric, half angel," and this attitude had somehow found its way into the scientific writing. Scientists seeking to justify this had "seized" upon the menstrual cycle as the probable source of the alleged "mystery" and "caprice of womankind." Once formulated, then, the dogma became cited as authority from author to author until the present day. A second possible explanation of the error was that physicians had not based their conclusions upon accurate evidence. She postulated that normal women did not come under the care and observations of physicians but rather only those with mental and physical diseases. Physicians generalized from these patients, and determined that women were chronically ill. Moreover, once these observations were accepted, experiments to disprove them were difficult since, until the end of the nineteenth century, all investigators were men and the taboo upon mention of the menstrual function made such research next to impossible.[37]

In actuality the explanation is probably far more complex than this. It is quite possible that physicians were simply blind to what was going on and were so prejudiced that they refused to see reality. There is also the possibility that during the nineteenth century young women did have more than their share of menstrual difficulties. One source of such problems was undoubtedly diet. It was generally believed a century ago that certain foods, especially highly flavored dishes and meats, aroused the sexual appetites. It was, accordingly, desirable to regulate the diets of young girls so as to protect them from unhealthy desires, and physicians found that protein deprivation was a successful cure for female masturbation.[38] Female boarding schools, to minimize sexual interest among their charges, were likely to follow such a prescribed vegetable diet. A study of female higher education in the 1890s deplored the low state of boarding school health, due, it was believed, to diet and lack of exercise, as well as the pressures of the curriculum.[39]

Clelia Mosher, whose research into menstruation among college women spanned several generations between 1890 and 1920, found that girls in the earlier period probably did have greater menstrual difficulties than those in the 1920s. She at first concluded that the reason for this was that during the nineteenth century girls were taught that they were going to be sick during menstruation and the result was a self-fulfilling prophecy. She also found, however, that there was a correlation between dress and menstrual difficulties. During the 1890s and the early years of the twentieth century most young women were put into tight corsets, banded clothing, and unsupported heavy skirts. This clothing interfered with the respiration, made the abdominal muscles flabby, restricted physical activity, and deformed the body on the same principle that the binding of feet in China did. The result was, Mosher held, chronic disturbances of the organs and prolonged menstrual flow.[40] She prepared tables correlating menstrual pain among college women with the width and weight of their skirts and the measurements of their waists. Her figures showed that as the skirt grew shorter and skimpier, and the waist larger, the functional health of women improved. In 1894, 19 percent of the college women were free from menstrual difficulties; in 1915–16, 68 percent considered their periods no problem. In the earlier period the average skirt was 13.5 feet around the hem, the average waist measurement was twenty inches, and the woman also wore several petticoats, some fifteen pounds of clothing hanging from a constricted waist. By the beginning of World War I women wore their skirts above the ankle, skirts were narrowed, petticoats fewer, and waist measurements had increased by 40 percent.[41]

Such studies did much to ease the traumas inflicted by some of the male medical writers of the last part of the nineteenth century. Increasing re-assurance came from the growth in numbers of college-educated and career women who seemed none the worse for their years of hard study or work. While the generation of Martha Thomas had been haunted by the "clanging chains of that gloomy little spector," Dr. Edward H. Clarke's *Sex in Education,* several generations of educated women tended to prove that "college women were not only not invalids, but that they [were] better physically than other women in their own class of life."[42] In part too, the development of the sanitary pad in the aftermath of World War I also freed women from some of the more confining aspects of menstruation. Not all physicians, however, adjusted their thinking to correspond with the latest scientific findings. At the beginning of the twentieth century most sex manuals warned against exciting lives and mental stimulation for pubertal girls.[43] Perhaps this was to be expected but, when the same sort of material was still being published thirty years later, it is possible to wonder what motivated the physicians who wrote it. William J. Robinson's book, for example, in 1931 in its twenty-second edition, still warned that only a minority of women were free from illness during their menstrual periods, and that most should rest at least two days, avoid dancing, cycling, riding, rowing, or any other·athletic exercises, and probably postpone travel by auto, train, or carriage.[44]

That some of the medical hesitation to change seems political, a hesitation to accept women as equals, is evident even in the 1970s. After all it was in 1970 that Edgar Berman, previously best known as the friend and physician of Hubert Humphrey, remarked that women could not fill leadership roles because of the influences of their periodicity, that is their menstrual cycles and menopause.[45] This statement cost him his position in the Democratic Party and made not only him but Humphrey an object of attack by the militant members of women's lib. That the belief still has currency is also indicated by the fact that the first issue of the new woman's magazine *Ms.* found it relevant enough to counter with an article on male cycles and gave hints to women on how to discover whether the men in their lives were ebbing or flowing.[46]

This is not the place to argue the existence of male cycles, however, but only to indicate that it is very possible for medical concepts to get mixed up with political and social beliefs. Perhaps this is inevitable since we are human, but it ought to make the physician a little more cautious in distinguishing his biases from his objective findings. In retrospect it does seem that the nineteenth-century physician grew somewhat more shrill in his emphasis on the instability of the female at the very time that women and their male allies were challenging the old stereotypes. A few physicians jumped into the controversy citing their own clinical observations as evidence in ways that today we can regard only as ludicrous. This in fact happened with a whole series of physiological functions and human activities but was particularly harmful when such sexual topics as menstruation, masturbation, or birth control were dealt with. Obviously women are anatomically different from men, and they do have monthly periods, but to generalize from this and a few isolated patients to a whole theory of female inferiority seems to be an example of poor medical theorizing. The difficulty with past medical theory, whether good or bad, however, is that it often remains a part of the popular ideology of a later generation. One of the things that women of today have to overcome is some of the mistaken concepts about menstruation and its effect.[47]

NOTES

This paper was presented at the 45th annual meeting of the American Association for the History of Medicine, Montreal, Canada, May 4, 1972. Research sponsored by the Erickson Educational Foundation, Baton Rouge, La.

1 John Power, *Essays on the Female Economy* (London: Burgess and Hill, 1831); G. F. Girdwood, "Theory of menstruation," *Lancet*, 1842–43, i: 825–30; J. Bennet, "On healthy and morbid menstruation," *Lancet*, 1852, i: 35, 65, 215, 328, 353.

2 Aristotle [pseud.], *The Works of Aristotle in Four Parts*, containing I. *His complete Master-piece; . . . II. His Experienced Midwife; . . . III. His Book of Problems; . . . IV. His Last Legacy . . .* (London: published for the bookseller, 1808), 126.

3 See M. M. Smith, "Menstruation and some of its effects upon the normal mentalization of woman," *Memphis Medical Monthly*, 1896, *16*: 393–99; C. Frederick Fluhmann, *Menstrual Disorders, Diagnosis and Treatment* (Philadelphia: W. B. Saunders, 1939), 17–26.

4 A. F. A. King, "A new basis for uterine pathology," *American Journal of Obstetrics*, 1875–76, *8*: 242–43.

5 E.F.W. Pflüger, *Ueber die Eierstöcke der Sügethiere und des Menschen* (Leipzig: Engelmann, 1863).

6 Thomas Woody, *A History of Women's Education in the United States*, 2 vols. (New York: The Science Press, 1929), 2: 137.

7 Benjamin Rush, *Essays, Literary, Moral and Philosophical* (Philadelphia: Thomas & Samuel Bradford, 1798), 75–92.

8 Woody, *History of Women's Education*, 2: 231.

9 See Vern Bullough and Bonnie Bullough, *Emergence of Modern Nursing* (New York: Macmillan, 1969), passim.

10 Edward H. Clarke, *Sex in Education; or, A Fair Chance for Girls* (Boston: James R. Osgood & Co., 1873), 37–38.

11 Ibid., 40–41.

12 Ibid., 63.

13 Ibid., 65–72.

14 Ibid., 133.

15 Ibid., 156–57.

16 Ibid., 162–81.

17 George F. Comfort and Anna Manning Comfort, *Woman's Education and Woman's Health* (Syracuse: Thomas W. Durston & Co., 1874), 154.

18 G. Stanley Hall, *Adolescence, Its Psychology and Its Relations to Physiology, Anthropology, Sociology, Sex, Crime, Religions and Education*, 2 vols. (New York: D. Appleton and Co., 1904), 2: 569.

19 T. S. Clouston, "Female education from a medical point of view," *Popular Science Monthly* 24 (Dec. 1883–Jan. 1884): 322–33.

20 John Dewey, "Health and sex in higher education," *Popular Science Monthly* 28 (March 1886): 606.

21 Annie G. Howes et al. *Health Studies of Women College Graduates: Report of a Special Committee of the Association of Collegiate Alumnae* (Boston: Wright & Potter, 1885), 9.

22 Dewey, "Health and sex in higher education," 611.

23 Henry Maudsley, *Sex in Mind and in Education* (Syracuse: C.W. Bardeen, 1884), 14.

24 John Goodman, "The menstrual cycle," *Transactions*, American Gynecological Society, 1877, *2*: 650–62; "The cyclical theory of menstruation," *American Journal of Obstetrics*, 1878. *11*: 673–94.

25 George J. Engelmann, "The American girl of today: the influence of modern education on functional development," *Transactions*, American Gynecological Society, 1900, *25*: 8–45.

26 J.H. Kellogg, *Plain Facts for Old and Young* (Burlington, Iowa: I. F. Segner, 1882), 83.

27 Ibid., 86.

28 F. W. Van Dyke, "Higher education a cause of phys-

ical decay in women," *Medical Records,* 1905, *67:* 296–98.

29 Ralph Wait Parsons, "The American girl *versus* higher education, considered from a medical point of view," *New York Medical Journal,* 1907, *85:* 116.

30 Ibid., 119.

31 Mary Roberts Smith, "Statistics of college and non-college women," *Publications,* American Statistical Association, 1900–1901, *7, nos. 49–56:* 1–26.

32 Hall, *Adolescence,* 1: 478.

33 Ibid., 1: 511.

34 Ibid., 2: 646.

35 Ibid., 2: 639.

36 M. Carey Thomas, "Present tendencies in women's college and university education," Feb., 1908, in *The Woman Movement: Feminism in the United States and England,* ed., William O'Neill (Chicago: Quadrangle Books, 1969), 168.

37 Leta Stetter Hollingworth, *Functional Periodicity: An Experimental Study of the Mental and Motor Abilities of Women during Menstruation,* Teachers College, Columbia University Contributions to Education, No. 69 (New York: Columbia University Press, 1914), 44, 66, 93, 95.

38 John Tompkins Walton, "Case of nymphomania

successfully treated," *American Journal of the Medical Sciences,* 1857, *33:* 47–50.

39 Anna C. Brackett, ed., *Women and the Higher Education* (New York: Harper, 1893), 90.

40 Clelia Duel Mosher, "Normal menstruation and some of the factors modifying it," *Johns Hopkins Hospital Bulletin,* 1901, *12:* 178–79.

41 Clelia Duel Mosher, *Woman's Physical Freedom* (New York: The Woman's Press, 1923), 1, 29.

42 Thomas, "Present tendencies in women's college and university education," 169.

43 See, for example, William H. Walling, *Sexology* (Philadelphia: Puritan Publishing co., 1904), 207.

44 William J. Robinson, *Woman: Her Sex and Love Life,* 22d ed. (New York: Eugenics Publishing Co., 1931), 80–81.

45 *New York Times,* July 26, 1970; *Los Angeles Times,* Feb. 21, 1972.

46 Estelle Ramey, "Men's cycles," *Ms.,* Spring 1972, 8–15.

47 For a survey of some recent research on the topic see Mary E. Luschen and David M. Pierce, "Menstrual cycle, mood and arousability," *Sex Research* 8 (February 1972): 41–47.

SEXUALITY

According to Victorian ideology, men were passionate and sexual and women were passionless and uninterested in sex. As Carl Degler relates, one British woman advising her daughter before her marriage is said to have told her to submit to her husband's needs and to "lie still and think of the Empire." Most physicians, however, recognized that women could and did enjoy sexual activity. But the medical profession had its own ideas about what was healthy for women sexually and what produced problems. In this section, Degler explores the ideology and the medical and women's response to it, and Nancy Cott responds to his interpretations with her own analysis of women's sexuality in the first half of the nineteenth century.

The dual "problem" of masturbation and homosexuality produced its own set of medical advice literature. Physicians and society in general did not sanction what they believed was abnormal and dangerous behavior, and yet, as Carroll Smith-Rosenberg and Leila J. Rupp illustrate, the society that could not condone homosexuality may have been harboring it. These historians, and others not represented here, explore women's intimate social world and posit that in the nineteenth and early twentieth centuries a version of lesbian relations may have flourished within women's domestic and separate culture. These historians reveal the homosocial (if not homosexual) relations that allowed emotional attachments between women to grow and provided an acceptable outlet for passionate feelings. The issue of labeling, as Rupp notes, may confuse our understanding of the past and should warn us to tread carefully when studying this sensitive and personal arena.

Sexuality, like menstruation, was a subject that most women did not write about explicitly or frequently. Thus the historian confronts the same dilemma of trying to understand a subject in the face of very few data. Degler's analysis of Clelia Mosher's survey provides some concrete evidence of women's perceptions of their sexuality, but the record remains silent for so many women that generalization is elusive. It may be impossible for historians ever to sort out and understand the role sexuality played in women's lives in the past, but from indirect evidence in advice manuals, physicians' records, and in women's personal writings to intimate friends and anonymous diaries, we can begin to piece together another dimension of people's personal lives that had signficant implications for the shape and quality of their lives in general.

3

What Ought to Be and What Was:
Women's Sexuality in the Nineteenth Century

CARL N. DEGLER

As every schoolgirl knows, the nineteenth century was afraid of sex, particularly when it manifested itself in women. Captain Marryat, in his travels in the United States, told of some American women so refined that they objected to the word "leg," preferring instead the more decorous "limb." Marryat also reported seeing this delicacy carried to extremes in a girls' school where a school mistress, in the interest of protecting the modesty of her charges, had dressed all four "limbs" of the piano "in modest little trousers with frills at the bottom of them!"[1] Women's alleged lack of passion was epitomized, too, in the story of the English mother who was asked by her daughter before her marriage how she ought to behave on her wedding night. "Lie still and think of the Empire," the mother advised.

This view of Victorian attitudes toward sexuality is captured in more than stories. Steven Marcus, writing about the attitudes of English Victorians toward sexuality, and Nathan Hale, Jr., summarizing the attitudes of Americans on the same subject, both quote at length from Dr. William Acton's *Functions and Disorders of the Reproductive Organs,* which went through several editions in England and the United States during the middle years of the nineteenth century.[2] Acton's book was undoubtedly one of the most widely quoted sexual advice books in the English-speaking world. The book summed up the medical literature on women's sexuality by saying that "the majority of women (happily for them) are not very much troubled with sexual feelings of any kind. What men are habitu-

ally, women are only exceptionally."[3] Theophilus Parvin, an American doctor, told his medical class in 1883, "I do not believe one bride in a hundred, of delicate, educated, sensitive women, accepts matrimony from any desire for sexual gratification; when she thinks of this at all, it is with shrinking, or even with horror, rather than with desire."[4]

Modern writers on the sexual life of women in the nineteenth century have echoed these contemporary descriptions. "For the sexual act was associated by many wives only with a duty," writes Walter Houghton, "and by most husbands with a necessary if pleasurable yielding to one's baser nature; by few, therefore, with any innocent and joyful experience."[5] Writing about late-nineteenth century America, David Kennedy quotes approvingly from Viola Klein when she writes that "in the whole Western world during the nineteenth century and at the beginning of the twentieth century it would have been not only scandalous to admit the existence of a strong sex urge in women, but it would have been contrary to all observation."[6] Nathan Hale, Jr., sums up his review of the sexual-advice literature at the turn of the century with a similar conclusion: "Many women came to regard marriage as little better than legalized prostitution. Sexual passion became associated almost exclusively with the male, with prostitutes, and women of the lower classes."[7] Most recently Ben Barker-Benfield has argued that male doctors were so convinced that women had no sexual interest that when it manifested itself drastic measures were taken to subdue it, including excision of the sexual organs. "Defining the absence of sexual desire in women as normal, doctors came to see its presence as disease. . . . Sexual appetite was a male quality (to be properly channelled of course). If a woman showed it, she resembled a man."[8]

CARL N. DEGLER is Margaret Byrne Professor of American History at Stanford University, Stanford, California.

Reprinted with permission of author. This article first appeared in *American Historical Review* 79 (1974): 1467–1490.

Despite the apparent agreement between the nineteenth-century medical writers and modern students of the period, it is far from clear that there was in the nineteenth century a consensus on the subject of women's sexuality or that women were in fact inhibited from acknowledging their sexual feelings. In examining these two issues I shall be concerned with an admittedly limited yet significant population, namely, women of the urban middle class in the United States. This was the class to which the popular medical advice books, of which William Acton's volume was a prime example, were directed. It is principally the women of this class upon whom historians' generalizations about women's lives in the nineteenth century are based. And though these women were not a numerical majority of the sex, they undoubtedly set the tone and provided the models for most women. The sources drawn upon are principally the popular and professional medical literature concerned with women and a hitherto undiscovered survey of married women's sexual attitudes and practices that was begun in the 1890s by Dr. Clelia D. Mosher.

Let me begin with the first question or issue. Was William Acton representative of medical writers when he contended that women were essentially without sexual passion? Rather serious doubts arise as soon as one looks into the medical literature, popular as well as professional, where it was recognized that the sex drive was so strong in woman that to deny it might well compromise her health. Dr. Charles Taylor, writing in 1882, said, "It is not a matter of indifference whether a woman live a single or a married life. . . . I do not for one moment wish to be understood as believing that an unmarried woman cannot exist in perfect health for I know she can. But the point is, that *she must take pains for it.*" For if the generative organs are not used, then "some other demand for the unemployed functions, must be established. Accumulated force must find an outlet, or disturbance first and weakness ultimately results." His recommendation was muscular exercise and education for usefulness. He also described cases of women who had denied their sexuality and even experienced orgasms without knowing it. Some women, he added, ended up, as a result, with impairment of movement or other physical symptoms.[9]

Other writers on medical matters were even more direct in testifying to the presence of sexual feelings in women. "Passion absolutely necessary in woman," wrote Orson S. Fowler, the phrenologist, in 1870. "Amativeness is created in the female head as universally as in the male. . . . That female passion exists, is as obvious as that the sun shines," he wrote. Without woman's passion, he contended, a fulfilled love could not occur.[10] Both sexes enjoy the sexual embrace, asserted Henry Chavasse, another popular medical writer, in 1866, but among human beings, as among the animals in general, he continued, "the male is more ardent and fierce, and . . . the desires of the female never reach that hight [*sic*] as to impel her to the commission of crime." Woman's pleasure, though it may be "less acute," is longer lasting than man's, Chavasse said. R. T. Trall, also a popular medical writer, counseled in a similar vein. "Whatever may be the object of sexual intercourse," he wrote, "whether intended as a love embrace merely, or a generative act, it is very clear that it should be as pleasurable as possible to *both parties.*"[11]

If one can judge the popularity of a guide for women by the number of its editions, then Dr. George Napheys's *The Physical Life of Woman: Advice to the Maiden, Wife, and Mother* (1869) must have been one of the leaders. Within two weeks of publication it went into a second printing, and within two years sixty thousand copies were in print. Napheys was a well-known Philadelphia physician. Women, he wrote, quoting an unnamed "distinguished medical writer," are divided into three classes. The first consists of those who have no sexual feelings, and it is the smallest group. The second is larger and comprises those who have "strong passion." The third is made up of "the vast majority of women, in whom the sexual appetite is as moderate as all other appetites." He went on to make his point quite clear. "It is a false notion and contrary to nature that this passion in a woman is a derogation to her sex. The science of physiology indicates most clearly its propriety and dignity." He then proceeded to denounce those wives who "plume themselves on their repugnance or their distaste for their conjugal obligations." Napheys also contended that authorities agree that "conception is more assured when the two individuals who co-operate in it participate at the same time in the transports of which it is the fruit." Napheys probably had no sound reason for this point, but the accuracy of his statement is immaterial. What is of moment is that as an adviser to women he was clearly convinced that women possessed sexual feelings, which ought to be cultivated rather than suppressed. Concerning sexual relations during pregnancy he wrote, "There is no reason why passions should not be gratified in moderation and with caution during the whole period of pregnancy." And since his book is directed to women, there is no question that the passion he is talking about here is that of women.[12]

In 1878 Dr. Ely Van de Warker of Syracuse, a fellow of the American Gynecological Society, described sexual passion in women as "the analogue of the subjective copulative sensations of man, . . . the acme of the sexual orgasm in woman is the sensory equivalent of emission in man, observing the distinction necessarily implied between the sexes—that in woman it is psychic and subjective, and that in man it has also a physical element and is objective," that is, it is accompanied by seminal emission. The principal purpose of Van de Warker's article was to deplore the fact that some women lacked sexual feeling, a state which he called "female impotency."[13] What is striking about his article is that he obviously considered such lack of feeling in women abnormal and worthy of medical attention, just as impotency in a man would cause medical concern.

Van de Warker's remarks, as well as his use of the word, make it evident that physicians were well aware that normal women experienced orgasms. Lest there be any doubt that their meaning of the word was the same as ours today, let me quote from a physician in 1883 who described in some detail woman's sexual response. He began by describing the preparatory stage, which, he said,

> may be reached by any means, bodily or mental, which, in the opposite sex, cause erection. Following upon this, then, is a stage of pleasurable excitement, gradually increasing and culminating in an acme of excitement, which may be called the state of consummation, and the analogue of which in the male is emission. This is followed in both sexes by a degree of nervous prostration, less marked, however, in the female, and . . . by a relief to the general congestion of all the genital organs which has existed, and

perhaps increased, from the beginning of the preparatory stage.[14]

All of this evidence, it seems to me, shows that there was a significant body of opinion and information quite different from that advanced on women's sexuality by William Acton and others of his outlook. Now it might be asked how widespread was this counter-Acton point of view? Was it not confined primarily to physicians writing for other physicians? Not at all. Napheys, Chavasse, and Fowler, to name three, were all writing their books for the large lay public that was interested in sexual matters. As we have seen, many of these marriage manuals, particularly Napheys's and Fowler's, were printed in several large editions.

Yet, in the end, there is a certain undeniable inconclusiveness in simply raising up one collection of writers against another, even if their existence does make the issue an open one, rather than the closed one that so many secondary writers have made it. It suggests, at the very least, that there was a sharp difference of medical opinion, rather than a consensus, on the nature of women's sexual feelings and needs. In fact there is some reason to believe, as we shall see, that the so-called Victorian conception of women's sexuality was more that of an ideology seeking to be established than the prevalent view of practice of even middle-class women, especially as there is a substantial amount of nineteenth-century writing about women that assumes the existence of strong sexual feelings in women. One of the historian's recognized difficulties in showing, through quotations from writers who assert a particular outlook, that a social attitude prevailed in the past is that one always wonders how representative and how self-serving the examples or quotations are. This is especially true in this case where medical opinion can be found on both sides of the question. When writers, however, assume the attitude in question to be prevalent while they are intent upon writing about something else, then one is not so dependent upon the tyranny of numbers in quoting from sources. For behind the assumption of prevalence lie many examples, so to speak. Such testimony, moreover, is unintended and therefore not self-serving. This kind of evidence, furthermore, helps us to answer the second question—to what extent were women in the nineteenth century inhibited from expressing their sexual feelings? For in assuming that women had sexual feelings, these writers are offering clear, if unintended, testimony to women's sexuality.

Medical writers like Acton may have asserted that women did not possess sexual feelings, but there were many doctors who clearly assumed not only that such feelings existed but that the repression of them caused illness. One medical man, for example, writing in 1877, traced a cause of insanity in women to the onset of sexuality. "Sexual development initiates new and extraordinary physical change," he pointed out. "The erotic and sexual impulse is awakened."[15] Another, writing ten years later, asserted that some of women's illnesses were due to a denial of sexual satisfaction. "Females feel often that they are not appreciated," wrote Dr. William McLaury in a medical journal, "that they have no one to confide in; then they become morose, angular, and disagreeable as a result of continual disappointment to their social and sexual longings. Even those married may become the victims of sexual starvation when the parties are mentally, magnetically, and physically antagonistic."[16] Henry Chavasse, writing for a popular audience, was also impressed by the need for sexual outlets for women. There may be some individuals "of phlegmatic temperament," he conceded, who are not injured by celibacy, but "absolute continence in the sanguine and ardent disposition predisposes to the gravest maladies." His listing of the resulting maladies, of which nymphomania was one, makes it clear that he was referring to women as well as men. These maladies, he went on, "are born as well of extreme restraint as of extreme excess. . . . Females seem to suffer even more than males . . . perhaps because their continence is more complete." (Presumably he was referring here to the absence of nocturnal emissions in women.) As a result, he continued, nunneries were notorious as places of fanaticism. "Hence the old proverb, 'The convent and the confessional are the cradles of hysteria and nymphomania.'"[17]

To Dr. Van de Warker women's sexuality was so obvious that he assumed men required it in order to achieve full sexual satisfaction for themselves. In marriage, he wrote, the husband

not only demands pleasure and satisfaction for himself, but he requires something much

more difficult to give—the appearance, if not the real existence, of satisfaction and pleasure in the object of his attentions. Unhappiness and suspicion are often the result of the absence of this pleasure [in women], and are sure to work to the material disadvantage of the weaker party. To show that this is really the case, I need but to remind physicians how often they are approached by husbands upon this subject; yet further, how often the coldness and indifference of wives are alleged as the excuse for conjugal infidelity.[18]

What is striking in this passage is that husbands complained to doctors about their wives' coldness, a fact that makes it quite evident that passion in wives was not only desired by men, but expected—why, otherwise, would they complain of its lack? Van de Warker, it is worth pointing out, was writing for his fellow physicians, who were in a position to verify his assertions from their own experience with patients.

Van de Warker's explanation for "impotency" in women is revealing, too. Ascribing it to "sexual incompatibility," he went on to say that "so far as my own observation extends, the husband is generally at fault. The more common cause is acute sexual irritability on the part of the husband."[19] Dr. William Goodell, writing in 1887, also asserted that mutual pleasure was essential to successful marital intercourse. In Goodell's mind, as in Van de Warker's, that meant men must recognize women's interests and sexual rhythm. "Destroy the reciprocity of the union," Goodell cautioned, "and marriage is no longer an equal partnership, but a sensual usurpation on the one side and a loathing submission on the other."[20] Another medical writer who also acknowledged women's pleasure in the sex act made the same point as Goodell and Van de Warker. Men must not force themselves upon women or "overpersuade, but await the wife's invitation at this time [during ovulation], when her husband is a hero in her eyes." In this way the husband "would enjoy more and suffer less," the physician predicted.[21] These writers, in short, were not only testifying to their knowledge that women possessed sexual feelings, they were also explaining how those feelings were sometimes denied legitimate satisfaction by inept husbands.

The assumption that women had sexual feelings which required satisfaction also comes through in the course of discussions about contraception. Generally, physicians and other writers on this subject in the nineteenth century strongly opposed contraception, though all recognized that it was widely practiced. One of the methods in common use was coitus interruptus, or withdrawal by the male prior to ejaculation. This method was condemned for a variety of reasons, but for our purposes it is significant that among the objections was its harmful effects upon women. This method, wrote Henry Chavasse, is "attended with disastrous consequences, most particularly to the female, whose nervous system suffers from ungratified excitement."[22] Dr. John Harvey Kellogg, a popular writer on medical matters, also warned against the method because of its effects upon women. He quoted at length from a French authority. Whenever this method is practiced, the authority wrote, all of women's genital organs "enter into a state of orgasm, a storm which is not appeased by the natural crisis; a nervous super excitation persists" after the act. The authority then compared the unreleased tension to that evoked in presenting food to a "famished man" and then snatching it away. "The sensibilities of the womb and the entire reproductive system are teased to no purpose." It is evident that in the minds of both writers women were assumed to have sexual feelings that were normally aroused during sexual intercourse.[23] Dr. Augustus Gardner, writing in 1870 also for a popular audience, quoted from the same French authority and for the same purpose as Kellogg.[24]

Anyone who has looked into the sexual history of the nineteenth century is immediately struck by the deep and anxious concern physicians as well as other people felt about masturbation. Although it is often thought that boys were the principal objects of that concern, the fact is that girls were just as much fretted about. That there were such concerns about girls' masturbating is in itself a sign and measure of the recognition of sexual feelings in women. In fact in 1866 one popular medical writer on women defined masturbation as "the mechanical irritation of the sexual organs in order to excite the same voluptuous sensations attendant upon natural intercourse."[25] Mary Wood-Allen, a leader in the Women's Christian Temperance Union and a writer of advice books for young women,

had no doubt that girls could be led into self-abuse. Even girls who would not use any mechanical means "to arouse sexual desire," she pointed out, nevertheless permitted themselves to fantasize or to have mental images that "arouse the spasmodic feelings of sexual pleasure."[26] Indeed from Wood-Allen's book one receives the message that women's sexual feelings were not only present but dangerously easy to arouse.

Discussion about masturbation in women reveals in another way how widely accepted was the idea that women possessed sexual desires. One physician, in the course of an article on the subject, said that the worst thing about masturbation in women was that a climax and resolution of tension were generally not achieved; hence the vice was persisted in. In response another doctor agreed that masturbation indeed gave rise to all the physical harm alleged in the article. But he disagreed with the assertion that in a woman sexual excitation could stop short of orgasm. "A commencement of the act, either of masturbation or coition," the letter writer contended, "*naturally* leads to its consummation, viz., an orgasm." Furthermore, he persisted, if "in the *healthy* female, an orgasm is not produced in the act of coition, she is not satisfied, and either will continue the act herself or with her coadjutor till such consummation does take place."[27]

Women's sexuality is also assumed in another class of medical concerns. When Dr. J. Marion Sims, the "founding father" of American gynecology, published *Clinical Notes on Uterine Surgery* in 1866, conception was only dimly understood. In explaining how it took place Sims revealed, in passing, that most people took for granted that women experienced sexual feelings. "It is the vulgar opinion, and the opinion of many savants," Sims remarked, "that, to ensure conception, sexual intercourse should be performed with a certain degree of completeness, that would give an exhaustive satisfaction to both parties at the same moment." This sounds like twentieth-century ideas on optimum sexual performance, for Sims then went on to note, again in passing, that husbands and wives strove for such simultaneity and were unhappy when they failed to have simultaneous orgasms. "How often do we hear husbands complain of coldness on the part of the wives; and attribute to this the failure to procreate. And sometimes wives are disposed to think, though they never complain, that the fault lies with the hasty ejaculation of the husband."[28] Sims's point, of course, was that conception did not depend upon either sexual arousal or satisfaction in the women. The important point for us, however, is that Sims, the medical readers he was addressing, and the patients he treated all believed women were naturally capable of sexual feelings. Napheys in his popular book of advice for women also alluded to the prevalent idea that conception and pleasure were connected. He said that many people erroneously believed that conception could be known from the "more than ordinary degree of pleasure" on the part of the woman during the sexual act.[29]

In the course of discussing other kinds of women's illnesses, physicians often made it clear that they not only recognized the existence of sexual feelings in women but expected them in normal women. As we have observed already, Dr. Van de Warker considered the lack of sexual feelings in a woman as an abnormality to be cured. He called such women "impotent," just as one would denominate a man who failed to have adequate sexual responses. To Van de Warker, women had to learn how to dislike sex; enjoyment of it was natural.[30] Napheys, too, saw frigidity as abnormal; its removal, he thought, was "so desirable."[31] One physician in 1882, in discussing a case of excessive masturbation, wrote that during an examination his female patient experienced "the most intense orgasm that I have ever witnessed,"[32] implying that he had witnessed others. Another physician listed among the pathological symptoms of one patient "an absence of all sexual desire"[33]—as if its presence were the normal condition of a woman. One medical doctor, in trying to show how intense was the pain a married patient experienced during intercourse, said that both partners had given up sexual relations "although both had usually violent animal passions."[34] In arguing against birth control Dr. Augustus Gardner told of a wife who, fearing pregnancy since she had borne seven children in seven years, was "otherwise very ardent."[35]

During the 1880s and 1890s, as surgeons became more skillful and antisepsis made abdominal operations safer, a number of doctors sought to alleviate otherwise incurable or obscure pelvic pains and nervous conditions in women through the removal of ovaries. This medical development is a complex one, especially as to the attitudes it might reveal on the part of doctors and society in general. This is not the place to pursue that question, however. It serves to explain, though, why ovariodectomies were a subject of considerable interest among gynecologists. One consequence of that interest was a report in 1890 by a surgeon who had removed forty-six pairs of ovaries. Significantly, he related that "the sexual instinct was always preserved. Three patients, virginal before operation, married later and lived in happy wedlock. The passions persist particularly when the operation is performed early on young persons," he concluded.[36] For us the significance of this report is not whether it is accurate; in fact I suspect that it is not. For as Dr. Van de Warker remarked on a different occasion, many women who suffered the pain or nervousness that caused them to submit to the operation in the first place probably had never felt any sexual pleasure. Consequently, to ask them after the operation whether there was any diminution in sexual feeling generally brought a denial. Moreover, the removal of the ovaries may well have reduced or eliminated hormonal secretions that may contribute to normal sexual feelings in women. In short, the physician's report suffers from his clear wish to put his series of operations in a good light. But that very wish is revealing, for what it tells us is that women were expected to have sexual feelings and it was undesirable for a surgeon or, presumably, anyone else, to eliminate or even reduce those feelings.

In the light of the foregoing it is difficult to accept the view that women were generally seen in the nineteenth century as without sexual feelings or drives. The question then arises as to how this widely accepted historical interpretation got established? Part of the reason, undoubtedly, is the result of the general reticence of the nineteenth century in regard to sex. The excessive gentility of the middle class has been read by historians as a sign of hostility toward sexuality, particularly in women. The whole cult of the home and women's allegedly exalted place in it was easily translated by some historians into an antisexual attitude.[37] But a good part of the explanation must also be attributable to the simple failure on the part of historians to survey fully the extant sources. The kind of statements quoted from medical writers in this article, for example, was either overlooked or ignored.

Another important part of the explanation is that the sources that were surveyed and quoted were taken to be descriptive of the sexual ideology of the time when in fact they were part of an effort by some other medical writers to establish an ideology, not to delineate an already accepted one. In other words, the medical literature that was emphasized by Steven Marcus, Oscar Handlin, or Nathan Hale, Jr., was really normative or prescriptive rather than descriptive.

This misinterpretation was easy enough to make since much nineteenth-century medical literature was often descriptive in form even though in fact it was seeking to set a new standard of sexual behavior. Sometimes, however, the normative concerns and purposes showed through the ostensible description. A close reading, for example, of William Acton's second edition of *The Functions and Disorders of the Reproductive Organs* reveals in several places his desire to establish a new and presumably "higher" standard of sexual attitude and behavior. After pointing out that publicists strongly condemn sexual relations outside marriage, he asks, "But should we stop there? I think not. The audience should be informed that, in the present state of society, the sexual appetites must not be fostered; and experience teaches those who have had the largest means of information on the matter, that self-control must be exercised." So far, he continues, no one has "dared publicly to advocate . . . this necessary regulation of the sexual feelings or training to continence." Or later, when he discusses women in particular, it is evident that he is arguing for a special attitude, not merely describing common practice. "The *best* mothers, wives, and managers of households know little or nothing of sexual indulgence. Love of home, children, and domestic duties are the only passions they feel," he writes.[38]

American writers of the time who followed the lead of Acton as well as quoting him display a similar mixture of prescription and description. Take Dr. John Kellogg's *Plain Facts for Old and Young*, which sold over three hundred thousand copies by 1910 and went through five editions. Kellogg, like Acton, made it clear that he thought sex was too dominant in the thoughts of people. As we look around us today, he wrote, "it would appear that the opportunity for sensual gratification has come to be, in the world at large, the chief attraction

between the sexes. If to these observations," he continued, "we add the filthy disclosures constantly made in police court and scandal suits, we have a powerful confirmation of the opinion."[39] It was this excess that he warns against, drawing upon quotations from Acton to support his arguments. He is at pains to show, too, that continence, especially in men, is not deleterious to health, as some contended. He admits that the medical profession is not in agreement on the amount of sexual indulgence permitted in marriage. "A very few hold that the sexual act should never be indulged except for the purpose of reproduction, and then only at periods when reproduction will be possible. Others, while equally opposed to the excesses . . . limit indulgence to the number of months in the year." Human beings, he advised, should take their cue from animals, who have intercourse only for procreation and then at widely spaced intervals. Instead of heeding this counsel, he writes, loosely quoting from Acton, "the lengths to which married people carry excesses is perfectly astonishing."[40]

Kellogg's reference to the behavior of animals as a worthy guideline for human behavior was echoed by other writers who sought to control sexuality. William Acton and Orson S. Fowler, for example, also used that standard of sexual behavior. Kellogg even went so far as to make an overt defense of the analogy. He carefully explained to his readers that in the modern age of biology these analogies were extremely helpful in getting at nature's purpose. "It is by this method of investigation," he remarked, "that most of the important truths of physiology have been developed; and the plan is universally acknowledged to be a proper and logical one." Then he launched into a condemnation of those men who use their wives as harlots, "having no other end but pleasure." For it was clear that among animals the end was reproduction only and then only at those one or two times a year when reproduction was possible. But by the time Kellogg reached the place in his book where he defended the analogy with animals he had already revealed that his purpose in invoking the analogy was reformist and normative, not simply scientific and logical. For in the early pages of his book, in making a different normative point—the need to protect children from premature sexuality—he told of a parent whose adolescent children often played games in the nude. When admonished for permitting this practice, the parent replied that it was only natural. "Perfectly harmless; just like little pigs!" Kellogg quoted the parent as saying. Kellogg's comment, however, was quite different from what he would advise later in his book: "as though pigs were models for human beings!"[41]

In the end Kellogg himself virtually admitted that his "plain facts" were hardly facts at all, but prescriptions and hopes. "There will be many," he wrote, "the vast majority, perhaps, who will not bring their minds to accept the truth which nature seems to teach, which would confine sexual acts to reproduction wholly." And so he was prepared to offer a compromise, that is, a method of contraception. It was not a very effective method, as he admitted—the so-called safe period—but again what is important is his frank recognition that only a minority among his readers confined their sexual activities to reproduction and that he hoped he would be able to induce more to do so.[42]

It would be a mistake, in short, to accept the prescriptive or normative literature, like that of Acton, Kellogg, and others,[43] as revealing very much about sexual behavior in the Victorian era. It may be possible to derive a sexual ideology from such writers, but it is a mistake to assume that the ideology thus delineated is either characteristic of the society or reflective of behavior. On the contrary, it is the argument of this article that the attitudes and behavior of middle-class women were only peripherally affected by the ideology. Not only did many medical writers, as we have seen, encourage women to express their sexuality, but there is a further, even more persuasive reason for believing that the prescriptive literature is not a reliable guide to either the sexual behavior or the attitudes of middle-class women. It is the testimony of women themselves.

Any systematic knowledge of the sexual habits of women is a relatively recent historical acquisition, confined to the surveys of women made in the 1920s and 1930s and culminating in the well-known Kinsey report.[44] Until recently no even slightly comparable body of evidence for nineteenth-century women was known to exist. In the Stanford University Archives, however, are questionnaires completed by a group of women testifying to their sexual habits. The questionnaires are part of the papers of Dr. Clelia Duel Mosher (1863–1940), a physi-

cian at Stanford University and a pioneer in the study of women's sexuality. Mosher began her work on the sexual habits of married women when she was a student at the University of Wisconsin prior to 1892. That year she transferred for her senior year to Stanford, where she received an A.B. degree in 1893 and an M.A. in 1894. In 1900 she earned an M.D. degree from Johns Hopkins University. After a decade of private practice she joined the Stanford faculty as a member of the department of hygiene and medical adviser of women students. Her published work dealt with the physical capabilities of women; she was a well-known advocate of physical exercise for women. Mosher's questionnaires are carefully arranged and bound in volume 10 of her unpublished work, "Hygiene and Physiology of Women." Mosher, however, apparently never drew more than a few impressionistic conclusions from the highly revealing questionnaires. She did not even publish the fact of their existence, and so far as can be ascertained no use has heretofore been made of this manuscript source. Yet the amount and kind of information on sexual habits and attitudes of married women in the late nineteenth century contained in these questionnaires are unique.

The project, which spanned some twenty years, was begun at the University of Wisconsin when Mosher was a student of biology in the early 1890s. She designed the questionnaire when asked to address the Mother's Club at the university on the subject of marriage. In later years she added to her cases and used the information when giving advice to women about sexual and hygienic matters.[45] This initiative, as well as the kind of questions she asked, reveals that Mosher was far ahead of her time. She amassed information on women's sexuality that none of the many nineteenth-century writers on the subject studied in any systematic way at all.

The questionnaire itself is quite lengthy, comprising twenty-five questions, each one of which is divided into several parts. Much of the questionnaire, it is true, is taken up with ascertaining facts about the parents and even the grandparents of the respondents, but over half of the questions deal directly with women's sexual behavior and attitudes.[46] The information contained in the questionnaires not only supports the interpretation of women's sexuality that already has been drawn from the published literature, both lay and medical, but also provides us with a means of measuring the degree to which the prescriptive marriage literature affected women's sexual behavior.

Since the evidence in this questionnaire, which I call the Mosher survey, has never been used before, it is first worthwhile to examine the social background of the women who answered the questionnaires. All told there are forty-six useable questionnaires, but since two of the questionnaires seem to have been filled out by the same woman at an interval of twenty-three years, the number of women actually surveyed is forty-five.[47] In the aggregates that follow I have counted only forty-five questionnaires. The questionnaires, it ought to be said, were not administered at the same time, but at three different periods at least; moreover the date of administration of nine questionnaires cannot be ascertained. Of those that do provide that information, seventeen were completed before 1900, fourteen were filled out between 1913 and 1917, and five were answered in 1920.

More important than the date of administration of the questionnaires are the birth dates of the respondents. All but one of the forty-four women who provided their dates of birth were born before 1890. In fact thirty-three, or 70 percent of the whole group, were born before 1870. And of these, seventeen, or slightly over half, were born before the Civil War. For comparative purposes it might be noted that in Alfred Kinsey's survey of women's sexuality the earliest cohort of respondents was born only in the 1890s. In short, the attitudes and practices to which the great majority of the women in the Mosher survey testify were those of women who grew up and married within the nineteenth century, regardless of when they may have completed the questionnaires.

An important consideration in evaluating the responses, of course, is the social origins of the women. From what class did they come, and from what sections of the country? The questionnaire, fortunately, provides some information here, but not with as much precision as one might like. Since the great majority of the respondents attended college or a normal school (thirty-four out of forty-five, with the education of three unknown), it is evident that the group is not representative of the population of the United States as a whole. The remainder of the group attended secondary school, either public or private, a pattern that is again not rep-

resentative of a general population in which only a tiny minority of young people attended secondary school. But for purposes of evaluating the impact of the prescriptive or marital advice literature upon American women this group is quite appropriate. For inasmuch as their educational background identifies them as middle- or upper-class women, it can be said that they were precisely those persons to whom that advisory literature was directed and upon whom its effects ought to be most evident.

In geographical origin the respondents to the Mosher survey seem to be somewhat more representative, if the location of parents, birthplaces, and colleges attended can be taken as a measure, albeit impressionistic, of geographical distribution. Unfortunately there is no other systematic or more reliable information on this subject. The colleges attended, for example, are located in the Northeast (Cornell [6], Smith, Wellesley, and Vassar [2]), in the Middle West (Ripon, Iowa State University, and Indiana), and in the Far West (Stanford [9], the University of California, and the University of the Pacific). The South is not represented at all among the colleges attended.

Although the emphasis upon prestigious colleges might make one think that these were women of the upper or even leisure class, rather than simply middle class, a further piece of information sugets that in fact they were not. One of the questions asked concerned working experience prior to marriage. Although seven of the respondents provided no data at all on this point, and eight reported that they had married immediately after completing their education, thirty of the women reported that they had worked prior to marriage. As a sidelight on the opportunities available to highly educated women in the late nineteenth century, it is worth adding that twenty-seven of the thirty worked as teachers. On the basis of their working experience it seems reasonable to conclude that the respondents were principally middle- or upper-middle-class women rather than members of a leisure class.

Despite the high level of education of these women, they confessed to having a pretty poor knowledge, by modern standards, of sexual physiology before marriage. Only eleven said that they had much knowledge on that subject, obtained from female relatives, books, or courses in college, while another thirteen said that they had some knowledge. The remainder—slightly over half—reported that they had very little or no knowledge. No guidelines were given in the questionnaire for estimating the amount of knowledge. The looseness of the definition is shown by the fact that three of the respondents who said that they had no knowledge at all named books on women's physiology that they had read. From other titles mentioned in passing it is clear that a number of these women had direct acquaintance with the prescriptive and advisory literature of the time. How did it affect their behavior? Did they repress their sexual impulses or deny them, as some of the prescriptive literature advised? Were they in fact without sexual desire? Or were they motivated toward personal sexual satisfaction as the medical literature quoted in this article advised?

The Mosher survey provides a considerable amount of evidence to answer these and other questions. To begin with, thirty-five of the forty-five women testified that they felt desire for sexual intercourse independent of their husband's interest, while nine said they never or rarely felt any such desire. What is more striking, however, is the number who testified to orgasmic experience. According to the standard view of women's sexuality in the nineteenth century, women were not expected to feel desire and certainly not to experience an orgasm. Yet it is striking that in constructing the questionnaire Dr. Mosher asked not only whether the respondents experienced an orgasm during intercourse but whether "you *always* have a venereal orgasm?" (my italics). Although that form of the question makes quite clear Mosher's own assumption that female orgasms were to be expected, it unfortunately confuses the meaning of the responses. (Incidentally, only two of the forty-five respondents failed to answer this question.) Five of the women, for instance, responded "no" without further comment. Given the wording of the question, however, that negative could have meant, "not always, but almost always" as well as "never" or any response in between these extremes. The ambiguity is further heightened when it is recognized that in answer to another question, three of the five negatives said that they had felt sexual desire, while a fourth said "sometimes but not often," and the fifth said sex was "usually a nuisance." Luckily, however, most of the women who responded to the question concerning orgasm

made more precise answers. The great majority of them said that they had experienced orgasms. The complete pattern of responses is set forth in Table 1.

In sum, thirty-four of the women experienced orgasm, with the possibility that the figure might be as high as thirty-seven if those who reported "no" but said they had felt sexual desire are categorized as "sometimes." (Interestingly enough, of nine women out of the forty-five who said they had never felt any sexual desire, seven said that they had experienced orgasms.) Moreover, sixteen or almost half of those who experienced orgasms did so either "always" or "usually." As we have seen, in the whole group of forty-five, all but two responded to the question asking if an orgasm was always experienced. Of those forty-three, thirty-four were born before 1875. Five answered "no" to that question without any further comment. One other woman responded "never," and two others said "once or twice." If the "noes" and the "never" are taken together, the proportion of women born before 1875 who experienced at least one orgasm is 82 percent. If the "noes" are taken to mean "sometimes" or "once or twice," as they might well be, given the wording of the question, then the proportion rises to 95 percent. For comparative purposes the figures for twentieth-century women provided in Kinsey's study are given in Table 2. Kinsey's proportions are arranged by age group and chronological period; hence they are not strictly comparable with those derived from Mosher's data. But the comparison is still suggestive, even when made with the women in the age group 26–30.[48]

Much more interesting and valuable than the bare statistics are the comments or rationales furnished

Table 1
Response to the Query:
"Do You Always Have a Venereal Orgasm?"

Response	Number	Percentage
No Response	2	4.4
"No" with no further comment	5	11.1
"Always"	9	20.0
"Usually"	7	15.5
"Sometimes," "Not always," or "No" with instances	18	40.0
"Once" or "Never"	4	8.8

Table 2
Percentage of Women Experiencing Orgasm
during Intercourse
(by decade of birth)

Women Born	Ages 21–25	Ages 26–30
Before 1900	72%	80%
1900–09	80%	86%
1910–19	87%	91%
1920–29	89%	93%

Source: Alfred C. Kinsey et al., *Sexual Behavior in the Human Female* (Philadelphia, 1953), 397, table 97.

by the women, which provide an insight into the sexual attitudes of middle-class women. As one might expect in a population by its own admission poorly informed on sexual physiology, the sexual adjustment of some of these women left something to be desired. Mosher, for example, in one of her few efforts at drawing conclusions from the survey, pointed out that sexual maladjustment within marriage sometimes began with the first intercourse. "The woman comes to this new experience of life often with no knowledge. The woman while she may give mental consent often shrinks physically." From her studies Mosher had also come to recognize that women's "slower time reaction" in reaching full sexual excitement was a source of maladjustment between husband and wife that could kill off or reduce sexual feelings in some women. Women, she recognized, because of their slower timing were left without "the normal physical response. This leaves organs of women over congested."[49] At least one of her respondents reported that for years intercourse was distasteful to her because of her "slow reaction," but "orgasm [occurs] if time is taken." On the other hand, the respondent continued, "when no orgasm, [she] took days to recover."[50] Another woman spoke of the absence of an orgasm during intercourse as "bad, even disastrous, nerve-wracking—unbalancing, if such conditions continue for any length of time." Still a third woman, presumably referring to the differences in the sexual rhythms of men and women, said, "Men have not been properly trained." One of the women in the Mosher survey testified in another way to her recognition of the differences in the sexuality of men and women. "Every wife submits when perhaps she is not in the mood," she wrote, "but I can see no bad effect. It is as if it

had not been. But my husband was absolutely considerate. I do not think I could endure a man who forced it." And her response to a question about the effects of an orgasm upon her corroborate her remark: "a general sense of well being, contentment and regard for husband. This is true Doctor," she earnestly wrote.[51]

Mosher's probing of the attitudes of women toward their sexuality went beyond asking about orgasms. Several of her questions sought to elicit the reactions of women to sexual intercourse. What is the purpose of sex, she asked? Is it a necessity for a man or for a woman? Is it for pleasure, or is it for reproduction?[52] Only two of the women failed to respond in some fashion to these questions. Nine thought sex was a necessity for men, while thirteen thought it was a necessity for both men and women. Fifteen of the respondents thought it was not a necessity for either sex. Twenty-four of the forty-five thought that it was a pleasure for both sexes, while only one thought it was exclusively a pleasure for men. Given the view generally held about sexual attitudes in the nineteenth century, it comes as something of a surprise to find that only thirty marked "reproduction" as the primary purpose of sex. In fact, as we shall see in a moment, some of the women thought reproduction was not as important a justification for intercourse as love.

As one might expect, this particular series of questions was usually answered with a good deal of explanation. One woman who emphasized reproduction as the principal justification took the opportunity to condemn those couples she apparently had heard of who did not want children. "I cannot recognize as true marriage that relation unaccompanied by a strong desire for children." She thought it was close to "legalized prostitution." She admitted that because of her love for her husband she "cultivated the passion to effect the 'compromise' in this direction that must come in every other [area] when people marry." She went on to say that she did not experience orgasm until the fifth or sixth year of her marriage and that even at the time of her response to the questionnaire—the early 1890s—she still did not reach a sexual climax half of the time. A second woman was also apparently out of phase with her husband's sexual interests, for she thought a woman's needs for sex occurred "half as often as a man's." It is revealing of her own feelings that though she said "half as often," the figures she used to illustrate her point—twice a week for a man and twice a month for a woman—are actually in the ratio of one to four rather than of one to two as she said. Her true attitude was also summed up in the remark that since she was always in good health and intercourse "did not hurt me, . . . I always meant to be obliging."[53]

But, as the earlier statistical breakdown makes evident, the women who only tolerated intercourse were in a decided minority. A frank and sometimes enthusiastic acceptance of sexual relations was the response from most of the women. Sexual intercourse "makes more normal people," said a woman born in 1857. She was not even sure that children were necessary to justify sexual relations within marriage. "Even if there are no children, men love their wives more if they continue this relation, and the highest devotion is based upon it, a very beautiful thing, and I am glad nature gave it to us." Since marriage should bring two people close together, said one woman born in 1855, sexual intercourse is the means that achieves that end. "Living relations have a right to exist between married people and these cannot exist in perfection without sexual intercourse to a moderate degree. This is the result of my experience," she added. A woman born in 1864 described sexual relations as "the gratification of a normal healthy appetite." The only respondent who was divorced and remarried testified in 1913 that at age fifty-three "my passionate feeling has declined somewhat and the orgasm does not always occur," but intercourse, she went on, was still "agreeable" to her.[54]

Several of the women even went so far as to reject reproduction as sufficient justification for sex. Said one woman, "I consider this appetite as ranking with other natural appetites and like them to be indulged legitimately and temperately; I consider it illegitimate to risk bringing children into the world under any but most favorable circumstances." This woman was born before the Compromise of 1850 and made her comment after she had been married ten years. Another woman, also born a decade before the Civil War, denied that reproduction "alone warrants it at all; I think it is only warranted as an expression of true and passionate love. This is the prime condition for a happy conception, I fancy." To her, too, the pleasure derived from sexual intercourse was "not sensual pleasure, but the pleasure of love."[55]

A third woman born before 1861 doubted that sex was a necessity in the same sense as food or drink, but she had no doubt that "the desire of both husband and wife for this expression of their union seems to me the first and highest reason for intercourse. The desire for offspring is a secondary, incidental, although entirely worthy motive but could never to me make intercourse right unless the mutual desire were also present." She saw a clear conflict between the pleasure of intercourse and reproduction. "My husband and I," she said in 1893,

> believe in intercourse for its own sake—we wish it for ourselves and spiritually miss it, rather than physically, when it does not occur, because it is the highest, most sacred expression of our oneness. On the other hand, even a slight risk of pregnancy, and then we deny ourselves the intercourse, feeling all the time that we are losing that which keeps us closest to each other.[56]

Another woman, in describing the ideal of sexual relations, said that she did not want intercourse to occur at any time when conception was likely, for conception should not occur by accident. Instead it ought to be the result of

> deliberate design on both sides in time and circumstances most favorable physically and spiritually for the accomplishment of an immensely important act. It amounts to separating times and objects of intercourse into (a) that of expression of love between man and woman (that act is frequently simply the extreme caress of love's passion, which it would be a pity to limit . . . to once in two or three years) and (b) that of carrying on a share in the perpetuation of the race, which should be done carefully and prayerfully.[57]

It seems evident that among these women sexual relations were neither rejected nor engaged in with distaste or reluctance. In fact for them sexual expression was a part of healthy living and frequently a joy. Certainly the prescriptive literature that denigrated sexual feelings or expression among women cannot be read as descriptive of the behavior or attitude of these women. Nevertheless this is not quite the same as saying that the marriage handbooks had no effect at all. To be sure, there is no evidence that the great majority of women in the Mosher survey felt guilty about indulging in sex because of what they were told in the prescriptive literature. But in two cases the literature seems to have left feelings of guilt. One woman said that sexual relations were "apparently a necessity for the *average* person" and that it was "only [the] superior individuals" who could be "independent of sex relations with no evident ill-results." To her, as to St. Paul and some of the marriage advice books, it was better to indulge than to burn, but it was evidently even better to be free from burning from the beginning. A more blatant sign of guilt over sex came from the testimony of a woman who quite frankly thought the pleasure of sex was a justification for intercourse, but she added "not necessarily a legitimate one."[58]

Dr. Mosher herself obliquely testified to the effects of the prescriptive literature. She attributed the difficulties some women experienced in reaching orgasm to the fact that "training has instilled the idea that any physical response is coarse, common and immodest which inhibits [women's] proper part in this relation."[59] That was the same point that some of the medical writers in the nineteenth century had made in explaining the coldness of some women toward their husbands.

The advice literature, for men as well as for women, generally warned against excessive sexual activity.[60] This emphasis upon limits is reflected in the remarks of some of the women in the Mosher survey. One woman said, for example, that "the pleasure is sufficient warrant" for sexual relations, but only if "people are extremely moderate and do not allow it to injure their health or degrade their best feelings toward each other." Another woman had concluded that "to the man and woman married from love," sexual intercourse "may be used temperately as one of the highest manifestations of love granted us by our Creator." A third woman, who had no doubt that sexual relations were "necessary to marital happiness," nonetheless said she believed in "temperance in it."[61] But temperance, another one of the women in the Mosher survey reminds us, should not be confused with repugnance or distaste. Although this respondent did not think the ideal sexual relation should occur more often than once a month, she did think it ought to take place "during the menstrual period . . . and in the daylight." The fact is this woman, in

answer to other questions, indicated that she experienced sexual desire about once a week, but with greatest intensity "before and during menses." She was, in short, restricting her own ideal to what she considered an acceptable frequency of indulgence. Her description of her feelings after orgasm suggests where she learned that limits on frequency might be desirable or expected: "Very sleepy and comfortable. No disgust, as I have heard it described."[62]

This examination of the literature, the popular advice books, and particularly the Mosher survey makes clear that the historians are ill advised to rely upon the marital advice books as descriptions either of the sexual behavior of women or of general attitudes toward women's sexuality. It is true that a literature as admittedly popular as much of the prescriptive or normative literature was could be expected to have some effect upon behavior as well as attitudes. But those effects were severely limited. Most people apparently did not follow the prescriptions laid down by the marriage and advice manuals. Indeed some undoubtedly found that advice wrong or misleading when measured against experience. Through some error or accident the same woman was apparently interviewed twice in the Mosher survey, twenty-three years apart. As a result we can compare her attitudes at the beginning of her marriage in 1896 and her attitude in 1920. After one year of marriage she thought that sexual relations ought to be confined to reproduction only, but when asked the same question in 1920, she said that intercourse ought not to be confined to reproduction, though she thought it should be indulged in only when not pressed with work and when there was time for pleasure.[63] Another woman in the Mosher survey changed her mind about sexual relations even earlier in her sexual life. She said,

> My ideas as to the reason for [intercourse] have changed materially from what they were before marriage. I then thought reproduction was the only object and that once brought about, intercourse should cease. But in my experience the habitual bodily expression of love has a deep psychological effect in making possible complete mental sympathy, and

perfecting the spiritual union that must be the lasting "marriage" after the passion of love has passed away with years.

These remarks were made in 1897 by a woman of thirty after one year of marriage.[64]

Her comments make clear once again that historians need to recognize that the attitudes of ordinary people are quite capable of resisting efforts to reshape or alter them. That there was an effort to deny women's sexual feelings and to deny them legitimate expression cannot be doubted in the light of the books written then and later about the Victorian conception of sexuality. But the many writings by medical men who spoke in a contrary vein and the Mosher survey should make us doubt that

the ideology was actually put into practice by most men or women of the nineteenth century, even among the middle class, though it was to this class in particular that the admonitions and ideology were directed. The women who responded to Dr. Mosher's questions were certainly middle- and upper-middle-class women, but they were, as a group, neither sexless nor hostile to sexual feelings. The great majority of them, after all, experienced orgasm as well as sexual desire. Their behavior in the face of the antisexual ideology pressed upon them at the time offers testimony to the truth of Alex Comfort's comment that "the astounding resilience of human commonsense against the anxiety makers is one of the really cheering aspects of history."[65]

NOTES

1 Captain Frederick Marryat, *A Diary in America, with Remarks on Its Institutions* (London, 1839), 2: 244–47. The story of the trousers on piano legs is taken seriously in John Duffy, "Masturbation and clitoridectomy: a nineteenth century view," *Journal of the American Medical Association* 1963, *186:* 246; G. Rattray Taylor, *Sex in History* (New York, 1954), 203; and Peter T. Cominos, "Innocent Femina sensualis in unconscious conflict," in *Suffer and Be Still: Women in the Victorian Age,* ed. Martha Vicinus (Bloomington, 1972), 157.

2 William Acton, *The Functions and Disorders of the Reproductive Organs in Youth, in Adult Age, and in Advanced Life: Considered in Their Physiological, Social, and Psychological Relations* (1857; 2d ed., London, 1858; expanded American ed., Philadelphia, 1865). For references to Acton's writings, see Steven Marcus, *The Other Victorians: A Study of Sexuality and Pornography in Mid-Nineteenth-Century England* (New York, 1966), chap. 1; and Nathan G. Hale, Jr., *Freud and the Americans: The Beginnings of Psychoanalysis in the United States, 1876–1917* (New York, 1971), 36–37.

3 Acton, *Functions and Disorders* (1865), 133.

4 Theophilus Parvin, "Hygiene of the sexual functions," *New Orleans Medical and Surgical Journal,* 1883–84, *n.s.11:* 607. Parvin also quotes at length from Acton's book.

5 Walter E. Houghton, *The Victorian Frame of Mind, 1830–1870* (New Haven, 1957), 353. Marcus presents a portrait of Victorian attitudes toward sex similar to that of Houghton, but he disclaims to be talking about behavior: "We need not pause to discuss the degree of truth or falsehood in these asser-

tions. What is of more immediate concern is that these assertions indicate a system of beliefs." *Other Victorians,* 32. Yet it is not clear what point there is in detailing a system of beliefs unless it has some behavioral consequences. Peter T. Cominos also relies upon Acton, in "Late Victorian sexual respectability and the social system," *International Review of Social History,* 1963, *8:* 18–48, 217–50. E. M. Sigsworth and T. J. Wyke doubt the pervasiveness in Victorian England of Acton's conception of women's sexuality. They write: "Victorian opinion on the innate sexuality of women was cloudy and divided"—a view about which more will be said in this article. "A study of Victorian prostitution and venereal disease," in Vicinus, *Suffer and Be Still,* 83.

6 Viola Klein, *The Feminine Character: History of an Ideology* (1946; reprint, Urbana, 1972), 85, as quoted in David M. Kennedy, *Birth Control in America: The Career of Margaret Sanger* (New Haven, 1970), 56–57.

7 Hale, *Freud and the Americans,* 31. Elsewhere Hale sums up the medical view as he sees it: "By 1906. . . .some physicians regarded the asexual female as the norm: 'It may be offered that the sexual appetite in the majority of American females is evoked only by the purest love. In many the appetite never asserts itself and, indeed, the only impulse thereto is in the desire to gratify the object of affection'" (pp. 39–40; quotation from Ferdinand C. Valentine, "Education in sexual subjects," *New York Medical Journal,* Feb. 10, 1906, 276).

8 Ben (G.J.) Barker-Benfield, "The spermatic economy: a nineteenth century view of sexuality," *Feminist Studies,* 1972, *1:* 54.

9 Charles Fayette Taylor, "Effect on women of imper-

fect hygiene of the sexual function," *American Journal of Obstetrics*, 1882, *15:* 175–76, 168–71, italics in original.

10 Orson S. Fowler, *Sexual Science; Including Manhood, Womanhood, and Their Mutual Interrelations, etc. . . .as Taught by Phrenology* (Philadelphia, 1870), 680.

11 P. Henry Chavasse, *Physical Life of Man and Woman; or, Advice to Both Sexes* (1866; reprint, New York, 1897), 291–92; quotation from Trall in Michael Gordon, "From an unfortunate necessity to a cult of mutual orgasm: sex in American marital education literature, 1830–1940," in *Studies in the Sociology of Sex*, ed. James M. Henslin (New York, 1971), 58, my italics.

12 George H. Napheys, *The Physical Life of Woman: Advice to the Maiden, Wife, and Mother* (1869; Philadelphia, 1871), 74–75, 180.

13 Ely Van de Warker, "Impotency in women," *American Journal of Obstetrics*, 1878, *11:* 47.

14 J. Milne Chapman, "On masturbation as an etiological factor in the production of gynic diseases," *American Journal of Obstetrics*, 1883, *16:* 454.

15 Montrose S. Pallen, "Some suggestions with regard to the insanities of females," *American Journal of Obstetrics, 1877, 10:* 209.

16 William M. McLaury, "Remarks on the Relation of the menstruation to the sexual functions," *American Journal of Obstetrics*, 1887, *20:* 161.

17 Chavasse, *Physical Life of Man and Woman*, 372–73.

18 Van de Warker, "Impotency in women," 38–39.

19 Ibid., 41. Today the complaint is called premature ejaculation.

20 William Goodell, *Lessons in Gynecology* (Philadelphia, 1887), 567, as quoted in Hale, *Freud and the Americans*, 40.

21 McLaury, "Remarks on the relation of the menstruation," 161.

22 Chavasse, *Physical Life of Man and Woman*, 424–25.

23 John Harvey Kellogg, *Plain Facts for Old and Young* (1879; Burlington, Iowa, 1881), 252.

24 Augustus K. Gardner, *Conjugal Sins against the Laws of Life and Health and Their Effects upon the Father, Mother, and Child* (New York, 1870), 98.

25 Chavasse, *Physical Life of Man and Woman*, 33.

26 Mary Wood-Allen, *What a Young Woman Ought to Know* (Philadelphia, 1905), 155.

27 Chapman, "On masturbation"; letter from S. E. McCully, *American Journal of Obstetrics*, 1883, *16:* 844, my italics.

28 James Marion Sims, *Clinical Notes on Uterine Surgery* (London, 1866), 369.

29 Napheys, *Physical Life of Woman*, 104–5. This belief, which other writers also speak of, may well have affected some women's attitudes toward orgasm, for

if a woman, under this view, could repress pleasure or climax, conception could be prevented.

30 Van de Warker, "Impotency in women," 39.

31 Napheys, *Physical Life of Woman*, 86.

32 Horatio Bigelow, "Aggravated instance of masturbation in the female," *American Journal of Obstetrics*, 1882, *15:* 437.

33 "A case of excision of both ovaries for fibrous tumors of the uterus, and a case of excision of the left ovary for chronic oöphoritis and displacement," reported by Dr. E. H. Trenholme in *Canada Lancet*, July 1876, *American Journal of Obstetrics*, 1876–77, *9:* 703.

34 "Case of vaginismus," reported by Dr. George Pepper, *American Journal of Obstetrics*, 1871, *3:* 322–24.

35 Gardner, *Conjugal Sins*, 97.

36 Summary of paper by Dr. Keppler, "The sexual life of the female after castration," given at the 10th International Medical Congress, *American Journal of Obstetrics*, 1890, *23:* 1155–56.

37 Not all historians, it should be noted, have assumed that nineteenth-century concerns about sex meant hostility toward women's sexuality. In tracing the history of the social purity movement after 1870, David J. Pivar is careful to distinguish between a concern with the exploitation of women's sexuality and an opposition to women's sexual feelings. See his *Purity Crusade: Sexual Morality and Social Control, 1868–1900* (Westport, 1973).

38 Acton, *Functions and Disorders* (1858), 8–9; (1865), 134, my italics.

39 Kellogg, *Plain Facts*, 178. Hale gives the figures on Kellogg's sales in *Freud and Americans*, 37.

40 Kellogg, *Plain Facts*, 206, 209, 247, 225–26. Kellogg also quoted Acton.

41 Ibid., 217, 221–25, 118.

42 Ibid., 265–66.

43 It is true that some of the advice and medical literature that recognized women's sexual feelings and from which I have been quoting was also prescriptive rather than merely descriptive. But for convenience and economy of words in subsequent pages when I refer to "prescriptive or normative literature" I mean only that which minimized or denied women's sexuality.

44 Among the largest and most significant of such surveys were Katherine B. Davis, *Factors in the Sex Life of Twenty-two Hundred Women* (New York, 1929); Robert Latou Dickinson and Lura Beam, *A Thousand Marriages: A Medical Study of Sex Adjustment* (Baltimore, 1931); and Alfred C. Kinsey et al., *Sexual Behavior in the Human Female* (Philadelphia, 1953). The first chapter of Robert Latou Dickinson and Lura Beam, *The Single Woman* (Baltimore, 1934),

concerns the sexual life of working girls in the 1890s, but it is based on forty-six cases, the typical patient being born "soon after 1870." I am indebted to David M. Kennedy of Stanford University for this reference.

45 Mosher, "Hygiene and Physiology of Woman," 10: xv, Mosher Papers, Stanford University Archives.

46 The principal questions dealing with women's sexual habits are: number of conceptions; number of conceptions by choice and by accident; frequency of intercourse; whether intercourse is participated in during pregnancy; whether intercourse is "agreeable"; whether an orgasm occurs; what effects from orgasm, or from failure to have one; purpose of intercourse; the ideal habit of sexual relations; whether there is desire for intercourse other than during pregnancy; whether contraception is used and method employed; whether wife sleeps in same bed with husband; knowledge of sexual physiology prior to marriage; and the character of menses: age of onset, pain, and amount.

47 The small number of women queried in the Mosher survey may cause some readers to discount almost entirely the significance of any conclusions drawn from it. While such a response may be understandable as a first reaction, in the end I think it would be unwise. So far as I know, this is the only survey of sexual attitudes and practices in the nineteenth century; historians' standard conception of women's sexual practices and attitudes in the nineteenth century has been derived from no previous survey at all. Certainly the systematic questioning of forty-five women at considerable length and their rationales for their answers ought to be at least as significant in shaping historians' conceptions of women's sexuality as the scraps of information from interested writers at the time, novels, and recollections, which have been the bases of our traditional picture of women's sexual attitudes and behavior in the nineteenth century. It is true that we do not know at the present time who these women were or how random their selection was. But there seems little reason to believe that the women were specifically chosen by Mosher, if only because the purpose of the original questionnaire as well as the use of the information gained from it was to help her in advising women students. Moreover, as an unmarried woman herself, it is very likely that the information from the questionnaires was Mosher's most valuable source of knowledge on women's sexuality. It is probably true, given the general reluctance of nineteenth-century people to discuss sex, that some women whom Mosher approached refused to answer the questionnaire. But it is worth recalling that

the value even of modern sex surveys, including Kinsey's, has been questioned on the grounds that the respondents were largely self-selected. Obviously the Mosher survey is not the final word on the sexual behavior and attitudes of women in the nineteenth century. But at the same time it ought not to be rejected because of its limited size; that would be applying a methodological standard quite inappropriate for a sensitive subject in which the evidence is always limited and fugitive.

48 A comparison of the sexual responses of the older and younger women in the Mosher survey did not reveal any greater interest in sex among the younger group, but the numbers involved were too small to be significant. The responses of fourteen women born before 1860 were compared with those of the eight women born after 1875. On the other hand, if the responses to the questions about desire for sex and about orgasmic experience are categorized by date at which the questionnaire was completed, regardless of the age of the respondent, there is a slight, if somewhat ambiguous, difference between the earlier and later respondents. Seventeen women completed the questionnaire before 1900; nineteen did so after 1912. Thirteen of the seventeen completed before 1900 responded to the question of whether they had experienced orgasm; four of the thirteen said they had not. Eighteen of the nineteen who completed the questionnaire after 1912 answered that question; only one out of eighteen failed to experience an orgasm. In themselves these data suggest that women who answered the questionnaire in the twentieth century achieved somewhat more satisfaction in their sexual experience than those who completed the questionnaire in the nineteenth century. But when a similar division by century is made of the questionnaires in regard to another question, that conclusion is not so clear. One of the questions asked whether the respondent felt sexual desire. Fourteen women answered the question prior to 1900, of whom only two said they had failed to feel desire. But out of the sixteen who responded to the same question after 1912, three said they lacked any feeling of desire. Here the proportion of sexuality was higher among the nineteenth- than the twentieth-century respondents.

49 Mosher, "Hygiene and physiology of women," 10: 1. Twelve of the women were asked how soon after marriage they engaged in intercourse. Six said within the first three days, while six said from ten days to a year after the ceremony.

50 Ibid., case no. 51. The case numbers have been assigned by Mosher herself and appear on each page of each questionnaire. Hereafter the citation of cases

56   I. THE HEALTH OF WOMEN

will carry only "Hygiene and physiology of women" and case number.

51 Ibid., case nos. 47, 40, 41.

52 Since each respondent could legitimately answer "yes" to all three suggested justifications for sexual relations, the totals here can go beyond forty-five, though not all questions were always answered.

53 Ibid., case nos. 24, 19.

54 Ibid., case nos. 41, 18, 2. It is worth noting that here, as elsewhere in the survey, no mention was made of religious reasons for or against intercourse. These women had almost entirely secularized their sexual ideology.

55 Ibid., case nos. 14, 12.

56 Ibid., case no. 15.

57 Ibid., case no. 22.

58 Ibid., case nos. 47, 30. Marcus found a comparable example of guilt arising out of the prescriptive literature against masturbation. In discussing the Victorian sexual autobiography *My Secret Life,* Marcus observes that the anonymous author gave full credence to the dangers described in the literature, yet he masturbated nonetheless. After doing so, however, the anonymous author reported he suffered from depression, guilt, fatigue, and general feelings of debilitation though he felt none of these symptoms after sexual intercourse. Marcus ascribes these feelings to an internalizing of social attitudes, presumably derived from the prescriptive literature against masturbation. *Other Victorians,* 112. It is significant, however, that the prescriptions did not stop the practice. Why it did not stop is suggested by a more recent study of sexual behavior. Masters

and Johnson report that most of their male subjects still believed the old tales of physical and psychical harm from masturbation, especially from "excessive" activity, but none of them desisted from the practice. The authors point out that no matter how active a subject was in this respect, he always defined "excessive" as more active than his own practice. William H. Masters and Virginia E. Johnson, *Human Sexual Response* (Boston, 1966), 201–2.

59 Mosher, "Hygiene and physiology of women," 10: 1.

60 Hale cites sources ranging in origin from 1830 to 1910 on the concern for conserving sexual energy. *Freud and the Americans,* 35. Oscar Handlin sums up the advice in this fashion: "Abstinence, repression, and self-restraint thus were the law; and violations were punished by the most hideous natural consequences, described in considerable graphic detail." Handlin's conclusion, however, that the readers of that literature "were overwhelmed by the guilt and shame the necessities of self-control imposed," seems unwarranted on the basis of present evidence. *Race and Nationality in American Life* (Garden City, 1957), 122–23.

61 Mosher, "Hygiene and physiology of women," case nos. 33, 10, 13.

62 Ibid., case no. 11.

63 Ibid., case nos. 30, 33. Mosher gives no indication that she knew the two questionnaires were from the same person.

64 Ibid., case no. 22.

65 Alex Comfort, *The Anxiety Makers: Some Curious Preoccupations of the Medical Profession* (London, 1967), 113.

4

Passionlessness: An Interpretation of Victorian Sexual Ideology, 1790–1850

NANCY F. COTT

In 1903 Havelock Ellis announced that the notion of women's sexual "anaesthesia," as he called it, was a nineteenth-century creation. He had researched literary and medical sources from ancient Greece to early modern Europe and discovered, to his own amazement, that women had generally been thought to desire and enjoy sexual relations more than men.[1] Ellis and his contemporaries initially sought the source of the idea that women lacked sexual passion in the generations immediately preceding their own. The late nineteenth century was an era of contention over female sexuality, physiology, health, dress, and exercise, and one in which medical opinion had become an authoritative sector of public opinion. Since investigators have found rich documentation on these controversies, particularly in medical sources, they have been little induced to look beyond them. Until quite recently, historians tended not only to follow Ellis's chronological bias but, like him, to associate the idea that women lacked sexual passion with social repression and dysfunction. Now that attitude has been challenged by the possibility that nineteenth-century sexual ideology held some definite advantages for women, and by the claim that ideology reflected or influenced behavior far less than had been thought.[2]

A full appraisal of the idea that women lacked sexual passion requires an investigation of its origins. My purpose is to offer a hypothesis, if not a proven case, regarding the initiation and reception of that central tenet of Victorian sexual ideology which I call "passionlessness." I use the term to convey the view that women lacked sexual aggres-

siveness, that their sexual appetites contributed a very minor part (if any at all) to their motivations, that lustfulness was simply uncharacteristic. The concept of passionlessness represented a cluster of ideas about the comparative weight of woman's carnal nature and her moral nature; it indicated more about drives and temperament than about actions and is to be understood more metaphorically than literally.

Obviously, a single conception of women's sexuality never wholly prevails. Western civilization up to the eighteenth century, as Ellis discovered, accentuated women's concupiscence: a fifteenth-century witch-hunters' guide warned, for instance, that "carnal lust . . . in women is insatiable."[3] But the Christian belief system that called unsanctified earthly women the devil's agents allowed, on the other hand, that women who embodied God's grace were more spiritual, hence less susceptible to carnal passion, than men. Nineteenth-century views of female sexuality were also double edged: notions of women's inherent licentiousness persisted, to be wielded against women manifesting any form of deviance under the reign of passionlessness. Acknowledging that notions of women's sexuality are never monolithic, I would nonetheless emphasize that there was a traditionally dominant Anglo-American definition of women as *especially* sexual which was reversed and transformed between the seventeenth and the nineteenth centuries into the view that women (although still primarily identified by their female gender) were *less* carnal and lustful than men.

The following pages focus on early appearances of the idea of female passionlessness, discuss its social context, and analyze if and why it was acceptable, especially to women. The documents in this test case are limited to New England; to apply

NANCY F. COTT is Associate Professor of History and American Studies at Yale University, New Haven, Connecticut.
Reprinted with permission from *Signs* 4 (1978): 219–236. © 1978 by The University of Chicago Press.

the interpretive paradigm to literate, Protestant, middle-class women elsewhere would require further testing. I have looked to women's public and private writings in order to put the women involved in the forefront and prevent viewing them as passive recipients of changing ideas. My other sources are largely didactic and popular works, especially religious ones, which influenced women. Most of what is known about sexual ideology before the twentieth century comes from "prescriptive" sources—those manuals, essays, and books that tried to establish norms of behavior. Although religious views, expressed in sermons and tracts, were the most direct and commanding "prescriptions" from the seventeenth through the early nineteenth century, they have not been so finely combed for evidence of sexual norms as has been medical advice, a comparable source of "prescriptions" for the later nineteenth century.[4] Religious opinion is particularly relevant to this inquiry because of the churches' hold on the female population. Women became a majority in the Protestant churches of America in the mid-seventeenth century and continued to increase their numerical predominance until, by the mid-nineteenth century, "Christian" values and virtues and "female" values and virtues were almost identical.[5] In my view, the ideology of passionlessness was tied to the rise of evangelical religion between the 1790s and the 1830s. Physicians' adoption of passionlessness was a second wave, so to speak, beginning at midcentury. By the time that physicians took up the question of passionlessness and attempted to reduce the concept to "scientific" and somatic quantities the idea had been diffused through the spiritual realm and had already engendered its own opposition.[6]

Early American prescriptive and legal documents suggest that the New England colonists expected women's sexual appetites to be comparable with men's, if not greater.[7] Calvinists assumed that men and women in their "fallen" state were equally licentious, that sexual drives were natural and God given in both sexes, and had their proper outlet in marriage. If anything, the daughters of Eve were considered more prone to excess of passion because their rational control was seen as weaker. And yet it was objectionable for women to exercise the sexual initiative; regardless of women's sexual drives, the religious and social context required female subordination. Puritan theology weakened but did not destroy the double standard of sexual morality. In colonial law, for example, fornication was punished equally in either sex, but adultery was defined by the participation of a married woman. A married man did not commit adultery but fornication—unless he took up with another man's wife. In Massachusetts until the Revolutionary period, a wife's adultery was always cause for her husband to divorce her, but wives had little success in freeing themselves from unfaithful husbands. Men also won suits to recover "damages" from their wives' lovers.[8] As Keith Thomas has put it, such suits reflected the underlying tenet of the double standard: "the view that men have property in women and that the value of this property is immeasurably diminished if the woman at any time has sexual relations with anyone other than her husband."[9] There was vast potential for sexual exploitation in a society in which women's sexual nature was considered primary and their social autonomy was slight.[10] The physical and biological consequences of sexual adventure also burdened women more heavily than men in an era lacking effective means to prevent conception or infection.

In the second century of colonial settlement one finds many more numerous prescriptions for the role of women. The reasons for this increase are diverse: new class concern for standards of distinction and taste, the spread of literacy, the growth of printing and journalism, and "enlightened" interest in reformulating social systems and personal relations in "natural," "rational," rather than scriptural, terms. Britain led in discussions of female character and place, setting sex role conventions for the literate audience.[11] Since British social ideals became more influential in the mid-eighteenth century with the decline in Puritanism, the diffusion of Protestant energies, and the growth of an affluent urban class in the colonies, British "prescriptions" must be taken into consideration. At least three phases of British opinion contributed to the development of the idea of passionlessness. In the beginning of the century when spokesmen for the new professional and commercial middle class began explicitly to oppose aristocratic pretension, vanity, and libertinism, reforming writers such as Daniel Defoe, Jeremy Collier, Richard Steele, and Samuel Richardson portrayed sexual promiscuity as one of those aristocratic excesses that threatened middle-class virtue and domestic security. Their kind of propriety led to an ideal of sexual self-control, verbal prudery, and opposition to the double standard of sexual morality (for the sake of purity for men rather than justice for women). Due to their influence, in part, "the eighteenth century witnessed a redefinition of virtue in primarily sexual terms," Ian Watt has pointed out. By elevating sexual control highest among human virtues the middle-class moralists made female chastity the archetype for human morality.[12]

Out of the upper class came a different prescriptive genre, the etiquette manual. The ones most available to middle-class women in America, such as George Savile's *A Lady's New Year's Gift* or John Gregory's *A Father's Legacy to His Daughters*, consistently held that woman was made for man's pleasure and service; woman was strong only insofar as she could use her own weakness to manipulate the opposite sex (within the bounds of social propriety).[13] These authors advised a great deal of restraint and affectation (not to mention deception) in women's behavior. At the same time, modesty and demureness took center stage among the female virtues enshrined. According to Keith Thomas, the idea of passionlessness emerged in this context as an extension of the ideal of chastity needed to protect men's property rights in women; it was a reification in "nature" of the double standard.[14] Yet it must be objected that in the nineteenth century women who believed in passionlessness usually rejected the double standard of sexual morality. Modesty was the quintessential female virtue in works such as Gregory's, but, amid the manipulative and affected tactics advised, it connoted only demure behavior—a good act—not, necessarily, passionlessness. Indeed, the underlying theme that women had to appeal to men turned modesty into a sexual ploy, emphasizing women's sex objectification.[15] John Gregory did hint that sexual desire was weaker in women, with their "superior delicacy," than in men. He was sure that nature had assigned to wives rather than husbands the "reserve" which would prevent "satiety and disgust" in marital relations.[16] But not until a third phase at the close of the century did emphasis move

implacably from modesty to passionlessness, under the Evangelical aegis.

The British Evangelicals were conservative reformers horrified at the French Revolution and its "godlessness"; they worked to regenerate Protestantism in order to secure social and political order. Like earlier middle-class moralists, the Evangelicals opposed aristocratic blasphemies and profligacy, cherished family life, and advocated chastity and prudence in both sexes. Because they observed women's greater piety, and hoped that women would influence men and the next generation, they focused much of their proselytizing zeal on women. In contrast to earlier eighteenth-century didacts, they harped on the theme that women were made for God's purposes, not man's. Thomas Gisborne, for example, clearly considered women moral beings responsible for themselves and to society. His call for self-conscious moral integrity on women's part directly opposed Gregory's insinuations about the shaping of women's behavior to men's tastes; he objected that such behavior was "not discretion, but art. It is dissimulation, it is deliberate imposition."[17] Evangelical works of the 1790s argued that aristocratic models of vanity, artifice, and irreligion had undermined and corrupted women's valuable potential. They claimed that female piety and sincerity would bring "effectual reformation . . . in every department of society," because "all virtues, all vices, and all characters are intimately connected with the manners, principles, and dispositions of our women."[18] The Evangelicals transformed the truism of etiquette books, that individual women influenced individual men's manners, into the proposition that the collective influence of women was an agency of moral reform.

More to the point, the Evangelicals linked moral agency to female character with a supporting link to passionlessness. Their insistence on sincerity or "simplicity," accompanying their emphasis on women's moral potential, caused them to imply that women were virtuous by nature. Continuing to stress the female virtue of modesty, Evangelicals could not (in contrast to Gregory) allow that modesty was a behavior assumed to suit society's conventions and men's preferences. If women were to act modestly and be sexually passive, and also act without affectation, then, logically, they must be passionless. Gisborne said women had "quicker feelings of native delicacy, and a stronger sense of shame" than men. The anonymous author of *Female Tuition* claimed the female sex was "naturally attached to purity."[19]

Hannah More's work perfected the transformation of woman's image from sexual to moral being. Her *Strictures on the Modern System of Female Education* called for the rescue of religion and morality and located her constituency among her own sex. She detailed further than any predecessor the power that women could command, first making clear that this was power derived from their moral and spiritual endowment, not from their winning or endearing (sexual) ways. "It is humbling to reflect," More began her *Strictures*, "that in those countries in which fondness for the mere persons of women is carried to the highest excess, *they are slaves;* and that their moral and intellectual degradation increases in direct proportion to the adoration which is paid to mere external charms."[20] More offered a resounding alternative to the idea that women were made for men's pleasure—but at the price of a new level of self-control. Since she believed that human nature was corrupt, her educational program consisted of repression as much as enhancement.[21] Her outlook revealed to women a source of power (in moral influence) and an independence of men (through reliance on God) in a female world view that inspired and compelled women throughout the nineteenth century.[22] In her refusal to see women as childish and affectedly weak beings, designed only "to gratify the appetite of man, or to be the upper servant," she agreed with her contemporary, Mary Wollstonecraft. Despite the spectrum of difference between More and Wollstonecraft in politics and personal behavior, they both abhorred "libertine notions of beauty" and "weak elegancy of mind" in women, wished to emphasize women's moral and intellectual powers rather than their "mere animal" capacities, and expected reformed women to reform the world.[23] Their two critiques rose from shared indignation that women were degraded by their sexual characterization.

The new focus on moral rather than sexual determinants of female character in didactic works at the end of the eighteenth century required a reversal in Protestant views of women. In Puritan ideology, earthly women were the inheritors of Eve's legacy of moral danger. By the mid-eighteenth century, however, New England ministers had discarded similes to Eve, probably in deference to their predominately female congregations, and portrayed women as more sensitive to the call of religion than men.[24] Nineteenth-century Protestantism relied on women for its prime exemplars and symbols. Between 1790 and 1820 particularly, as an evangelical united front spread across the United States and Britain, the clergy intensified their emphasis on women as crucial advocates of religion.[25] Evangelical Protestants constantly reiterated the theme that Christianity had raised women from slaves in status to moral and intellectual beings.[26] The tacit condition for that elevation was the suppression of female sexuality. Christian women were "exalted above human nature, raised to that of angels"; proper understanding of the gospel enabled women to dismiss the earthly pride or sensuality that subjected them to men's whims.[27] The clergy thus renewed and generalized the idea that women under God's grace were more pure than men, and they expected not merely the souls but the bodies of women to corroborate that claim.

The pastors had a double purpose in training their eyes on the moral rather than the sexual aspect of woman's being. It enabled them to welcome women as worthy allies and agents of Protestantism, which seemed more and more essential as men's religious commitment dissipated. Second, a world view in which woman's sexual nature was shadowed behind her moral and spiritual endowment eclipsed her primitive and original power over men, the power of her sexuality.[28] The evangelical view, by concentrating on women's spiritual nature, simultaneously elevated women as moral and intellectual beings and disarmed them of their sexual power. Passionlessness was on the other side of the coin which paid, so to speak, for women's admission to moral equality.

The correlation between passionlessness and a distinctly improved view of women's character and social purpose begins to suggest the appeal of the concept to women. By replacing sexual with moral motives and determinants, the ideology of passionlessness favored women's power and self-respect. It reversed the tradition of Christian mistrust based on women's sexual treacherousness. It elevated women above the weakness of animal nature, stressing instead that they were "formed for exalted purity, felicity, and glory."[29] It postulated that woman's influence was not ensnaring but disinterested. It routed women out of the cul-de-sac of education for attractiveness, thus allowing more intellectual breadth.[30] To women who wanted means of self-preservation and self-control, this view of female nature may well have appealed, as Hannah More's views appealed. It remains to be seen in what social circumstances such views came to the fore.

There was extraordinary turbulence in sexual patterns and definitions in the late eighteenth century. The traditional system under which parents exercised authority over their children's marriage choices was breaking down.[31] This change might seem to imply greater freedom for youth of both sexes in choosing their spouses. Since men conventionally exercised the sexual/marital initiative, however, the demise of parental control probably meant a relative decline in the leverage available to marriageable women, who no longer had their parents operating openly on their behalf and could not assume that role themselves. Eliza Southgate, an articulate and well-to-do eighteen-year-old of Maine, remarked in 1800 that women sensed their "inequality of privilege" most grievously "in the liberty of choosing a partner in marriage; true, we have the liberty of refusing those we don't like, but not of selecting those we do."[32] Owing primarily to the changing sex ratio, the average age at which women first married rose from a low of about twenty years in the early colonies to about twenty-three by the Revolutionary period, while men's age at first marriage fell slightly. The proportion of women who never married rose appreciably in the same period, and the remarriage rate of widows dropped. One might interpret these statistics favorably to mean that "those who wed may have taken longer to consider the implications of such actions and the alternatives," or even that it was now "possible for unmarried men and women to find a satisfying role."[33] But since marriage was the principal means women had of supporting themselves, one could argue that the number of desperate and exploitable women multiplied. While marriage was the likeliest source for economic security for a woman, marital subjection remained the living symbol of women's general subjection to men. In Abigail Adams's famous request to her husband, John, in

1776 to "remember the ladies," her central complaint was not women's political disenfranchisement but husbands' legal exercise of "unlimited power" over their wives. Turning Revolutionary rhetoric to marital relations, Abigail reminded John that "all men would be tyrants if they could," and urged that a new law code "put it out of the power of the vicious and lawless to use us with cruelty and indignity with impunity."[34] Her objections evoke the double spectres, of sharper victimization or greater equity, borne before women's eyes during these Revolutionary years. Did women's marital status trouble her because it had become, of late, more abject, or did some hints of improvement in women's marital power precipitate her demand for further change?

During the same decades, the prebridal pregnancy rate rose dramatically. At peak years between 1760 and 1800, one-third to one-half of all recorded legitimate first births were the result of premarital sexual intercourse in several New England towns where the same measure was one-tenth or one-twentieth in the seventeenth century.[35] Again, numerous and contradictory interpretations can be drawn from these figures. The increase in prebridal pregnancy could be ascribed to a general increase in premarital sexual activity, which in itself could possibly represent greater individual and sexual freedom for both sexes, or just as possibly indicate greater vulnerability and exploitation of women. Or, premarital sexual activity could have remained constant but have led more frequently to marriage and legitimation.[36] The continued reign of a double standard of sexual morality made it unlikely that sexual "freedom" came without cost to women. A content analysis of nine New England magazines between 1777 and 1794 has shown that characters in both fiction and nonfiction regularly advocated punishment or ostracism for the male partner in illicit sex and sympathy for the female as the victim of force or misguided ignorance. In actual portrayals of illicit sexual encounters, however, the males involved escaped scot-free and the women almost always suffered punishment or ostracism.[37] On this injustice the young wife of a lawyer in Haverhill, Massachusetts, reflected in 1802: "Man boasts superior strength of mind, I would have him prove it, by avoiding or conquering temptation; but man disgraces his godlike reason, and yields to a thousand follies, to give them no harsher name—and passes through the world in high repute, such conduct would blast the reputation of poor weak women. . . . 'tis an unrighteous custom, which gives such license to our lords of the creation." She was not alone in protesting men's combination of sexual license with their claim to righteous social power. On the eve of her marriage, Sarah Connell of Concord, New Hampshire, lamented a local instance of seduction and betrayal, empathizing with the many unprotected girls who had "fallen victim to the baseness of those who call themselves lords of the Creation."[38]

The sexual exploitation possible in contemporary disruption of marital and sexual patterns was probably more obvious to women because of heightened expectations on their part. The clergy, adopting a more positive image of women in their sermons, no longer presented marriage as a hierarchical relationship but stressed that women were complementary, and piously influential, marriage partners. The rhetoric of the American Revolution glorified women's role further by connecting it with the success of the national experiment. In an abrupt reversal in 1773, Massachusetts women were victorious if they petitioned their governor and council for divorce on account of their husbands' adulteries; and women's overall success in obtaining divorce was almost equal to men's in the decade after 1776.[39] If not the most isolated farmers' wives, then literate women, living in populated areas sharing in the commerce of goods and ideas, were particularly likely to anticipate better treatment.[40]

A vision of sexual equity arising from awareness of sexual injustice brought feminist writers into the open during the same years. Judith Sargent Murray of Gloucester, Massachusetts, began criticizing female education in the 1770s, anticipating the themes of More and Wollstonecraft. Under the pseudonym "Constantia" she argued that men's presumed superiority in rationality was due to their superior education and continued advantages, not to any inherent preeminence. She demanded that women have opportunity to cultivate other means than sexual attraction. Pointing out that the typical upbringing of girls trivialized their minds and made them rely on physical beauty, she urged women to develop aspirations, a "reverence of self," moral and intellectual integrity, and the capacity for self-

fulfillment.[41] Constantia put her hopes in the female academies springing up. Another pseudonymous feminist, an "aged matron" of Connecticut who published *The Female Advocate* in 1801, wished to disabuse the world of the idea that woman was inferior to man or made for men's uses. God and Nature, she claimed, had given the two sexes "equality of talents, of genius, of morals, as well as intellectual worth," and only male arrogance had invaded that equality. Men had deprived women of education and experience while they themselves "engross[ed] all the emoluments, offices, honors and merits, of church and state." In her eyes the sexual double standard epitomized male usurpation of power, because it allowed a man to flaunt the arts of seduction without losing public esteem while it condemned a woman forever if she once succumbed to a deceiver. *The Female Advocate*'s images of women's powerlessness and vulnerability contrasted with its portrayal of men's aggrandizement of power and seductive wiles. Yet its author was optimistic that "well informed mind[s]" would be "the means of enabling us [women] to possess some command over ourselves."[42]

Polite ladies' magazines, which first appeared in the 1780s with the growth of a literate female audience, unintentionally paraded the contemporary controversy over sexual definitions. They celebrated female intellectual accomplishments and aimed not to cater to homemakers' tastes but to "improve and amuse" ladies' minds. In this "polite" entertainment, the subjects of fornication, prostitution, adultery, seduction, and betrayal were legion.[43] By and large, the stories and essays in these magazines broadcast the view that women's modus operandi was sexual, and consisted in manipulating men. But they also gave the impression that women met victimization and downfall more often than they gained influence and happiness through the solicitation of men's passions. The sexual definition of women could undermine their control of encounters with men, as Patty Rogers, a young woman of Exeter, New Hampshire, discovered for herself and confided to her diary.[44] Some writers in ladies' magazines were restless or indignant with the sexual characterization of women. A "Fragment on Prostitutes" argued that so-called women of pleasure were really women of grief and suffering, who had been betrayed by their seducers and abandoned by unsympathetic kin. The author railed against the injustice of prostitutes' being punished by laws made by men, their seducers.[45] Another author, opposing "what is called Amiable Weakness in women," asserted that women deserved the chance to cultivate their knowledge, intelligence, and self-discipline, because they were moral beings and not merely decorative objects or household drudges. A serious "Scheme for Increasing the Power of the Ladies" called on women to end the double standard by refusing to tolerate fashionable "rakes"; like Hannah More, the writer emphasized that it was up to women to reverse their complaisance with and degradation under the existing code. Sarah Connell concluded her account of her acquaintance's seduction with similar sentiment: "Did every virtuous female show her detestation of the libertine by wholly renouncing his society, there would be a much smaller number of them."[46]

Only a handful of New England women at this time questioned the political inequities of their situation, but sexual and marital subjection—unequal sexual prerogatives—seem to have rankled a much larger population. As *The Female Advocate* pointed out, women had to conform to male tastes and wait to be chosen but resist seduction or suffer ostracism for capitulating; men, meanwhile, were free to take the first step, practice flattery, and escape the consequences of illicit sexual relations. In sexual encounters women had more than an even chance to lose, whether by censure under the double standard, unwanted pregnancy and health problems, or ill-fated marriage. In this perspective, women might hail passionlessness as a way to assert control in the sexual arena—even if that "control" consisted in denial. Some scholars have claimed that women adhered to the ideology of passionlessness to bolster their position in a disadvantageous marriage market, that is, to play "hard to get" with conviction.[47] More essentially, passionlessness served women's larger interests by downplaying altogether their sexual characterization, which was the cause of their exclusion from significant "human" (i.e., male) pursuits.[48] The positive contribution of passionlessness was to replace that sexual/carnal characterization of women with a spiritual/moral one, allowing women to develop their human faculties and their self-esteem. The belief that women lacked carnal motivation was the

cornerstone of the argument for women's moral superiority, used to enhance women's status and widen their opportunities in the nineteenth century. Furthermore, acceptance of the idea of passionlessness created sexual solidarity among women; it allowed women to consider their love relationships with one another of higher character than heterosexual relationships because they excluded (male) carnal passion. "I do not believe that men can ever feel so pure an enthusiasm for women as we can feel for one another," Catherine Sedgwick recorded in her diary of 1834, upon meeting Fanny Kemble, "—ours is nearest to the love of angels."[49] "Love is spiritual, only passion is sexual," Mary Grew wrote at the end of the century to vindicate her intense and enduring friendship with Margaret Burleigh. That sense of the angelic or spiritual aspect of female love ennobled the experience of sisterhood which was central to the lives of nineteenth-century women and to the early woman's rights movement.[50] Women considered passionlessness an important shared trait which distinguished them favorably from men.[51]

It must not be assumed that women who internalized the concept of passionlessness necessarily shunned marriage. The pervasive ideology of romantic love, and also the evangelical conflation of the qualities of earthly and spiritual love, bridged the gap and refuted the ostensible contradiction between passionlessness and marriage. On a practical level, belief in female passionlessness could aid a woman to limit sexual intercourse within marriage and thus limit family size. Daniel Scott Smith has postulated a direct relation between women's exertion of that sort of power within the family, which he calls "domestic feminism," and the decline of the birthrate during the nineteenth century.[52] The conviction and the demand that it was woman's right to control reproduction, advocated by health reformers in the 1850s and promulgated in the movement for "voluntary motherhood" in subsequent decades, depended on the ideology of female passionlessness. Linda Gordon has shown the feminist basis of the argument for voluntary motherhood in the claim that women had the right to refuse their husband's sexual demands, despite the legal and customary requirements of submission to marital "duty."[53]

The degree to which a woman might incorporate the idea of passionlessness is revealed in an

1845 letter of Harriet Beecher Stowe to her husband. Responding to his revelations about "licentiousness" on the part of certain clergymen, she wrote: "What terrible temptations lie in the way of your sex—till now I never realized it—for tho I did love you with an almost insane love before I married you I never knew yet or felt the pulsation which showed me that I could be tempted in that way—there never was a moment when I felt anything by which you could have drawn me astray—for I loved you as I now love God."[54] Angelina Grimké's passionless attitude was a feminist affirmation of woman's dignity in revulsion from male sexual domination. To the man who would become her husband she revealed her judgment "that men in general, the vast majority, believe most seriously that women were made to gratify their animal appetites, *expressly* to minister to their pleasure—yea Christian men too." She continued: "My soul abhors such a base letting down of the high dignity of my nature as a woman. How I have feared the possibility of ever being married to one who regarded *this* as the *end*—the great design of marriage. In truth I may say that I never was reconciled to the compound [relat]ions of marriage until I read Combe on the Constitution of man this winter."[55]

Yet a belief so at odds with the traditional appreciation of female sexuality, and one which seems to mid-twentieth-century sensibilities so patently counterproductive, so symbolic of the repression and subordination of women, cannot be interpreted simply. Historians' frequent assumption that men devised the ideology of female passionlessness to serve their own interests—"to help gentlemen cope with the problem of controlling their own sexuality"—is partial (in both senses of the word) but not illogical.[56] An ideal of male continence, of virtuous and willed repression of existing carnal desires (as distinct from passionlessness, which implied absence of carnal motivation), figures in nineteenth-century directions for men's respectability and achievement in the bustling new world of industrial capitalism.[57] In one aspect, female passionlessness was a keystone in men's construction of their own self-control. But Howard Gadlin has underlined the paradox of the ideology, as well as reason for its diffusion and rootedness, in his remark that "the nineteenth-century double standard was the vehicle for a desexualization desired by both men and women for opposing

purposes. Men wanted to desexualize relationships to maintain their domination; women wanted to desexualize relationships to limit male domination."[58]

Both women's participation in the creation of Victorian sexual standards and the place of passionlessness in the vanguard of feminist thought deserve more recognition. The serviceability of passionlessness to women in gaining social and familial power should be acknowledged as a primary reason that the ideology was quickly and widely accepted. Yet feminists were the first to question and oppose the ideology once it was entrenched. When prudery became confused with passionlessness, it undermined women physically and psychologically by restricting their knowledge of their own sexual functioning. From the first, women health reformers and moral reformers rejected this injurious implication while fostering the positive meanings of passionlessness.[59] Feminist opposition arose when the medical establishment adopted passionlessness and moved the grounds for judging the concept from the spiritual to the somatic. When female passionlessness came to be insisted upon literally, more than one woman reacted as Rebecca Harding Davis did: "In these rough and tumble days, we'd better give [women] their places as flesh and blood, with exactly the same wants and passions as men." Mary Gove Nichols claimed: "A healthy and loving woman is impelled to material union as surely, often as strongly, as man. . . . The apathy of the sexual instinct is caused by the enslaved and unhealthy condition in which she lives."[60] Several woman's rights activists of the later part of the century, including Isabella Beecher Hooker, Alice Stockham, and Elizabeth Cady Stanton, discussed among themselves their belief in the existence and legitimacy of female sexual drives, even while the movement of which they were part banked on women's superior morality and maternal instinct as chief supports.[61] Consistent with the general conflicts and contradictions in sexual ideology after 1860, feminists perceived oppression in prudery while clinging to the promises that passionlessness held out.

The ideology of passionlessness, conceived as self-preservation and social advancement for women, created its own contradictions: on the one hand, by exaggerating sexual propriety so far as to immobilize women and, on the other, by allowing claims of women's moral influence to obfuscate the need for other sources of power. The assertion of moral integrity within passionlessness had allowed women to retrieve their identity from a trough of sexual vulnerability and dependence. The concept could not assure women full autonomy—but what transformation in sexual ideology alone could have done so?

NOTES

I am grateful to the friends who have kindly read and criticized one or another version of this essay over the past several years. I would especially like to thank Sacvan Bercovitch, Mari Jo Buhle, Laurie Crumpacker, John Demos, David B. Davis, Ellen Dubois, David H. Fischer, Linda Gordon, James R. Green, Jean Humez, Janet W. James, Carol Karlsen, Ann Margolis, Michael McGiffert, Mary Beth Norton, and Kathryn Kish Sklar. In addition, the anonymous readers were exceptionally helpful in bringing the essay to its final form.

1 Havelock Ellis, *Studies in the Psychology of Sex*, 2d ed., rev. (1903; Philadelphia: F. A. Davis Co., 1913), 3: 193–94.

2 On the former challenge, see Carroll Smith-Rosenberg, "Beauty, the Beast, and the militant woman," *American Quarterly*, 1971, *23:* 562–84, and "The female world of love and ritual," below; Linda Gordon, "Voluntary motherhood: the beginnings of feminist birth control ideas in the United States," in this volume, and *Woman's Body, Woman's Right* (New York: Grossman Publishers, 1976); John S. Haller, Jr., and Robin M. Haller, *The Physician and Sexuality in Victorian America* (Urbana: University of Illinois Press, 1974), esp. xii; Daniel Scott Smith, "Family limitation, sexual control and domestic feminism in Victorian America," in *Clio's Consciousness Raised*, ed. Mary Hartman and Lois Banner (New York: Harper Torchbook, 1974), and Randall Collins, "A conflict theory of sexual stratification," *Social Problems* 19 (Summer 1971): 7, 13–19. The latter point has been raised most recently by Carl N. Degler, "What ought to be and what was: women's sexuality in the nineteenth century," in this volume. Historians' focus on the later part of the nineteenth century in discussions of sexual ideology is evident in Haller and Haller's and Degler's works as well as in Peter T. Cominos, "Innocent Femina sensualis in unconscious conflict," in *Suffer and Be Still*, ed. Martha Vicinus (Bloomington: University of Indiana Press, 1972), and "Late Victorian sexual respectability and the social system," *International Review of Social History*, 1963, *8:* 18–48, 216–50; Nathan G. Hale, Jr., *Freud and the Americans* (New York: Oxford University Press, 1971); and Charles E. Rosenberg and Carroll Smith-Rosenberg, "The female animal: medical and biological views of woman and her role in nineteenth-century America," in this volume.

Daniel Scott Smith, "The dating of the American sexual revolution: evidence and interpretation," in *The American Family in Social-Historical Perspective*, ed. Michael Gordon (New York: St. Martin's Press, 1974), 328–32, and Michael Gordon, "From an unfortunate necessity to a cult of mutual orgasm: sex in marital education literature, 1830–1940," in *Studies in the Sociology of Sex*, ed. James Henslin (New York: Appleton-Century-Crofts, 1971), note conflict and change in sexual opinion in the last third of the century.

3 Quoted from *Malleus Maleficarum* in Deirdre English and Barbara Ehrenreich, *Witches, Midwives and Nurses: A History of Women Healers* (Oyster Bay, N.Y.: Glassmountain Pamphlets, 1972), 10. I remain indebted to Eleanor McLaughlin for conversations, at Wellesley in 1974, about medieval views of women and passionlessness.

4 Historians have noted that doctors took over the advisory role of ministers in the late nineteenth century (see Haller and Haller, *The Physician and Sexuality*, x–xi; Gordon, *Woman's Body*, 170; Barbara Sicherman, "The uses of diagnosis: doctors, patients, and neurasthenia," *Journal of the History of Medicine and Allied Sciences* 32 [January 1977]: 53–54). The new function of doctors as spiritual counselors highlights the shift of moral authority from religion to science during the course of the century.

5 See Barbara Welter, "The feminization of American religion," in Hartman and Banner, *Clio's Consciousness;* and Nancy F. Cott, *The Bonds of Womanhood: 'Woman's Sphere' in New England, 1780–1835* (New Haven, Conn.: Yale University Press, 1977), chap. 4.

6 Degler, "What ought to be," in this volume, 40–56, cites numerous conflicts within medical opinion. Physicians were never of one mind, and the British physician William Acton, who announced in the 1850s that "the majority of women . . . are not very much troubled with sexual feeling of any kind," represented one end of the range of opinion (see Gordon, "From an unfortunate necessity," 57–58).

7 See Edmund Morgan, "The Puritans and sex," *New England Quarterly*, 1942, *15:* 592–93, and *The Puritan Family*, rev. ed. (New York: Harper Torchbooks, 1966), 37–42; and Otho T. Beall, Jr., "Aristotle's

MasterPiece in America: a landmark in the folklore of medicine," *William and Mary Quarterly*, 1963, *3d ser. 20:* 216–20.

8 George E. Howard, *A History of Matrimonial Institutions* (1904; New York: Humanities Press, 1964), 2: 169–70, 173, 331, 348, 351, 354; John P. Demos, *A Little Commonwealth* (New York: Oxford University Press, 1970), 96–97; Nancy F. Cott, "Eighteenth-century family and social life revealed in Massachusetts divorce records," *Journal of Social History* 10 (Fall 1976): 34–35, and "Divorce and the changing status of women in eighteenth-century Massachusetts," *William and Mary Quarterly*, 3d ser. 33 (October 1976): 586–614.

9 Keith Thomas, "The double standard," *Journal of the History of Ideas*, 1959, *20:* 210.

10 See Morgan, "Puritans and sex," 594–600, for examples.

11 On the sex role distinctions employed in British and American writings, see Mary S. Benson, *Women in Eighteenth-Century America* (New York: Columbia University Press, 1935), 37–39. Frank L. Mott notes, in his *History of American Magazines, 1741–1850* (Cambridge, Mass.: Belknap Press, 1957), 64–65, that titles such as "Advice to the Fair" and "Counsel upon Female Virtues" became "sickeningly frequent" in the last quarter of the eighteenth century.

12 Ian Watt, "The New Woman: Samuel Richardson's *Pamela*," in *The Family: Its Structure and Functions*, ed. Rose L. Coser (New York: St. Martin's Press, 1964), 281–82. On the rise of middle-class morality, see also Watt, 286–88; Thomas "Double standard," 204; Gordon Rattray Taylor, *The Angel-Makers: A Study in the Psychological Origins of Historical Change, 1750–1850* (London: William Heinemann, 1958), 12–24; Christopher Hill, "Clarissa Harlowe and her times," *Essays in Criticism*, 1955, *5:* 320. Samuel Richardson's *Pamela* (1742) first portrayed a heroine whose delicacy verged on passionlessness. On the American attention paid to these British moralists and novelists, see Lawrence A. Cremin, *American Education: The Colonial Experience* (New York: Harper Torchbooks, 1970), 366–67, 371; Benson, *Women in Eighteenth-Century America*, 46; and Robert Palfrey Utter and Gwendolyn B. Needham, *Pamela's Daughters* (New York: Macmillan Publishing Co., 1936).

13 [George Savile, Marquis of Halifax], *The Lady's New Year's Gift; or, Advice to a Daughter* (London: Randal Taylor, 1688); Dr. [John] Gregory, *A Father's Legacy to His Daughters* (London: J. Sharpe, 1822). James Fordyce, *Sermons to Young Women*, new ed. (Philadelphia: Thomas Dobson, 1787), should be grouped with these although it was not an etiquette book in

the traditional sense. Savile's book, which went through fifteen British editions, circulated in the colonies during the first two-thirds of the eighteenth century. Fordyce's work was first published in England in 1765 and was reprinted in America by 1787; it was then frequently excerpted in magazines and reprinted in entirety. Gregory's appeared in England in 1774, was published in Philadelphia the following year, and had sixteen more editions in the United States before 1794 plus selections in compilations and serials. Editions continued to appear into the nineteenth century. See Julia C. Spruill, *Women's Life and Work in the Southern Colonies* (1935; New York: W. W. Norton & Co., 1969), 215–25, and Benson, *Women in Eighteenth-Century America*, 60–61, on the circulation of these books. Direct evidence of Gregory's readership in America appears in the manuscript diaries of Ruth Henshaw of Leicester, Mass., July 1, 1792, and Sally Ripley of Greenfield, Mass., December 1, 1799, both in the collection of the American Antiquarian Society, Worcester, Mass. American essayists frequently echoed the themes of the British didactic works (see, e.g., *Gentleman's and Lady's Town and Country Magazine* [Boston] 1 [May 1784]: 28; and Noah Webster's *American Magazine* [1788], quoted in Mott, *History of American Magazines*, 64).

14 Thomas, "Double standard," 214.

15 The eighteenth-century prescriptive work which made the connection between modesty and sexual ploy most obvious was Rousseau's *Emile* (1762), book 5, on the character of the ideal woman.

16 Gregory, *A Father's Legacy*, 11, 36, 72, 83.

17 Thomas Gisborne, *An Enquiry into the Duties of the Female Sex* (London; reprint ed. Philadelphia: J. Humphreys, 1798), 2–3, 187, 193. On the British Evangelicals, see Charles I. Foster, *An Errand of Mercy: The Evangelical United Front, 1790–1837* (Chapel Hill: University of North Carolina Press, 1960); and M. G. Jones, *Hannah More* (Cambridge: Cambridge University Press, 1952).

18 Quotations from *Female Tuition; or, An Address to Mothers, on the Education of Daughters* (London: J. Murray, 1784), preface, and 34; see also 2–3, 42–47; and Gisborne, *An Enquiry*, chaps. 2, 4, 7, 9; *The Female Aegis* (London: J. Ginger, 1798) an anonymous plagiarism of Gisborne's book; Thomas Branagan, *The Excellency of the Female Character Vindicated* (1807; Harrisburg, Pa.: Francis Wyeth, 1828), chap. 2; Hannah More, *Strictures on the Modern System of Female Education*, 9th ed. (1799; London: T. Cadell & W. Davies, 1801), 1: 70–72, 75–79, 111–12, 256–57.

19 Gisborne, *An Enquiry*, 183; *Female Tuition*, 243. On

"simplicity" see, e.g., Gisborne, *An Enquiry*, 104–11, 187, 193; *Female Tuition*, 112–75.

20   More, *Strictures*, 1: 3 (quotation) and passim. Her *Strictures* followed upon her two other successful critiques of aristocratic manners, *Thoughts on the Importance of the Manners of the Great* (1788) and *An Estimate of the Religion of the Fashionable World* (1790) (see Jones, *Hannah More*, on her life and work).

21   More, *Strictures*, see esp. 17–18, 29, 32–33, 137–38, 154–55.

22   During the first several decades of the nineteenth century all sorts of literate women—farm-bred daughters, society girls, schoolteachers, and matrons, from rural towns to commercial seaports—read and quoted Hannah More. For examples see *The Writings of Nancy Maria Hyde* (Norwich, Conn.: Russell Hubbard, 1816), diary entry for June 14, 1812; manuscript journal of Margaret Searle, August 22, 1812, Curson Family Papers, Houghton Library, Harvard University; manuscript book of extracts of Lucinda Read, 1815–16, Massachusetts Historical Society, Boston; manuscript journal of Mehitable May Dawes, June 12, 1815, May-Goddard Papers, Schlesinger Library, Radcliffe College. Jones, *Hannah More*, 193, states that More's novel *Coelebs in Search of a Wife* (which personified her ideals for female character) sold out thirty editions in the United States between 1808 and 1834. The British visitor Harriet Martineau was mightily impressed, in the 1830s, with the impact More had on American women; her comments and others are cited by Keith Melder, "Ladies Bountiful," *New York History* 48 (July 1967): 233–34, 254n. Jill K. Conway assembles other evidence of More's wide-ranging influence on American women in "Evangelical Protestantism and its influence on women in North America, 1790–1860" (paper read at the American Historical Association Convention, New Orleans, December 1972).

23   Mary Wollstonecraft, *A Vindication of the Rights of Women* (1792), ed. Charles W. Hagelman, Jr. (New York: W. W. Norton & Co., 1967), 34–35, 49–72, 77, 84, 91–92, 191–92, 206–10.

24   Lonna Myers Malmsheimer, "New England funeral sermons and changing attitudes toward women, 1692–1792" (Ph.D. diss., University of Minnesota, 1973), esp. 178–79.

25   See Cott, *Bonds of Womanhood*, 128–35, 146–48; Foster, *Errand of Mercy*, 92–100, 115–32.

26   See Cott, *Bonds of Womanhood*, 130.

27   *The Female Friend, or, the Duties of Christian Virgins* (Baltimore: H. S. Keatinge, 1809), 40–42; Samuel Worcester, *Female Love to Christ* (Salem, Mass.: Pool & Palfrey, 1809), 12–13.

28   See Karen Horney, "The dread of woman," *International Journal of Psychoanalysis*, 1932, *13:* 348–60; and H. R. Hays, *The Dangerous Sex: The Myth of Feminine Evil* (New York: Putnam Books, 1966).

29   Worcester, *Female Love*, 12–13.

30   Cf. Emma Willard's protest, in her *Plan for Improving Female Education* (1819; reprint ed., Middlebury, Vt.: Middlebury College, 1918), 14–15, that current female education was far too attuned to pleasing the opposite sex.

31   Daniel Scott Smith, "Parental power and marriage patterns—an analysis of historical trends in Hingham, Massachusetts," *Journal of Marriage and the Family*, 1973, *35:* 326.

32   Eliza Southgate to Moses Porter, 1800, reprinted in *A Girl's Life Eighty Years Ago*, ed. Clarence Cook (New York: Scribner's, 1887).

33   Robert V. Wells, "Quaker marriage patterns in a colonial perspective," *William and Mary Quarterly*, 1972, *3d ser. 29:* 437–39 (quotations); and Daniel Scott Smith, personal communication. Wells's figures for the proportion of women never marrying, and for remarriage of widows, are based on a New Jersey population; those on age at marriage reflect both the New England and the middle colonies population.

34   Abigail Adams to John Adams, March 31, 1776, reprinted in *The Feminist Papers*, ed. Alice Rossi (New York: Bantam Books, 1974), 10–11.

35   Daniel Scott Smith and Michael S. Hindus, "Premarital pregnancy in America: an overview and interpretation," *Journal of Interdisciplinary History*, 1975, *5:* 537–71; cf. David H. Flaherty, "Law and the enforcement of morals in early America," *Perspectives in American History*, 1971, *5:* 246–47.

36   If premarital sexual activity remained constant while bridal pregnancy increased then illegitimate births would have decreased. This is unlikely. Although the figures for illegitimacy in early America are not known, as Smith and Hindus point out, illegitimacy and bridal pregnancy usually rise and fall together. Another factor affecting the rise and fall of bridal pregnancy is nutrition, but Smith and Hindus tend to discount its relevance in this case.

37   Herman R. Lantz et al., "Preindustrial patterns in the colonial family in America: a content analysis of colonial magazines," *American Sociological Review*, 1968, *33:* 422–23.

38   Manuscript diary of Mary Orne Tucker, May 7, 1802, James Duncan Phillips Library, Essex Institute, Salem, Mass.; Sarah Connell to Susan Kittredge, March 13, 1810, in *Diary of Sarah Connell Ayer* (Portland, Me.: n.p., 1910), 372–73.

39   Malmsheimer, *New England Funeral Sermons*, 138–

79; Gordon S. Wood, *The Creation of the American Republic* (New York: W. W. Norton & Co., 1969), 65–70, 123–24; Cott, "Divorce and the changing status of women."

40 Kenneth R. Lockridge, *Literacy in Colonial New England* (New York: W. W. Norton & Co., 1974), 38–42, 57–58, estimates that half of New England women were literate in the 1780s (see also Cott, "Divorce and the changing status of women," 595–96; and Richard D. Brown, "The emergence of urban society in rural Massachusetts, 1760–1830," *Journal of American History* 61 [June 1974]: 29–51).

41 Constantia, "On the equality of the sexes," *Massachusetts Magazine* 2 (March 1790): 32–35, reprinted in *Up from the Pedestal* ed. Aileen S. Kraditor (Chicago: Quadrangle Books, 1968), 31–33; "Desultory thoughts upon the utility of encouraging a degree of self-complacency, especially in female bosoms," *Gentleman's and Lady's Town and Country Magazine* 1 (October 1784): 251–53.

42 *The Female Advocate*, Written by a Lady (New Haven, Conn.: Thomas Green & Son, 1801), 6, 13–17, 22, 27–28.

43 My discussion is based on *Gentleman's and Lady's Town and Country Magazine*, Boston, 1784; *Gentleman's and Ladies' Town and Country Magazine*, Boston, 1789–90; *Lady's Magazine and Repository of Entertaining Knowledge*, Philadelphia, 1792–93; *Lady* [sic] *and Gentleman's Pocket Magazine of Literary and Polite Amusement*, New York, 1796; *Ladies' Museum*, Philadelphia, 1800–1801; *Lady's Magazine and Musical Repository*, New York, 1801; *Ladies' Monitor*, New York, 1801–2; *Ladies' Miscellany, or the Weekly Visitor*, New York, 1802–5; *Ladies' Visitors*, Boston, 1806–7; *Ladies' Weekly Miscellany*, New York, 1805–8.

44 Manuscript diary of Polly [Patty] Rogers, August 4, September 14, September 21, 1785, in the collection of the American Antiquarian Society.

45 *Weekly Visitor*, vol. 2 (January 21, 1804).

46 *Lady and Gentleman's Pocket Magazine* (October 1796), 174–79; *Lady's Magazine* (June 1792); *Diary of Sarah Connell Ayer*, 373.

47 See D. S. Smith "Family limitation," 129–31; Collins, "Conflict theory," 7, 13–19; Watt, "New Woman."

48 Cf. Harriot Hunt's defensive line of argument in her application for admission to the Harvard Medical School in 1850: "In opening your doors to woman, it is mind that will enter the lecture room, it is intelligence that will ask for food; sex will never be felt where science leads for the atmosphere of thought will be around every lecture" (quoted in Mary Roth Walsh, *Doctors Wanted: No Women Need Apply* [New Haven, Conn.: Yale University Press, 1977], 31).

49 Manuscript diary of Catherine Maria Sedgwick, May 16, 1834, Massachusetts Historical Society, Boston.

50 Mary Grew to Isabel Howland, April 27, 1892, quoted in Carroll Smith-Rosenberg, "The female world of love and ritual," an essay which describes in rich detail female friendships during the nineteenth century, in this volume, 70. See also Cott, *Bonds of Womanhood*, chap. 5.

51 At the end of her life Sarah Grimké opined to Elizabeth Smith Miller that "the sexual passion in man is ten times stronger than in woman," and that woman was innately man's superior (quoted in Ronald G. Walters, "The erotic South: civilization and sexuality in American abolitionism," *American Quarterly* 25 [May 1973]: 196).

52 See Smith, "Family limitation."

53 Gordon, *Woman's Body*, 103.

54 Quoted in Edmund Wilson, *Patriotic Gore* (New York: Oxford University Press, 1966), 22. I am indebted to Kathryn Kish Sklar for bringing this letter to my attention.

55 Angelina Grimké to Theodore Dwight Weld, March 4, 1838, in *Letters of Theodore Dwight Weld, Angelina Grimké Weld, and Sarah Grimké*, ed. Gilbert Barnes and D. L. Dumond (New York: D. Appleton-Century, 1934), 2: 587. "Combe" is the Scottish phrenologist Andrew Combe.

56 Cominos, "Innocent Femina sensualis," 162 and passim.

57 See Charles E. Rosenberg, "Sexuality, class and role in nineteenth-century America," *American Quarterly* 1973, *25*: 131–53; and Stephen Nissenbaum, "Sex, reform, and social change, 1830–1840" (paper delivered at the annual meeting of the Organization of American Historians, Washington, D.C., April 6, 1972).

58 Howard Gadlin, "Private lives and public order: a critical view of the history of intimate relations in the U.S.," *Massachusetts Review* 17 (Summer 1976): 318.

59 See Catharine E. Beecher, *Letters to the People on Health and Happiness* (New York: Harper & Bros., 1855); Smith-Rosenberg, "Beauty, the Beast," 571; Walsh, *Doctors Wanted*, 40–41.

60 Rebecca Harding Davis, "Paul Blecker," *Atlantic Monthly* (June/July 1863), quoted in introduction by Tillie Olsen to Davis's *Life in the Iron Mills* (New York: Feminist Press, 1972), 168n; Mary Gove Nichols (with T. L. Nichols), *Marriage: Its History, Character and Results* . . . (New York: T. L. Nichols, 1854), quoted in Nancy F. Cott, ed., *Root of Bitterness*, (New York: E. P. Dutton & Co., 1972), 286. Cf. Elizabeth Cady Stanton's response to Walt Whitman's poem "There Is a Woman Waiting for Me" in her diary of

1883: "Whitman seems to understand everything in nature but woman. . . . He speaks as if the female must be forced to the creative act, apparently ignorant of the great natural fact that a healthy woman has as much passion as a man, that she needs nothing stronger than the law of attraction to draw her to the male" (quoted in *Feminist Papers*, 393).

61 Gordon, *Woman's Body*, 98–100, 183.

5

The Female World of Love and Ritual: Relations between Women in Nineteenth-Century America

CARROLL SMITH-ROSENBERG

The female friendship of the nineteenth century, the long-lived intimate, loving friendship between two women, is an excellent example of the type of historical phenomena which most historians know something about, which few have thought much about, and which virtually no one has written about.[1] It is one aspect of the female experience which consciously or unconsciously we have chosen to ignore. Yet an abundance of manuscript evidence suggests that eighteenth- and nineteenth-century women routinely formed emotional ties with other women. Such deeply felt, same-sex friendships were casually accepted in American society. Indeed, from at least the late eighteenth through the mid-nineteenth century, a female world of varied and yet highly structured relationships appears to have been an essential aspect of American society. These relationships ranged from the supportive love of sisters, through the enthusiasms of adolescent girls, to sensual avowals of love by mature women. It was a world in which men made but a shadowy appearance.[2]

Defining and analyzing same-sex relationships involves the historian in deeply problematical questions of method and interpretation. This is especially true since historians, influenced by Freud's libidinal theory, have discussed these relationships almost exclusively within the context of individual psychosexual developments or, to be more explicit, psychopathology.[3] Seeing same-sex relationships in terms of a dichotomy between normal and abnormal, they have sought the origins of such apparent

deviance in childhood or adolescent trauma and detected the symptoms of "latent" homosexuality in the lives of both those who later became "overtly" homosexual and those who did not. Yet theories concerning the nature and origins of same-sex relationships are frequently contradictory or based on questionable or arbitrary data. In recent years such hypotheses have been subjected to criticism from both within and without the psychological professions. Historians who seek to work within a psychological framework, therefore, are faced with two hard questions: Do sound psychodynamic theories concerning the nature and origins of same-sex relationships exist? If so, does the historical datum exist which would permit the use of such dynamic models?

I would like to suggest an alternative approach to female friendships—one which would view them within a cultural and social setting rather than from an exclusively individual psychosexual perspective. Only by thus altering our approach will we be in the position to evaluate the appropriateness of particular dynamic interpretations. Intimate friendships between men and men and women and women existed in a larger world of social relations and social values. To interpret such friendships more fully they must be related to the structure of the American family and to the nature of sex-role divisions and of male-female relations both within the family and in society generally. The female friendship must not be seen in isolation; it must be analyzed as one aspect of women's overall relations with one another. The ties between mothers and daughters, sisters, female cousins and friends, at all stages of the female life cycle constitute the most suggestive framework for the historian to begin an analysis of intimacy and affection between women.

CARROLL SMITH-ROSENBERG is Professor of History at the University of Pennsylvania, Philadelphia, Pennsylvania.
Reprinted with permission from *Signs* 1 (1975): 1–29.

Such an analysis would not only emphasize general cultural patterns rather than the internal dynamics of a particular family or childhood; it would shift the focus of the study from a concern with deviance to that of defining configurations of legitimate behavioral norms and options.[4]

This analysis will be based upon the correspondence and diaries of women and men in thirty-five families between the 1760s and the 1880s. These families, though limited in number, represented a broad range of the American middle class, from hard-pressed pioneer families and orphaned girls to daughters of the intellectual and social elite. It includes families from most geographic regions, rural and urban, and a spectrum of Protestant denominations ranging from Mormon to orthodox Quaker. Although scarcely a comprehensive sample of America's increasingly heterogeneous population, it does, I believe, reflect accurately the literate middle class to which the historian working with letters and diaries is necessarily bound. It has involved an analysis of many thousands of letters written to women friends, kin, husbands, brothers, and children at every period of life from adolescence to old age. Some collections encompass virtually entire life spans; one contains over a hundred thousand letters as well as diaries and account books. It is my contention that an analysis of women's private letters and diaries which were never intended to be published permits the historian to explore a very private world of emotional realities central both to women's lives and to the middle-class family in nineteenth-century America.[5]

The question of female friendships is peculiarly elusive; we know so little or perhaps have forgotten so much. An intriguing and almost alien form of human relationship, they flourished in a different social structure and amidst different sexual norms. Before attempting to reconstruct their social setting, therefore, it might be best first to describe two not atypical friendships. These two friendships, intense, loving, and openly avowed, began during the women's adolescence and, despite subsequent marriages and geographic separation, continued throughout their lives. For nearly half a century these women played a central emotional role in each other's lives, writing time and again of their love and of the pain of separation. Paradoxically to twentieth-century minds, their love appears to have been both sensual and platonic.

Sarah Butler Wister first met Jeannie Field Musgrove while vacationing with her family at Stockbridge, Massachusetts, in the summer of 1849.[6] Jeannie was then sixteen, Sarah fourteen. During two subsequent years spent together in boarding school, they formed a deep and intimate friendship. Sarah began to keep a bouquet of flowers before Jeannie's portrait and wrote complaining of the intensity and anguish of her affection.[7] Both young women assumed noms de plume, Jeannie a female name, Sarah a male one; they would use these secret names into old age.[8] They frequently commented on the nature of their affection: "If the day should come," Sarah wrote Jeannie in the spring of 1861, "when you failed me either through your fault or my own, I would forswear all human friendship, thenceforth." A few months later Jeannie commented: "Gratitude is a word I should never use toward you. It is perhaps a misfortune of such intimacy and love that it makes one regard all kindness as a matter of course, as one has always found it, as natural as the embrace in meeting."[9]

Sarah's marriage altered neither the frequency of their correspondence nor their desire to be together. In 1864, when twenty-nine, married, and a mother, Sarah wrote to Jeannie: "I shall be entirely alone [this coming week]. I can give you no idea how desperately I shall want you. . . ." After one such visit Jeannie, then a spinster in New York, echoed Sarah's longing: "Dear darling Sarah! How I love you & how happy I have been! You are the joy of my life. . . . I cannot tell you how much happiness you gave me, nor how constantly it is all in my thoughts. . . . My darling how I long for the time when I shall see you. . . ." After another visit Jeannie wrote: "I want you to tell me in your next letter, to assure me, that I am your dearest. . . . I do not doubt you, & I am not jealous but I long to hear you say it once more & it seems already a long time since your voice fell on my ear. So just fill a quarter page with caresses & expressions of endearment. Your silly Angelina," Jeannie ended one letter: "Goodbye my dearest, dearest lover—ever, your own Angelina." And another, "I will go to bed . . . [though] I could write all night—A thousand kisses—I love you with my whole soul—your Angelina."

When Jeannie finally married in 1870 at the age of thirty-seven, Sarah underwent a period of extreme anxiety. Two days before Jeannie's marriage

Sarah, then in London, wrote desperately: "Dearest darling—How incessantly have I thought of you these eight days—all today—the entire uncertainty, the distance, the long silence—are all new features in my separation from you, grevious to be borne. . . . Oh Jeannie, I have thought & thought & yearned over you these two days. Are you married I wonder? My dearest love to you wherever and *who*ever you are."[10] Like many other women in this collection of thirty-five families, marriage brought Sarah and Jeannie physical separation; it did not cause emotional distance. Although at first they may have wondered how marriage would affect their relationship, their affection remained unabated throughout their lives, underscored by their loneliness and their desire to be together.[11]

During the same years that Jeannie and Sarah wrote of their love and need for each other, two slightly younger women began a similar odyssey of love, dependence, and—ultimately—physical, though not emotional, separation. Molly and Helena met in 1868 while both attended the Cooper Institute School of Design for Women in New York City. For several years these young women studied and explored the city together, visited each other's families, and formed part of a social network of other artistic young women. Gradually, over the years, their initial friendship deepened into a close intimate bond which continued throughout their lives. The tone in the letters which Molly wrote to Helena changed over these years from "My dear Helena," and signed "your attached friend," to "My dearest Helena," "My Dearest," "My Beloved," and signed "Thine always" or "thine Molly."[12]

The letters they wrote to each other during these first five years permit us to reconstruct something of their relationship together. As Molly wrote in one early letter:

I have not said to you in so many or so few words that I was happy with you during those few so incredibly short weeks but surely you do not need words to tell you what you must know. Those two or three days so dark without, so bright with firelight and contentment within I shall always remember as proof that, for a time, at least—I fancy for quite a long time—we might be sufficient for each other. We know that we can amuse each other for many idle hours together and now we know

that we can also work together. And that means much, don't you think so?

She ended: "I shall return in a few days. Imagine yourself kissed many times by one who loved you so dearly."

The intensity and even physical nature of Molly's love was echoed in many of the letters she wrote during the next few years, as, for instance in this short thank-you note for a small present: "Imagine yourself kissed a dozen times my darling. Perhaps it is well for you that we are far apart. You might find my thanks so expressed rather overpowering. I have that delightful feeling that it doesn't matter much what I say or how I say it, since we shall meet so soon and forget in that moment that we were ever separated. . . . I shall see you soon and be content."[13]

At the end of the fifth year, however, several crises occurred. The relationship, at least in its intense form, ended, though Molly and Helena continued an intimate and complex relationship for the next half-century. The exact nature of these crises is not completely clear, but it seems to have involved Molly's decision not to live with Helena, as they had originally planned, but to remain at home because of parental insistence. Molly was now in her late twenties. Helena responded with anger and Molly became frantic at the thought that Helena would break off their relationship. Though she wrote distraught letters that made despairing attempts to see Helena, the relationship never regained its former ardor—possibly because Molly had a male suitor.[14] Within six months Helena had decided to marry a man who was, coincidentally, Molly's friend and publisher. Two years later Molly herself finally married. The letters toward the end of this period discuss the transition both women made to having male lovers—Molly spending much time reassuring Helena, who seemed depressed about the end of their relationship and with her forthcoming marriage.[15]

It is clearly difficult from a distance of a hundred years and from a post-Freudian cultural perspective to decipher the complexities of Molly and Helena's relationship. Certainly Molly and Helena were lovers—emotionally if not physically. The emotional intensity and pathos of their love become apparent in several letters Molly wrote Helena during their crisis: "I wanted so to put my arms round my girl of all the girls in the world and tell her . . . I love her as wives do love their husbands, as *friends* who have taken each other for life—and believe in her as I believe in my God. . . . If I didn't love you do you suppose I'd care about anything or have ridiculous notions and panics and behave like an old fool who ought to know better. I'm going to hang on to your skirts. . . . You can't get away from [my] love." Or as she wrote after Helena's decision to marry: "You know dear Helena, I really was in love with you. It was a passion such as I had never known until I saw you. I don't think it was the noblest way to love you." The theme of intense female love was one Molly again expressed in a letter she wrote to the man Helena was to marry: "Do you know sir, that until you came along I believe that she loved me almost as girls love their lovers. *I know I loved her so.* Don't you wonder that I can stand the sight of you." This was in a letter congratulating them on their forthcoming marriage.[16]

The essential question is not whether these women had genital contact and can therefore be defined as heterosexual or homosexual. The twentieth-century tendency to view human love and sexuality within a dichotomized universe of deviance and normality, genitality and platonic love, is alien to the emotions and attitudes of the nineteenth century and fundamentally distorts the nature of these women's emotional interaction. These letters are significant because they force us to place such female love in a particular historical context. There is every indication that these four women, and their husbands and families—all eminently respectable and socially conservative—considered such love both socially acceptable and fully compatible with heterosexual marriage. Emotionally and cognitively, their heterosocial and their homosocial worlds were complementary.

One could argue, on the other hand, that these letters were but an example of the romantic rhetoric with which the nineteenth century surrounded the concept of friendship. Yet they possess an emotional intensity and a sensual and physical explicitness that is difficult to dismiss. Jeannie longed to hold Sarah in her arms; Molly mourned her physical isolation from Helena. Molly's love and devotion to Helena, the emotions that bound Jeannie and Sarah together, while perhaps a phenomenon of nineteenth-century society were not the less real for their Victorian origins. A survey of the correspondence and diaries of eighteenth- and nineteenth-century women indicates that Molly, Jeannie, and Sarah represented one very real behavioral and emotional option socially available to nineteenth-century women.

This is not to argue that individual needs, personalities, and family dynamics did not have a significant role in determining the nature of particular relationships. But the scholar must ask if it is historically possible and, if possible, important to study the intensely individual aspects of psychosexual dynamics. Is it not the historian's first task to explore the social structure and the world view which made intense and sometimes sensual female love both a possible and an acceptable emotional option? From such a social perspective a new and quite different series of questions suggests itself. What emotional function did such female love serve? What was its place within the hetero- and homosocial worlds which women jointly inhabited? Did a spectrum of love-object choices exist in the nineteenth century across which some individuals, at least, were capable of moving? Without attempting to answer these questions it will be difficult to understand either nineteenth-century sexuality or the nineteenth-century family.

Several factors in American society between the mid-eighteenth and the mid-nineteenth centuries may well have permitted women to form a variety of close emotional relationships with other women. American society was characterized in large part by rigid gender role differentiation within the family and within society as a whole, leading to the emotional segregation of women and men. The roles of daughter and mother shaded imperceptibly and ineluctably into each other, while the biological realities of frequent pregnancies, childbirth, nursing, and menopause bound women together in physical and emotional intimacy. It was within just such a social framework, I would argue, that a specifically female world did indeed develop, a world built around a generic and unselfconscious pattern of single-sex or homosocial networks. These supportive networks were institutionalized in social conventions or rituals which accompanied virtually every important event in a woman's life, from birth to death. Such female relationships were frequently supported and paralleled by severe social restrictions on intimacy between young men and women. Within such a world of emotional richness and complexity devotion to and love of other women became a plausible and socially accepted form of human interaction.

An abundance of printed and manuscript sources exists to support such a hypothesis. Etiquette books, advice books on child rearing, religious sermons, guides to young men and young women, medical texts, and school curricula all suggest that late-eighteenth- and most nineteenth-century Americans assumed the existence of a world composed of distinctly male and female spheres, spheres determined by the immutable laws of God and nature.[17] The unpublished letters and diaries of Americans during this same period concur, detailing the existence of sexually segregated worlds inhabited by human beings with different values, expectations, and personalities. Contacts between men and women frequently partook of a formality and stiffness quite alien to twentieth-century America and which today we tend to define as "Victorian." Women, however, did not form an isolated and oppressed subcategory in male society. Their letters and diaries indicate that women's sphere had an essential integrity and dignity that grew out of women's shared experiences and mutual affection and that, despite the profound changes which affected American social structure and institutions between the 1760s and the 1870s, retained a constancy and predictability. The ways in which women thought of and interacted with each other remained unchanged. Continuity, not discontinuity, characterized this female world. Molly Hallock's and Jeannie Field's words, emotions, and experiences have direct parallels in the 1760s and the 1790s.[18] There are indications in contemporary sociological and psychological literature that female closeness and support networks have continued into the twentieth-century—not only among ethnic and working-class groups but even among the middle class.[19]

Most eighteenth- and nineteenth-century women lived within a world bounded by home, church, and the institution of visiting—that endless trooping of women to each other's homes for social purposes. It was a world inhabited by children and by other women.[20] Women helped each other with domestic chores and in times of sickness, sorrow, or trouble. Entire days, even weeks, might be spent almost exclusively with other women.[21] Urban and town women could devote virtually every day to visits, teas, or shopping trips with other women. Rural women developed a pattern of more extended visits that lasted weeks and sometimes months, at times even dislodging husbands from their beds and bedrooms so that dear friends might spend every hour of every day together.[22] When husbands traveled, wives routinely moved in with other women, invited women friends to teas and suppers, sat together sharing and comparing the letters they had received from other close women friends. Secrets were exchanged and cherished, and the husband's return at times viewed with some ambivalence.[23]

Summer vacations were frequently organized to permit old friends to meet at water spas or share a country home. In 1848, for example, a young matron wrote cheerfully to her husband about the delightful time she was having with five close women friends whom she had invited to spend the summer with her; he remained at home alone to face the heat of Philadelphia and a cholera epidemic.[24] Some ninety years earlier, two young Quaker girls commented upon the vacation their aunt had taken alone with another woman; their remarks were openly envious and tell us something of the emotional quality of these friendships: "I hear Aunt is gone with the Friend and wont be back for two weeks, fine times indeed I think the old friends had, taking their pleasure about the country ... and have the advantage of that fine woman's conversation and instruction, while we poor young girls must spend all spring at home. . . . What a disappointment that we are not together. . . ."[25]

Friends did not form isolated dyads but were normally part of highly integrated networks. Knowing each other, perhaps related to each other, they played a central role in holding communities and kin systems together. Especially when families became geographically mobile women's long visits to each other and their frequent letters filled with discussions of marriage and births, illness and deaths, descriptions of growing children, and reminiscences of times and people past provided an important sense of continuity in a rapidly changing society.[26] Central to this female world was an inner core of kin. The ties between sisters, first cousins, aunts, and nieces provided the underlying structure upon which groups of friends and their network of female relatives clustered. Although most of the women within this sample would appear to be living within isolated nuclear families, the emotional ties between nonresidential kin were deep and binding and provided one of the fundamental existential realities of women's lives.[27] Twenty years after Parke Lewis Butler moved with her husband to Louisiana, she sent her two daughters back to Virginia to attend school, live with their grandmother and aunt, and be integrated back into Virginia society.[28] The constant letters between Maria Inskeep and Fanny Hampton, sisters separated in their early twenties when Maria moved with her husband from New Jersey to Louisiana, held their families together, making it possible for their daughters to feel a part of their cousins' network of friends and interests.[29] The Ripley daughters, growing up in western Massachusetts in the early 1800s, spent months each year with their mother's sister and her family in distant Boston; these female cousins and their network of friends exchanged gossip-filled letters and gradually formed deeply loving and dependent ties.[30]

Women frequently spent their days within the social confines of such extended families. Sisters-in-law visited each other and, in some families, seemed to spend more time with each other than with their husbands. First cousins cared for each other's babies—for weeks or even months in times of sickness or childbirth. Sisters helped each other with housework, shopped and sewed for each other. Geographic separation was borne with difficulty. A sister's absence for even a week or two could cause loneliness and depression and would be bridged by frequent letters. Sibling rivalry was hardly unknown, but with separation or illness the theme of deep affection and dependency reemerged.[31]

Sisterly bonds continued across a lifetime. In her old age a rural Quaker matron, Martha Jefferis, wrote to her daughter Anne concerning her own half-sister, Phoebe: "In sister Phoebe I have a real friend—she studies my comfort and waits on me like a child. . . . She is exceedingly kind and this to all other homes (set aside yours) I would prefer—it is next to being with a daughter." Phoebe's own letters confirmed Martha's evaluation of her feel-

ings. "Thou knowest my dear sister," Phoebe wrote, "there is no one . . . that exactly feels [for] thee as I do, for I think without boasting I can truly say that my desire is for thee."[32]

Such women, whether friends or relatives, assumed an emotional centrality in each other's lives. In their diaries and letters they wrote of the joy and contentment they felt in each other's company, their sense of isolation and despair when apart. The regularity of their correspondence underlines the sincerity of their words. Women named their daughters after one another and sought to integrate dear friends into their lives after marriage.[33] As one young bride wrote to an old friend shortly after her marriage: "I want to see you and talk with you and feel that we are united by the same bonds of sympathy and congeniality as ever."[34] After years of friendship one aging woman wrote of another: "Time cannot destroy the fascination of her manner . . . her voice is music to the ear. . . ."[35] Women made elaborate presents for each other, ranging from the Quakers' frugal pies and breads to painted velvet bags and phantom bouquets.[36] When a friend died, their grief was deeply felt. Martha Jefferis was unable to write to her daughter for three weeks because of the sorrow she felt at the death of a dear friend. Such distress was not unusual. A generation earlier a young Massachusetts farm woman filled pages of her diary with her grief at the death of her "dearest friend" and transcribed the letters of condolence other women sent her. She marked the anniversary of Rachel's death each year in her diary, contrasting her faithfulness with that of Rachel's husband who had soon remarried.[37]

These female friendships served a number of emotional functions. Within this secure and empathetic world women could share sorrows, anxieties, and joys, confident that other women had experienced similar emotions. One mid-nineteenth-century rural matron in a letter to her daughter discussed this particular aspect of women's friendships: "To have such a friend as thyself to look to and sympathize with her—and enter into all her little needs and in whose bosom she could with freedom pour forth her joys and sorrows—such a friend would very much relieve the tedium of many a wearisome hour. . . ." A generation later Molly more informally underscored the importance of this same function in a letter to Helena:

"Suppose I come down . . . [and] spend Sunday with you quietly," she wrote Helena ". . . that means talking all the time until you are relieved of all your latest troubles, and I of mine. . . ."[38] These were frequently troubles that apparently no man could understand. When Anne Jefferis Sheppard was first married, she and her older sister Edith (who then lived with Anne) wrote in detail to their mother of the severe depression and anxiety which they experienced. Moses Sheppard, Anne's husband, added cheerful postscripts to the sisters' letters—which he had clearly not read—remarking on Anne's and Edith's contentment. Theirs was an emotional world to which he had little access.[39]

This was, as well, a female world in which hostility to and criticism of other women were discouraged, and thus a milieu in which women could develop a sense of inner security and self-esteem. As one young woman wrote to her mother's long-time friend: "I cannot sufficiently thank you for the kind unvaried affection & indulgence you have ever shown and expressed both by words and actions for me. . . . Happy would it be did all the world view me as you do, through the medium of kindness and forbearance."[40] They valued each other. Women, who had little status or power in the larger world of male concerns, possessed status and power in the lives and worlds of other women.[41]

An intimate mother-daughter relationship lay at the heart of this female world. The diaries and letters of both mothers and daughters attest to their closeness and mutual emotional dependency. Daughters routinely discussed their mothers' health and activities with their own friends, expressed anxiety in cases of their mothers' ill health and concern for their mothers' cares.[42] Expressions of hostility which we would today consider routine on the part of both mothers and daughters seem to have been uncommon indeed. On the contrary, this sample of families indicates that the normal relationship between mother and daughter was one of sympathy and understanding.[43] Only sickness or great geographic distance was allowed to cause extended separation. When marriage did result in such separation, both viewed the distance between them with distress.[44] Something of this sympathy and love between mothers and daughters is evident in a letter Sarah Alden Ripley, at age sixty-nine, wrote her youngest and recently married daughter: "You do not know how much I miss you,

not only when I struggle in and out of my mortal envelop and pump my nightly potation and no longer pour into your sympathizing ear my senile gossip, but all the day I muse away, since the sound of your voice no longer rouses me to sympathy with your joys and sorrows. . . . You cannot know how much I miss your affectionate demonstrations."[45] A dozen aging mothers in this sample of over thirty families echoed her sentiments.

Central to these mother-daughter relations is what might be described as an apprenticeship system. In those families where the daughter followed the mother into a life of traditional domesticity, mothers and other older women carefully trained daughters in the arts of housewifery and motherhood. Such training undoubtedly occurred throughout a girl's childhood but became more systematized, almost ritualistic, in the years following the end of her formal education and before her marriage. At this time a girl either returned home from boarding school or no longer divided her time between home and school. Rather, she devoted her energies to two tasks: mastering new domestic skills and participating in the visiting and social activities necessary to finding a husband. Under the careful supervision of their mothers and of older female relatives, such late-adolescent girls temporarily took over the household management from their mothers, tended their young nieces and nephews, and helped in childbirth, nursing, and weaning. Such experiences tied the generations together in shared skills and emotional interaction.[46]

Daughters were born into a female world. Their mothers' life expectations and sympathetic network of friends and relations were among the first realities in the life of the developing child. As long as the mother's domestic role remained relatively stable and few viable alternatives competed with it, daughters tended to accept their mothers' world and to turn automatically to other women for support and intimacy. It was within this closed and intimate female world that the young girl grew toward womanhood.

One could speculate at length concerning the absence of that mother-daughter hostility today considered almost inevitable to an adolescent's struggle for autonomy and self-identity. It is possible that taboos against female aggression and hostility were sufficiently strong to repress them even between mothers and their adolescent daughters. Yet these letters seem so alive and the interest of daughters in their mothers' affairs so vital and genuine that it is difficult to interpret their closeness exclusively in terms of repression and denial. The functional bonds that held mothers and daughters together in a world that permitted few alternatives to domesticity might well have created a source of mutuality and trust absent in societies where greater options were available for daughters than for mothers. Furthermore, the extended female network—a daughter's close ties with her own older sisters, cousins, and aunts—may well have permitted a diffusion and a relaxation of mother-daughter identification and so have aided a daughter in her struggle for identity and autonomy. None of these explanations are mutually exclusive; all may well have interacted to produce the degree of empathy evident in those letters and diaries.

At some point in adolescence, the young girl began to move outside the matrix of her mother's support group to develop a network of her own. Among the middle class, at least, this transition toward what was at the same time both a limited autonomy and a repetition of her mother's life seemed to have most frequently coincided with a girl's going to school. Indeed education appears to have played a crucial role in the lives of most of the families in this study. Attending school for a few months, for a year, or longer, was common even among daughters of relatively poor families, while middle-class girls routinely spent at least a year in boarding school.[47] These school years ordinarily marked a girl's first separation from home. They served to wean the daughter from her home, to train her in the essential social graces, and, ultimately, to help introduce her into the marriage market. It was not infrequently a trying emotional experience for both mother and daughter.[48]

In this process of leaving one home and adjusting to another, the mother's friends and relatives played a key transitional role. Such older women routinely accepted the role of foster mother; they supervised the young girl's deportment, monitored her health, and introduced her to their own network of female friends and kin.[49] Not infrequently women, friends from their own school years, arranged to send their daughters to the same school so that the girls might form bonds paralleling those their mothers had made. For years Molly and

Helena wrote of their daughters' meeting and worried over each other's children. When Molly finally brought her daughter east to school, their first act on reaching New York was to meet Helena and her daughters. Elizabeth Bordley Gibson virtually adopted the daughters of her school chum, Eleanor Custis Lewis. The Lewis daughters soon began to write Elizabeth Gibson letters with the salutation "Dearest Mama." Eleuthera DuPont, attending boarding school in Philadelphia at roughly the same time as the Lewis girls, developed a parallel relationship with her mother's friend, Elizabeth McKie Smith. Eleuthera went to the same school and became a close friend of the Smith girls and eventually married their first cousin. During this period she routinely called Mrs. Smith "Mother." Indeed Eleuthera so internalized the sense of having two mothers that she casually wrote her sisters of her "Mamma's" visits at her "mother's" house—that is at Mrs. Smith's.[50]

Even more important to this process of maturation than their mothers' friends were the female friends young women made at school. Young girls helped each other overcome homesickness and endure the crises of adolescence. They gossiped about beaux, incorporated each other into their own kinship systems, and attended and gave teas and balls together. Older girls in boarding school "adopted" younger ones, who called them "Mother."[51] Dear friends might indeed continue this pattern of adoption and mothering throughout their lives; one woman might routinely assume the nurturing role of pseudomother, the other the dependency role of daughter. The pseudomother performed for the other woman all the services which we normally associate with mothers; she went to absurd lengths to purchase items her "daughter" could have obtained from other sources, gave advice and functioned as an idealized figure in her "daughter's" imagination. Helena played such a role for Molly, as did Sarah for Jeannie. Elizabeth Bordley Gibson bought almost all Eleanor Parke Custis Lewis's necessities—from shoes and corset covers to bedding and harp strings—and sent them from Philadelphia to Virginia, a procedure that sometimes took months. Eleanor frequently asked Elizabeth to take back her purchases, have them redone, and argue with shopkeepers about prices. These were favors automatically asked and complied with. Anne Jefferis Sheppard made the analogy very explicitly in a letter to her own mother written shortly after Anne's marriage, when she was feeling depressed about their separation: "Mary Paulen is truly kind, almost acts the part of a mother and trys to aid and *comfort me*, and also to *lighten my new cares.*"[52]

A comparison of the references to men and women in these young women's letters is striking. Boys were obviously indispensable to the elaborate courtship ritual girls engaged in. In these teenage letters and diaries, however, boys appear distant and warded off—an effect produced both by the girls' sense of bonding and by a highly developed and deprecatory whimsy. Girls joked among themselves about the conceit, poor looks, or affectations of suitors. Rarely, especially in the eighteenth and early nineteenth centuries, were favorable remarks exchanged. Indeed, while hostility to and criticism of other women were so rare as to seem almost tabooed, young women permitted themselves to express a great deal of hostility toward peer group men.[53] When unacceptable suitors appeared, girls might even band together to harass them. When one such unfortunate came to court Sophie DuPont she hid in her room, first sending her sister Eleuthera to entertain him and then dispatching a number of urgent notes to her neighboring sister-in-law, cousins, and a visiting friend who all came to Sophie's support. A wild female romp ensued, ending only when Sophie banged into a door, lacerated her nose, and retired, with her female cohorts, to bed. Her brother and the presumably disconcerted suitor were left alone. These were not the antics of teenagers but of women in their early and mid-twenties.[54]

Even if young men were acceptable suitors, girls referred to them formally and obliquely: "The last week I received the unexpected intelligence of the arrival of a friend in Boston," Sarah Ripley wrote in her diary of the young man to whom she had been engaged for years and whom she would shortly marry. Harriet Manigault assiduously kept a lively and gossipy diary during the three years preceding her marriage, yet did not once comment upon her own engagement or indeed make any personal references to her fiance—who was never identified as such but always referred to as Mr. Wilcox.[55] The point is not that these young women were hostile

to young men. Far from it; they sought marriage and domesticity. Yet in these letters and diaries men appear as an other or out group, segregated into different schools, supported by their own male network of friends and kin, socialized to different behavior, and coached to a proper formality in courtship behavior. As a consequence, relations between young women and men frequently lacked the spontaneity and emotional intimacy that characterized the young girls' ties to each other.

Indeed, in sharp contrast to their distant relations with boys, young women's relations with each other were close, often frolicsome, and surprisingly long lasting and devoted. They wrote secret missives to each other, spent long solitary days with each other, curled up together in bed at night to whisper fantasies and secrets.[56] In 1862 one young woman in her early twenties described one such scene to an absent friend: "I have sat up to midnight listening to the confidences of Constance Kinney, whose heart was opened by that most charming of all situations, a seat on a bedside late at night, when all the household are asleep & only oneself & one's confidante survive in wakefulness. So she has told me all her loves and tried to get some confidences in return but being five or six years older than she, I know better. . . ."[57] Elizabeth Bordley and Nelly Parke Custis, teenagers in Philadelphia in the 1790s, routinely secreted themselves until late each night in Nelly's attic, where they each wrote a novel about the other.[58] Quite a few young women kept diaries, and it was a sign of special friendship to show their diaries to each other. The emotional quality of such exchanges emerges from the comments of one young girl who grew up along the Ohio frontier:

> Sisters CW and RT keep diaries & allow me the inestimable pleasure of reading them and in turn they see mine—but O shame covers my face when I think of it; theirs is so much better than mine, that every time. Then I think well now I *will* burn mine but upon second thought it would deprive me the pleasure of reading theirs, for I esteem it a very great privilege indeed, as well as very improving, as we lay our hearts open to each other, it heightens our love & helps to cher-

ish & keep alive that sweet soothing friendship and endears us to each other by that soft
attraction.[59]

Girls routinely slept together, kissed and hugged
each other. Indeed, while waltzing with young men
scandalized the otherwise flighty and highly fashionable Harriet Manigault, she considered waltzing with other young women not only acceptable
but pleasant.[60]

Marriage followed adolescence. With increasing
frequency in the nineteenth century, marriage involved a girl's traumatic removal from her mother
and her mother's network. It involved, as well, adjustment to a husband, who, because he was male,
came to marriage with both a different world view
and vastly different experiences. Not surprisingly,
marriage was an event surrounded with supportive, almost ritualistic, practices. (Weddings are one
of the last female rituals remaining in twentieth-
century America.) Young women routinely spent
the months preceding their marriage almost exclusively with other women—at neighborhood sewing
bees and quilting parties or in a round of visits to
geographically distant friends and relatives. Ostensibly they went to receive assistance in the practical preparations for their new home—sewing and
quilting a trousseau and linen—but of equal importance, they appear to have gained emotional
support and reassurance. Sarah Ripley spent over
a month with friends and relatives in Boston and
Hingham before her wedding; Nelly Parke Custis
Lewis exchanged visits with her aunts and first
cousins throughout Virginia.[61] Anne Jefferis, who
married with some hesitation, spent virtually half
a year in endless visiting with cousins, aunts, and
friends. Despite their reassurance and support,
however, she would not marry Moses Sheppard
until her sister Edith and her cousin Rebecca moved
into the groom's home, met his friends, and explored his personality.[62] The wedding did not take
place until Edith wrote to Anne: "I can say in truth
I am entirely willing thou shouldst follow him even
away in the Jersey sands believing if thou are not
happy in thy future home it will not be any fault
on his part. . . ."[63]

Sisters, cousins, and friends frequently accompanied newlyweds on their wedding night and

wedding trip, which often involved additional family
visiting. Such extensive visits presumably served to
wean the daughter from her family of origin. As
such they often contained a note of ambivalence.
Nelly Custis, for example, reported homesickness
and loneliness on her wedding trip. "I left my Beloved and revered Grandmamma with sincere regret," she wrote Elizabeth Bordley. "It was sometime before I could feel reconciled to traveling
without her." Perhaps they also functioned to reassure the young woman herself, and her friends
and kin, that though marriage might alter it would
not destroy old bonds of intimacy and familiarity.[64]

Married life, too, was structured about a host of
female rituals. Childbirth, especially the birth of
the first child, became virtually a *rite de passage*,
with a lengthy seclusion of the woman before and
after delivery, severe restrictions on her activities,
and finally a dramatic reemergence.[65] This seclusion was supervised by mothers, sisters, and loving
friends. Nursing and weaning involved the advice
and assistance of female friends and relatives. So
did miscarriage.[66] Death, like birth, was structured
around elaborate unisexed rituals. When Nelly
Parke Custis Lewis rushed to nurse her daughter
who was critically ill while away at school, Nelly
received support, not from her husband, who remained on their plantation, but from her old school
friend, Elizabeth Bordley. Elizabeth aided Nelly in
caring for her dying daughter, cared for Nelly's
other children, played a major role in the elaborate
funeral arrangements (which the father did not
attend), and frequently visited the girl's grave at
the mother's request. For years Elizabeth continued to be the confidante of Nelly's anguished recollections of her lost daughter. These memories,
Nelly's letters make clear, were for Elizabeth alone.
"Mr. L. knows nothing of this," was a frequent
comment.[67] Virtually every collection of letters and
diaries in my sample contained evidence of women
turning to each other for comfort when facing the
frequent and unavoidable deaths of the eighteenth
and nineteenth centuries.[68] While mourning for
her father's death, Sophie DuPont received elaborate letters and visits of condolence—all from
women. No man wrote or visited Sophie to offer
sympathy at her father's death.[69] Among rural
Pennsylvania Quakers, death and mourning ritu-

als assumed an even more extreme same-sex form, with men or women largely barred from the death-beds of the other sex. Women relatives and friends slept with the dying woman, nursed her, and prepared her body for burial.[70]

Eighteenth- and nineteenth-century women thus lived in emotional proximity to each other. Friendships and intimacies followed the biological ebb and flow of women's lives. Marriage and pregnancy, childbirth and weaning, sickness and death involved physical and psychic trauma which comfort and sympathy made easier to bear. Intense bonds of love and intimacy bound together those women who, offering each other aid and sympathy, shared such stressful moments.

These bonds were often physical as well as emotional. An undeniably romantic and even sensual note frequently marked female relationships. This theme, significant throughout the stages of a woman's life, surfaced first during adolescence. As one teenager from a struggling pioneer family in the Ohio Valley wrote in her diary in 1808: "I laid with my dear R[ebecca] and a glorious good talk we had until about 4[A.M.]—O how hard I do *love* her. . . ."[71] Only a few years later Bostonian Eunice Callender carved her initials and Sarah Ripley's into a favorite tree, along with a pledge of eternal love, and then waited breathlessly for Sarah to discover and respond to her declaration of affection. The response appears to have been affirmative.[72] A half-century later urbane and sophisticated Katherine Wharton commented upon meeting an old school chum: "She was a great pet of mine at school & I thought as I watched her light figure how often I had held her in my arms—how dear she had once been to me." Katie maintained a long intimate friendship with another girl. When a young man began to court this friend seriously, Katie commented in her diary that she had never realized "how deeply I loved Eng and how fully." She wrote over and over again in that entry: "Indeed I love her!" and only with great reluctance left the city that summer since it meant also leaving Eng with Eng's new suitor.[73]

Peggy Emlen, a Quaker adolescent in Philadelphia in the 1760s, expressed similar feelings about her first cousin, Sally Logan. The girls sent love poems to each other (not unlike the ones Elizabeth Bordley wrote to Nelly Custis a generation later), took long solitary walks together, and even haunted the empty house of the other when one was out of town. Indeed Sally's absences from Philadelphia caused Peggy acute unhappiness. So strong were Peggy's feelings that her brothers began to tease her about her affection for Sally and threatened to steal Sally's letters, much to both girls' alarm. In one letter that Peggy wrote the absent Sally she elaborately described the depth and nature of her feelings: "I have not words to express my impatience to see My Dear Cousin, what would I not give just now for an hours sweet conversation with her, it seems as if I had a thousand things to say to thee, yet when I see thee, everything will be forgot thro' joy. . . . I have a very great friendship for several Girls yet it dont give me so much uneasiness at being absent from them as from thee. . . . [Let us] go and spend a day down at our place together and there unmolested enjoy each others company."[74]

Sarah Alden Ripley, a young, highly educated woman, formed a similar intense relationship, in this instance with a woman somewhat older than herself. The immediate bond of friendship rested on their atypically intense scholarly interests, but it soon involved strong emotions, at least on Sarah's part. "Friendship," she wrote Mary Emerson, "is fast twining about her willing captive the silken hands of dependence, a dependence so sweet who would renounce it for the apathy of self-sufficiency?" Subsequent letters became far more emotional, almost conspiratorial. Mary visited Sarah secretly in her room, or the two women crept away from family and friends to meet in a nearby woods. Sarah became jealous of Mary's other young woman friends. Mary's trips away from Boston also thrust Sarah into periods of anguished depression. Interestingly, the letters detailing their love were not destroyed but were preserved and even reprinted in a eulogistic biography of Sarah Alden Ripley.[75]

Tender letters between adolescent women, confessions of loneliness and emotional dependency, were not peculiar to Sarah Alden, Peggy Emlen, or Katie Wharton. They are found throughout the letters of the thirty-five families studied. They have, of course, their parallel today in the musings of many female adolescents. Yet these eighteenth- and nineteenth-century friendships lasted with undiminished, indeed often increased, intensity throughout the women's lives. Sarah Alden Ripley's first child was named after

Mary Emerson. Nelly Custis Lewis's love for and dependence on Elizabeth Bordley Gibson only increased after her marriage. Eunice Callender remained enamored of her cousin Sarah Ripley for years and rejected as impossible the suggestion by another woman that their love might some day fade away.[76] Sophie DuPont and her childhood friend, Clementina Smith, exchanged letters filled with love and dependency for forty years while another dear friend, Mary Black Couper, wrote of dreaming that she, Sophie, and her husband were all united in one marriage. Mary's letters to Sophie are filled with avowals of love and indications of ambivalence toward her own husband. Eliza Schlatter, another of Sophie's intimate friends, wrote to her at a time of crisis: "I wish I could be with you present in the body as well as the mind & heart—I would turn your *good husband out of bed*—and snuggle into you and we would have a long talk like old times in Pine St.—I want to tell you so many things that are not *writable*. . . ."[77]

Such mutual dependency and deep affection is a central existential reality coloring the world of supportive networks and rituals. In the case of Katie, Sophie, or Eunice—as with Molly, Jeannie, and Sarah—their need for closeness and support merged with more intense demands for a love which was at the same time both emotional and sensual. Perhaps the most explicit statement concerning women's lifelong friendships appeared in the letter abolitionist and reformer Mary Grew wrote about the same time, referring to her own love for her dear friend and lifelong companion, Margaret Burleigh. Grew wrote, in response to a letter of condolence from another woman on Burleigh's death: "Your words respecting my beloved friend touch me deeply. Evidently . . . you comprehend and appreciate, as few persons do . . . the nature of the relation which existed, which exists, between her and myself. Her only surviving niece . . . also does. To me it seems to have been a closer union than that of most marriages. We know there have been other such between two men and also between two women. And why should there not be. Love is spiritual, only passion is sexual."[78]

How then can we ultimately interpret these long-lived intimate female relationships and integrate them into our understanding of Victorian sexuality? Their ambivalent and romantic rhetoric presents us with an ultimate puzzle: where to place the relationship along the spectrum of human emotions between love, sensuality, and sexuality.

One is tempted, as I have remarked, to compare Molly, Peggy, or Sophie's relationships to the friendships adolescent girls in the twentieth century routinely form—close friendships of great emotional intensity. Helena Deutsch and Clara Thompson have both described these friendships as emotionally necessary to a girl's psychosexual development. But, they warn, such friendships might shade into adolescent and postadolescent homosexuality.[79]

It is possible to speculate that in the twentieth century a number of cultural taboos evolved to cut short the homosocial ties of girlhood and to impel the emerging women of thirteen or fourteen toward heterosexual relationships. In contrast, nineteenth-century American society did not taboo close female relationships but rather recognized them as a socially viable form of human contact—and, as such, acceptable throughout a woman's life. Indeed it was not these homosocial ties that were inhibited but rather heterosexual leanings. While closeness, freedom of emotional expression, and uninhibited physical contact characterized women's relationships with each other, the opposite was frequently true of male-female relationships. One could thus argue that within such a world of female support, intimacy, and ritual it was only to be expected that adult women would turn trustingly and lovingly to each other. It was a behavior they had observed and learned since childhood. A different type of emotional landscape existed in the nineteenth century, one in which Molly and Helena's love became a natural development.

Of perhaps equal significance are the implications we can garner from this framework for the understanding of heterosexual marriages in the nineteenth century. If men and women grew up as they did in relatively homogeneous and segregated sexual groups, then marriage represented a major problem in adjustment. From this perspective we could interpret much of the emotional stiffness and distance that we associate with Victorian marriage as a structural consequence of contemporary sex role differentiation and gender role socialization. With marriage both women and men had to adjust to life with a person who was, in essence, a member of an alien group.

I have thus far substituted a cultural or psycho-social for a psychosexual interpretation of women's emotional bonding. But there are psychosexual implications in this model which I think it only fair to make more explicit. Despite Sigmund Freud's insistence on the bisexuality of us all or the recent American Psychiatric Association decision on homosexuality, many psychiatrists today tend explicitly or implicitly to view homosexuality as a totally alien or pathological behavior—as totally unlike heterosexuality. I suspect that in essence they may have adopted an explanatory model similar to the one used in discussing schizophrenia. As a psychiatrist can speak of schizophrenia and of a borderline schizophrenic personality as both ultimately and fundamentally different from a normal or neurotic personality, so they also think of both homosexuality and latent homosexuality as states totally different from heterosexuality. With this rapidly dichotomous model of assumption, "latent homosexuality" becomes the indication of a disease in progress—seeds of a pathology which belie the reality of an individual's heterosexuality.

Yet at the same time we are well aware that cultural values can affect choices in the gender of a person's sexual partner. We, for instance, do not necessarily consider homosexual object choice among men in prison, on shipboard, or in boarding schools a necessary indication of pathology. I would urge that we expand this relativistic model and hypothesize that a number of cultures might well tolerate or even encourage diversity in sexual and nonsexual relations. Based on my research into this nineteenth-century world of female intimacy, I would further suggest that rather than seeing a gulf between the normal and the abnormal we view sexual and emotional impulses as part of a continuum or spectrum of affect gradations strongly affected by cultural norms and arrangements, a continuum influenced in part by observed and thus learned behavior. At one end of the continuum lies committed heterosexuality, at the other uncompromising homosexuality; between, a wide latitude of emotions and sexual feelings. Certain cultures and environments permit individuals a great deal of freedom in moving across this spectrum. I would like to suggest that the nineteenth century was such a cultural environment. That is, the supposedly repressive and destructive Victorian sexual ethos may have been more flexible and responsive to the needs of particular individuals than that of the mid-twentieth century.

NOTES

Research for this paper was supported in part by a grant from the Grant Foundation, New York, and by National Institutes of Health trainee grant 5 FO3 HD48800–03. I would like to thank several scholars for their assistance and criticism in preparing this paper: Erving Goffman, Roy Schafer, Charles E. Rosenberg, Cynthia Secor, Anthony Wallace. Judy Breault, who has just completed a biography of an important and introspective nineteenth-century feminist, Emily Howland, served as a research assistant for this paper and her knowledge of nineteenth-century family structure and religious history proved invaluable.

1   The most notable exception to this rule is now eleven years old: William R. Taylor and Christopher Lasch, "Two 'kindred spirits': sorority and family in New England, 1839–1846," *New England Quarterly*, 1963, *36:* 25–41. Taylor has made a valuable contribution to the history of women and the history of the family with his concept of "sororial" relations. I do not, however, accept the Taylor-Lasch thesis that female friendships developed in the mid-nineteenth century because of geographic mobility and the breakup of the colonial family. I have found these friendships as frequently in the eighteenth century as in the nineteenth and would hypothesize that the geographic mobility of the mid-nineteenth century eroded them as it did so many other traditional social institutions. Helen Vendler (Review of *Notable American Women, 1607–1950*, ed. Edward James and Janet James, *New York Times* [November 5, 1972]: sec. 7) points out the significance of these friendships.

2   I do not wish to deny the importance of women's relations with particular men. Obviously, women were close to brothers, husbands, fathers, and sons. However, there is evidence that despite such closeness relationships between men and women differed in both emotional texture and frequency from those between women. Women's relations with each other, although they played a central role in the American family and American society, have been so seldom examined either by general social historians or by historians of the family that I wish in this article simply to examine their nature and analyze their implications for our understanding of so-

cial relations and social structure. I have discussed some aspects of male-female relationships in two articles: "Puberty to menopause: the cycle of femininity in nineteenth-century America," *Feminist Studies*, 1973, *1*: 58–72, and, with Charles Rosenberg, "The female animal: medical and biological views of woman and her role in 19th-Century America," in this volume.

3 See Freud's classic paper on homosexuality, "Three essays on the theory of sexuality," in *The Standard Edition of the Complete Psychological Works of Sigmund Freud*, trans. James Strachey (London: Hogarth Press, 1953), 7:135–72. The essays originally appeared in 1905. Prof. Roy Shafer, Department of Psychiatry, Yale University, has pointed out that Freud's view of sexual behavior was strongly influenced by nineteenth-century evolutionary thought. Within Freud's schema, genital heterosexuality marked the height of human development (Schafer, "Problems in Freud's psychology of women," *Journal of the American Psychoanalytic Association*, 1974, *22*: 459–85).

4 For a novel and most important exposition of one theory of behavioral norms and options and its application to the study of human sexuality, see Charles Rosenberg, "Sexuality, class and role," *American Quarterly*, 1973, *25*: 131–53.

5 See, e.g., the letters of Peggy Emlen to Sally Logan, 1768–72, Wells Morris Collection, Box 1, Historical Society of Pennsylvania, Philadelphia; and the Eleanor Parke Custis Lewis Letters, Historical Society of Pennsylvania.

6 Sarah Butler Wister was the daughter of Fanny Kemble and Pierce Butler. In 1859 she married a Philadelphia physician, Owen Wister. The novelist Owen Wister is her son. Jeannie Field Musgrove was the half-orphaned daughter of constitutional lawyer and New York Republican politician David Dudley Field. Their correspondence (1855–98) is in the Sarah Butler Wister Papers, Wister Family Papers, Historical Society of Pennsylvania.

7 Sarah Butler, Butler Place, S.C., to Jeannie Field, New York, September 14, 1855.

8 See, e.g., Sarah Butler Wister, Germantown, Pa., to Jeannie Field, New York, September 25, 1862, October 21, 1863; or Jeannie Field, New York, to Sarah Butler Wister, Germantown, July 3, 1861, January 23 and July 12, 1863.

9 Sarah Butler Wister, Germantown, to Jeannie Field, New York, June 5, 1861, February 29, 1864; Jeannie Field to Sarah Butler Wister, November 22, 1861, January 4 and June 14, 1863.

10 Sarah Butler Wister, London, to Jeannie Field Musgrove, New York, June 18 and August 3, 1870.

11 See, e.g., two of Sarah's letters to Jeannie: December 21, 1873, July 16, 1878.

12 This is the 1868–1920 correspondence between Mary Hallock Foote and Helena, a New York friend (the Mary Hallock Foote Papers are in the Manuscript Division, Stanford University). Wallace E. Stegner has written a fictionalized biography of Mary Hallock Foote (*Angle of Repose* [Garden City, N.Y.: Doubleday & Co., 1971]). See, as well, her autobiography: Mary Hallock Foote, *A Victorian Gentlewoman in the Far West: The Reminiscences of Mary Hallock Foote*, ed. Rodman W. Paul (San Marino, Calif.: Huntington Library, 1972). In many ways these letters are typical of those women wrote to other women. Women frequently began letters to each other with salutations such as "Dearest," "My Most Beloved," "You Darling Girl," and signed them "tenderly" or "to my dear dear sweet friend, goodbye." Without the least self-consciousness, one woman in her frequent letters to a female friend referred to her husband as "my other love." She was by no means unique. See, e.g., Annie to Charlena Van Vleck Anderson, Appleton, Wis., June 10, 1871, Anderson Family Papers, Manuscript Division, Stanford University; Maggie to Emily Howland, Philadelphia, July 12, 1851, Howland Family Papers, Phoebe King Collection, Friends Historical Library, Swarthmore College; Mary Jane Burleigh to Emily Howland, Sherwood, N.Y., March 27, 1872, Howland Family Papers, Sophia Smith Collection, Smith College; Mary Black Couper to Sophia Madeleine DuPont, Wilmington, Del., n.d. [1834] (two letters), Samuel Francis DuPont Papers, Eleutherian Mills Foundation, Wilmington, Del.; Phoebe Middleton, Concordiville, Pa., to Martha Jefferis, Chester County, Pa., February 22, 1848; and see in general the correspondence (1838–49) between Rebecca Biddle of Philadelphia and Martha Jefferis, Chester County, Pa., Jefferis Family Correspondence, Chester County Historical Society, West Chester, Pa.; Phoebe Bradford Diary, June 7 and July 13, 1832, Historical Society of Pennsylvania; Sarah Alden Ripley to Abba Allyn, Boston, n.d. [1818–20], and Sarah Alden Ripley to Sophia Bradford, November 30, 1854, in the Sarah Alden Ripley Correspondence, Schlesinger Library, Radcliffe College; Fanny Canby Ferris to Anne Biddle, Philadelphia, October 11 and November 19, 1811, December 26, 1813, Fanny Canby to Mary Canby, May 27, 1801, Mary R. Garrigues to Mary Canby, five letters n.d. [1802–8], Anne Biddle to Mary Canby, two letters n.d., May 16, July 13, and November 24, 1806, June 14, 1807, June 5, 1808, Anne Sterling Biddle Family Papers, Friends Historical

Society, Swarthmore College; Harriet Manigault Wilcox Diary, August 7, 1814, Historical Society of Pennsylvania. See as well the correspondence between Harriet Manigault Wilcox's mother, Mrs. Gabriel Manigault, Philadelphia, and Mrs. Henry Middleton, Charleston, S.C., between 1810 and 1830, Cadwalader Collection, J. Francis Fisher Section, Historical Society of Pennsylvania. The basis and nature of such friendships can be seen in the comments of Sarah Alden Ripley to her sister-in-law and long-time friend, Sophia Bradford: "Hearing that you are not well reminds me of what it would be to lose your loving society. We have kept step together through a long piece of road in the weary journey of life. We have loved the same beings and wept together over their graves" (Mrs. O. J. Wister and Miss Agnes Irwin, eds., *Worthy Women of Our First Century* [Philadelphia: J. B. Lippincott & Co., 1877], 195).

13 Mary Hallock [Foote] to Helena, n.d. [1869–70], n.d. [1871–72], Folder 1, Mary Hallock Foote Letters, Manuscript Division, Stanford University.

14 Mary Hallock [Foote] to Helena, September 15 and 23, 1873, n.d. [October 1873], October 12, 1873.

15 Mary Hallock [Foote] to Helena, n.d. [January 1874], n.d. [Spring 1874].

16 Mary Hallock [Foote] to Helena, September 23, 1873; Mary Hallock [Foote] to Richard, December 13, 1873. Molly's and Helena's relationship continued for the rest of their lives. Molly's letters are filled with tender and intimate references, as when she wrote, twenty years later and from 2,000 miles away: "It isn't because you are good that I love you—but for the essence of you which is like perfume" (n.d. [1890s?]).

17 I am in the midst of a larger study of adult gender roles and gender role socialization in America, 1785–1895. For a discussion of social attitudes toward male and female roles, see Barbara Welter, "The cult of true womanhood: 1820–1860," *American Quarterly* 18 (Summer 1966): 151–74; Ann Firor Scott, *The Southern Lady: From Pedestal to Politics, 1830–1930* (Chicago: University of Chicago Press, 1970), chaps. 1–2; Smith-Rosenberg and Rosenberg, "The female animal," in this volume, 12–27.

18 See, e.g., the letters of Peggy Emlen to Sally Logan, 1768–72, Wells Morris Collection, Box 1, Historical Society of Pennsylvania; and the Eleanor Parke Custis Lewis Letters, Historical Society of Pennsylvania.

19 See esp. Elizabeth Botts, *Family and Social Network* (London: Tavistock Publications, 1957); Michael Young and Peter Willmott, *Family and Kinship in East London,* rev. ed. (Baltimore: Penguin Books, 1964).

20 This pattern seemed to cross class barriers. A letter that an Irish domestic wrote in the 1830s contains seventeen separate references to women and but only seven to men, most of whom were relatives and two of whom were infant brothers living with her mother and mentioned in relation to her mother (Ann McGrann, Philadelphia, to Sophie M. DuPont, Philadelphia, July 3, 1834, Sophie Madeleine DuPont Letters, Eleutherian Mills Foundation).

21 Harriet Manigault Diary, June 28, 1814, and passim; Jeannie Field, New York, to Sarah Butler Wister, Germantown, April 19, 1863; Phoebe Bradford Diary, January 30, February 19, March 4, August 11, and October 14, 1832, Historical Society of Pennsylvania; Sophie M. DuPont, Brandywine, to Henry DuPont, Germantown, July 9, 1827, Eleutherian Mills Foundation.

22 Martha Jefferis to Anne Jefferis Sheppard, July 9, 1843; Anne Jefferis Sheppard to Martha Jefferis, June 28, 1846; Anne Sterling Biddle Papers, passim, Biddle Family Papers, Friends Historical Society, Swarthmore College; Eleanor Parke Custis Lewis, Virginia, to Elizabeth Bordley Gibson, Philadelphia, November 24 and December 4, 1820, November 6, 1821, Historical Society of Pennsylvania.

23 Phoebe Bradford Diary, January 13, November 16–19, 1832, April 26 and May 7, 1833; Abigail Brackett Lyman to Mrs. Catling, Litchfield, Conn., May 3, 1801, collection in private hands; Martha Jefferis to Anne Jefferis Sheppard, August 28, 1845.

24 Lisa Mitchell Diary, 1860s, passim, Manuscript Division, Tulane University; Eleanor Parke Custis Lewis to Elizabeth Bordley [Gibson] February 5, 1822; Jeannie McCall, Cedar Park, to Peter McCall, Philadelphia, June 30, 1849, McCall Section, Cadwalader Collection, Historical Society of Pennsylvania.

25 Peggy Emlen to Sally Logan, May 3, 1769.

26 For a prime example of this type of letter, see Eleanor Parke Custis Lewis to Elizabeth Bordley Gibson, passim, or Fanny Canby to Mary Canby, Philadelphia, May 27, 1801; or Sophie M. DuPont, Brandywine, to Henry DuPont, Germantown, February 4, 1832.

27 Place of residence is not the only variable significant in characterizing family structure. Strong emotional ties and frequent visiting and correspondence can unite families that do not live under one roof. Demographic studies based on household structure alone fail to reflect such emotional and even economic ties between families.

28 Eleanor Parke Custis Lewis to Elizabeth Bordley Gibson, April 20 and September 25, 1848.

29 Maria Inskeep to Fanny Hampton Correspondence, 1823–60, Inskeep Collection, Tulane University Library.

30 Eunice Callender, Boston, to Sarah Ripley [Stearns],

September 24 and October 29, 1803, February 16, 1805, April 29 and October 9, 1806, May 26, 1810, Schlesinger Library, Radcliffe College.

31 Sophie DuPont filled her letters to her younger brother Henry (with whom she had been assigned to correspond while he was at boarding school) with accounts of family visiting (see, e.g., December 13, 1827, January 10 and March 9, 1828, February 4 and March 10, 1832; also Sophie M. DuPont to Victorine DuPont Bauday, September 26 and December 4, 1827, February 22, 1828; Sophie M. DuPont, Brandywine, to Clementina B. Smith, Philadelphia, January 15, 1830; Eleuthera DuPont, Brandywine, to Victorine DuPont Bauday, Philadelphia, April 17, 1821, October 20, 1826; Evelina DuPont [Biderman] to Victorine DuPont Bauday, October 18, 1816). Other examples, from the Historical Society of Pennsylvania, are Harriet Manigault [Wilcox] Diary, August 17, September 8, October 19 and 22, December 22, 1814; Jane Zook, West Town School, Chester County, Pa., to Mary Zook, November 13, December 7 and 11, 1870, February 26, 1871; Eleanor Parke Custis [Lewis] to Elizabeth Bordley [Gibson], March 30, 1796, February 7 and March 20, 1798; Jeannie McCall to Peter McCall, Philadelphia, November 12, 1847; Mary B. Ashew Diary, July 11 and 13, August 17, Summer and October 1858, and, from a private collection, Edith Jefferis to Anne Jefferis Sheppard, November 1841, April 5, 1842; Abigail Brackett Lyman, Northampton, Mass., to Mrs. Catling, Litchfield, Conn., May 13, 1801; Abigail Brackett Lyman, Northampton, to Mary Lord, August 11, 1800. Mary Hallock Foote vacationed with her sister, her sister's children, her aunt, and a female cousin in the summer of 1874; cousins frequently visited the Hallock farm in Milton, N.Y. In later years Molly and her sister Bessie set up a joint household in Boise, Idaho (Mary Hallock Foote to Helena, July [1874?] and passim). Jeannie Field, after initially disliking her sister-in-law, Laura, became very close to her, calling her "my little sister" and at times spending virtually every day with her (Jeannie Field [Musgrove] New York, to Sarah Butler Wister, Germantown, March 1, 8, and 15, and May 9, 1863).

32 Martha Jefferis to Anne Jefferis Sheppard, January 12, 1845; Phoebe Middleton to Martha Jefferis, February 22, 1848. A number of other women remained close to sisters and sisters-in-law across a long lifetime (Phoebe Bradford Diary, June 7, 1832, and Sarah Alden Ripley to Sophia Bradford, cited in Wister and Irwin, *Worthy Women*, 195).

33 Rebecca Biddle to Martha Jefferis, 1838–49, passim; Martha Jefferis to Anne Jefferis Sheppard, July 6, 1846; Anne Jefferis Sheppard to Rachael Jef-

feris, January 16, 1865; Sarah Foulke Farquhar [Emlen] Diary, September 22, 1813, Friends Historical Library, Swarthmore College; Mary Garrigues to Mary Canby [Biddle], 1802–8, passim; Anne Biddle to Mary Canby [Biddle], May 16, July 13, and November 24, 1806, June 14, 1807, June 5, 1808.

34 Sarah Alden Ripley to Abba Allyn, n.d., Schlesinger Library, Radcliffe College.

35 Phoebe Bradford Diary, July 13, 1832.

36 Mary Hallock [Foote] to Helena, December 23 [1868 or 1869]; Phoebe Bradford Diary, December 8, 1832; Martha Jefferis and Anne Jefferis Sheppard letters, passim.

37 Martha Jefferis to Anne Jefferis Sheppard, August 3, 1849; Sarah Ripley [Stearns] Diary, November 12, 1808, January 8, 1811. An interesting note of hostility or rivalry is present in Sarah Ripley's diary entry. Sarah evidently deeply resented the husband's rapid remarriage.

38 Martha Jefferis to Edith Jefferis, March 15, 1841; Mary Hallock Foote to Helena, n.d. [1874–75?]; see also Jeannie Field, New York, to Sarah Butler Wister, Germantown, May 5, 1863; Emily Howland Diary, December 1879, Howland Family Papers.

39 Anne Jefferis Sheppard to Martha Jefferis, September 29, 1841.

40 Frances Parke Lewis to Elizabeth Bordley Gibson, April 29, 1821.

41 Mary Jane Burleigh, Mount Pleasant, S.C., to Emily Howland, Sherwood N.Y., March 27, 1872, Howland Family Papers; Emily Howland Diary, September 16, 1879, January 21 and 23, 1880; Mary Black Couper, New Castle, Del., to Sophie M. DuPont, Brandywine, April 7, 1834.

42 Harriet Manigault Diary, August 15, 21, and 23, 1814, Historical Society of Pennsylvania; Polly [Simmons] to Sophie Madeleine DuPont, February 1822; Sophie Madeleine DuPont to Victorine Bauday, December 4, 1827; Sophie Madeleine DuPont to Clementina Beach Smith, July 24, 1828, August 19, 1829; Clementina Beach Smith to Sophie Madeleine DuPont, April 29, 1831; Mary Black Couper to Sophie Madeleine DuPont, December 24, 1828, July 21, 1834. This pattern appears to have crossed class lines. When a former Sunday school student of Sophie DuPont's (and the daughter of a worker in her father's factory) wrote to Sophie she discussed her mother's health and activities quite naturally (Ann McGrann to Sophie Madeleine DuPont, August 25, 1832; see also Elizabeth Bordley to Martha, n.d. [1797], Eleanor Parke Custis [Lewis] to Elizabeth Bordley [Gibson], May 13, 1796, July 1, 1798; Peggy Emlen to Sally Logan, January 8, 1786. All but the Emlen/Logan letters are in the

Eleanor Parke Custis Lewis Correspondence, Historical Society of Pennsylvania).

43 Mrs. S. S. Dalton, "Autobiography," (Circle Valley, Utah, 1876), 21–22, Bancroft Library, University of California, Berkeley; Sarah Foulke Emlen Diary, April 1809; Louisa G. Van Vleck, Appleton, Wis., to Charlena Van Vleck Anderson, Göttingen, n.d. [1875]; Harriet Manigault Diary, August 16, 1814, July 14, 1815; Sarah Alden Ripley to Sophy Fisher [early 1860s], quoted in Wister and Irwin, *Worthy Women*, 212. The Jefferis family papers are filled with empathetic letters between Martha and her daughters, Anne and Edith. See, e.g., Martha Jefferis to Edith Jefferis, December 26, 1836, March 11, 1837, March 15, 1841; Anne Jefferis Sheppard to Martha Jefferis, March 17, 1841, January 17, 1847; Martha Jefferis to Anne Jefferis Sheppard, April 17, 1848, April 30, 1849. A representative letter is this of March 9, 1837, from Edith to Martha: "My heart can fully respond to the language of my own precious Mother, that absence has not diminished our affection for each other, but has, if possible, strengthened the bonds that have united us together & I have had to remark how we had been permitted to mingle in sweet fellowship and have been strengthened to bear one another's burdens. ..."

44 Abigail Brackett Lyman, Boston, to Mrs. Abigail Brackett (daughter to mother), n.d.[1797], June 3, 1800, private collection; Sarah Alden Ripley wrote weekly to her daughter, Sophy Ripley Fisher, after the latter's marriage (Sarah Alden Ripley Correspondence, passim); Phoebe Bradford Diary, February 25, 1833, passim, 1832–33; Louisa G. Van Vleck to Charlena Van Vleck Anderson, December 15, 1873, July 4, August 15 and 29, September 19, and November 9, 1875. Eleanor Parke Custis Lewis's long correspondence with Elizabeth Bordley Gibson contains evidence of her anxiety at leaving her foster mother's home at various times during her adolescence and at her marriage, and her own longing for her daughters, both of whom had married and moved to Louisiana (Eleanor Parke Custis [Lewis] to Elizabeth Bordley [Gibson], October 13, 1795, November 4, 1799, passim, 1820s and 1830s). Anne Jefferis Sheppard experienced a great deal of anxiety on moving two days' journey from her mother at the time of her marriage. This loneliness and sense of isolation persisted through her marriage until, finally a widow, she returned to live with her mother (Anne Jefferis Sheppard to Martha Jefferis, April 1841, October 16, 1842, April 2, May 22, and October 12, 1844, September 3, 1845, January 17, 1847, May 16, June 3, and October 31,

1849; Anne Jefferis Sheppard to Susanna Lightfoot, March 23, 1845, and to Joshua Jefferis, May 14, 1854). Daughters evidently frequently slept with their mothers—into adulthood (Harriet Manigault [Wilcox] Diary, February 19, 1815; Eleanor Parke Custis Lewis to Elizabeth Bordley Gibson, October 10, 1832). Daughters also frequently asked mothers to live with them and professed delight when they did so. See, e.g., Sarah Alden Ripley's comments to George Simmons, October 6, 1844, in Wister and Irwin, *Worthy Women*, 185: "It is no longer 'Mother and Charles came out one day and returned the next,' for mother is one of us: she has entered the penetratice, been initiated into the mystery of the household gods, ... Her divertissement is to mend the stockings ... whiten sheets and napkins, ... and take a stroll at evening with me to talk of our children, to compare our experiences, what we have learned and what we have suffered, and, last of all, to complete with pears and melons the cheerful circle about the solar lamp." We did find a few exceptions to this mother-daughter felicity (M.B. Ashew Diary, November 19, 1857, April 10 and May 17, 1858). Sarah Foulke Emlen was at first very hostile to her stepmother (Sarah Foulke Emlen Diary, August 9, 1807), but they later developed a warm supportive relationship.

45 Sarah Alden Ripley to Sophy Thayer, n.d. [1861].

46 Mary Hallock Foote to Helena [winter 1873] (no. 52); Jossie, Stevens Point, Wis., to Charlena Van Vleck [Anderson], Appleton, Wis., October 24, 1870; Pollie Chandler, Green Bay, Wis., to Charlena Van Vleck [Anderson], Appleton, n.d. [1870]; Eleuthera DuPont to Sophie DuPont, September 5, 1829; Sophie DuPont to Eleuthera DuPont, December 1827; Sophie DuPont to Victorine Bauday, December 4, 1827; Mary Gilpin to Sophie DuPont, September 26, 1827; Sarah Ripley Stearns Diary, April 2, 1809; Jeannie McCall to Peter McCall, October 27 [late 1840s]. Eleanor Parke Custis Lewis's correspondence with Elizabeth Bordley Gibson describes such an apprenticeship system over two generations—that of her childhood and that of her daughters. Indeed Eleanor Lewis's own apprenticeship was quite formal. She was deliberately separated from her foster mother in order to spend a winter of domesticity with her married sisters and her remarried mother. It was clearly felt that her foster mother's (Martha Washington) home at the nation's capital was not an appropriate place to develop domestic talents (October 13, 1795, March 30, May 13, and [summer] 1796, March 18 and April 27, 1797, October 1827).

47 Education was not limited to the daughters of the

well-to-do. Sarah Foulke Emlen, the daughter of an Ohio Valley frontier farmer, for instance, attended day school for several years during the eary 1800s. Sarah Ripley Stearns, the daughter of a shopkeeper in Greenfield, Mass., attended a boarding school for but three months, yet the experience seemed very important to her. Mrs. S. S. Dalton, a Mormon woman from Utah, attended a series of poor country schools and greatly valued her opportunity, though she also expressed a great deal of guilt for the sacrifices her mother made to make her education possible (Sarah Foulke Emlen Journal, Sarah Ripley Stearns Diary, Mrs. S. S. Dalton, "Autobiography").

48   Maria Revere to her mother [Mrs. Paul Revere], June 13, 1801, Paul Revere Papers, Massachusetts Historical Society. In a letter to Elizabeth Bordley Gibson, March 28, 1847, Eleanor Parke Custis Lewis from Virginia discussed the anxiety her daughter felt when her granddaughters left home to go to boarding school. Eleuthera DuPont was very homesick when away at school in Philadelphia in the early 1820s (Eleuthera DuPont, Philadelphia, to Victorine Bauday, Wilmington, Del., April 7, 1821; Eleuthera DuPont to Sophie Madeleine DuPont, Wilmington Del., February and April 3, 1821).

49   Elizabeth Bordley Gibson, a Philadelphia matron, played such a role for the daughters and nieces of her lifelong friend, Eleanor Parke Custis Lewis, a Virginia planter's wife (Eleanor Parke Custis Lewis to Elizabeth Bordley Gibson, January 29, 1833, March 19, 1826, and passim through the collection). The wife of Thomas Gurney Smith played a similar role for Sophie and Eleuthera DuPont (see, e.g., Eleuthera DuPont to Sophie Madeleine DuPont, May 22, 1825; Rest Cope to Philema P. Swayne [niece], West Town School, Chester County, Pa., April 8, 1829, Friends Historical Library, Swarthmore College). For a view of such a social pattern over three generations, see the letters and diaries of three generations of Manigault women in Philadelphia: Mrs. Gabrielle Manigault, her daughter, Harriet Manigault Wilcox, and granddaughter, Charlotte Wilcox McCall. Unfortunately the papers of the three women are not in one family collection (Mrs. Henry Middleton, Charleston, S.C., to Mrs. Gabrielle Manigault, n.d. [mid 1800s]; Harriet Manigault Diary, vol. 1, December 1, 1813, June 28, 1814; Charlotte Wilcox McCall Diary, vol. 1, 1842, passim. All in Historical Society of Philadelphia).

50   Frances Parke Lewis, Woodlawn, Va., to Elizabeth Bordley Gibson, Philadelphia, April 11, 1821, Lewis Correspondence; Eleuthera DuPont, Philadelphia to Victorine DuPont Bauday, Brandywine, December 8, 1821, January 31, 1822; Eleuthera DuPont, Brandywine, to Margaretta Lammont [DuPont], Philadelphia, May 1823.

51   Sarah Ripley Stearns Diary, March 9 and 25, 1810; Peggy Emlen to Sally Logan, March and July 4, 1769; Harriet Manigault [Wilcox] Diary, vol. 1, December 1, 1813, June 28 and September 18, 1814, August 10, 1815; Charlotte Wilcox McCall Diary, 1842, passim; Fanny Canby to Mary Canby, May 27, 1801, March 17, 1804; Deborah Cope, West Town School, to Rest Cope, Philadelphia, July 9, 1828, Chester County Historical Society, West Chester, Pa.; Anne Zook, West Town School, to Mary Zook, Philadelphia, January 30, 1866, Chester County Historical Society, West Chester, Pa.; Mary Gilpin to Sophie Madeleine DuPont, February 25, 1829; Eleanor Parke Custis [Lewis] to Elizabeth Bordley [Gibson], April 27, July 2, and September 8, 1797, June 30, 1799, December 29, 1820; Frances Parke Lewis to Elizabeth Bordley Gibson, December 20, 1820.

52   Anne Jefferis Sheppard to Martha Jefferis, March 17, 1841.

53   Peggy Emlen to Sally Logan, March 1769, Mount Vernon, Va.; Eleanor Parke Custis [Lewis] to Elizabeth Bordley [Gibson], Philadelphia, April 27, 1797, June 30, 1799; Jeannie Field, New York, to Sarah Butler Wister, Germantown, July 3, 1861, January 16, 1863, Harriet Manigault Diary, August 3 and 11–13, 1814; Eunice Callender, Boston, to Sarah Ripley [Stearns], Greenfield, May 4, 1809. I found one exception to this inhibition of female hostility. This was the diary of Charlotte Wilcox McCall, Philadelphia (see, e.g., her March 23, 1842, entry).

54   Sophie M. DuPont and Eleuthera DuPont, Brandywine, to Victorine DuPont Bauday, Philadelphia, January 25, 1832.

55   Sarah Ripley [Stearns] Diary and Harriet Manigault Diary, passim.

56   Sophie Madeleine DuPont to Eleuthera DuPont, December 1827; Clementina Beach Smith to Sophie Madeleine DuPont, December 26, 1828; Sarah Foulke Emlen Diary, July 21, 1808, March 30, 1809; Annie Hethroe, Ellington, Wis., to Charlena Van Vleck [Anderson], Appleton, Wis., April 23, 1865; Frances Parke Lewis, Woodlawn, Va., to Elizabeth Bordley [Gibson], Philadelphia, December 20, 1820; Fanny Ferris to Debby Ferris, West Town School, Chester County, Pa., May 29, 1826. An excellent example of the warmth of women's comments about each other and the reserved nature of their references to men are seen in two entires in Sarah Ripley Stearn's diary. On January 8, 1811, she commented about a young woman friend: "The amiable Mrs. White of Princeton . . . one of the loveliest most in-

teresting creatures I ever knew, young fair and
blooming ... beloved by everyone ... formed to
please & to charm. ...." She referred to the man she
ultimately married always as "my friend" or "a
friend" (February 2 or April 23, 1810).

57 Jeannie Field, New York, to Sarah Butler Wister,
Germantown, April 6, 1862.

58 Elizabeth Bordley Gibson, introductory statement
to the Eleanor Parke Custis Lewis Letters [1850s],
Historical Society of Pennsylvania.

59 Sarah Foulke [Emlen] Diary, March 30, 1809.

60 Harriet Manigault Diary, May 26, 1815.

61 Sarah Ripley [Stearns] Diary, May 17 and October
2, 1812; Eleanor Parke Custis Lewis to Elizabeth
Bordley Gibson, April 23, 1826; Rebecca Ralston,
Philadelphia, to Victorine DuPont [Bauday], Brandywine, September 27, 1813.

62 Anne Jefferis to Martha Jefferis, November 22 and
27, 1840, January 13 and March 17, 1841; Edith
Jefferis, Greenwich, N.J., to Anne Jefferis, Philadelphia, January 31, February 6 and February 1841.

63 Edith Jefferis to Anne Jefferis, January 31, 1841.

64 Eleanor Parke Custis Lewis to Elizabeth Bordley,
November 4, 1799. Eleanor and her daughter Parke
experienced similar sorrow and anxiety when Parke
married and moved to Cincinnati (Eleanor Parke
Custis Lewis to Elizabeth Bordley Gibson, April 23,
1826). Helena DeKay visited Mary Hallock the
month before her marriage; Mary Hallock was an
attendant at the wedding; Helena again visited Molly
about three weeks after her marriage; and then
Molly went with Helena and spent a week with
Helena and Richard in their new apartment (Mary
Hallock [Foote] to Helena DeKay Gilder [Spring
1874] (no. 61), May 10, 1874 [May 1874], June 14,
1874 [Summer 1874]. See also Anne Biddle, Phila-
delphia, to Clement Biddle (brother), Wilmington,
March 12 and May 27, 1827; Eunice Callender,
Boston, to Sarah Ripley [Stearns], Greenfield, Mass.,
August 3, 1807, January 26, 1808; Victorine Du-
Pont Bauday, Philadelphia, to Evelina DuPont
[Biderman], Brandywine, November 25 and 26,
December 1, 1813; Peggy Emlen to Sally Logan, n.d.
[1769–70?]; Jeannie Field, New York, to Sarah But-
ler Wister, Germantown, July 3, 1861).

65 Mary Hallock to Helena DeKay Gilder [1876] (no.
81), n.d. (no. 83), March 3, 1884; Mary Ashew Diary,
vol. 2, September–January, 1860; Louisa Van Vleck
to Charlena Van Vleck Anderson, n.d. [1875]; Sophie DuPont to Henry DuPont, July 24, 1827; Benjamin Ferris to William Canby, February 13, 1805;
Benjamin Ferris to Mary Canby Biddle, December
20, 1825; Anne Jefferis Sheppard to Martha Jefferis, September 15, 1884; Martha Jefferis to Anne
Jefferis Sheppard, July 4, 1843, May 5, 1844, May

3, 1847, July 17, 1849; Jeannie McCall to Peter
McCall, November 26, 1847, n.d. [late 1840s]. A
graphic description of the ritual surrounding a first
birth is found in Abigail Lyman's letter to her husband Erastus Lyman, October 18, 1810.

66 Fanny Ferris to Anne Biddle, November 19, 1811;
Eleanor Parke Custis Lewis to Elizabeth Bordley
Gibson, November 4, 1799, April 27, 1827; Martha
Jefferis to Anne Jefferis Sheppard, January 31, 1843,
April 4, 1844; Martha Jefferis to Phoebe Sharpless
Middleton, June 4, 1846; Anne Jefferis Sheppard
to Martha Jefferis, August 20, 1843, February 12,
1844; Maria Inskeep, New Orleans, to Mrs. Fanny
G. Hampton, Bridgeton, N.J., September 22, 1848;
Benjamin Ferris to Mary Canby, February 14, 1805;
Fanny Ferris to Mary Canby [Biddle], December 2,
1816.

67 Eleanor Parke Custis Lewis to Elizabeth Bordley
Gibson, October–November 1820, passim.

68 Emily Howland to Hannah, September 30, 1866;
Emily Howland Diary, February 8, 11, and 27, 1880;
Phoebe Bradford Diary, April 12 and 13, and Au-
gust 4, 1833; Eunice Callender, Boston, to Sarah
Ripley [Stearns], Greenwich, Mass., September 11,
1802, August 26, 1810; Mrs. H. Middleton,
Charleston, to Mrs. Gabrielle Manigault, Philadel-
phia, n.d. [mid 1800s]; Mrs. H. C. Paul to Mrs.
Jeannie McCall, Philadelphia, n.d. [1840s]; Sarah
Butler Wister, Germantown, to Jeannie Field [Mus-
grove], New York, April 22, 1864; Jeannie Field
[Musgrove] to Sarah Butler Wister, August 25, 1861,
July 6, 1862; S. B. Randolph to Elizabeth Bordley
[Gibson], n.d. [1790s]. For an example of similar
letters between men, see Henry Wright to Peter
McCall, December 10, 1852; Charles McCall to Pe-
ter McCall, January 4, 1860, March 22, 1864; R.
Mercer to Peter McCall, November 29, 1872.

69 Mary Black [Couper] to Sophie Madeleine DuPont,
February 1827, [November 1, 1834], November 12,
1834, two letters [late November 1834]; Eliza
Schlatter to Sophie Madeleine DuPont, November
2, 1834.

70 For a few of the references to death rituals in the
Jefferis papers see: Martha Jefferis to Anne Jefferis
Sheppard, September 28, 1843, August 21 and
September 25, 1844, January 11, 1846, summer
1848, passim; Anne Jefferis Sheppard to Martha
Jefferis, August 20, 1843; Anne Jefferis Sheppard
to Rachel Jefferis, March 17, 1863, February 9, 1868.
For other Quaker families, see Rachel Biddle to
Anne Biddle, July 23, 1854; Sarah Foulke Far-
quhar [Emlen] Diary, April 30, 1811, February 14,
1812; Fanny Ferris to Mary Canby, August 31, 1810.
This is not to argue that men and women did not
mourn together. Yet in many families women aided

and comforted women and men men. The same-sex death ritual was one emotional option available to nineteenth-century Americans.

71 Sarah Foulke [Emlen] Diary, December 29, 1808.

72 Eunice Callender, Boston, to Sarah Ripley [Stearns] Greenfield, Mass., May 24, 1803.

73 Katherine Johnstone Brinley [Wharton] Journal, April 26, May 30, and May 29, 1856, Historical Society of Pennsylvania.

74 A series of roughly fourteen letters written by Peggy Emlen to Sally Logan (1768–71) has been preserved in the Wells Morris Collection, Box 1, Historical Society of Pennsylvania (see esp. May 3 and July 4, 1769, January 8, 1768).

75 The Sarah Alden Ripley Collection, the Arthur M. Schlesinger, Sr., Library, Radcliffe College, contains a number of Sarah Alden Ripley's letters to Mary Emerson. Most of these are undated, but they extend over a number of years and contain letters written both before and after Sarah's marriage. The eulogistic biographical sketch appeared in Wister and Irwin, *Worthy Women*. It should be noted that Sarah Butler Wister was one of the editors who sensitively selected Sarah's letters.

76 See Sarah Alden Ripley to Mary Emerson, November 19, 1823. Sarah Alden Ripley routinely, and one must assume ritualistically, read Mary Emerson's letters to her infant daughter, Mary. Eleanor Parke Custis Lewis reported doing the same with Elizabeth Bordley Gibson's letters, passim. Eunice Callender, Boston, to Sarah Ripley [Stearns], October 19, 1808.

77 Mary Black Couper to Sophie M. DuPont, March 5, 1832. The Clementina Smith–Sophie DuPont correspondence of 1,678 letters is in the Sophie DuPont Correspondence. The quotation is from Eliza Schlatter, Mount Holly, N.J., to Sophie DuPont, Brandywine, August 24, 1834. I am indebted to Anthony Wallace for informing me about this collection.

78 Mary Grew, Providence, R.I., to Isabel Howland, Sherwood, N.Y., April 27, 1892, Howland Correspondence, Sophia Smith Collection, Smith College.

79 Helena Deutsch, *Psychology of Women* (New York: Grune & Stratton, 1944), vol. 1, chaps. 1–3; Clara Thompson, *On Women*, ed. Maurice Green (New York: New American Library, 1971).

6

"Imagine My Surprise":
Women's Relationships in Historical Perspective

LEILA J. RUPP

When Carroll Smith-Rosenberg's article "The Female World of Love and Ritual" appeared in the
pages of *Signs* in 1975, it revolutionized the way in
which women's historians look at nineteenth-century
American society and even served notice on the
historical profession at large that women's relationships would have to be taken into account in
any consideration of Victorian society.[1] Since then
we have learned more about relationships between
women in the past, but we have not reached consensus on the issue of characterizing these relationships.[2] On the one hand, Smith-Rosenberg's work
has increasingly been misused to deny the sexual
aspect of relationships between prominent women
in the past. On the other hand, feminist scholars
have responded to such distortions by bestowing
the label "lesbian" on women who would themselves not have used the term. The issue goes beyond labels, however, because the very nature of
women's relationships is so complex. I would like
to consider here the issue of women's relationships
in historical perspective by reviewing the conflicting approaches, by presenting examples of different kinds of women's relationships from my own
research on the American women's movement in
the 1940s and 1950s, and finally, by suggesting a
conceptual approach that recognizes the complexity of women's relationships without denying the
common bond shared by all women who have committed their lives to other women in the past.

Looking first at what Blanche Cook proclaims
"the historical denial of lesbianism," we find the

most recent, most publicized, and most egregious
example in Doris Faber's *The Life of Lorena Hickok:
E. R.'s Friend,* the story of the relationship of Eleanor
Roosevelt and reporter Lorena Hickok.[3]

The Hickok book would make fascinating material for a case study of homophobia. Author Doris
Faber presents page after page of evidence that
delineates the growth and development of a love
affair between the two women, yet she steadfastly
maintains that a woman of Eleanor Roosevelt's
"stature" could not have *acted* on the love which
she expressed for Hickok. This attitude forces Faber to go to great lengths with the evidence before
her. For example, she quotes a letter Roosevelt wrote
to Hickok and asserts that it is "particularly susceptible to misinterpretation." Roosevelt's wish to "lie
down beside you tonight & take you in my arms,"
Faber claims, represents maternal—"albeit rather
extravagantly" maternal—solicitude. For Faber,
"there can be little doubt that the final sentence of
the above letter does not mean what it appears to
mean."[4]

Faber's interpretation, unfortunately, is not an
isolated one. She acknowledges an earlier "sensitive" and "fine" book, *Miss Marks and Miss Woolley,*
for reinforcing her own views "regarding the unfairness of using contemporary standards to characterize the behavior of women brought up under
almost inconceivably different standards."[5] Anna
Mary Wells, the author of the Marks and Woolley
book, set out originally to write a biography of
Mary Woolley and almost abandoned the plan when
she discovered the love letters of the two women.
Ultimately Wells went ahead with a book about the
relationship, but only after she decided, as she explains in the preface, that there was no physical
relationship between them. Comforted by this conviction, Wells paints a detailed picture of the joys

LEILA J. RUPP is Associate Professor of History and Wom-
en's Studies at Ohio State University, Columbus, Ohio.

This article originally appeared in *Frontiers: A Journal
of Women's Studies,* Volume V, No. 3 (Fall 1980), pp. 61–
70. Reprinted with permission from the author and publisher.

and sorrows of their life together, even acknowledging the role that hostility toward their relationship played in the careers of both women.

Another famous women's college president, M. Carey Thomas of Bryn Mawr, receives the same sort of treatment in a book that appeared at the same time as the Hickok book, but to less fanfare.[6] The discovery of the Woolley-Marks letters sparked a mild panic among Mount Holyoke alumnae and no doubt created apprehension about what might lurk in Thomas's papers, which were about to be microfilmed and opened to the public.[7] But Marjorie Dobkin, editor of *The Making of a Feminist: Early Journals and Letters of M. Carey Thomas*, insists that there is nothing to worry about. Thomas admittedly fell for women throughout her life. At fifteen, she wrote: "I think I must feel towards Anna for instance like a boy would, for I admire her so. Not any particular thing but just an undefined sense of admiration and then I like to touch her and the other morning I woke up and she was asleep and I admired her hair so much that I kissed it. I never felt so much with anybody else." And at twenty: "One night we had stopped reading later than usual and obeying a sudden impulse I turned to her and asked. 'Do you love me?' She threw her arms around me and whispered, 'I love you passionately.' She did not go home that night and we talked and talked." At twenty-three, Thomas wrote to her mother: "If it were only possible for women to elect women as well as men for a 'life's love!' . . . It *is* possible but if families would only regard it in that light!"[8]

Thomas did in fact choose women for her "life's loves," but Dobkin, who finds it "hard to understand why anyone should very much care" about personal and private behavior and considers the question of lesbianism "a relatively inconsequential matter," assures us that "physical contact" unquestionably played a part in Thomas's relationships with women, but "sexuality" just as unquestionably did not.[9] Along with this labored distinction between "physical contact" and "sexuality," Dobkin presents a battery of reasons why Thomas was not a lesbian: she never expressed the desire to be a man; she expressed a strong aversion to heterosexual intercourse when she learned the "facts of life" from a book at the age of twenty-one, an aversion, Dobkin insists, that would have applied even more strongly to homosexual sex; she was conventional

in everything but her feminism; she once loved a man—or was at least unable to stop thinking about him—and considered marrying him (Dobkin, with evident relief, devotes the middle section of the book to this relationship); Thomas established mother-daughter relationships with the two women with whom she lived (one moved in when the first eloped with a man); the women known at the time to be lesbians whom Thomas included among her friends traveled with her only after Thomas was already approaching old age; and, finally, Thomas expressed negative attitudes toward homosexuality, including the fear that public discussion of it would make it difficult for women who lived together. Dobkin's ignorance about lesbianism is staggering; on no other topic would a scholar so unfamiliar with the relevant literature forge ahead with the sort of assumptions she reveals.

The authors of these three books are determined to give us an "acceptable" version of women's relationships in the past, and they seize gratefully on Smith-Rosenberg's work to do it. But even Doris Faber's feverish denials could not eliminate public speculation about Eleanor Roosevelt's "sexual orientation." An article about the Hickok book was even carried in the *National Enquirer* which, for a change, probably presented the material more accurately, if more leeringly, than the respectable press.[10] Arthur Schlesinger, Jr., in the *New York Times Book Review*, for example, notes that the big question in "some people's minds" will be whether Hickok and Roosevelt were "lovers in the physical sense."[11] Schlesinger, like Dobkin, finds this an "issue of stunning inconsequence," but he "reluctantly" supposes that it must be discussed. After devoting the rest of his review to a subject he evidently finds distasteful, he cites Smith-Rosenberg's work and concludes that the two women were "children of the Victorian age" which accepted celibate love between women; they were "wounded women, doomed by chaotic childhoods to the unceasing quest for unattainable emotional security." Schlesinger is emphasizing here the incompatibility of our modern heterosexual-homosexual dichotomy with the sensibility of an earlier age. As Blanche Cook points out in her review of Faber's book, however, it is absurd to pretend that the years 1932 to 1962 now belong to the nineteenth century.[12] Although it is vitally important not to impose modern concepts and standards on the past,

I believe that we have gone entirely too far with the notion of an idyllic Victorian age in which chaste love between people of the same sex was possible and acceptable. A recent review in the *New York Times Book Review,* for example, discusses a biography of J. M. Barrie, the creator of Peter Pan, and almost congratulates Barrie for his "innocent, asexual, natural and dignified" love for the five boys who were both subjects and recipients of his stories. Despite the fact that Barrie was fond of photographing the boys, as the reviewer says, "*tout nu,* often bottoms up," he insists that there was nothing sexual about this love.[13] I think that we are naive to believe this.

It is not surprising, in light of such denials of sexuality, that many feminist scholars choose to claim as lesbians all women who have loved women in the past. Blanche Cook concludes firmly that "women who love women, who choose women to nurture and support and to create a living environment in which to work creatively and independently, are lesbians."[14] Cook names as lesbians Jane Addams, the founder of Hull House, who lived for forty years with Mary Rozet Smith; Lillian Wald, also a settlement house pioneer, who left evidence of a series of intense relationships with women; and Jeannette Marks and Mary Woolley. All, Cook says, were lesbians, and in the homophobic society in which we live must be claimed as such.

As it now stands, we are faced with a choice between, on the one hand, labeling women lesbians who might violently reject the label, or, on the other hand, glossing over the significance of women's relationships by labeling them Victorian, and therefore innocent of our post-Freudian sexual awareness. Although I understand and share the political perspective that leads Cook to claim women like Jane Addams as lesbians, I feel we need to see more precision in the use of the term. I would like to illustrate the diversity of women's relationships in the past—and complexity of those relationships—with evidence from the American women's movement in the late 1940s and 1950s.

I have found evidence of a variety of relationships in collections of women's papers and in the records of women's organizations from this period. I do not have enough information about many of these relationships to characterize them in any definitive way, nor can I even offer much information about some of the women. But we cannot afford to overlook whatever evidence women have left us, however fragmentary. I believe that it is important simply to present some of these relationships, because they illustrate the complexity of women's relationships in the past and the problems that confront us if we attempt any simple categorization. Since my research focuses on feminist activities, the women I discuss here are by no means a representative group of women. All of them are white, educated, and middle or upper class. The women's movement in the period after the Second World War was composed primarily of white, middle-class women, in part because of the racism and classism of the movement, and in part because black women and working-class women involved in social movement activity most often organized around issues of race and class, respectively, not gender.

Within the women's movement were two distinct phenomena—couple relationships and intense devotion to a charismatic leader—that help clarify the problems that face us if we attempt to define these relationships in any cut-and-dried fashion. None of the women who lived in couple relationships and belonged to the women's movement in the postwar period would, as far as can be determined, have identified themselves as lesbians. They did, however, often live together in long-term committed relationships, which were accepted in the movement, and they did sometimes build a community with other women like themselves. Descriptions of a few relationships that come down to us in the sources provide some insight into their nature.

Jeannette Marks and Mary Woolley, subjects of the biography mentioned earlier, met at Wellesley College in 1895 when Marks began her college education and Woolley arrived at the college as a history instructor. Less than five years later they made "a mutual declaration of ardent and exclusive love" and "exchanged tokens, a ring and a jeweled pin, with pledges of lifelong fidelity."[15] They spent the rest of their lives together, including the many years at Mount Holyoke where Woolley served as president and Marks taught English. Mary Woolley worked in the American Association of University Women and the Women's International League for Peace and Freedom. Jeannette Marks committed herself to suffrage and, later, through the National Woman's Party, to the Equal Rights Amendment. It is clear from Marks's correspondence with women in the movement that their relationship was accepted as a primary commitment. Few letters to Marks in the 1940s fail to inquire about Woolley, whose serious illness clouded Marks's life and work. One married woman, who found herself forced to withdraw from Woman's Party work because of her husband's health, acknowledged in a letter to Marks the centrality of Marks's and Woolley's commitment when she compared her own reasons for "pulling out" to "those that have bound you to Westport," the town in which the two women lived.[16] Mary Woolley died in 1947, and Jeannette Marks lived on until 1964, devoting herself to a biography of Woolley.

Lena Madesin Phillips, the founder of both the National and International Federations of Business and Professional Women's Clubs, lived for some thirty years with Marjory Lacey-Baker, an actress whom she first met in 1919. In an unpublished autobiography included in Phillips's papers, she straightforwardly wrote about her lack of interest in men and marriage. As a young girl, she wrote that she "cared little for boys," and at the age of seven she wrote a composition for school that explained: "There are so many little girls in the school and the thing i like about it there are no boys in school. i like that about it."[17] She noted that she had never taken seriously the idea of getting married. "Only the first of the half dozen proposals of marriage which came my way had any sense of reality to me. They made no impression because I was wholly without desire or even interest in the matter." Phillips seemed unperturbed by possible Freudian and/or homophobic explanations of her attitudes and behavior. She explained unabashedly that she wanted to be a boy and suffered severe disappointment when she learned that, contrary to her father's stories, there was no factory in Indiana that made girls into boys—and seemed impervious as well to the charges of lesbianism that her memories might provoke. She mentioned in her autobiography the "crushes" she had on girls at the Jessamine Female Institute—nothing out of the ordinary for a young woman of her generation, but perhaps a surprising piece of information chosen for inclusion in the autobiography of a woman who continued to devote her emotional energies to women.

In 1919, Phillips attended a pageant in which Lacey-Baker performed, and she inquired about the identity of the woman who had "[t]he most beautiful voice I ever heard."[18] Phillips "lost her heart to the sound of that voice," and the two women moved in together in the 1920s. In 1924, according to notes that Lacey-Baker recorded for a biography of Phillips, the two women went different places for Easter; recording this caused Lacey-Baker to quote from *The Prophet*: "Love knows not its own depth until the hour of separation."[19] Phillips described Lacey-Baker in her voluminous correspondence as "my best friend," or noted that she "shares a home with me."[20] Phillips's friends and acquaintances regularly mentioned Lacey-Baker. One male correspondent, for example, commented that Phillips's "lady-friend" was "so lovely, and so devoted to you and cares for you."[21] Phillips happily described the tranquility of their life together to her many friends: "Marjory and I have had a lovely time, enjoying once more our home in summertime. . . . Marjory would join in the invitation of this letter and this loving greeting if she were around. Today she is busy with the cleaning woman, while I sit with the door closed working in my study."[22] "We have had a happy winter, with good health for both of us. We have a variety of interests and small obligations, but really enjoy most the quiet and comfort of Apple Acres."[23] "We read and talk and work."[24]

Madesin Phillips's papers suggest that she and Marjory Lacey-Baker lived in a world of politically active women friends. Phillips had devoted much of her energy to international work with women, and she kept in touch with European friends through her correspondence and through her regular trips to Europe accompanied by Lacey-Baker. Gordon Holmes, of the British Federation of Business and Professional Women, wrote regularly to "Madesin and Maggie." In a 1948 letter she teased Phillips by reporting that "two other of our oldest & closest Fed officers whom you know could get married but are refusing—as they are both more than middle-aged (never mind their looks) it suggests 50–60 is about the new dangerous age for women (look out for Maggie!)."[25] Phillips reported to Holmes on their social life: "With a new circle of friends around us here and a good many of our overseas members coming here for luncheon or tea with us the weeks slip by."[26] The integral relationship between Phillips's social life and her work in the movement is suggested by Lacey-Baker's analysis of Phillips's personal papers from the year 1924: "There is the usual crop of letters to LMP following the Convention [of the BPW] from newly-met members in hero-worshipping mood—most of whom went on to be her good friends over the years."[27] Lacey-Baker was a part of Phillips's movement world, and their relationship received acceptance and validation throughout the movement, both national and international.

The lifelong relationship between feminist biographer Alma Lutz and Marguerite Smith began when they roomed together at Vassar in the early years of the twentieth century. From 1918 until Smith's death in 1959, they shared a Boston apartment and a summer home, Highmeadow, in the Berkshires. Lutz and Smith, a librarian at the Protestant Zion Research Library in Brookline, Massachusetts, worked together in the National Woman's Party. Like Madesin Phillips, Lutz wrote to friends in the movement of their lives together: "We are very happy here in the country—each busy with her work and digging in the garden."[28] They traveled together, visiting Europe several times in the 1950s. Letters to one of them about feminist work invariably included greetings or love to the other. When Smith died in 1959, Lutz struggled with her grief. She wrote to her acquaintance Florence Kitchelt, in response to condolences: "I am at Highmeadow trying to get my bearings. . . . You will understand how hard it is. . . . It has been a very difficult anxious time for me."[29] She thanked another friend for her note and added: "It's a hard adjustment to make, but one we all have to face in one way or another and I am remembering that I have much to be grateful for."[30] In December she wrote to one of her regular correspondents that she was carrying on but it was very lonely for her.[31]

The fact that Lutz and Smith seemed to have many friends who lived in couple relationships with other women suggests that they had built a community of women within the women's movement. Every year Mabel Vernon, a suffragist and worker for peace, and her friend and companion, Consuelo Reyes, whom Vernon had met through her work with the Inter-American Commission on Women, spent the summer at Highmeadow. Vernon, one of Alice Paul's closest associates during the suffrage struggle, had met Reyes two weeks after her arrival in the United States from Costa Rica in 1942. They began to work together in Ver-

non's organization, People's Mandate, in 1943, and they shared a Washington apartment from 1951 until Vernon's death in 1975.[32] Reyes received recognition in Vernon's obituaries as her "devoted companion" or "nurse-companion."[33] Two other women who also maintained a lifelong relationship, Alice Morgan Wright and Edith Goode, also kept in contact with Lutz, Smith, Vernon, and Reyes. Sometimes they visited Highmeadow in the summer.[34] Wright and Goode had met at Smith and were described as "always together" although they did not live together.[35] Like Lutz and Smith, they worked together in the National Woman's Party, traveled together, and looked after each other as old age began to take its toll.[36]

These examples illustrate what the sources provide: the bare outlines of friendship networks made up of woman-committed women. Much of the evidence must be pieced together, and it is even scantier when the women did not live together. Alma Lutz's papers, for example, do not include any personal correspondence from the postwar period, so what we know about her relationship with Marguerite Smith comes from the papers of her correspondents. Sometimes a relationship surfaces only upon the death of one of the women. For example, Agnes Wells, chairman of the National Woman's Party in the late 1940s, explained to an acquaintance in the party that her "friend of forty-one years and house-companion for twenty-eight years" had just died.[37] When Mabel Griswold, executive secretary of the Woman's Party, died in 1955, a family member suggested that the party send the telegram of sympathy to Elsie Wood, the woman with whom Griswold had lived.[38] This kind of reference tells us little about the nature of the relationship involved, but we do get a sense of the nature of couple relationships within the women's movement.

A second important phenomenon found in the women's movement—the charismatic leader who attracts intense devotion—also adds to our understanding of the complexity of women's relationships. Alice Paul, the founder and leading light of the National Woman's Party, inspired devotion that bordered on worship. One woman even addressed her as "My Beloved Deity."[39] But, contrary to both the ideal type of the charismatic leader and the portrait of Paul as it exists now in the historical scholarship, Paul maintained close relationships with a number of women she had first met in the suffrage struggle.[40] Paul's correspondence in the National Woman's Party papers does not reveal much about the nature of her relationships, but it does make it clear that her friendships provided love and support for her work.

It is true that many of the expressions of love, admiration, and devotion addressed to Paul seem to have been one-sided, from awestruck followers, but this is not the only side of the story.

Paul maintained close friendships with a number of women discussed earlier who lived in couple relationships with other women. She had met Mabel Vernon when they attended Swarthmore College together, and they maintained contact throughout the years, despite Vernon's departure from the Woman's Party in the 1930s.[41] Of Alice Morgan Wright, she said that, when they first met, they "just became sisters right away."[42] Jeannette Marks regularly sent her love to "dear Alice" until a conflict in the Woman's Party ruptured their relationship.[43] Other women, too, enjoyed a closer relationship than the formal work-related one for which Paul is so well known.

Paul obviously cared deeply, for example, for her old friend Nina Allender, the cartoonist of the suffrage movement. Allender, who lived alone in Chicago, wrote to Paul in 1947 of her memories of their long association: "No words can tell you what that [first] visit grew to mean to me & to my life. . . . I feel now as I did then—only more intensely—I have never changed or doubted—but have grown more inspired as the years have gone by. . . . There is no use going into words. I believe them to be unnecessary between us."[44] Paul wrote that she thought of Allender often and sent her "devoted love."[45] She worried about Allender's loneliness and gently encouraged her to come to Washington to live at Belmont House, the Woman's Party headquarters, where she would be surrounded by loving friends who appreciated the work she had done for the women's movement.[46] Paul failed to persuade her to move, however. Two years later Paul responded to a request from Allender's niece for help with the costs of a nursing home with a $100 check and a promise to contact others who might be able to help.[47] But Allender died, within a month, at the age of eighty-five.

Paul does not seem to have formed an intimate relationship with any one woman, but she did live and work within a close-knit female world. When in Washington, she lived, at least some of the time, at Belmont House; when away she lived either alone or with her sister, Helen Paul, in Vermont and later Connecticut. Helen Paul, through her relationship with Alice, often played a major role in Woman's Party work. It is clear that Alice Paul's ties—whether to her sister or to close friends or to admirers—served as a bond that knit the Woman's Party together. That Paul and her network could also tear the movement asunder is obvious from the stormy history of the Woman's Party.

Alice Paul is not the only example of a leader who inspired love and devotion among women in the movement. One senses from Marjory Lacey-Baker's comment, quoted above—that "newly-met members in hero-worshipping mood" wrote to Lena Madesin Phillips after every BPW convention—that Phillips too had a charismatic aura. But the best and most thoroughly documented example of a charismatic leader is Anna Lord Strauss of the League of Women Voters, an organization that opted out of the women's movement.

Strauss, the great-granddaughter of Lucretia Mott, came from an old and wealthy family; she was prominent and respected, a staunch liberal and an anti- or at best a nonfeminist. She never married and her papers leave no evidence of intimate relationships outside her family. Yet Strauss was the object of some very strong feelings on the part of the women with whom she worked. She, like Alice Paul and Madesin Phillips, received numerous hero-worshiping letters from awestruck followers. But in her case we also have evidence that some of her co-workers fell deeply in love with her. It is hard to know how the following women would have interpreted their relationship with Strauss. The two women who expressed their feelings explicitly were both married women, and in one case Strauss obviously had a cordial relationship with the woman's husband and children. Yet there can be no question that this League officer fell in love with Strauss. She found Strauss "the finest human being I had ever known," and knowing her "the most beautiful and profound experience I have ever had."[48] Loving Strauss—she asked permission to say it—made the earth move and "the whole landscape of human affairs and nature" take on a new appearance.[49] Being with Strauss made "the tone and fiber" of her day different; although she could live without her, she could see no reason for having to prove it all the time.[50] She tried to "ration and control" her thoughts of Strauss, but it was small satisfaction.[51] When Strauss was recovering from an operation, this woman wrote: "I love you! I can't imagine the world without you. . . . I love you. I need you."[52]

Although our picture of this relationship is completely one-sided—for Strauss did not keep copies of most of her letters—it is clear that Strauss did not respond to such declarations of love. This woman urged Strauss to accept her and what she had to say without "the slightest sense of needing to be considerate of me because I feel as I do." She understood the "unilateral character" of her feelings, and insisted that she had more than she deserved by simply knowing Strauss at all.[53] But her hurt, and her growing suspicion that Strauss shunned intimacy, escaped on occasion. She asked: "And how would it hurt you to let someone tell you sometime how beautiful—how wonderful you are? Did you ever let anyone have a decent chance to try?"[54] She realized that loving someone did not always make things easier—that sometimes, in fact, it made life more of a struggle—but she believed that to withdraw from love was to withdraw from life. In what appears to have been a hastily written note, she expressed her understanding—an understanding that obviously gave her both pain and comfort—that Strauss was not perfect after all: "Way back there in the crow's nest (or at some such time) you decided not to become embroiled in any intimate human relationship, except those you were, by birth, committed to. I wonder. . . . There is something you haven't mastered. Something you've been afraid of after all."[55]

This woman's perception that Strauss avoided intimacy is confirmed elsewhere in Strauss's papers. One old friend was struck, in 1968, by Strauss's ability to "get your feelings out & down on paper!" She continued:"I know you so well that I consider this great progress in your own inner state of mental health. It is far from easy for you to express your feelings. . . ."[56] This aspect of Strauss's personality fits with the ideal type of the charismatic leader. The other case of a woman's falling in love with Strauss that emerges clearly from her papers reinforces this picture. This woman, also a League officer, wrote in circuitous fashion of her intense pleasure at receiving Strauss's picture. In what was

certainly a reference to lesbianism, she wrote that she hoped Strauss would not think that she was "one of those who had never outgrown the emotional extravaganzas of the adolescent." Before she got down to League business, she added:

> But, Darling, as I softly close the door on all this—as I should and as I want to—and as I must since all our meetings are likely to be formal ones in a group—as I go back in the office correspondence to "Dear Miss Strauss" and "Sincerely yours," . . . as I put myself as much as possible in the background at our March meeting in order to share you with the others who have not been with you as I have—as all these things happen, I want you to be very certain that what is merely under cover is still there—as it most surely will be— and that if all the hearts in the room could be exposed there'd be few, I'm certain, that would love you more than. . .[I].[57]

Apparently Strauss never responded to this letter, for a month later, this woman apologized for writing it: "I have had qualms, dear Anna, about that letter I wrote you. (You knew I would eventually of course!)." Continuing in a vein that reinforces the above-quoted perception of Strauss's inability to be intimate, she wrote of imagining the "recoil . . . embarrassment, self-consciousness and general discomfort" her letter must have provoked in such a "reserved person." She admitted that the kind of admiration she had expressed, "at least in certain classes of relationships (of which mine to you is one)—becomes a bit of moral wrong-doing."[58] She felt ashamed and asked forgiveness. It is not at all clear what she meant by all of this, and I quote it here without speculating on the nature of their relationship.

What is clear is that this was a momentous and significant relationship to at least one of the parties. Almost twenty years later, this woman wrote of her deep disappointment in missing Strauss's visit to her city. She had allowed herself to dream that she could persuade Strauss to stay with her awhile, even though she knew that others would have prior claims on Strauss's time. She wrote:

> I have not seen you since that day in Atlantic City when you laid the gavel of the League of Women Voters down. . . . I do not look

back on that moment of ending with any satisfaction for my own behavior, for I passed right by the platform on which you were still standing talking with one of the last persons left in the room and shyness at the thought of expressing my deep feeling about your going—*and* the fact that you were talking with someone else led me to pass on without even a glance in your direction as I remember though you made some move to speak to me!. . . . But if I gave you a hurt it is now a very old one and forgotten, I'm sure—as well as understood.[59]

Whatever the interpretation these two women would have devised to explain their feelings for Strauss, it is clear that the widely shared devotion to this woman leader could sometimes grow into something more intense. Strauss's reserve and her inability to express her feelings may or may not have had anything to do with her own attitude toward intimate relationships between women. One tantalizing letter from a friend about to be married suggests that Strauss's decision not to marry had been made early: "I remember so well your answer when I pressed you, once, on why you had never married. . . . Well, it is very true, one does not marry unless one can see no other life."[60] A further fragment, consisting of entries in the diary of Doris Stevens—a leading suffragist who took a sharp swing to the right in the postwar period—suggests that at least some individuals suspected Strauss of lesbianism. Stevens, by this time a serious red-baiter and, from the evidence quoted here, a "queer-baiter" as well, apparently called a government official in 1953 to report that Strauss was "not a bit interested in men."[61] She seemed to be trying to discredit Strauss, far too liberal for her tastes, with a charge of "unorthodox morals."[62]

Stevens had her suspicions about other women in the movement as well. She recorded in her diary a conversation with a National Woman's Party member about Jeannette Marks and Mary Woolley, noting that the member, who had attended Wellesley with Marks, "Discreetly indicated there was 'talk.'"[63] At another point she reported a conversation with a different Woman's Party member who had grown disillusioned about Alice Paul. Stevens noted that her informant related "weird goings on at Wash. hedquts wherein it was clear she thought

Paul a devotee of Lesbos & afflicted with Jeanne d'Arc identification."[64]

Stevens's charges suggest that the intensity of women's relationships and the existence of woman-committed women in women's organizations had the potential, particularly during the McCarthy years, to attract ridicule or denunciation. Stevens wrote to the viciously right-wing and anti-Semitic columnist Westbrook Pegler to "thank you for knowing I'm not a queerie."[65] This would suggest that, at least in certain circles, participation in the women's movement was highly suspect.

What exactly should we make of all this? In one way it is terribly frustrating to have such tantalizingly ambiguous glimpses into women's lives. In another way, it is exciting to find out so much about women's lives in the past. I think it is enormously important *not* to read into these letters what we want to find, or what we think we should find. At the same time, we cannot dismiss what little evidence we have as insufficient when it is all we have; nor can we continue to contribute to the conspiracy of silence that urges us to ignore what is not perfectly straightforward. Thus, although it is tempting to try to speculate about the relationships I have described here in order to impose some analysis on them, I would rather simply lay them out, fragmentary as they are, in order to suggest a conceptual approach that recognizes the complexities of the issue.

It is clear, I think, that none of these relationships can be easily categorized. There were women who lived their entire adult lives in couple relationships with other women, and married women who fell in love with other women. Were they lesbians? Probably they would be shocked to be identified in that way. Alice Paul, for example, spoke scornfully of *Ms.* magazine as "all about homosexuality and so on."[66] Another woman who lives in a couple relationship distinguished between the (respectable) women involved in the ERA struggle in the old days and the "lesbians and bra-burners" of the contemporary movement.[67] Sasha Lewis, in *Sunday's Women*, reports an incident we would do well to remember here. One of her informants, a lesbian, went to Florida to work against Anita Bryant and stayed with an older cousin who had lived for years in a marriagelike relationship with another woman. When Lewis's informant saw the way the two women lived—sharing everything, including a bedroom—she said something to them about the danger of Bryant's campaign for their lives. They were aghast that she would think them lesbians, since, they said, they did not do anything sexual together.[68] If even women who lived with or maintained close attachments to other women would reject the label "lesbian," what about the married women, or the women who avoided intimate relationships?

The fact that the three recent historical studies discussed here misuse the concept of women's culture to proclaim that their subjects did not have sexual relationships with other women makes it imperative that historians pull back the veil that has too often shrouded love between women in the past. But it is equally important that we not obscure the enormous significance, from both an individual and historical perspective, of the formation of a lesbian identity. Recent research on the history of homosexuality shows that the concept of a homosexual identity or role emerged only in relatively recent times.[69] Paradoxically, as Smith-Rosenberg points out, the nineteenth century permitted a great deal of freedom in moving along the sexual and emotional continuum that ranges from heterosexuality to homosexuality. The twentieth century has not. What is important here is that we can begin to speak of a "lesbian identity" in American society by the twentieth century.[70] Passionate love between women has always existed, but it has not always been named. Since it *has* been named in the twentieth century, we need to distinguish between women who identify as lesbians and/or who are part of a lesbian culture, where one exists, and a broader category of woman-committed women who would not identify as lesbians but whose primary commitment, in emotional and practical terms, was to other women. It is especially important, in considering twentieth-century women, that we not sloppily apply the label "Victorian." In the 1950s there *was* such a thing as a lesbian culture— in local communities, in the bars, in the military. There is an important difference between women who put themselves in such a culture on the very fringes of society and women like Eleanor Roosevelt and the women whose relationships I have described here. Similarly, there is an important difference today between a politically active lesbian feminist and a "maiden aunt" who has lived her entire life with another woman but would reject any suggestions of lesbianism.

Identity, and not sexual behavior, is the crucial factor in the discussion.[71] There are lesbians who have never had a sexual relationship with another woman, and there are women who have had sexual experiences with women but do not identify as lesbians. This is not to suggest that there is no difference between women who loved each other and lived together but did not make love (although even that can be difficult to define, since sensuality and sexuality, "physical contact" and "sexual contact," have no distinct boundaries) and those who did. But sexual behavior—something about which we rarely have historical evidence anyway—is only one of a number of relevant factors in a relationship. Blanche Cook has said everything that needs to be said about the inevitable question of evidence: "Genital 'proofs' to confirm lesbianism are never required to confirm the heterosexuality of men and women who live together for 20, or 50, years." Cook reminds us of the recently publicized relationship of General Eisenhower and Kay Summersby during the Second World War: they "were passionately involved with each other. They looked ardently into each others' eyes. They held hands. They cantered swiftly across England's countryside. They played golf and bridge and laughed. They were inseparable. But they never 'consummated' their love in the acceptable, traditional, sexual manner. Now does that fact render Kay Summersby and Dwight David Eisenhower somehow less in love? Were they not heterosexual?"[72]

Of course, emphasizing identity rather than proof of genital contact does not make everything simple. At this point, I think, the best we can do is to describe carefully and sensitively what we do know about a woman's relationships, keeping in mind both the historical development of a lesbian identity (Did such a thing as a lesbian identity exist? Was there a lesbian culture?), and the individual process that we now identify as "coming out" (Did a woman feel attachment to another woman or women? Did she act on this feeling in some positive way? Did she recognize the existence of other women with the same commitment? Did she express solidarity with those women?).[73] Using this approach allows us to make distinctions among women's relationships in the past—intimate friendships, supportive relationships growing out of common political work, couple relationships—without denying their significance or drawing fixed boundaries. We can recognize the importance of friendships among a group of women who, like Alma Lutz, Marguerite Smith, Mabel Vernon, Consuelo Reyes, Alice Morgan Wright, and Edith Goode, built a community of women but did not identify it as a lesbian community. We can do justice to both the woman-committed woman who would angrily reject any suggestion of lesbianism and the self-identified lesbian without distorting their common experiences.

This approach does not solve all the problems of dealing with women's relationships in the past, but it is a beginning. The greatest problem remains the weakness of sources. Not only have women who loved women in the past been wisely reluctant to leave evidence of their relationships for the prying eyes of a homophobic society, but what evidence they did leave was often suppressed or destroyed.[74] Furthermore, as the three books discussed above show, even the evidence saved and brought to light can be savagely misinterpreted.

How do we know if a woman felt attachment, acted on it, recognized the existence of other women like her, or expressed solidarity? There is no easy answer to this, but it is revealing, I think, that both Doris Faber and Anna Mary Wells are fairly certain that Lorena Hickok and Jeannette Marks, respectively, *did* have "homosexual tendencies" (although Faber insists that even Hickok cannot fairly be placed in the "contemporary gay category"), even if the admirable figures in each book, Eleanor Roosevelt and Mary Woolley, certainly did not. That is, both of these authors, as hard as they try to deny lesbianism, find evidence that forces them to discuss it, and both cope by pinning the "blame" on the women they paint as unpleasant—fat, ugly, pathetic Lorena Hickok and nasty, tortured, arrogant Jeannette Marks.

And, of course, despite censorship, we do know about women in the past who acted on their feelings for other women and who created lesbian communities. Consider the French lesbian culture of the late-nineteenth–early-twentieth century, the

world depicted in Radclyffe Hall's *The Well of Loneliness*.[75] And we are beginning to learn more about working-class and middle-class lesbian communities in the 1950s as well—in the closet, in the bars, and in the military.[76]

Using this approach, then, allows us to make distinctions among different sorts of women's relationships in the past without denying their significance or assigning fixed categories. Returning to the relationships described in this paper, we can differentiate between the intimate and supportive friendships, the couple relationships with other women that some women formed, and the feelings of falling in love that others expressed. I think it is important to state here that these relationships, whatever their nature, are not simply a side issue for the history of feminism and the women's movement. Blanche Cook has argued that the existence of female support networks has been vital to women's political activism; Smith-Rosenberg and others have shown how nineteenth-century "women's culture" both led to, and ultimately limited, organizing and public activity among middle-class women.[77] I believe that women's relationships have been absolutely central to the success of feminist activity throughout history. Woman-committed women have had the emotional commitment, the support, and often the time to devote their lives to a cause, as did many of the women I have discussed.

It is important that nineteenth-century American women sought and found emotional support in a homosocial world. It is also important that throughout history there have been women who chose other women for the primary relationship in their lives. It is important that some of these women would have been shocked to be labeled lesbians, and it is important that some of them claimed their lesbianism and built a culture and community around it with other lesbians. It is imperative that we not deny the reality of any of these women's historical experiences by blurring the distinctions among them. At the same time, recognition of the common bond of commitment to women shared by diverse women throughout history strengthens our struggle against those who attempt to divide and defeat us.

NOTES

Holly Near's song "Imagine My Surprise" celebrates the discovery of women's relationships in the past. The song is recorded on the album *Imagine My Surprise*, Redwood Records. I am grateful to Holly Near and Redwood Records for their permission to use the title here.

1 Carroll Smith-Rosenberg, "The female world of love and ritual: relations between women in nineteenth-century America," in this volume, 70–89.

2 Nancy F. Cott, *The Bonds of Womanhood* (New Haven: Yale University Press, 1977), chap. 5; Nancy Sahli, "Smashing: women's relationships before the Fall," *Chrysalis*, 1979, *no. 8:* 17–27; Blanche Wiesen Cook, "Female support networks and political activism: Lillian Wald, Crystal Eastman and Emma Goldman," *Chrysalis*, 1977, *no. 3:* 43–61; and Blanche W. Cook, "The historical denial of lesbianism," *Radical History Review*, 1979, *20:* 60–65. See especially the Lesbian History issue of *Frontiers*, vol. 4, no. 3 (Fall 1979); see also, Judith Schwarz, "*Yellow Clover:* Katharine Lee Bates and Katharine Coman," *Frontiers*, vol. 4 no. 1 (Spring 1979), 59–67.

3 Doris Faber, *The Life of Lorena Hickok: E. R.'s Friend* (New York: William Morrow and Co., 1980).

4 Faber, *Lorena Hickok*, 176.

5 Anna Mary Wells, *Miss Marks and Miss Woolley* (Boston: Houghton Mifflin, 1978); Faber, *Lorena Hickok*, 354. Cook, "Historical denial," is a review of the Wells book.

6 Marjorie Housepian Dobkin, *The Making of a Feminist: Early Journals and Letters of M. Carey Thomas* (Kent, Ohio: Kent State University Press, 1980). See the review by Helen Vendler, "Carey Thomas of Bryn Mawr," *New York Times Book Review*, February 24, 1980, 24–25. Vendler accuses Dobkin of psychological naiveté in her portrait of Thomas.

7 *New York Times*, August 21, 1976, 22.

8 Dobkin, *Making of a Feminist*, 72, 118, 229.

9 Ibid., 79, 86.

10 Edward Sigall, "Eleanor Roosevelt's secret romance—the untold story," *National Enquirer*, November 13, 1979, 20–21.

11 Arthur Schlesinger, Jr., "Interesting women," *New York Times Book Review*, February 17, 1980, 31.

12 Blanche Wiesen Cook, review of *The Life of Lorena Hickok*, *Feminist Studies*, 1980, *6:* 511–16.

13 Morton N. Cohen, "Love story, Victorian-style" (review of Andrew Birkin's *J. M. Barrie and the Lost Boys*), *New York Times Book Review*, January 13, 1980, 3.

14 Cook, "Female support networks," 48.

15 Wells, *Miss Marks*, 56.

16 Caroline Babcock to Jeannette Marks, February 12, 1947, Babcock Papers, Box 8(105), Schlesinger Library, Radcliffe College, Cambridge, Massachusetts. I am grateful to the Schlesinger Library for permission to use the material quoted here.

17 "The unfinished autobiography of Lena Madesin Phillips," Phillips Papers, Schlesinger Library.

18 "Chronological record of events and activities for the biography of Lena Madesin Phillips, 1881–1955," Phillips Papers.

19 Ibid.

20 Lena Madesin Phillips to Audrey Turner, January 21, 1948, Phillips Papers, Schlesinger Library; Lena Madesin Phillips to Olivia Rossetti Agresti, April 26, 1948, Phillips Papers.

21 Robert Heller to Lena Madesin Phillips, September 26, 1948, Phillips Papers.

22 Lena Madesin Phillips to Mary C. Kennedy, August 20, 1948, Phillips Papers.

23 Lena Madesin Phillips to Gordon Holmes, March 28, 1949, Phillips Papers.

24 Lena Madesin Phillips to [Ida Spitz], November 13, 1950, Phillips Papers.

25 Gordon Holmes to Madesin & Maggie, December 15, 1948, Phillips Papers.

26 Lena Madesin Phillips to Gordon Holmes, March 28, 1949, Phillips Papers.

27 "Chronological record of events and activities for the biography of Lena Madesin Phillips, 1881–1955," Phillips Papers.

28 Alma Lutz to Florence Kitchelt, July 1, 1948, Kitchelt Papers, Box 6 (177), Schlesinger Library.

29 Alma Lutz to Florence Kitchelt, July 29, 1959, Kitchelt Papers, Box 7 (178).

30 Alma Lutz to Florence Armstrong, August 26, 1959, Armstrong Papers, Box 1 (17), Schlesinger Library.

31 Alma Lutz to Rose Arnold Powell, December 14, 1959, Powell Papers, Box 3 (43), Schlesinger Library.

32 Mabel Vernon, "Speaker for suffrage and petitioner for peace," an oral history conducted in 1972 and 1973 by Amelia R. Fry, Regional Oral History Office, University of California, 1976.

33 Press release from Mabel Vernon Memorial Committee, in Vernon, "Speaker for suffrage"; obituary in the *Wilmington Morning News*, September 3, 1975, in Vernon, "Speaker for suffrage."

34 Alice Morgan Wright to Anita Pollitzer, July 9, 1946, National Woman's Party Papers, Reel 89. The National Woman's Party papers have been microfilmed and are distributed by the Microfilming

Corporation of America. I am grateful to the National Woman's Party for permission to quote the material used here.

35 Alice Paul, "Conversations with Alice Paul: woman suffrage and the Equal Rights Amendmet," an oral history conducted in 1972 and 1973 by Amelia R. Fry, Regional Oral History Office, University of California, 1976, 614. Courtesy, the Bancroft Library. Nora Stanton Barney to Alice Paul, n.d. (received May 10, 1945), National Woman's Party Papers, Reel 86.

36 Alice Morgan Wright to Caroline Babcock, June 28, 1945, National Woman's Party Papers, Reel 86; Edith Goode to Caroline Babcock, July 10, 1946, Babcock Papers, Box 7 (98), Schlesinger Library; Edith Goode to Emma Guffey Miller, December 23, 1963, National Woman's Party Papers, Reel 108; Edith Goode to Jacques Sichel, March 22, 1967, National Woman's Party Papers, Reel 110; Paul, "Conversations," 614.

37 Agnes Wells to Anita Pollitzer, August 24, 1946, National Woman's Party Papers, Reel 89.

38 Alice Paul to Dorothy Griswold, February 2, 1955, National Woman's Party Papers, Reel 101.

39 Lavinia Dock to Alice Paul, May 9, 1945, National Woman's Party Papers, Reel 86.

40 See, for example, Susan D. Becker, "An intellectual history of the National Woman's Party, 1920–1941," Phd. diss., Case Western Reserve University, 1975.

41 Vernon, "Speaker for suffrage."

42 Paul, "Conversation," 197.

43 Jeannette Marks to Alice Paul, March 25, 1945, National Woman's Party Papers, Reel 85; Jeannette Marks to Alice Paul, March 30, 1945, National Woman's Party Papers, Reel 85; Jeannette Marks to Alice Paul, April 27, 1945, National Woman's Party Papers, Reel 85.

44 Nina Allender to Alice Paul, January 5, 1947, National Woman's Party Papers, Reel 90.

45 Alice Paul to Nina Allender, March 9, 1950, National Woman's Party Papers, Reel 96.

46 Alice Paul to Nina Allender, November 20, 1954, National Woman's Party Papers, Reel 100; Kay Boyle to Alice Paul, December 5, 1954, National Woman's Party Papers, Reel 100; Alice Paul to Nina Allender, December 6, 1954, National Woman's Party Papers, Reel 100.

47 Kay Boyle to Alice Paul, February 13, 1957, National Woman's Party Papers, Reel 103; Alice Paul to Kay Boyle, March 5, 1957, National Woman's Party Papers, Reel 103.

48 Letter to Anna Lord Strauss, December 22, 1945, Strauss Papers, Box 6 (118), Schlesinger Library. Because of the possibly sensitive nature of the material reported here, I am not using the names of the women involved.

49 Letter to Anna Strauss, September 19, 1946, Strauss Papers, Box 6 (119), Schlesinger Library.

50 Letter to Anna Lord Strauss, May 9, 1947, Strauss Papers, Box 6 (121).

51 Letter to Anna Lord Strauss, June 28, 1948, Strauss Papers, Box 6 (124).

52 Letter to Anna Lord Strauss, February 26, 1951, Strauss Papers, Box 1 (15).

53 Letter to Anna Lord Strauss, December 22, 1945, Strauss Papers, Box 6 (118).

54 Letter to Anna Lord Strauss, May 9, 1947, Strauss Papers, Box 6 (121).

55 "Stream of consciousness," March 10, 1948, Strauss Papers, Box 6 (124).

56 Augusta Street to Anna Lord Strauss, n.d. [1968], Strauss Papers, Box 7 (135).

57 Letter to Anna Lord Strauss, February 11, 1949, Strauss Papers, Box 6 (125).

58 Letter to Anna Lord Strauss, March 3, 1949, Strauss Papers, Box 6 (125).

59 Letter to Anna Lord Strauss, March 8, 1968, Strauss Papers, Box 7 (135).

60 Lilian Lyndon to Anna Lord Strauss, April 23, 1950, Strauss Papers, Box 1 (14).

61 Diary entries, August 30, 1953 and September 1, 1953, Doris Stevens Papers, Schlesinger Library.

62 Diary entry, August 24, 1953, Doris Stevens Papers.

63 Diary entry, February 4, 1946, Doris Stevens Papers.

64 Diary entry, December 1, 1945, Doris Stevens Papers.

65 Doris Stevens to Westbrook Pegler, May 3, 1946, Stevens Papers.

66 Paul, "Conversations," 195–96.

67 Interview conducted by Verta Taylor and Leila Rupp, December 10, 1979.

68 Sasha Gregory Lewis, *Sunday's Women: A Report on Lesbian Life Today* (Boston: Beacon Press, 1979), 94.

69 Mary McIntosh, "The homosexual role," *Social Problems*, 1968, *16, no. 2:* 182–91; Jeffrey Weeks, *Coming Out: Homosexual Politics in Britain, from the Nineteenth Century to the Present* (London: Quartet Books, 1977); Bert Hansen, "The historical construction of homosexuality," *Radical History Review,* 1979, *20:* 66–73.

70 See Vern Bullough and Bonnie Bullough, "Lesbianism in the 1920s and 1930s: a newfound study," *Signs,* 1977, *2, no. 4:* 895–904; Lewis, *Sunday's Women;* and Madeline Davis, Liz Kennedy, and Avra Michelson, "Aspects of the Buffalo lesbian community in the fifties," Buffalo Women's Oral History Project, paper presented at the National Women's Studies

Association Conference, Bloomington, Indiana, May 1980. Local research projects are beginning to explore the history of gay and lesbian culture in the pre-gay liberation and women's movement years in a number of cities in addition to Buffalo. Such projects currently exist in Boston, Chicago, New York, Philadelphia, and San Francisco.

71 Much of the recent literature on lesbianism emphasizes this crucial distinction between identity and experience. See, for example, Barbara Ponse, *Identities in the Lesbian World: The Social Construction of Self* (Westport, Conn.: Greenwood Press, 1978); and E. M. Ettore, *Lesbians, Women and Society* (London: Routledge & Kegan Paul, 1980).

72 Cook, "Historical denial," 64.

73 On coming out as a process, see Ponse, *Identities;* Ettore, *Lesbians;* Julia Penelope Stanley and Susan J. Wolfe, *The Coming Out Stories* (Watertown, Mass.: Persephone Press, 1980); and Margaret Cruikshank, *The Lesbian Path* (Monterey, Ca.: Angel Press, 1980).

74 The Mount Holyoke administration closed the Marks-Woolley papers when Wells discovered the love letters, and the papers are open to researchers now only because an American Historical Association committee, including Blanche Cook as one of its members, applied pressure to keep the papers open after Wells, to her credit, contacted them. Faber describes her unsuccessful attempts to persuade the archivists at the FDR Library to close the Lorena Hickok papers.

75 See Dolores Klaich, *Woman + Woman* (1974; rpt. New York: Morrow-Quill, 1979), 129–215; and Barbara Grier and Coletta Reid, *Lesbian Lives: Biographies of Women from the Ladder* (Baltimore: Diana Press, 1976).

76 Lewis, *Sunday's Women;* Davis, Kennedy, and Michelson, "Buffalo lesbian community."

77 Cook, "Female support networks"; Smith-Rosenberg, "Female world"; Cott, *Bonds of Womanhood;* Mary P. Ryan, "The power of women's networks: a case study of female moral reform in antebellum America," *Feminist Studies,* 1979, *5:* 66–85; Carroll Smith-Rosenberg, "Beauty, the Beast and the militant woman: a case study of sex roles and social stress in Jacksonian America," *American Quarterly,* 1971, *23,* no. *4:* 562–84. See Ellen DuBois et al., "Politics and culture in women's history," *Feminist Studies,* 1980, *6:* 26–64.

BIRTH CONTROL

Women have tried to limit the number of their offspring, using different methods and with varying intensity and success, throughout history. The historians in this section, all of whom have written books on the subject, examine three parts of the American response. Linda Gordon analyzes a nineteenth-century feminist movement that aimed to increase women's control over their bodies through sexual restraint. James Mohr reviews the increasing use of abortion in the nineteenth century, first mostly by unmarried and poor women and then also by the more affluent and frequently married women, and the medical profession's response to these trends. James Reed studies the social context out of which the medical profession slowly came to accept its role in dispensing advice about the means by which women could begin to control their conceptions.

As with their attitudes toward menstruation and sexuality, women did not find it easy to reveal their feelings about birth control. Yet because of the public manifestation of success or failure of birth control methods—in variations in the birthrate—the issue of family limitation and discussion of various methods by which it could be accomplished form a fairly visible part of the recoverable historical record. Historians have documented not only the methods women and men used to engage in heterosexual intercourse and limit conception but also personal and political motivations for using contraception and abortion.

The questions of which sexual partner made decisions about controlling number of offspring and how this changed through history can be particularly revealing of women's position within the family. Some methods, such as withdrawal or condoms, rested in male control; others, like abortion, could be controlled by women; and still others, like abstinence, encouraged cooperation between both partners. By examining the patterns of use of the more popular methods, historians can learn the extent to which women in any given historical period wanted to or could control their own reproductive capacities.

The physicians' role in controlling, monitoring, or ignoring birth control practices has been, and remains today, particularly controversial. The three historians here either directly or indirectly address this question, and their collective evidence suggests that the medical profession's response could not always be predicted. The interests of this group changed considerably over time, sometimes reflecting society's values about which social groups should be reproducing at the greatest rates, sometimes reflecting the state of medical knowledge, sometimes reflecting individual male physicians' views as husbands and fathers, and sometimes reflecting purely professional goals. One conclusion seems certain from the record: before the mid-twentieth century, the women whose bodies and lives were most intimately affected by birth control decisions only rarely found themselves in alliance with the physicians.

7

Voluntary Motherhood: The Beginnings of Feminist Birth Control Ideas in the United States

LINDA GORDON

Voluntary motherhood was the first general name for a feminist birth control demand in the United States in the late nineteenth century.[1] It represented an initial response of feminists to their understanding that involuntary motherhood and child raising were important parts of woman's oppression. In this paper, I would like to trace the content and general development of "voluntary motherhood" ideas and to situate them in the development of the American birth control movement.

The feminists who advocated voluntary motherhood were of three general types: suffragists; people active in such moral reform movements as temperance and social purity, in church auxiliaries, and in women's professional and service organizations (such as Sorosis); and members of small, usually anarchist, Free Love groups. The Free Lovers played a classically vanguard role in the development of birth control ideas. Free Love groups were always small and sectarian, and they were usually male dominated, despite their extreme ideological feminism. They never coalesced into a movement. On the contrary, they were the remnants of a dying tradition of utopian socialist and radical Protestant religious dissent. The Free Lovers, whose very self-definition was built around commitments to iconoclasm and to isolation from the masses, were precisely the group that could offer intellectual leadership in formulating the shocking arguments that birth control in the nineteenth century required.[2]

LINDA GORDON is Professor of History at the University of Massachusetts, Boston, Massachusetts.

Reprinted with the permission of the author from *Feminist Studies* 1 (1973): 5–22.

The suffragists and moral reformers, concerned to win mass support, were increasingly committed to social respectability. As a result, they did not generally advance very far beyond prevalent standards of propriety in discussing sexual matters publicly. Indeed, as the century progressed the social gap between them and the Free Lovers grew, for the second and third generations of suffragists were more concerned with respectability than the first. In the 1860s and 1870s the great feminist theoreticians had been much closer to the Free Lovers, and at least one of these early giants, Victoria Woodhull, was for several years a member of both the suffrage and the Free Love camps. But even respectability did not completely stifle the mental processes of the feminists, and many of them said in private writings—in letters and diaries—what they were unwilling to utter in public.

The similar views of Free Lovers and suffragists on the question of voluntary motherhood did not bridge the considerable political distance between the groups, but did show that their analyses of the social meaning of reproduction for the women were converging. The sources of that convergence, the common grounds of their feminism, were their similar experiences in the changing conditions of nineteenth-century America. Both groups were composed of educated, middle-class Yankees responding to severe threats to the stability, if not dominance, of their class position. Both groups were disturbed by the consequences of rapid industrialization—the emergence of great capitalists in a clearly defined financial oligarchy, and the increased immigration which threatened the dignity and economic security of the middle-class Yankee. Free Lovers and suffragists, as feminists, looked forward to a decline in patriarchal power within the family, but worried, too, about the possible disintegration of the family and the loosening of sexual morality. They saw reproduction in the context of these larger social changes, and in a movement for women's emancipation; and they saw that movement as an answer to some of these large social problems. They hoped that giving political power to women would help to reinforce the family, to make the government more just and the economy less monopolistic. In all these attitudes there was something traditional as well as something progressive; the concept of voluntary motherhood reflected this duality.

Since we all bring a twentieth-century understanding to our concept of birth control, it may be best to make it clear at once that neither Free Lovers nor suffragists approved of contraceptive devices. Ezra Heywood, patriarch and martyr, thought "artificial" methods "unnatural, injurious, or offensive." Tennessee Claflin wrote that the "washes, teas, tonics and various sorts of appliances known to the initiated" were a "standing reproach upon, and a permanent indictment against, American women.... No woman should ever hold sexual relations with any man from the possible consequences of which she might desire to escape." *Woodhull and Claflin's Weekly* editorialized: "The means they [women] resort to for . . . prevention is sufficient to disgust every natural man."[3]

On a rhetorical level, the main objection to contraception[4] was that it was "unnatural," and the arguments reflected a romantic yearning for the "natural," rather pastorally conceived, that was typical of many nineteenth-century reform movements. More basic, however, particularly in women's arguments against contraception, was an underlying fear of the promiscuity that it could permit. The fear of promiscuity was associated less with fear for one's virtue than with fear of other women—the perhaps mythical "fallen" women—who might threaten a husband's fidelity.

To our twentieth-century minds a principle of voluntary motherhood that rejects the practice of contraception seems so theoretical as to have little real impact. What gave the concept substance was that it was accompanied by another, potentially explosive, conceptual change: the reacceptance of female sexuality. As with birth control, the most open advocates of female sexuality were the Free Lovers, not the suffragists; nevertheless both groups based their ideas on the traditional grounds of the "natural." Free Lovers argued, for example, that celibacy was unnatural and dangerous—for men and women alike. "Pen cannot record, nor lips express, the enervating, debauching effect of celibate life upon young men and women."[5] Asserting the existence, legitimacy, and worthiness of female sexual drive was one of the Free Lovers' most important contributions to sexual reform; it was a logical correlate of their argument from the "natural" and of their appeal for the integration of body and soul.

Women's rights advocates, too, began to demand recognition of female sexuality. Isabella Beecher Hooker wrote to her daughter: "Multitudes of women in all the ages who have scarce known what sexual desire is—being wholly absorbed in the passion of maternity, have sacrificed themselves to the beloved husbands as unto God—and yet these men, full of their human passion and defending it as righteous & God-sent lose all confidence in womanhood when a woman here and there betrays her similar nature & gives herself soul & body to the man she adores."[6] Alice Stockham, a Spiritualist Free Lover and feminist physician, lauded sexual desire in men and women as "the prophecy of attainment." She urged that couples avoid reaching sexual "satiety" with each other, in order to keep their sexual desire constantly alive, for she considered desire pleasant and healthful.[7] Elizabeth Cady Stanton, commenting in her diary in 1883 on the Whitman poem "There Is a Woman Waiting for Me," wrote: "he speaks as if the female must be forced to the creative act, apparently ignorant of the fact that a healthy woman has as much passion as a man, that she needs nothing stronger than the law of attraction to draw her to the male."[8] Still, she loved Whitman, and largely because of that openness about sex that made him the Free Lovers' favorite poet.

According to the system of ideas then dominant, women, lacking sexual drives, submitted to sexual intercourse (and notice how Beecher Hooker continued the image of a woman "giving herself," never taking) in order to please their husbands and to conceive children. The ambivalence underlying this view was expressed in the equally prevalent notion that women must be protected from exposure to sexuality lest they "fall" and become depraved, lustful monsters. This ambivalence perhaps came from a subconscious lack of certainty about the reality of the sexless woman, a construct laid only thinly on top of the conception of woman as highly sexed, even insatiably so, that prevailed up to the eighteenth century. Victorian ambivalence on this question is nowhere more tellingly set forth than in the writings of physicians, who viewed woman's sexual organs as the source of her being, physical and psychological, and blamed most mental derangements on disorders of the reproductive organs.[9] Indeed, they saw it as part of the nature of things, as Rousseau had written, that men were male only part of the time, but women were female always.[10] In a system that deprived women of the opportunity to make extrafamilial contributions to culture, it was inevitable that they should be more strongly identified with sex than men were. Indeed, females were frequently called "the sex" in the nineteenth century.

The concept of maternal instinct helped to smooth the contradictory attitudes about woman's sexuality. In many nineteenth-century writings we find the idea that the maternal instinct was the female analogue of the male sex instinct; it was as if the two instincts were seated in analogous parts of the brain, or soul. Thus to suggest, as feminists did, that women might have the capacity for sexual impulses of their own automatically tended to weaken the theory of the maternal instinct. In the fearful imaginations of self-apppointed protectors of the family and of womanly innocence, the possibility that women might desire sexual contact not for the sake of pregnancy—that they might even desire it at a time when they positively did not want pregnancy—was a wedge in the door to denying that women had any special maternal instinct at all.

Most of the feminists did not want to open that door either. Indeed, it was common for nineteenth-century women's rights advocates to use the presumed "special motherly nature" and "sexual purity" of women as arguments for increasing their freedom and status. It is no wonder that many of them chose to speak their subversive thoughts about the sexual nature of women privately, or at least softly. Even among the more outspoken Free Lovers, there was a certain amount of hedging. Lois Waisbrooker and Dora Forster, writing for a Free Love journal in the 1890s, argued that while men

and women both had an "amative" instinct, it was much stronger in men; and that women—only women—also had a reproductive, or "generative" instinct. "I suppose it must be universally conceded that men make the better lovers," Forster wrote. She thought that it might be possible that "the jealousy and tyranny of men have operated to suppress amativeness in women, by constantly sweeping strongly sexual women from the paths of life into infamy and sterility and death," but she thought also that the suppression, if it existed, had been permanently inculcated in woman's character.[11]

Modern birth control ideas rest on a full acceptance, at least quantitatively, of female sexuality. Modern contraception is designed to permit sexual intercourse as often as desired without the risk of pregnancy. Despite the protestations of sex counselors that there are no norms for the frequency of intercourse, in the popular view there are such norms. Most people in the mid-twentieth century think that "normal" couples have intercourse several times a week. By twentieth-century standards, then, the Free Lovers' rejection of artificial contraception and "unnatural" sex seems to preclude the possibility of birth control at all. Nineteenth-century sexual reformers, however, had different sexual norms. They did not seek to make an infinite number of sterile sexual encounters possible. They wanted to make it possible for women to avoid pregnancy if they badly needed to do so for physical or psychological reasons, but they did not believe that it was essential for such women to engage freely in sexual intercourse.

In short, for birth control, they recommended periodic or permanent abstinence. The proponents of voluntary motherhood had in mind two distinct contexts for abstinence. One was the mutual decision of a couple. This could mean continued celibacy, or it could mean following a form of the rhythm method. Unfortunately all the nineteenth-century writers miscalculated women's fertility cycle. (It was not until the 1920s that the ovulation cycle was correctly plotted, and until the 1930s it was not widely understood among American doctors.)[12] Ezra Heywood, for example, recommended avoiding intercourse from six to eight days before menstruation until ten to twelve days after it. Careful use of the calendar could also provide control over the sex of a child, Heywood believed: conception in the first half of the menstrual cycle would produce girls, in the second half, boys.[13] These misconceptions functioned, conveniently, to make practicable Heywood's and others' ideas that celibacy and contraceptive devices should *both* be avoided.

Some of the Free Lovers also endorsed male continence, a system practiced and advocated by the Oneida community, in which the male avoids climax entirely.[14] (There were other aspects of the Oneida system that antagonized the Free Lovers, notably the authoritarian quality of John Humphrey Noyes's leadership.)[15] Dr. Stockham developed her own theory of continence called "Karezza," in which the female as well as the male was to avoid climax. Karezza and male continence were whole sexual systems, not just methods of birth control. Their advocates expected the self-control involved to build character and spiritual qualities, while honoring, refining, and dignifying the sexual functions; and Karezza was reputed to be a cure for sterility as well, since its continued use was thought to build up the resources of fertility in the body.[16]

Idealizing sexual self-control was characteristic of the Free Love point of view. It was derived mainly from the thought of the utopian communitarians of the early nineteenth century,[17] but Ezra Heywood elaborated the theory. Beginning with the assumption that people's "natural" instincts, left untrammeled, would automatically create a harmonious, peaceful society—an assumption certainly derived from liberal philosophical faith in the innate goodness of man—Heywood applied it to sexuality, arguing that the natural sexual instinct was innately moderated, self-regulating. He did not imagine, as did Freud, a powerful, simple libido that could be checked only by an equally powerful moral and rational will. Heywood's theory implicitly contradicted Freud's description of inner struggle and constant tension between the drives of the id and the goals of the super-ego; Heywood denied the social necessity of sublimation.

On one level Heywood's theory may seem inadequate as a psychology, since it cannot explain such phenomena as repression and the strengthening of self-control with maturity. It may, however, have a deeper accuracy. It argues that society and its attendant repressions have distorted the animal's natural self-regulating mechanism, and have thereby created excessive and obsessive sexual drives. It offers a social explanation for the phenomena that Freud described in psychological terms, and thus holds out the hope that they can be changed.

Essentially similar to Wilhelm Reich's theory of "sex-economy," the Heywood theory of self-regulation went beyond Reich's in providing a weapon against one of the ideological bastions of male supremacy. Self-regulation as a goal was directed against the prevalent attitude that male lust was an uncontrollable urge, an attitude that functioned as a justification for rape specifically and for male sexual irresponsibility generally. We have to get away from the tradition of "man's necessities and woman's obedience to them," Stockham wrote.[18] The idea that men's desires are irrepressible is merely the other face of the idea that women's desires are nonexistent. Together, the two created a circle that enclosed woman, making it her exclusive responsibility to say No, and making pregnancy her God-imposed burden if she didn't, while denying her both artificial contraception and the personal and social strength to rebel against male sexual demands.

Heywood developed his theory of natural sexual self-regulation in answer to the common anti–Free Love argument that the removal of social regulation of sexuality would lead to unhealthy promiscuity: "in the distorted popular view, Free Love tends to unrestrained licentiousness, to open the flood gates of passion and remove all barriers in its desolating course; but it means just the opposite; it means the *utilization of animalism*, and the triumph of Reason, Knowledge, and Continence."[19] He applied the theory of self-regulation to the problem of birth control only as an afterthought, perhaps when women's concerns with that problem reached him. Ideally, he trusted, the amount of sexual intercourse that men and women desired would be exactly commensurate with the number of children that were wanted. Since sexual repression had had the boomerang effect of intensifying our sexual drives far beyond "natural" levels, effective birth control now would require the development of the inner self-control to contain and repress sexual urges. But in time he expected that sexual moderation would come about naturally.

Heywood's analysis, published in the mid-1870s, was concerned primarily with excessive sex drives in men. Charlotte Perkins Gilman, one of the lead-

ing theoreticians of the suffrage movement, reinterpreted that analysis two decades later to emphasize its effects on women. The economic dependence
of woman on man, in Gilman's analysis, made her
sexual attractiveness necessary not only for winning a mate, but as a means of getting a livelihood
too. This is the case with no other animal. In the
human female it had produced "excessive modification to sex," emphasizing weak qualities characterized by humans as "feminine." She made an
analogy to the milk cow, bred to produce far more
milk than she would need for her calves. But Gilman agreed completely with Heywood about the
effects of exaggerated sex distinction on the male;
it produced excessive sex energy and excessive indulgence to an extent debilitating to the whole species. Like Heywood she also believed that the path
of progressive social evolution moved toward mo-
nogamy and toward reducing the promiscuous sex
instinct.[20]

A second context for abstinence, in addition to
mutual self-regulation by a couple, was the right
of the wife unilaterally to refuse her husband. This
idea is at the heart of voluntary motherhood. It
was a key substantive demand in the mid-nineteenth
century when both law and practice made sexual
submission to her husband a woman's duty.[21] A
woman's right to refuse is clearly the fundamental
condition of birth control—and of her independence and personal integrity.

In their crusade for this right of refusal the voices
of Free Lovers and suffragists were in unison. Ezra
Heywood demanded "Woman's Natural Right to
ownership and control over her own body-self—a
right inseparable from Woman's intelligent existence."[22] Paulina Wright Davis, at the National
Woman Suffrage Association in 1871, attacked the
law "which makes obligatory the rendering of marital rights and compulsory maternity." When, as a
result of her statement, she was accused of being a
Free Lover, she responded by accepting the description.[23] Isabella Beecher Hooker wrote her
daughter in 1869 advising her to avoid pregnancy
until "you are prepared in body and soul to receive
and cherish the little one."[24] In 1873 she gave similar advice to women generally, in her book *Womanhood*.[25] Elizabeth Cady Stanton had characteristically used the same phrase as Heywood: woman

owning her own body. Once asked by a magazine
what she meant by it, she replied: "womanhood is
the primal fact, wifehood and motherhood its incidents . . . must the heyday of her existence be
wholly devoted to the one animal function of bearing children? Shall there be no limit to this but
woman's capacity to endure the fearful strain on
her life?"[26]

The insistence on women's right to refuse often
took the form of attacks on men for their lusts and
their violence in attempting to satisfy them. In their
complaints against the unequal marriage laws, chief
or at least loudest among them was the charge that
they legalized rape.[27] Victoria Woodhull raged, "I
will tell the world, so long as I have a tongue and
the strength to move it, of all the infernal misery
hidden behind this horrible thing called marriage,
though the Young Men's Christian Association sentence me to prison a year for every word. I have
seen horrors beside which stone walls and iron bars
are heaven."[28] Angela Heywood attacked men incessantly and bitterly; if one were to ignore the
accuracy of her charges, she could well seem ill-
tempered. "Man so lost to himself and woman as
to invoke legal *violence* in these sacred nearings,
*should have solemn meeting with, and look serious at his
own penis until he is able to be lord and master of it,
rather than it should longer rule, lord and master, of him
and of the victims he deflowers*."[29] Suffragists spoke
more delicately, but not less bitterly. Feminists organized social purity organizations and campaigns,
their attacks on prostitution based on a critique of
the double standard, for which their proposed
remedy was that men conform to the standards
required of women.[30]

A variant of this concern was a campaign against
"sexual abuses"—a Victorian euphemism for de-
viant sexual practices, or simply excessive sexual
demands, not necessarily violence or prostitution.
The Free Lovers, particularly, turned to this cause,
because it gave them an opportunity to attack marriage. The "sexual abuses" question was one of the
most frequent subjects of correspondence in Free
Love periodicals. For example, a letter from Mrs.
Theresa Hughes of Pittsburgh described:

> . . . a girl of sixteen, full of life and health
> when she became a wife. . . . She was a slave
> in every sense of the word, mentally and sex-

ually, never was she free from his brutal outrages, morning, noon and night, up almost to the very hour her baby was born, and before she was again strong enough to move about. . . . Often did her experience last an hour or two, and one night she will never forget, the outrage lasted exactly four hours.[31]

Or from Lucinda Chandler, well-known moral reformer:

This useless sense gratification has demoralized generation after generation, till monstrosities of disorder are common. Moral education, and healthful training will be requisite for some generations, even after we have equitable economics, and free access to Nature's gifts. The young man of whom I knew who threatened his bride of a week with a sharp knive in his hand, to compel her to perform the office of 'sucker,' would no doubt have had the same disposition though no soul on the planet had a want unsatisfied or lacked a natural right.[32]

From an anonymous woman in Los Angeles:

I am nearly wrecked and ruined by . . . nightly intercourse, which is often repeated in the morning. This and nothing else was the cause of my miscarriage . . . he went to work like a man a-mowing, and instead of a pleasure as it might have been, it was most intense torture. . . .[33]

Clearly these remarks reflect a level of hostility toward sex. The observation that many feminists hated sex has been made by several historians,[34] but they have usually failed to perceive that feminists' hostility and fear of it came from the fact that they were women, not that they were feminists. Women in the nineteenth century were, of course, trained to repress their own sexual feelings, to view sex as a duty. But they also resented what they experienced, which was not an abstraction, but a particular, historical kind of sexual encounter—intercourse dominated by and defined by the male in conformity with his desires and in disregard of what might bring pleasure to a woman. (That this might have resulted more from male ignorance than malevolence could not change

women's experiences.) Furthermore, sexual intercourse brought physical danger. Pregnancy, childbirth, and abortions were risky, painful, and isolating experiences in the nineteenth century; venereal diseases were frequently communicated to women by their husbands. Elmina Slenker, a Free Lover and novelist, wrote, "I'm getting a host of stories (truths) about women so starved sexually as to use their dogs for relief, and finally I have come to the belief that a CLEAN dog is better than a drinking, tobacco-smelling, venereally diseased man!"[35]

"Sex-hating" women were not just misinformed, or priggish, or neurotic. They were often responding rationally to their material reality. Denied the possibility of recognizing and expressing their own sexual needs, denied even the knowledge of sexual possibilities other than those dictated by the rhythms of male orgasm, they had only two choices: passive and usually pleasureless submission, with high risk of undesirable consequences, or rebellious refusal. In that context abstinence to ensure voluntary motherhood was a most significant feminist demand.

What is remarkable is that some women recognized that it was not sex per se, but only their husbands' style of making love, that repelled them. One of the women noted above who complained about her treatment went on to say: "I am undeveloped sexually, never having desires in that direction; still, with a husband who had any love or kind of feelings for me and one less selfish it *might* have been different, but he cared nothing for the torture to *me* as long as *he* was gratified."[36]

Elmina Slenker herself, the toughest and crustiest of all these "sex haters," dared to explore and take seriously her own longings, thereby revealing herself to be a sex lover in disguise. As the editor of the *Water-Cure Journal,* and a regular contributor to *Free Love Journal,*[37] she expounded a theory of "Dianaism, or Non-procreative Love," sometimes called "Diana-love and Alpha–abstinence." It meant free sexual contact of all sorts except intercourse.

We want the sexes to love more than they do; we want them to love openly, frankly, earnestly; to enjoy the caress, the embrace, the glance, the voice, the presence & the very step of the beloved. We oppose no form or act of love between any man & woman. Fill the world as full of genuine sex love as you can . . . but forbear to rush in where generations yet unborn may suffer for your unthinking, uncaring, unheeding actions.[38]

Comparing this to the more usual physical means of avoiding conception—coitus interruptus and male continence—reveals how radical it was. In modern history, public endorsement of nongenital sex, and of forms of genital sex beyond standard "missionary position" intercourse, has been a recent, post-Freudian, even post-Masters-and-Johnson phenomenon. The definition of sex as heterosexual intercourse has been one of the oldest and most universal cultural norms. Slenker's alienation from existing sexual possibilities led her to explore alternatives with a bravery and a freedom from religious and psychological taboos extraordinary for a nineteenth-century Quaker reformer.

In the nineteenth century, neither Free Lovers nor suffragists ever relinquished their hostility to contraception. But among the Free Lovers, free speech was always an overriding concern, and for that reason Ezra Heywood agreed to publish some advertisements for a vaginal syringe, an instrument the use of which for contraception he personally deplored, or so he continued to assure his readers. Those advertisements led to Heywood's prosecution for obscenity, and he defended himself with characteristic flair by making his position more radical than ever before. Contraception was moral, he argued, when it was used by women as the only means of defending their rights, including the right to voluntary motherhood. Although "artificial means of preventing conception are not generally patronized by Free Lovers," he wrote, reserving for his own followers the highest moral ground, still he recognized that not all women were lucky enough to have Free Lovers for their sex partners.[39]

Since Comstockism makes male will, passion and power absolute to *impose* conception, I stand with women to resent it. The man who would legislate to choke a woman's vagina with semen, who would force a woman to retain his seed, bear children when her own reason and conscience oppose it, would waylay her, seize her by the throat and rape her person.[40]

Angela Heywood enthusiastically pushed this new political line.

Is it "proper," "polite," for men, to go to Washington to say, by penal law, fines and imprisonment, whether woman may continue her natural right to wash, rinse, or wipe her own vaginal body opening—as well legislate when she may blow her nose, dry her eyes, or nurse her babe. . . . Whatever she may have been pleased to receive, from man's own, is his gift and her property. Women do not like rape, and have a right to resist its results.[41]

Her outspokenness, vulgarity in the ears of most of her contemporaries, came from a substantive, not merely a stylistic, sexual radicalism. Not even the heavy taboos and revulsion against abortion stopped her: "To cut a child up in woman, procure abortion, is a most fearful, tragic deed; but *even that* does not call for man's arbitrary jurisdiction over woman's womb."[42]

It is unclear whether Heywood, in this passage, was actually arguing for legalized abortion; if she was, she was alone among all nineteenth-century sexual reformers in saying it. Other feminists and Free Lovers condemned abortion, and argued that the necessity of stopping its widespread practice was a key reason for instituting voluntary motherhood by other means. The difference on the abortion question between sexual radicals and sexual conservatives was in their analysis of its causes and remedies. While doctors and preachers were sermonizing on the sinfulness of women who obtained abortions,[43] the radicals pronounced abortion itself an undeserved punishment, and a woman who had one a helpless victim. Woodhull and Claflin wrote about Madame Restell's notorious abortion "factory" in New York City without moralism, arguing that only voluntary conception would put it out of business.[44] Elizabeth Cady Stanton also sympathized with women who had abortions, and used the abortion problem as an example of women's victimization by laws made without their consent.[45]

Despite stylistic differences, which stemmed from differences in goals, nineteenth-century American Free Lovers and women's rights advocates shared the same basic attitudes toward birth control: they opposed contraception and abortion, but endorsed voluntary motherhood achieved through periodic abstinence; they believed that women should always have the right to decide when to bear a child: and they believed that women and men both had natural sex drives and that it was not wrong to indulge those drives without the intention of conceiving children. The two groups also shared the same appraisal of social and political significance of birth control. Most of them were favorably inclined toward neo-Malthusian reasoning (at least until the 1890s, when the prevailing concern shifted to the problem of underpopulation rather than overpopulation).[46] They were also interested, increasingly, in controlling conception for eugenic purposes.[47] They were hostile to the hypocrisy of the sexual double standard and, beyond that, shared a general sense that men had become oversexed and that sex had been transformed into something disagreeably violent.

But above all their commitment to voluntary motherhood expressed their larger commitment to women's rights. Elizabeth Cady Stanton thought voluntary motherhood so central that on her lecture tours in 1871 she held separate afternoon meetings for *women only* (a completely unfamiliar practice at the time) and talked about "the gospel of fewer children & a healthy, happy maternity."[48] "What radical thoughts I then and there put into their heads & as they feel untrammelled, these thoughts are permanently lodged there! That is all I ask."[49] Only Ezra Heywood had gone so far as to defend a particular contraceptive device—the syringe. But the principle of woman's rights to choose the number of children she would bear and when was accepted in the most conservative sections of the women's rights movement. At the First Congress of the Association for the Advancement of Women in 1873, a whole session was devoted to the theme "Enlightened Motherhood," which had voluntary motherhood as part of its meaning.[50]

The general conviction of the feminist community that women had a right to choose when to conceive a child was so strong by the end of the nineteenth century that it seems odd that they were unable to overcome their scruples against artificial contraception. The basis for the reluctance lies in their awareness that a consequence of effective contraception would be the separation of sexuality from reproduction. A state of things that permit-

ted sexual intercourse to take place normally, even frequently, without the risk of pregnancy, inevitably seemed to nineteenth-century middle-class women as an attack on the family, as they understood the family. In the mid-Victorian sexual system, men normally conducted their sexual philandering with prostitutes; accordingly prostitution, far from being a threat to the family system, was a part of it and an important support of it. This was the common view of the time, paralleled by the belief that prostitutes knew of effective birth control techniques. This seemed only fitting, for contraception in the 1870s was associated with sexual immorality. It did not seem, even to the most sexually liberal, that contraception could be legitimized to any extent, even for the purposes of family planning for married couples, without licensing extramarital sex. The fact that contraception was not morally acceptable to respectable women was, from a woman's point of view, a guarantee that those women would not be a threat to her own marriage.

The fact that sexual intercourse often leads to conception was also a guarantee that men would marry in the first place. In the nineteenth century women needed marriage far more than men. Lacking economic independence, women needed husbands to support them, or at least to free them from a usually more humiliating economic dependence on fathers. Especially in the cities, where women were often isolated from communities, deprived of the economic and psychological support of networks of relatives, friends and neighbors, the prospect of dissolving the cement of nuclear families was frightening. In many cases children, and the prospect of children, provided that cement. Man's responsibilities for children were an important pressure for marital stability. Women, especially middle-class women, were also dependent on their children to provide them with meaningful work. The belief that motherhood was a woman's fulfillment had a material basis: parenthood was often the only creative and challenging activity in a woman's life, a key part of her self-esteem.

Legal, efficient birth control would have increased men's freedom to indulge in extramarital sex without greatly increasing women's freedom to do so. The pressures enforcing chastity and marital fidelity on middle-class women were not only fear of illegitimate conception but a powerful combination of economic, social, and psychological factors, including economic dependence, fear of rejection by husband and social support networks, internalized taboos and, hardly the least important, a socially conditioned lack of interest in sex that may have approached functional frigidity. The double standard of the Victorian sexual and family system, which had made men's sexual freedom irresponsible and oppressive to women, left most feminists convinced that increasing, rather than releasing, the taboos against extramarital sex was in their interest, and they threw their support behind social purity campaigns.

In short, we must forget the twentieth-century association of birth control with a trend toward sexual freedom. The voluntary motherhood propaganda of the 1870s was associated with a push toward a more restrictive, or at least a more rigidly enforced, sexual morality. Achieving voluntary motherhood by a method that would have encouraged sexual license was absolutely contrary to the felt interests of the very group that formed the main social basis for the cause—middle-class women. Separating these women from the early-twentieth-century feminists, with their interests in sexual freedom, were nearly four decades of significant social and economic changes and a general weakening of the ideology of the Lady. The ideal of the Free Lovers—responsible, open sexual encounters between equal partners—was impossible in the 1870s because men and women were not equal. A man was a man whether faithful to his wife or not. But women's sexual activities divided them into two categories—wife or prostitute. These categories were not mere ideas, but were enforced in reality by severe social and economic sanctions. The fact that so many, indeed most, Free Lovers in practice led faithful, monogamous, legally married lives is not insignificant in this regard. It suggests that they understood that Free Love was an ideal not to be realized in that time.

As voluntary motherhood was an ideology intended to encourage sexual purity, so it was also a pro-motherhood ideology. Far from debunking motherhood, the voluntary motherhood advocates consistently continued the traditional Victorian mystification and sentimentalization of the mother. It is true that at the end of the nineteenth century an increasing number of feminists and elite women—that is, still a relatively small group—were

choosing not to marry or become mothers. That was primarily because of their increasing interest in professional work, and the difficulty of doing such work as a wife and mother, given the normal uncooperativeness of husbands and the lack of social provisions for child care. Voluntary motherhood advocates shared the general belief that mothers of young children ought not to work outside their homes but should make mothering their full-time occupation. Suffragists argued both to make professions open to women and to ennoble the task of mothering; they argued for increased rights and opportunities for women *because* they were mothers.

The Free Lovers were equally pro-motherhood; they wanted only to separate motherhood from legal marriage.[51] They devised pro-motherhood arguments to bolster their case against marriage. Mismated couples, held together by marriage laws, made bad parents and produced inferior offspring, Free Lovers said.[52] In 1870 *Woodhull and Claflin's Weekly* editorialized, "Our marital system is the greatest obstacle to the regeneration of the race."[53]

This concern with eugenics was characteristic of nearly all feminists of the late nineteenth century. At the time eugenics was mainly seen as an implication of evolutionary theory and was picked up by many social reformers to buttress their arguments that improvement of the human condition was possible. Eugenics had not yet become a movement in itself. Feminists used eugenics arguments as if they instinctively felt that arguments based solely on women's rights had not enough power to conquer conservative and religious scruples about reproduction. So they combined eugenics and feminism to produce evocative, romantic visions of perfect motherhood. "Where boundless love prevails. . . ." *Woodhull and Claflin's Weekly* wrote, "the mother who produces an inferior child will be dishonored and unhappy . . . and she who produces superior children will feel proportionately pleased. When woman attains this position, she will consider superior offspring a necessity and be apt to procreate only with superior men."[54] Free Lovers and suffragists alike used the cult of motherhood to argue for making motherhood voluntary. Involuntary motherhood, wrote Harriot Stanton Blatch, daughter of Elizabeth Cady Stanton and a prominent suffragist, is a prostitution of the maternal instinct.[55] Free Lover Rachel Campbell cried out that motherhood was being "ground to dust under the misrule of masculine ignorance and superstition."[56]

Not only was motherhood considered an exalted, sacred profession, and a profession exclusively woman's responsibility, but for a woman to avoid it was to choose a distinctly less noble path. In arguing for the enlargement of woman's sphere, feminists envisaged combining motherhood with other activities, not rejecting motherhood. Victoria Woodhull and Tennessee Claflin wrote:

Tis true that the special and distinctive feature of woman is that of bearing children, and that upon the exercise of her function in this regard the perpetuity of race depends. It is also true that those who pass through life failing in this special feature of their mission cannot be said to have lived to the best purposes of woman's life. But while maternity should always be considered the most holy of all the functions woman is capable of, it should not be lost sight of in devotion to this, that there are as various spheres of usefulness outside of this for woman as there are for man outside of the marriage relation.[57]

Birth control was not intended to open the possibility of childlessness, but merely to give women leverage to win more recognition and dignity. Dora Forster, a Free Lover, saw in the fears of underpopulation a weapon of blackmail for women:

I hope the scarcity of children will go on until maternity is honored at least as much as the trials and hardships of soldiers campaigning in wartime. It will then be worth while to supply the nation with a sufficiency of children . . . every civilized nation, having lost the power to enslave woman as mother, will be compelled to recognize her voluntary exercise of that function as by far the most important service of any class of citizens.[58]

"Oh, women of the world, arise in your strength and demand that all which stands in the path of true motherhood shall be removed from your path," wrote Lois Waisbrooker, a Free Love novelist and moral reformer.[59] Helen Gardener based a plea for women's education entirely on the argument

that society needed educated mothers to produce able sons (not children, sons).

Harvard and Yale, not to mention Columbia, may continue to put a protective tariff on the brains of young men: but so long as they must get those brains from the proscribed sex, just so long will male brains remain an "infant industry" and continue to need this protection. Stupid mothers never did and stupid mothers never will, furnish this world with brilliant sons.[60]

Clinging to the cult of motherhood was part of a broader conservatism shared by Free Lovers and suffragists—acceptance of traditional sex roles. Even the Free Lovers rejected only one factor—legal marriage—of the many that defined woman's place in the family. They did not challenge conventional conceptions of woman's passivity and limited sphere of concern.[61] In their struggles for equality the women's rights advocates never suggested that men should share responsibility for child raising, housekeeping, nursing, cooking. When Victoria Woodhull in the 1870s and Charlotte Perkins Gilman in the early 1900s suggested socialized child care, they assumed that only women would do the work.[62] Most feminists wanted economic independence for women, but most, too, were reluctant to recommend achieving this by turning women loose and helpless into the economic world to compete with men.[63] This attitude was conditioned by an attitude hostile to the egoistic spirit of capitalism; but the attitude was not transformed into a political position and usually appeared as a description of women's weakness, rather than an attack on the system. Failing to distinguish, or even to indicate awareness of a possible distinction between, women's conditioned passivity and their equally conditioned distaste for competition and open aggression, these feminists also followed the standard Victorian rationalization of sex roles, the idea that women were morally superior. Thus the timidity and self-effacement that were the marks of women's powerlessness were made into innate virtues. Angela Heywood, for example, praised women's greater ability for self-control, and, in an attribution no doubt intended to jar and titillate the reader, branded men inferior on account of their lack of sexual temperance.[64] Men's refusal to accept women as human beings she identified, similarly, as a mark of men's incapacity: "man has not yet achieved himself to realize and meet a PERSON in woman."[65] In idealistic, abstract terms, no doubt such male behavior is an incapacity. Yet that conceit failed to remark on the power and privilege over women that the supposed "incapacity" gave men.

This omission is characteristic of the cult of motherhood. Indeed, what made it a cult was its one-sided failure to recognize the privileges men received from women's exclusive responsibility for parenthood. The "motherhood" of the feminists' writings was not merely the biological process of gestation and birth, but a package of social, economic, and cultural functions. Although many of the nineteenth-century feminists had done substantial analysis of the historical and anthropological origins of woman's social role, they nevertheless agreed with the biological determinist point of view that women's parental capacities had become implanted at the level of instinct, the famous "maternal instinct." That concept rested on the assumption that the qualities that parenthood requires—capacities for tenderness, self-control and patience, tolerance for tedium and detail, emotional supportiveness, dependability and warmth— were not only instinctive but sex linked. The concept of the maternal instinct thus also involved a definition of the normal instinctual structure of the male that excluded these capacities, or included them only to an inferior degree; it also carried the implication that women who did not exercise these capacities, presumably through motherhood, remained unfulfilled, untrue to their destinies.

Belief in the maternal instinct reinforced the belief in the necessary spiritual connection for women between sex and reproduction, and limited the development of birth control ideas. But the limits were set by the entire social context of women's lives, not by the intellectual timidity of their ideas. For women's "control over their own bodies" to lead to a rejection of motherhood as the *primary* vocation and measure of social worth required the existence of alternative vocations and sources of worthiness. The women's rights advocates of the 1870s and 1880s were fighting for those other opportunities, but a significant change had come only to a few privileged women, and most women faced essentially the same options that existed fifty years earlier. Thus voluntary motherhood in this period remained almost exclusively a tool for women to strengthen their positions within conventional marriages and families, not to reject them.

NOTES

1   The word "feminist" must be underscored. Since the early nineteenth century, there had been developing a body of population control writings, which recommended the use of birth control techniques to curb nationwide or worldwide populations; usually called neo-Malthusians, these writers were not concerned with the control of births as a means by which women could gain control over their own lives, except, very occasionally, as an auxiliary argument. And of course birth control practices date back to the most ancient societies on record.

2   There is no space here to compensate for the general lack of information about the Free Lovers. There is is a fuller discussion of them in my *Woman's Body, Woman's Right: A Social History of Birth Control* (New York: Viking, Penguin, 1976). Some of the major Free Love writings include: R.D. Chapman, *Freelove a Law of Nature* (New York: author, 1881).
Tennessee Claflin, *The Ethics of Sexual Equality* (New York: Woodhull & Claflin, 1873).
Tennessee Claflin, *Virtue, What It Is and What It Isn't;*

Seduction, What It Is and What It Is Not (New York: Woodhull & Claflin, 1872).
Ezra Heywood, *Cupid's Yokes; or, The Binding Force of Conjugal Life* (Princeton, Mass.: Cooperative Publishing Co., n.d., probably 1876).
Ezra Heywood, *Uncivil Liberty: An Essay to Show the Injustice and Impolicy of Ruling Woman without Her Consent* (Princeton, Mass.: Cooperative Publishing Co., 1872).
C.L. James, *The Future Relation of the Sexes* (St. Louis: author, 1872).
Juliet Severance, *Marriage* (Chicago: M. Harman, 1901).
Victoria Claflin Woodhull, *The Scare-Crows of Sexual Slavery* (New York: Woodhull & Claflin, 1874).
Victoria Claflin Woodhull, *A Speech on the Principles of Social Freedom* (New York: Woodhull & Claflin, 1872).
Victoria Claflin Woodhull, *Tried as by Fire; or, The True and the False Socially* (New York: Woodhull & Claflin, 1874).

3   Heywood, *Cupid's Yokes,* 20; Claflin, *The Ethics of Sex-*

ual Equality, 9–10; *Woodhull & Claflin's Weekly,* 1870, *1, no. 6:* 5.

4 Contraception will be used to refer to artificial devices used to prohibit conception during intercourse, while birth control will be used to mean anything, including abstinence, which limits pregnancy.

5 Heywood, *Cupid's Yokes,* 17–18.

6 Letter to her daughter Alice, 1874, in the Isabella Beecher Hooker Collection, Beecher Stowe Mss, Stowe–Day Library, Hartford, Conn. This reference was brought to my attention by Ellen Dubois of SUNY-Buffalo.

7 Alice B. Stockham, M.D., *Karezza: Ethics of Marriage* (Chicago: Alice B. Stockham & Co., 1898), 84, 91–92.

8 Theodore Stanton and Harriot Stanton Blatch, eds., *Elizabeth Cady Stanton as Revealed in Her Letters, Diary and Reminiscences* (New York: Harper & Bros., 1922), 2:210 (Diary, 9–6–1883).

9 Ben Barker-Benfield, "The spermatic economy: a nineteenth century view of sexuality," *Feminist Studies,* 1, no. 1 (Summer 1972): 53.

10 J.J. Rousseau, *Emile* (New York: Columbia University Teachers College, 1967), 132. Rousseau was, after all, a chief author of the Victorian revision of the image of woman.

11 Dora Forster, *Sex Radicalism as Seen by an Emancipated Woman of the New Time* (Chicago: M. Harman, 1905), 40.

12 Norman E. Himes, *Medical History of Contraception* (New York: Gamut Press, 1963).

13 Heywood, *Cupid's Yokes,* 19–20, 16.

14 Ibid., 19–20; *Woodhull & Claflin's Weekly* 1, no. 18 (September 10, 1870): 5.

15 Heywood, *Cupid's Yokes, 14–15.*

16 Stockham, *Karezza,* 82–83, 53.

17 See for example, *Free Enquirer,* ed. Robert Owen and Frances Wright, May 22, 1830, 235–36.

18 Stockham, *Karezza,* 86.

19 Heywood, *Cupid's Yokes,* 19.

20 Charlotte Perkins Gilman, *Women and Economics* (New York: Harper Torchbooks, 1966), 38–39, 43–44, 42, 47–48, 209.

21 In England, for example, it was not until 1891 that the courts first held against a man who forcibly kidnaped and imprisoned his wife when she left him.

22 Ezra Heywood, *Free Speech: Report of Ezra H. Heywood's Defense before the United States Court, in Boston, April 10, 11, and 12, 1883* (Princeton, Mass.: Cooperative Publishing Co., n.d.), 16.

23 Quoted in Nelson Manfred Blake, *The Road to Reno: A History of Divorce in the United States* (New York: Macmillan, 1962), 108, from the *New York Tribune,* May 12, 1871, and July 20, 1871.

24 Letter of August 29, 1869, in Hooker Collection, Beecher Stowe Mss. This reference was brought to my attention by Ellen Dubois of SUNY-Buffalo.

25 Isabella Beecher Hooker, *Womanhood: Its Sanctities and Fidelities* (Boston: Lee and Shepard, 1873), 26.

26 Elizabeth Cady Stanton Mss., no. 11, Library of Congress, undated. This reference was brought to my attention by Ellen Dubois of SUNY-Buffalo.

27 See, for example, *Lucifer, The Light-Bearer,* ed. Moses Harman (Valley Falls, Kansas, 1894–1907) 18, no. 6 (October 1889): 3.

28 Victoria Woodhull, *The Scare-Crows,* 21. Her mention of the YMCA is a reference to the fact that Anthony Comstock, author and chief enforcer for the U.S. Post Office of the antiobscenity laws, had begun his career in the YMCA.

29 *The Word* (Princeton, Mass.) 20, no. 9 (March 1893): 2–3. Emphasis in original.

30 See for example, the National Purity Congress of 1895, sponsored by the American Purity Alliance.

31 *Lucifer,* April 26, 1890, 1–2.

32 N.a., *Next Revolution; or, Woman's Emancipation from Sex Slavery* (Valley Falls, Kansas: Lucifer Publishing Co., 1890), 49.

33 Ibid., 8–9.

34 Linda Gordon et al., "Sexism in American historical writing," *Women's Studies* 1, no. 1 (Fall 1972).

35 *Lucifer* 15, no. 2 (September 1886): 3.

36 *The Word,* 1892–93, *20.*

37 (Slenker) *Lucifer,* May 23, 1907; *Cyclopedia of American Biography,* 8: 488.

38 See for example *Lucifer* 18, no. 8 (December 1889): 3; 18, no. 6 (October 1889): 3; 18, no. 8 (December 1889): 3.

39 Heywood, *Free Speech,* 17, 16.

40 Ibid., 3–6. "Comstockism" also is a reference to Anthony Comstock. Noting the irony that the syringe was called by Comstock's name, Heywood continued: "To name a really good thing 'Comstock' has a sly, sinister, wily look, indicating vicious purpose; in deference to its N.Y., venders, who gave that name, the Publishers of *The Word* inserted an advertisement . . . which will hereafter appear as 'the Vaginal Syringe'; for its intelligent, humane and worthy mission should no longer be libelled by forced association with the pious scamp who thinks Congress gives him legal right of way to and control over every American Woman's Womb." At this trial, Heywood's second, he was acquitted. At his first trial, in 1877, he had been convicted, sentenced to two years, and served six months; at his third, in 1890, he was sentenced to and served two years at hard labor, an ordeal which probably caused his death a year later.

41 *The Word* 10, no. 9 (March 1893): 2–3.

42 Ibid.

43 See for example Horatio Robinson Storer, M.D., *Why Not? A Book for Every Woman* (Boston: Lee and Shepard, 1868). Note that this was the prize essay in a contest run by the AMA in 1865 for the best antiabortion tract.

44 Claflin, *Ethics;* Emanie Sachs, *The Terrible Siren, Victoria Woodhull, 1838–1927* (New York: Harper & Bros., 1928), 139.

45 Elizabeth Cady Stanton, Susan Anthony, Matilda Gage, eds., *History of Woman Suffrage,* 1:597–598.

46 Heywood, *Cupid's Yokes,* 20; see also *American Journal of Eugenics,* ed. M. Harman, 1, no. 2 (September 1907); *Lucifer* (February 15, 1906; June 7, 1906; March 28, 1907; and May 11, 1905).

47 I deal with early feminists' ideas concerning eugenics in my book. See note 2.

48 Elizabeth Cady Stanton to Martha Wright, June 19, 1871, Stanton Mss. This reference was brought to my attention by Ellen Dubois of SUNY-Buffalo; see also Stanton, *Eight Years After: Reminiscences, 1815–1897* (New York: Schocken, 1971), 262, 297.

49 Stanton and Blatch, *Stanton as Revealed in Her Letters, 132–33.*

50 *Papers and Letters,* Association for the Advancement of Women, 1873. The AAW was a conservative group formed in opposition to the Stanton-Anthony tendency. Nevertheless Chandler, a frequent contributor to Free Love journals, spoke here against undesired maternity and the identification of woman with her maternal function.

51 *Woodhull & Claflin's Weekly* 1, no. 20 (October 1, 1870): 10.

52 Woodhull, *Tried As by Fire,* 37; Lillian Harman, *The Regeneration of Society,* Speech before Manhattan Liberal Club, March 31, 1898 (Chicago: Light Bearer Library, 1900).

53 *Woodhull & Claflin's Weekly* 1, no. 20 (October 1, 1870): 10.

54 Ibid.

55 Harriot Stanton Blatch, "Voluntary motherhood," *Transactions,* National Council of Women of 1891, ed. Rachel Foster Avery (Philadelphia: J.B. Lippincott, 1891), 280.

56 Rachel Campbell, *The Prodigal Daughter; or, The Price of Virtue* (Grass Valley, Calif., 1885), 3. An essay read to the New England Free Love League, 1881.

57 *Woodhull & Claflin's Weekly* 1, no. 14 (August 13, 1870): 4.

58 In addition to the biography by Sachs mentioned above, see also Johanna Johnston, *Mrs. Satan* (New York: G.P. Putnam's Sons, 1967), and M.M. Marberry, *Vicky: A Biography of Victoria C. Woodhull* (New York: Funk & Wagnalls, 1967).

59 From an advertisement for her novel, *Perfect Motherhood: or, Mabel Raymond's Resolve* (New York: Murray Hill, 1890), in the *Next Revolution.*

60 Helen Hamilton Gardner, *Pulpit, Pew and Cradle* (New York: Truth Seeker Library, 1891), 22.

61 Even the most outspoken of the Free Lovers had conventional, role-differentiated images of sexual relations. Here is Angela Heywood, for example: "Men must not emasculate themselves for the sake of 'virtue,' they must, they will, recognize manliness and the life element of manliness as the fountain source of good manners. Women and girls demand strong, well-bred, generative, vitalizing sex ability. Potency, virility, is the grand basic principle of man, and it holds him clean, sweet and elegant, to the delicacy of his counterpart," From *The Word* 14, no. 2 (June 1885):3.

62 Woodhull, *The Scare-Crows;* Charlotte Perkins Gilman, *Concerning Children* (Boston: Small, Maynard, 1900).

63 See for example Blatch, "Voluntary motherhood," 283–84.

64 *The Word* 20, no. 8 (February 1893): 3.

65 Ibid.

8

Patterns of Abortion and the Response of American Physicians, 1790–1930

JAMES C. MOHR

Abortion has been practiced in the United States since the founding of the republic, though both its social character and its demographic impact have varied considerably. In the late eighteenth century, Americans viewed abortion primarily as the recourse of women who wanted to rid themselves of pregnancies that resulted from illicit relationships. Medical guides contained abortion-related information and abortifacient recipes, and physicians could and did terminate pregnancies when confronted with various sorts of medical situations or with requests from their patients. But it is unlikely that abortion played a significant role in regulating the fertility of American women prior to 1800.[1] Indeed, it is unlikely that anything played a significant role in regulating the fertility of American women prior to 1800, for birthrates in the United States at the end of the eighteenth century exceeded any ever recorded in Europe. As Americans began to reduce those record high rates, however, the place of abortion in American life changed dramatically.

The most striking change was a sharp rise in the incidence of abortion in the United States after 1830, as the nation underwent a demographic transition to lower birthrates that has since become recognized as quite typical of modernizing societies. Demographers point out that abortion has often played a key in these transitions during the twentieth century. Abdel Omran, for example, basing his opinion on the experiences of Japan and Chile, has observed "that when developing societies are highly motivated to accelerate their transition from high to low fertility, induced abortion becomes such a popular method of fertility control that it becomes a kind of epidemic."[2] Students of

JAMES C. MOHR is Professor of History at the University of Maryland Baltimore County, Baltimore, Maryland.

the modernization of Europe have alluded to similar trends there as well.[3] The testimony of scores of nineteenth-century observers now indicates conclusively that the United States was no exception to this common pattern. Contemporaries repeatedly asserted that abortion was a quantitatively significant factor in the reduction of American birthrates during the middle decades of the nineteenth century, and they would almost certainly have agreed with Omran's use of the word "epidemic."

The exact dimensions of that "epidemic" cannot be calculated with precision. Historians must rely upon indirect evidence and contemporary estimates. But the best-informed and most systematic observers at the time were convinced that American women were aborting at least one of every five pregnancies by midcentury.[4] Many analysts considered that ratio too conservative and placed the incidence of abortion much higher. Contemporaries also agreed that most of the women who were practicing abortion by the middle decades of the nineteenth century were married, white, and native born. Prominent among them were young wives who wished to delay childbearing and middle-aged women who already had as many children as they wanted. In short, abortion had shifted from being a marginal practice of the desperate few to being a quantitatively significant factor in the effort of American women to regulate their own fertility.[5]

Abortion was certainly not the only, or even the primary, factor in America's demographic transition. Recent research confirms the fact that contraceptive information was also being widely disseminated throughout the United States after 1830, and that some of the techniques advocated were at least partially effective even by modern standards.[6] Yet modern demographers have noticed the paradox that an increased use of contraceptive techniques has frequently led to an increase rather than a decrease in abortion rates, at least in the short run. This is explained by the theory that people beginning to use contraceptive techniques have made a commitment to limit the size of their families, but lack experience with the methods of contraception they have decided to try. The result is a high rate of "mistakes," or unwanted conceptions, and a consequent turning to abortion to erase them. This has occurred in twentieth-century societies, even when the contraceptive techniques themselves were extremely effective once mastered.[7]

In the United States during the nineteenth century several successive generations of Americans were introduced to new contraceptive techniques over a period of several decades and were making mistakes with them. They were also burdened with the additional handicap that the techniques themselves were frequently unreliable even when mastered. This must have greatly extended the period of reliance on abortion as a quantitatively significant backstop for women who sought to limit the number or to determine the spacing of their children in nineteenth-century America. Consequently, the gradual commitment of Americans to contraceptive practices after the 1830s paradoxically increases, rather than decreases, the likelihood that contemporary observers who testified to the existence of a great upsurge of abortion in the United States during the middle decades of the nineteenth century were right.

Further evidence of the widespread practice of abortion in the United States during the nineteenth century can be found in the fact that it became commercialized as early as the 1840s. Specialists advertised in the daily press their willingness to provide abortion services. Pharmaceutical firms competed with one another in the lucrative marketplace of purported abortifacients. Local apothecaries did a brisk business in such substances as cottonroot, which was never prescribed in regular medical practice but had a popular reputation as a mild and effective emmenagogue.[8]

Underlying the increased practice of abortion in nineteenth-century America lay two important factors. The first was the nearly universal adherence among Americans to the old common law notion of quickening. The vast majority of American women did not consider a prequickened fetus

a distinct human being with a separate existence of its own. The historical evidence in support of this point is overwhelming. Both those who accepted the new role of abortion in American life and those who abhorred it concurred in this judgment. The great dividing line in the minds of most Americans was set at quickening, the perception of fetal movement near the midpoint of gestation, not at conception. Abortions accomplished before quickening were on a continuum extending back through the various forms of contraception, not on a continuum reaching forward toward the various degrees of murder. Legislators often reflected this popular attitude by linking abortion and contraception together in the regulatory statutes they began to pass near midcentury.[9]

The second factor, closely related to the first, was the legal status of abortion in the United States prior to the Civil War. A few states, frightened by the nation's declining birthrates, had moved to discourage the practice, but not to outlaw it. A few others, offended by the commercialization of abortion services, had enacted antiadvertising laws, but they were pitifully weak. And several states had put forward criminal statutes designed to punish abortionists who harmed their patients. But the quickening doctrine remained in effect in every jurisdiction in the United States as late as 1860, essentially unchanged from the days of British and colonial common law. Under this doctrine, the performance of an abortion, provided it took place prior to quickening and provided the woman was not injured, was not an indictable action.[10]

The second of these factors was the first to change. The nation's regular physicians, those who favored formal education and scientific research, mounted a major campaign to stamp out the epidemic of abortion in America. They undertook their crusade for a number of complex, interrelated, and overlapping reasons. First, they knew that gestation was a continuous process and that quickening was a relatively unimportant event in the development of a fetus. In the absence of any other dramatic event, they decided that the interruption of gestation at any given point after conception, even early in a pregnancy, was just as logically unjustifiable, and hence immoral, as interruption at any other given point, including late in pregnancy. Second, they considered themselves the supreme champions of life as an absolute value, including fetal life. This was an important part of their ideology, and it was embodied in the Hippocratic oath to which they were pledged. They were bitterly disappointed that the nation's mainstream Protestant denominations quietly but consistently rebuffed their pleas to join the antiabortion crusade of the post–Civil War era; right through the early decades of the twentieth century medical journals would remain full of grumbling about the reluctance of Protestant clergymen to denounce abortions as sinful under any circumstances. Third, many regular physicians tended to be both nativistic and antifeminist; they attacked abortion with "race suicide" arguments and "women's place" arguments. Finally, regular physicians recognized in antiabortion statutes a way to deploy the powers of the state against their irregular rivals in the medical field, especially midwives, botanics, and folk healers. In short, the abortion issue combined for many nineteenth-century physicians both their ideological world view and their professional self-interest.[11]

Organized under the auspices of the American Medical Association and its affiliates at the state and local level, and coordinated by a Harvard-trained obstetrician, Horatio Robinson Storer, this campaign peaked in the late 1860s and early 1870s. Using their organizational skills, their political influence, and their social standing, the physicians persuaded many state legislators to drop traditional quickening rules from their criminal codes, to revoke common law immunities for women undergoing abortions, and to enlist the peripheral powers of the state, such as the definition of what was obscene, in support of the physicians' great crusade to reverse the surging incidence of abortion in the United States. The effect was to proscribe most, but not all, types of abortions as illegal actions carrying criminal penalties. Many of the statutes passed by the separate states during the post–Civil War period remained literally unchanged through the 1960s; others were altered only in legal phraseology, not in basic philosophy. Taken as a whole, those laws established the official policies toward the practice of abortion that most Americans would live with through the first two-thirds of the twentieth century.[12]

Official policy, however, does not always reflect public practice. This, to put it mildly, seems to have been the case with abortion in the United States. A series of events in Chicago neatly illustrated the situation during the first decade of the twentieth century. There, fired by the embarrassing and disturbing anomaly that their city was both the recognized abortion center of the Midwest and headquarters to the American Medical Association, which had spearheaded the drive to outlaw abortion in the United States, members of the Chicago Medical Society voted in January 1904 to explore what might be done to eliminate the practice in their area. Their president-elect believed that some ten thousand abortions were being performed annually in his city, despite prohibitive legislation that dated from 1867 and 1872.

As its first major step, the medical society staged a symposium on the problem of abortion in Chicago. It was held November 23, 1904, at the public library and proved highly successful. Leading legal scholars, the coroner of Cook County, and a spokesman for the city's Catholic hierarchy joined the physicians in offering papers; the assistant state's attorney, the registrar of vital statistics, the superintendent of the Chicago Home and Aid Society, and chief counsel for the Woman's Protective Association were among the participating discussants. All agreed that abortion was every bit as prevalent as the physicians feared, all agreed that something should be done about it, and all agreed to cooperate with the physicians in their efforts to enforce the state's antiabortion laws.

During the early months of 1905, members of the Chicago Medical Society, working with the Woman's Protective Association, persuaded some of the city's newspapers to drop the thinly disguised abortion-related advertisements they had been carrying. With the help of the state's attorney, the medical society also initiated prosecutions of two suspected abortionists in test cases. On the strength of these early successes the physicians decided to make their campaign an ongoing project, and they formally amended the constitution of the Chicago Medical Society in February 1906, to establish the Committee on Criminal Abortion as a permanent standing committee with "the right to co-operate with the proper legal authorities and with similar committees from other organizations whose purpose is the betterment of social conditions." Dr. Rudolph Weiser Holmes, a thirty-five-year-old obstetrician and gynecologist, became the committee's first permanent chairman. In May, the doctors agreed to back Holmes's effort financially, should private contributions fail to cover his committee's expenses.

Holmes increased the pressure on Chicago's newspapers by visiting the editorial offices of each one accompanied by an attorney from the Legal Aid Society, a Paulist father, and the medical society's own special counsel, Joseph I. Kelly. Their moral suasion induced a few more dailies to suspend abortifacient advertisements, and a postal "stop order" that Kelly obtained April 21, 1907, coerced the rest. In May of that year the Holmes committee triumphantly reported to the medical society that "the lay press had eliminated from their columns all advertisements pertaining to criminal abortion." Working with the coroner, the Cook County grand jury, and their own special counsel, the Holmes committee had also helped indict six more of the city's most notorious abortionists. Actions were pending against others. At the June meeting of the medical society, there was talk of persuading the governor to appoint a special assistant state's attorney, whose sole function would be to carry on the physicians' campaign against abortion in Chicago.[13]

But no special assistant state's attorney was ever appointed. Instead, abortion-related advertisements began to reappear in the daily press, and one paper claimed those advertisements were worth some $50,000 per paper per year in revenue. Indictments were dropped for lack of evidence; juries usually refused to convict in the few cases that were carried forward. The press alleged that city officials had begun again to accept payoffs from abortionists in exchange for protection and immunity. A state legislator was said to be financially involved in one of Chicago's largest abortion hospitals. When it became clear that many of Chicago's abortions were being performed by medical society members, for whatever reasons, most physicians began to close ranks and to testify to one another's good standing and sound medical judgment. The permanent Committee on Criminal Abortion stopped reporting regularly to the medical society. In short, the crusade that seemed so successful in June 1907 was nearly defunct by 1908, four years after it began.

Holmes himself explained what had happened. Responding to a paper on criminal abortion that

was read to the American Medical Association convention in 1908, Holmes minced no words:

> I have had the misfortune for three years to be a sort of mentor on criminal abortion work in Chicago. During this period I have presided over a committee of the Chicago Medical Society to investigate, and to attempt to eradicate the evil; I have come to the conclusion that the public does not want, the profession does not want, the women in particular do not want, any aggressive campaign against the crime of abortion.

Holmes's fellow Chicagoan, Dr. R. S. Yarros, supported the same contention. "To formulate laws and have them enacted is comparatively easy," observed Yarros. "To enforce a law is an entirely different thing. You can not enforce laws, as some of the speakers have already said, with which the public has little sympathy."[14] A prominent attorney told the Chicago Gynecological Society in 1910 that the nation's antiabortion laws were almost invariably enforced for murder, rather than for abortion per se; "the authorities ordinarily do not wake up unless the victim dies." The United States, he concluded, was simply "hypocritical" on the subject of abortion.[15]

Reports from elsewhere around the country confirmed the experience of Chicago's physicians. In St. Louis, for example, the commissioner of health assigned his assistant commissioner the job of cracking down on the continued practice of abortion. In November 1907, the assistant commissioner obtained a bench order similar to the one issued seven months earlier in Chicago that temporarily banned abortion-related advertising in the local press, and he organized a committee of physicians who agreed to help the district attorney prosecute some of the city's most flagrant practitioners.[16] But by the end of 1908, everyone involved had given up the effort. A member of the physicians' committee of St. Louis complained that he "had wasted much time in court without results. . . . The average jury does not seem inclined to convict" even the most outrageous abortionist.[17]

Dr. William R. Nicholson of Philadelphia, addressing a joint meeting of the Obstetrical Societies of Philadelphia and New York, explained the lack of progress against abortion in his city on the grounds that the practice was "enshrined in the affections of a very large portion of the community" and it was "not considered as evil by them."[18] A colleague from New York agreed:

> I would say to Doctor Nicholson that over here in New York, not only is abortion a national failing, but it is becoming a Metropolitan characteristic. In fact, my experience indicates to me, that it is a very profitable and persistent pursuit for a great many physicians, and so much so, that they are successful professionally and financially, and are very much respected members of the community. I do not expect to tell you how we get after the abortionists over here, but I am glad to tell you how popular abortionists are with the public, and also to tell you with what measure of success we have met in punishing them. . . . In the last ten years we have managed to convict and sentence three abortionists. One of them was caught red-handed, was convicted, received six months and served them. The other two, in this County, were "framed-up." . . . All three of those gentlemen, however, such was their influence and experience (one of them had two former District Attorneys to represent him) were pardoned by the Governor. That is the net result of our prosecution.[19]

Other members of the New York society concurred, citing examples of the unwillingness of juries to convict persons indicted for performing an abortion unless the person was simply incompetent.[20] Physicians in Ohio had reached a similar conclusion by 1914. It was "more or less futile for doctors and lawyers to discuss this question," said Dr. J. W. Rowe. "Criminal abortion is performed all the time . . . and the law does not convict."[21]

Perhaps H. N. Hawkins, an attorney from Denver, assessed the situation best. His local medical society had called a symposium in 1903 to discuss criminal abortion, and the society asked Hawkins for advice. In essence, Hawkins told the physicians not to waste their time. Abortion was rampant in Colorado, he explained, despite adequate prohibitions, because "the people do not really feel very harshly toward the abortionist. It is only when a

bungling job is done, where a woman is killed, that public outcry is heard."[22]

Hawkins's opinion remained a reasonably accurate assessment of American attitudes for the next half-century. There is a great deal of evidence that the nation's criminal statutes on the subject of abortion were invoked during the first half of the twentieth century almost exclusively against those who harmed women; invoked, in other words, to *regulate* the practice of abortion, not to eliminate it. Even then, sanctions were usually brought against midwives or renegades, rarely against regular physicians. Cynics might even see such highly selective enforcement as a form of quality control, consciously or unconsciously condoned by the physicians, the public authorities, and the people. In any event, beneath the veil of illegality and prohibition, Americans continued to seek and receive abortion services. And there is also a great deal of evidence that most of those services were provided by regular private physicians, notwithstanding the official public position of the American Medical Association and its constituent societies.[23] This is not to say that the social character of abortion did not change in the twentieth century as the result of late-nineteenth-century legislation. The practice was no longer so commercially visible in the American press, for example, and few voices defended the practice publicly as some of the nation's irregular medical practitioners had done in the nineteenth century. But abortion certainly did not disappear in the United States as a result of the statutes designed to outlaw it.

The most significant social shifts in the historical role of abortion that did take place in the early twentieth century probably had less to do with official proscription than with two related demographic factors. The first was the spread of contraceptive sophistication among those groups that had accounted for the increased incidence of abortion since the middle decades of the nineteenth century: married, white, native-born women. The economic demographers Paul David and Warren Sanderson, for example, discovered that "native born white women of native parentage living in Rhode Island, Cleveland and Minneapolis had lower cumulative fertility in 1900 than did similar women in the United States in 1970."[24] Contemporaries and historians agreed that those low rates were attributable primarily to the increased use and effectiveness of contraception. To put it differently, as contraceptive techniques improved, abortion declined as a primary method of family limitation among native-born American women. For most of those people, abortion once again took on the character it had at the outset of the nineteenth century; it was a discreet way to terminate an indiscreet pregnancy. The net result, based upon contemporary observations and impressions, appears to have been a leveling off, and perhaps a modest decrease, in the rate of abortion in the country as a whole during the first three decades of the twentieth century. The most thorough analyst of abortion patterns in the United States between 1900 and 1936, Dr. Frederick Taussig of Washington University, believed that the ratio of abortions in the United States had fallen to fewer than one for every seven confinements by the turn of the twentieth century, and, significantly, that illegitimacy was "the dominant factor" among those who continued to have abortions.[25]

The second factor involves the somewhat contradictory observation that abortion rates, even while leveling off in the nation as a whole, probably increased among lower-class, especially immigrant, women in the United States during the first third of the twentieth century. Again, contemporary observers certainly believed that this was the case, as anyone familiar with the career of Margaret Sanger will quickly remember.[26] Moreover, demographers have witnessed similar patterns in other societies. To quote Omran once again:

> In the early stage of transition [to low birthrates], the socially mobile, upper stratum of society adopts small family-size norms more readily and frequently resorts to induced abortion to limit births. With a rise in educational levels and a stabilization of family-size norms, this group turns increasingly to contraception. Yet while the need to resort to abortion decreases for the upper stratum, the abortion wave is maintained, often at epidemic level, because each of the lower strata cohorts also pass [sic] through a state of abortion proneness.[27]

The final significant shift in the historical character of abortion in the United States prior to World War II took place at the onset of the great depression. Taussig amassed data that indicate a gradual increase in abortion rates from 1900 through 1928, with a temporary peak during the hard years right after World War I, followed by a sharp and dramatic upsurge as soon as the Depression struck. By the mid-1930s Taussig calculated that there was one abortion for every four pregnancies in the United States, and he pointed out that 90 percent of those abortions were being performed upon married women. Abortion had once again become a significant factor in regulating fertility generally, and marital fertility specifically, in the United States.[28]

Among the explanations offered for the resurgence of abortion in America during the 1930s, two stand out. One was the obvious fact that far more women found themselves in the plight immigrants had faced two decades before. It was as if Omran's "wave" hit bottom and began to well back up through the social structure. It is unlikely, however, that the increase in abortion during the 1930s represents a conscious choice to abandon contraception as a prime means of fertility control. It is more reasonable to assume that the difference between abortion rates in the 1920s and those in the 1930s approximates the national "mistake rate" in the use of contraception. During the 1920s, many women may have been willing, however reluctantly, to accept many of those "mistakes," so abortion rates remained low. In the 1930s, however, they were too desperate to continue to be willing to do so, and took action to erase the mistakes, thus raising the national abortion rates.

The second factor was the shifting role of women in American society. Recent research and modern experience both confirm Taussig's insightful suggestion that the changing place of abortion in the United States, as early as the 1930s, was also related to what he called "the revolt of womankind against the age-long domination of man" and "to the right of women to control their own bodies."[29] In short, two of the underlying historical patterns that would help produce a shift in official policy during the 1960s and 1970s, the renewed importance of abortion as a method of fertility control and the desire of women to determine for themselves without state interference when they wished to carry a pregnancy to term, had already been established by World War II.

NOTES

1 James C. Mohr, *Abortion in America: the Origins and Evolution of National Policy 1800–1900* (New York, 1978), 3–19.

2 Abdel R. Omran, "Abortion in the demographic transition," in *Rapid Population Growth: Consequences and Policy Implications,* report of a study committee of the National Academy of Sciences (Baltimore, 1971), 481.

3 See, for example, David V. Glass, *Population Policies and Movements in Europe* (New York, [1940] 1967), 278–82; and Edward Shorter, "Female emancipation, birth control, and fertility in European history," *American Historical Review* 78, no. 3 (June 1973): 605–40.

4 Horatio R. Storer and Franklin Fiske Heard, *Criminal Abortion: Its Nature, Its Evidence, and Its Law* (Cambridge, Mass., 1868) and Edwin M. Hale, *A Systematic Treatise on Abortion* (Chicago, 1866).

5 Mohr, *Abortion in America,* 46–118.

6 James Reed, *From Private Vice to Public Virtue: The Birth Control Movement and American Society since 1830* (New York, 1978).

7 Omran, "Abortion in the demographic transition," 508–11.

8 Mohr, *Abortion in America,* 46–118.

9 Ibid., passim.

10 Ibid., 119–46.

11 Ibid., 147–99. For twentieth-century examples of physicians' disgust with the clergy, see remarks of W. H. Wathen and J. A. Stucky in *Kentucky Medical Journal* 2, no. 4 (Sept. 1904), 98–99 and Walter B. Dorsett, "Criminal abortion in its broadest sense," *Journal of the American Medical Association* 51, no. 12 (Sept. 1908): 957.

12 Mohr, *Abortion in America,* 200–245.

13 The foregoing activities of the Chicago Medical Society are documented from their own Minutes, 1904–7, which are in the Manuscript Division of the Chicago Historical Society. I am indebted to Archie Motley and Edna Vanek for their help in surveying this unpublished material.

14 Discussion, *Journal of the American Medical Association,* 51, no. 2 (Sept. 19, 1908): 960–61.

15 Sigmond Zeisler, "The legal and moral aspects of abortion," *Surgery, Gynecology, and Obstetrics,* 1910, *10:* 539.

16 William B. Winn, "Midwifery in its relation to abortion and the laws of the state of Missouri," *Weekly Bulletin of the St. Louis Medical Society* 3, no. 5 (February 4, 1909): 58–61, 64.

17 Discussion of Dr. Ehrenfest, ibid., no. 7 (February 18, 1909): 87.

18 William R. Nicholson, "When, under the present code of medical ethics, is it justifiable to terminate pregnancy, before the third month; what should our attitude be toward a patient upon whom a criminal operation has been performed; what should be our attitude toward those suspected of the performance of criminal operations?" *American Journal of Obstetrics,* 1914, *69:* 1010.

19 Discussion of A. C. Vandiver, ibid., 1027.

20 Ibid., 125–35.

21 Discussion of J. W. Rowe following William Gillespie, "Abortion: with special reference to its medicolegal aspects," *Lancet-Clinic* 113, no. 4 (January 23, 1915): 140.

22 H. N. Hawkins, "The practical working of the law against criminal abortion," *Colorado Medical Journal* 9, no. 4 (April 1903): 153–56.

23 Frederick J. Taussig, *Abortion, Spontaneous and Induced: Medical and Social Aspects* (St. Louis, 1936).

24 Paul A. David and Warren C. Sanderson, "Contraceptive technology and fertility control in Victorian America: from facts to theories," Memorandum No. 202, Center for Research in Economic Growth, Stanford University, June 1976.

25 Taussig, *Abortion,* 388 and 391.

26 David M. Kennedy, *Birth Control in America: The Career of Margaret Sanger* (New Haven, 1970) and Mohr, *Abortion in America,* 238–45.

27 Omran, "Abortion in the Demographic Transition," 512.

28 Taussig, *Abortion,* 361–96, 438–41.

29 Ibid., 390.

9

Doctors, Birth Control, and Social Values, 1830–1970

JAMES REED

The history of medical attitudes toward birth control in the United States provides a stark example of the extent to which social values sometimes shape medical practice regardless of the knowledge and technology available to the profession. From the 1830s, when the practice of family limitation first became a subject of broad public debate, until the marketing of the birth control pill in the early 1960s, the majority of doctors viewed the desire for fewer children as a problem rather than as an opportunity to provide a medical service. They associated birth control with threats to the social order that they served and to their profession.[1]

Beginning in the late nineteenth century, generation after generation of Americans had progressively fewer children despite the wails of social leaders that they were shirking their patriotic duty, committing "race suicide," sinning against nature.[2] Before the 1960s, "the population problem," in the United States was a dearth of people of the "right kind."[3] Doctors, like other social arbiters, persistently complained of the low birth rate among the middle classes, a result, they claimed, of the selfish hedonism of the socially ambitious. While the "best" people too often avoided parenthood, the poor and foreign born seemed to multiply with abandon, raising the spectre of a tragic decline in the quality of the population. By the early 1930s, Americans were reproducing at a rate that would have resulted in a stationary or declining population, if it had continued. The end of population growth seemed to be at hand, and with it the prospect of

economic stagnation and national decline. Americans regained the will to multiply with wartime prosperity, but in 1960, as in 1830, the healthy woman was defined as a willing mother who wanted to do her part to bolster the sagging population growth rate. The unwilling mother was sick or confused, and her reluctance to procreate a sad commentary on social conditions.

Despite the dominant pronatalist values of American culture, large numbers of married Americans learned to control their fertility. Their restrictive behavior reflected decisions made within the family, for private reasons, in the absence of broadly recognized social justification or public sanction for family limitation. The great majority of would-be contraceptors succeeded or failed without the aid of a doctor. Businessmen who promoted powders and appliances for "feminine hygiene," marginal physicians, and quacks filled the void left by the indifference of medical leaders to the widespread, if semi-licit, demand for contraceptive advice. Birth control became associated with the patent medicine business and irregular practice, and with the threat which they posed to the economic and social status of the ethical physician. The reluctance of physicians to provide contraceptive services was not, however, a result of the association of birth control with quackery. Rather, medical leaders left birth control to the second-rate and the disreputable because of their commitment to the maintenance of social order as they understood it. The association of birth control with quackery was a result, rather than a cause, of the physicians' reluctance to provide services.[4]

If nineteenth-century medical men had wanted to provide reliable contraceptive means to the public, the requisite technology and knowledge of the process of conception were available. Historians

JAMES REED is Associate Professor of History at Rutgers University, New Brunswick, New Jersey.

Reprinted with permission from *The Therapeutic Revolution: Essays in the Social History of Human Medicine* ed. by Morris J. Vogel and Charles E. Rosenberg (Philadelphia: University of Pennsylvania Press, 1979), pp. 109–134.

have sometimes asserted that there were no "scientific" birth control methods available in the nineteenth century, but by 1865 rubber condoms, vaginal diaphragms, spermicidal douches, and the "infertile period" had all been described in popular medical manuals that were sold to the public.[5] Although Margaret Sanger led a successful campaign to popularize the spring-loaded diaphragm in the 1920s, there were no fundamental advances in contraceptive technology from the middle of the nineteenth century until the marketing of the birth control pill in 1960.[6] Sanger's crusade° for birth control was necessary because the great majority of physicians did not perceive contraception as an important problem. Their attitudes had little to do with the birth control means available. Birth control methods were damned as unreliable and unsafe because of their association with apparent threats to stable family life—specifically, the growing hedonism of a consumer society, the dissatisfaction of middle-class women with the social roles assigned to them, and the decline in birthrates among the "fit."

While attitudes toward sex, women, and the family were the most important determinants of medical opinion on contraception, doctors shared these attitudes with the great majority of respectable people. Since the integrity of any profession depends on public support, doctors could not have taken radical public positions on any sexual question without endangering their status. Before the rise of modern medicine, the physician's central role was to comfort and to reassure by interpreting the natural order, by explaining the sources of disease in the individual's failure to observe the laws of nature and of society.[7] Since his professional position depended on this essentially priestly function, he could hardly question the prevailing standards of sexual morality. Duty dictated, in fact, that he provide disease sanctions for them.[8]

The development of a somatic pathology, anesthesia, antisepsis, and bacteriology during the nineteenth century improved the physician's ability to prevent and to cure disease, but these gains did not lessen his profession's dependence on community support. If the new doctor was to be a scientist, then huge sums of money would have to be raised to subsidize medical education, and the new university-affiliated medical schools would need access to public hospitals and to the patients who provided subjects for both student and researcher. The newly rich found medical education and research especially attractive because these endeavors seemed to be unquestionable public benefits, philanthropies that minimized the risk of criticism for misusing the power represented by money. The continuing flow of philanthropic dollars into the new medical establishment depended, however, on a reputation for social service rather than criticism, especially not criticism of "civilized morality." It was appropriate that "the" man in gynecology at Johns Hopkins, during its era as the symbol of scientific medicine, was Howard Kelly, a Christian gentleman, well known for his piety and prudery, who had no interest in contraception or any kind of sex research.[9]

The demands of Margaret Sanger and other sexual reformers that physicians learn contraceptive technique and engage in contraceptive research were anathema to most physicians on two counts. First, they offended the sensibilities of medical men as social arbiters who wholeheartedly shared their society's values and who were reticent about birth control, not because of moral cowardice, as Sanger claimed, but because they, along with other respectable people, thought that women needed to have more children. Second, sexual reform threatened physicians as professionals who were dependent on the public's goodwill for the legislation and institutional support required if standards of education and practice were to be raised.

The career of James Marion Sims, the founder of American gynecology, illustrates the close relationship between the social attitudes of medical leaders and the services that they offered. Sims gained international fame in the 1850s by developing an operation for repair of tears in the bladder (vesicovaginal fistula), a common childbirth injury that had formerly doomed thousands of women to live out their lives continuously soaked with urine. He devoted a large part of his practice, however, to the treatment of sterility, and most of his classic *Clinical Notes on Uterine Surgery* (1866) was devoted to the dozens of elaborate, ingenious, and sometimes painful methods that he developed to help women conceive. He shared the prevailing sexual ideology which viewed all healthy women as willing mothers, and he ignored contraceptive technique. In an age when hysterectomy was a high-risk procedure, even the great surgeons like Sims relied heavily on pessaries in the treatment of uterine prolapse, and Sims described dozens of pessaries for various purposes, including a spring-loaded rubber ring that resembled in all but contraceptive intent the vaginal diaphragms used in twentieth-century birth control clinics. The popular medical journalist Edward Bliss Foote provided his lay readers with a description of a contraceptive "womb veil" (essentially a diaphragm) in *Medical Common Sense* (1864), but Sims, like most specialists in women's diseases, devoted himself solely to helping women become mothers, leaving contraception to the second-rate or the quack. As an expert in the fitting of pessaries, Sims was, if anything, more capable of designing and fitting a contraceptive diaphragm than physicians of the 1920s, when this device began to be widely used by American women. He chose not to, largely, it appears, because he did not feel that his society needed efficient contraception.[10]

After the passage of the Comstock Act (1873), it was illegal to give contraceptive advice, and the subject was omitted from post-1873 editions of many books in which it had originally been given space. Some physicians were prosecuted under the Comstock Act, but the suppression of birth control information was but a small part of a great crusade to make American cities safe for middle-class families through the suppression of commercial vice.[11] Some medical leaders were in sympathy with the purity crusaders. Others clashed with them, suffered humiliating defeats, and learned that it was the duty of their profession to defend the highest moral standards of the community. In 1874, Sims, president of the American Medical Association (AMA), recommended a national system of regulation for prostitution as a means of controlling venereal disease, but the effort to mobilize the medical profession for regulation was defeated by purity lobbyists who argued that the only acceptable venereal disease prophylaxis was a moral one, a single high standard for all, male and female. By 1894 the president of the New York Academy of Medicine endorsed efforts to collect physicians' signatures on a petition stating that chastity was in accord with the laws of health. The "new abolitionists" had taught doctors that sexual matters were to be treated with great seriousness.[12]

It is difficult, however, to estimate just how large an impact Comstockery had on medical behavior. Physicians seem to have been much more concerned over the apparently rising tide of marital unhappiness that they witnessed and by the low birthrate among their paying customers than with either the safety or legality of birth control.[13] In 1898, the Physicians Club of Chicago sponsored a symposium on "sexual hygiene" in order to provide a forum for a frank exchange of information that would help local doctors to become better marriage counselors. One of the participants explained, "Outside the medical profession it is taken for granted that the doctors know all about these things [sex]. But within our ranks we are aware that this is not true. The text-books omit this department." The public increasingly turned to physicians instead of to the clergy for sex advice, but some doctors were willing to admit, at least among themselves, that they had insufficient knowledge of the subject. An edited transcript of the symposium was published as a "for doctors only" handbook, entitled *Sexual Hygiene*, in an effort to meet the need for information.[14]

The editors of *Sexual Hygiene* believed that husbands bore a major share of the blame for the marital unhappiness that seemed to be reaching epidemic proportions. Too many of them were ignorant of, or ignored, the sexual needs of their wives. Husbands had to be taught that "the god-given relation is two-sided, and that without harmony and mutual enjoyment it becomes a mere masturbation to the body and mind of the one who alone is gratified." Perhaps better marital sex would lower the divorce rate and keep both husbands and wives at home, where they belonged.[15]

One chapter of *Sexual Hygiene* was devoted to contraception. Contributors ignored the illegality of contraceptive advice and accepted birth control as a necessary means, in some cases, of reconciling the economic and personal interests of husbands and wives. They knew of numerous methods, but birth control information had to be given with discretion. There were situations in which it should be kept from patients. "We all know perfectly the difference between the dragged-out woman on the verge of consumption . . . and the society belle who mistakenly thinks she does not want babies when every fiber of her being is crying out for this means of bringing her back to healthy thought."[16]

This ambiguous attitude toward birth control was

most strikingly revealed in a long discussion of contraceptive methods. The strong willed might try "limiting intercourse to the period from the sixteenth day after menstruation to the twenty-fifth." Men could practice withdrawal or use condoms. The condom was very effective, "if the best are used, but we all know that rubber is a non-conductor of electricity, and this is a factor that I think should not be lost sight of. They are not the easiest thing in the world to put on either."[17]

While a highly effective and safe contraceptive was mocked because it interfered with male pleasure, female methods received indiscriminate endorsement. "The little sponge in a silk net with string attached is a familiar sight in drug stores. If this is moistened with some acid or antiseptic solution before use and rightly placed it is very safe and harmless." In addition to the sponge, would-be female contraceptors might choose either douching, or "a vaginal suppository of cocoa butter and ten per cent of boric and tannic acids," or "the womb veil with eighty grams of quinine mutate to an ounce of petrolatum." All seemed to work well enough. The chief complaint against intra-uterine stem pessaries was that "there are many women who cannot place them." A final bit of advice was offered for the women who wanted to avoid having children without good reason. "Get a divorce and vacate the position for some other woman, who is able and willing to fulfill all a wife's duties as well as to enjoy her privileges."[18]

Although these physicians knew of many female methods, they expressed no concern with making distinctions between them or for the problems that women might have in using them. Systematic clinical evaluation of birth control would not begin until the 1920s, when minor improvements in the "womb veil" or vaginal diaphragm would provide the most effective female method available until the marketing of the anovulant pill in 1960. Serious study of birth control methods might have begun in the late nineteenth century, since, as the discussion of birth control methods in *Sexual Hygiene* makes clear, both the necessary technology and knowledge of sexual anatomy were available, but doctors did not make any major efforts to improve contraceptive means. Since the family might be weakened if sex was too easily separated from procreation, doctors believed that they had a social obligation to carefully manage the dissemination

of birth control. Indeed, in the case of the "society belle" or other healthy woman who did not want children, their duty was to force "her back to healthy thought." In this context doctors were not greatly concerned over the failure rates of birth control regimens.[19]

The major impetus for change in the status of contraception came during the first half of the twentieth century from lay women rather than from within the medical profession, but they were aided by some allies among medical men, most notably Robert Latou Dickinson.[20] Organized medicine could never accept demands from lay women, especially not from Margaret Sanger, a sexual reformer and biting critic of the profession. Dickinson played the role of mediator through whom organized medicine finally made its peace with the birth control movement. His personal lobbying led to a 1937 AMA resolution recognizing that informing patients about contraceptive methods was an important medical subject that should be taught in medical schools.

While Dickinson enjoyed considerable success in the role of medical educator, his own efforts to organize contraceptive research failed. Ironically, he was forced to depend on data from clinical investigations organized and directed by Margaret Sanger in his campaign to change medical opinion on birth control. His successful efforts during the 1920s to organize contraceptive research revealed the deep antagonism among his colleagues toward sexual reform and the barriers that even a distinguished gynecologist faced in attempting to study contraception.

Dickinson's social background and personal contacts were important sources of strength in his campaign to win medical support for birth control. His parents were prominent members of Brooklyn's social elite during the Gilded Age. He attended private schools in Europe, finished high school at Brooklyn Polytechnic, and began medical study at Long Island College Hospital in 1879, at the age of nineteen. He became the protégé of Alexander Skene, the modern discoverer of the paraurethral ducts in women ("Skene's glands"). Dickinson's artistic ability led to a job as illustrator for Skene's textbook, *Treatise on Diseases of Women* (1888), which dominated the American textbook market in gynecology for a decade.

Educated at a proprietary medical school in a

pre–Flexner Report system, Dickinson plunged into the business of ordinary practice upon graduation from Long Island College Hospital, in 1881, and found time to write only through driving self-discipline. He gradually won recognition as one of the country's leading specialists in the diseases of women and published prodigiously on questions of concern to the working practitioner of the art of medicine. He shed light on topics ranging from surgical technique to how to keep office records, but made no important contributions to the new science of obstetrics championed by J. Whitridge Williams of Johns Hopkins.[21]

Dickinson's lasting contributions to his specialty were made not as a surgeon or clinician, however, but as a sex researcher and reformer. Early in his career he became concerned over the contrast between his culture's genteel code of sexual morality and the behavior that he daily encountered as a doctor. In one of his early case histories, he wrote "Pregnant, have not asked particulars. I would never have believed it of this girl. My mother often praised her. . . ." He noticed frequent enlargements of the labia minora among his patients and traced deviations from normal sexual anatomy to masturbation, a practice that he found to be present among women of all classes and ages and not necessarily associated with any kind of antisocial behavior. Experience taught that there were probably as many induced abortions as live births in Brooklyn and that sexual incompatibility destroyed many marriages even when it did not lead to divorce. Dickinson responded to this sexual nightmare as a Christian gentleman with an empirical bent, by gathering information, consulting colleagues, and cautiously reporting his opinions through the proper channels. The correctness of his social and professional attitudes helped him to obtain a tolerant reception for his unorthodox work. His sex research always kept the goal of happy marriage in view. If sexual adjustment could be improved, then the family might be strengthened.[22]

Before he retired from active practice Dickinson published relatively little on sex, but the records he made of female sex anatomy in its diverse normal and pathological forms were unique in their quantity and accuracy. He recorded his observations in minute detail and then carefully compared and classified the specimens. Eventually providing a series stretching over forty years of practice, these records were a medical natural history and the essential source on which he later drew in founding American medical sex research.

Dickinson boasted that he always kept the perspective of the family physician, and his 1920 address as president of the American Gynecological Society (AGS) provides a sharp contrast with the scathing presidential rebuke delivered to the society by J. Whitridge Williams in 1914.[23] During the first decades of the century specialists in what Dickinson liked to call "uterology" (obstetrics and gynecology) were much concerned over the future of their group. The obstetrician had to compete with midwives and general practitioners, while general surgeons were performing the operations pioneered by gynecologists. Williams argued that the future of the speciality lay in basic research, in developing knowledge upon which a specialist's therapeutics could securely rest. Williams's attack on the generally "casuistical" and "sometimes puerile" publications of AGS members was self-conscious propaganda for the Johns Hopkins ideal and might be read as an attack on the tradition of education and practice that Dickinson exemplified. Dickinson lacked training in basic research but admitted no need to apologize for a career of healing and sexual counseling. He had devoted his life to "the study of womankind," and, like all great naturalists, he knew what could be discovered by the naked eye about his subject. In his 1920 presidential address, Dickinson argued that the future of the specialty depended on informed sexual counseling, and on modernizing the physician's traditional priestly role. He already had data in his own records to answer the rhetorical questions that he posed. What about the "distasteful" but burning issue of contraception? "What, indeed, is normal sex life?" He made a new career for himself. Retiring from active practice in 1920, Dickinson lived his own recommendation that "uterologists" take an "interest in sociological problems" falling within their domain and give serious attention to the social pathology caused by the conflict between the ideal and the real in the sexual realm.[24]

In 1916, Dickinson had urged a group of Chicago physicians to begin a clinical investigation of the safety and effectiveness of birth control methods. "We as a profession should take hold of this matter and not let it go to the radicals, and not let it receive harm by being pushed in any undignified or improper manner." When Margaret Sanger asked for his endorsement, he politely refused, but he believed that contraception was essential if normal marital relations were to be improved, so birth control was first on his agenda of topics that needed him. Having secured a grant from one of Sanger's disaffected supporters, in 1923 he began a search for institutional sponsorship for contraceptive research. The New York Obstetrical Society turned him down, but he was able to recruit some distinguished colleagues to serve on a Committee on Maternal Health, with temporary headquarters in Dickinson's apartment.[25]

Dickinson hoped that his Committee on Maternal Health would conduct authoritative investigations that would command the respect of the medical and philanthropic establishments and provide guidelines for ordered change. In January of 1923, Sanger opened the first physician-staffed birth control clinic in the United States, next door to the offices of the American Birth Control League, but the medical community was militantly opposed to the delivery of health care in "special" or extramural clinics, and Dickinson believed that the most efficient source for clinical data would be hospital outpatient departments. He hoped that the Committee on Maternal Health could provide contraceptive supplies and honorariums to the hospital clinic directors and then simply collect the records that would surely exceed those of Sanger's clinic in both quality and quantity.[26]

The first hitch in Dickinson's plan came when the diaphragms which he had ordered from Germany were confiscated by United States Customs despite a "gentlemen's agreement" that they would be allowed to pass. Sanger smuggled hers in. Since the committee forswore illegal activity, it could not provide clients with the most promising female contraceptive device. Finally, Sanger agreed to sell the committee diaphragms at cost from her own meagre supply.[27]

The second problem that stymied Dickinson's research was a lack of patients. His committee made up a rigid set of procedures that met all of the requirements of the New York law, which, thanks to a 1919 court decision engineered by Sanger, permitted contraceptive advice by a physician, but only "to cure or prevent disease." Thus, the committee required that all patients treated under its auspices have a written description from a gyne-

cologist of the medical indications justifying contraceptive advice. This requirement caused hospital physicians who were being paid by the committee to refer patients to them to send their patients to the Sanger clinic. One doctor explained, "However positive he might be that a certain patient would be in very grave danger if she conceived, yet he doubted whether he would be willing to put his name to a recommendation for contraceptive advice to be handed the patient, for fear of the use that might be put to such a paper." The committee even decided not to give slips of printed instructions to patients because they "might be copied or lost or other-wise convey information where it should not be available."[28]

Even with these stringent safeguards, hospital doctors refused to cooperate, despite generous monthly honorariums. One doctor received $125 and handed in six cases. In all, $1,500 brought only twenty-three patient records. Fitting diaphragms was just difficult enough to require special training and a willingness to devote time to work from which no professional prestige would result. With no glamor and some risk attached to this work, it was much easier to refuse advice or to send patients to the Sanger clinic, where female general practitioners were developing considerable skill in contraceptive technique.[29]

Dickinson finally gave up the effort to collect his own records and began a campaign to get Sanger to give control of her clinic to the committee. Sanger had never been able to obtain a dispensary license for the Birth Control Clinic Research Bureau, and she agreed to allow Dickinson to take over the bureau if he could obtain a license. The Rockefeller-funded Bureau of Social Hygiene provided a $10,000 grant for the first year of this arrangement. Dickinson recruited a staff of eminent medical men to serve as directors of the proposed Maternity Research Council, and only a dispensary license from the State Board of Charities was lacking to put the plan into effect. The Board of Charities admitted that all standard requirements had been met for a license but demanded a waiver from representatives of the Jewish, Protestant, and Roman Catholic faiths. Dickinson obtained waivers from Jewish and Protestant leaders but could get no response from the Catholic hierarchy of New York.[30]

Dickinson tried to get the Committee on Maternal Health to go ahead with the plan without a license, but the whole purpose of taking over the Sanger clinic had been to conduct a completely legal and ethical investigation, and the committee voted not to pursue further the plan to cooperate with Sanger. Sanger, however, had agreed to cooperate only on the condition that Dickinson provide what she could not—a license.

Although the clinic, staffed as it was by female general practitioners, had no specialists in gynecology, it did provide good records for analysis. By 1927, Dr. Hannah Stone, the clinic's medical director, had data to prove that the vaginal diaphragm was a safe and effective contraceptive. Dickinson was instrumental in getting these records published in 1928, although, characteristically, he promised more than he could deliver when he guaranteed Sanger that, if she would delay private publication, he would get Stone's article "Therapeutic Contraception" into either the *Journal of the American Medical Association* or the *American Journal of Obstetrics and Gynecology.* Both journals refused the article because the research was sponsored by Sanger. Stone's article finally appeared in the *Medical Journal and Record*, with a preface by Dickinson.[31]

Under Dickinson's direction it is doubtful that the Sanger clinic would have been able to find many women in the certified mortal danger required to meet the letter of the New York law. It was fortunate in this respect that Dickinson failed in his effort to capitalize on Sanger's goodwill with the fertile women of New York by taking control of her clinic. His frustrated adventure in clinical research under the auspices of the Committee on Maternal Health demonstrated, however, that it was impossible to conduct a clinical investigation of contraception that met all of the requirements of the law and of medical ethics.[32]

The rejection of Dr. Stone's pioneering analysis of the Birth Control Clinical Research Bureau's records by the AMA's *Journal* and by the leading journal in gynecology is not surprising, in view of the social values of their editors, Morris Fishbein and George Kosmak. Fishbein had included an intemperate attack on birth control advocates in his *Medical Follies* (1925). In the shrill tone characteristic of his treatment of all heresy, from faith healing to the Sheppard-Towner Act (1923), a law which provided modest federal subsidies for state pro-

grams to improve infant and maternal health, Fishbein unequivocally asserted that "no method of birth control is physiologically, psychologically and biologically sound in both principle and practice." One historian has explained Fishbein's diatribe against the "ardent economists, biologists, sociologists and philosophers who favor birth control" as part of his larger concern with the defense of a profession just coming into its own after years of struggle with quackery and with public indifference to the needs of the ethical practitioner. Yet Fishbein's categorical rejection of contraception was logically, if not emotionally, inconsistent with the brand of medicine which he claimed to be defending in *Medical Follies*.[33]

One of the most objectionable traits of quack systems of medicine, in Fishbein's view, was the oversimplification of complex issues, the a priori rejection of empirical treatment, and the exaggeration of the effectiveness of simplistic therapeutics. Fishbein stood for a sane positivism based on both science and common sense. Contraception certainly represented an area of social and medical practice which needed the empirical, common sense treatment provided by Hannah Stone, and in which Fishbein claimed to believe. Fishbein, however, justified his rejection of birth control on the grounds that the effectiveness of the known methods ranged from 10 to 90 percent. "Moreover some of them may have produced irritation of the tissues and grave consequences, including cancer. Little need be said of their psychological effects." Having raised the spectre of cancer and refused to distinguish between methods, or to recognize that medicine might have a responsibility to improve what was available, Fishbein saw sterilization by X-ray or the development of a spermatoxin as possible future sources of relief, but concluded that the only safe birth control method was continence.[34]

The inconsistency in his attitude was pointed out by James F. Cooper, the medical director of the American Birth Control League, in *Technique of Contraception* (1928). Cooper noted that there was a "great deal of thoughtless talk about 'no one hundred per cent method.'"

It is fair then to ask, have we any one hundred per cent methods in medicine, or surgery, or serum, or vaccine therapy? . . . The only ethical attitude a physician can take is to guarantee nothing. He can only promise to do his best.

This being true, how clearly absurd it is to single out one department of medical practice, namely contraception, for criticism on the ground that it is not one hundred per cent perfect and for that reason to regard it with indifference! If all physicians had adopted the same general attitude toward every other brand of medicine and surgery, their profession long since would have discontinued its activities.

As a matter of fact, there are very few fields indeed in the practice of medicine where such uniformly good results can be obtained as in contraception. It is a fact that the method recommended . . . in this book [vaginal diaphragm with spermicidal jelly] is safe, simple, and when properly followed, almost uniformly reliable.[35]

Fishbein's treatment of birth control had less to do with "professionalism" than with his attitudes toward women. He was reacting not as a scientist or physician but as a conservative who despised feminists almost as much as medical socialism.[36]

George Kosmak, editor of the *American Journal of Obstetrics and Gynecology,* also rejected Stone's "Therapeutic Contraception." Dickinson recruited his old friend Kosmak for the Committee on Maternal Health because he wanted it to be representative of medical opinion, but Kosmak was a practicing Catholic and proved a difficult ally. In 1936, he candidly admitted, "whenever a young wife fails in her contraceptive practice one thanks God that she did."[37] An inveterate foe of socialized medicine, whether in the form of national health insurance or birth control clinics, Kosmak fretted constantly over the low birthrate among the middle classes, believed that most women who could legally qualify for contraception were in such bad health that they should not have sex anyway, and, in 1939, told the delegates to the AMA convention that birth control propaganda was responsible "for the lack of sexual restraint which has become so evident."[38]

Kosmak agreed to join Dickinson's committee, in 1923, because it provided an opportunity to investigate and to condemn Sanger's activities. He wanted medical control of the dissemination of birth control information because that, he felt, was infinitely better than its free availability in any form. Proponents of birth control aroused public sympathy through tales of gravely ill women who could not obtain contraceptive advice, and Kosmak wanted contraception taught in medical schools, so that no woman with serious medical reasons for avoiding pregnancy would be unable to obtain advice from a private practitioner. In this way, charges of negligence could be disproved and the justification for clinics sponsored by lay groups undermined. But most important, medical students would learn "proper" attitudes toward contraception, along with techniques.[39]

If the antagonism toward birth control of two key leaders such as Kosmak and Fishbein was at all representative of their constituency, how did an affirmative resolution on birth control finally get through an AMA convention in 1937? It was not easy, but Dickinson managed, through persistent lobbying in a changing social context. Lay birth control advocates, with the cooperation of a few medical allies, had established a nationwide chain of several hundred birth control clinics, by the middle of the 1930s. The data from these clinics, reported in many authoritative publications, including Dickinson's *Control of Conception* (1931), demonstrated that safe and effective contraceptive practice was possible. Vague references to contraceptive-induced cancer and to psychological trauma had gradually lost their credibility.[40]

Social conservatives found contraception less offensive as supporters of birth control began to exploit the issue of skyrocketing welfare costs during the Depression; the reformers now talked less of women's controlling their bodies and more of the need to "democratize" contraceptive practice. Since the middle classes were clearly not going to stop practicing contraception, many of those who were concerned over differential fertility between classes believed that their best hope for altering dysgenic population trends lay in birth control for the poor.[41]

By the early thirties the "feminine hygiene" racket, supported by unscrupulous advertising, and flourishing in the absence of any medically recognized standards for discriminating among methods and products, began to arouse public attention, including that of doctors. Birth control was a $250 million-a-year business, "slightly bigger than the barbershop business and very slightly smaller than the jewelry business," but a business without any rational public regulation. In 1937, Americans spent an estimated $200 million for douche powders and other "feminine hygiene" products, $38 million on condoms, and nearly $1 million on diaphragms. Concern over this situation led to the creation of an AMA Committee on Contraception in 1935.[42]

Dickinson's initial optimism turned to chagrin when this committee, which included George Kosmak, issued its first report in 1936. The report denied that any safe or effective birth control methods existed; found no evidence that the federal or state Comstock laws had "interfered with any medical advice which a physician has felt called upon to furnish his patients"; and criticized the lay birth control leagues and "the support of such agencies by members of the medical profession." The AMA House of Delegates instructed the committee to continue its investigation.[43]

At this point, federal appeals court judge Augustus Hand and Robert Dickinson, acting independently, took decisive actions that led to a 1937 AMA report on contraception which seems hardly compatible with the 1936 document. Judge Hand confronted the task of making sense of the Comstock Act's prohibition of contraceptives in the changed social environment of the 1930s. A shipment of experimental diaphragms intended for Dr. Hannah Stone had been seized by United States Customs. Stone sued. Hand ruled that while the language of the Comstock Act was uncompromising with regard to contraceptive devices and information, if Congress had had available in 1873 the clinical data on the dangers of pregnancy and the safety of contraceptive practice that were available in 1936, birth control would not have been classified as obscenity. As Morris Ernst, Stone's lawyer, observed, "the law process is a simple one, it is a matter of educating judges to the mores of the day." Judge Hand's decision opened the mails to contraception materials intended for physicians and definitely established their right to give information, at least as far as federal law was concerned.[44]

Dickinson seized the opportunity provided by the Hand decision. Several key members of the AMA Committee on Contraception attended the American Gynecological Society meeting at Atlantic City in May 1936, where Dickinson spent three days with committee chairman Carl Davis, member

E. D. Plass, and Kosmak, refuting the committee's report point by point. The committee requested that he provide it with a detailed brief. Before the next meeting of the Committee on Contraception in February 1937, Dickinson's Committee on Maternal Health supplied "a voluminous amount of data . . . bearing on clinical prescription and success of contraception in this country."[45]

The Committee on Maternal Health also received a request for information on the "safe period" from another member of the AMA committee, John Rock, a Harvard gynecologist. Rock was a devout Catholic, and his views on contraception were far from those he later expressed in *The Time Has Come* (1963), where he argued that the pill was the "natural" contraceptive that Catholics had been waiting for, and that the population explosion provided another compelling reason for a liberalization of Catholic doctrine on birth control. Dickinson invited Rock to a dinner sponsored by the Committee on Maternal Health and a round table discussion on the topic "Should the Newly Married Practice Contraception?" in December 1936.[46]

Rock happily accepted the invitation because he "objected to the emphasis on *contra*-ception" and wanted "a more positive approach to fertility." There was, Rock stated at the meeting, only one valid reason for birth control: definite medical contraindications to pregnancy. But such situations should not arise, for "those with medical contraindications should not get married." The purpose of sex was procreation. Marriage existed to provide support for woman so that she could fulfill her nature. "Nature intended motherhood to be woman's career, and her proper career, she should start right away. . . . Anything which diverts her from her prime purpose is socially wrong." Economic arguments about the burden of children were "9/10s subterfuge and distortion of value. . . . Cases come to mind of wives supporting husbands' scholastic activities; far better to let the man take off [from school] so that she can have her baby, and then go back to his educational work." Finally, sex could not "be made an end in itself without dire consequences," yet that was the result of most decisions to postpone pregnancy in early marriage.[47]

Some sarcasm had crept into earlier discussions by the Committee on Maternal Health of Catholic doctrine on birth control. When told of support for the rhythm method at the 1934 AMA convention, Dickinson wanted to know, "Did they give out jelly with the calendars?"[48] But when Dr. Rock came to call, all was sweetness and light. His views were politely received and criticism was gentle. The eugenicist Frederick Osborn pointed out that birth control was "an accomplished fact which will not disappear, but which will spread." Regina Stix, of the Milbank Memorial Fund, argued that her studies with Raymond Pearl showed that contraception had "very little to do with the . . . advice of physicians," and that medical influence in this area waited on a better-informed profession. Another participant in the meeting observed that Rock's "view was, of course, not a biological but a philosophical one." Rock, he said, "failed to mention that his view makes of the physician a deus ex machina controlling the masses through enforced ignorance. Decisions should not be based upon ignorance, but upon knowledge." Dr. Sophia Kleegman made it clear that there was "no evidence that the early use of contraception leads to a diminution in desire for children," or the functional inability to have them when medically supervised. Finally,

> Dr. Dickinson pointed out that the National Committee on Maternal Health thirteen years ago stressed the positive side of birth control. When the first child comes too soon, the second may come never. Early marriage and shorter period of engagement are necessary; yet they are impractical unless contraception may be employed. Anyone who thinks young people do not want children is wrong.[49]

The Committee on Contraception's second report of February 1937 is all the more remarkable in that Rock and Kosmak remained on the committee. An AMA-sponsored study of techniques and standards was recommended, along with the promotion of instruction in medical schools. Significantly, criticism of lay-backed organizations in the field, and of their medical allies, was omitted. Finally, the committee declared that contraception advice should be given by the physican "largely on the judgment and wishes of individual patients."[50]

Although proponents of birth control were able to organize some major experiments in the mass delivery of contraceptives between 1937 and 1960, the prospect of spreading contraceptive practice beyond the middle class seemed to be profoundly limited by a lack of technology for birth control

methods that required less motivation from the user than the diaphragm or condom. Clarence James Gamble, a Harvard M.D. (1920) and researcher in experimental pharmacology at the University of Pennsylvania from 1923 to 1937, devoted a large part of his considerable ingenuity and wealth (from the soap fortune) to a search for a better contraceptive. Under the auspices of the Committee on Maternal Health, Gamble conducted a number of pioneer experiments in the mass delivery of simple contraceptives such as lactic acid jelly, but few medical men shared his interest in improving birth control techniques and technology.[51] Most first-class investigators, such as Earl Engle and Howard Taylor, Jr., both members of the Committee on Maternal Health, and colleagues on the Columbia medical school faculty, believed that real progress would have to wait for fundamental advances in knowledge of human sexual physiology. They opposed further experimentation with simple methods by the committee. As Engle bluntly explained in 1946, "We don't give a damn about contraception. We want a study of basic factors in human reproduction."[52] Basic researches were being conducted which would eventually make technological innovation possible, but it is significant that when Dr. George Corner of the University of Rochester, who in 1930 had been, along with his colleague Willard Allen, the first to demonstrate the specific effects of progesterone, reviewed the prospects for clinical use of the hormone in 1947, he did not mention suppression of ovulation as one of its potential uses.[53]

In the middle 1950s, the average physician had little more interest in contraception than in the 1930s. Only one doctor in five, among a sample interviewed by Columbia's Bureau of Applied Social Research in 1957, thought that most married couples got contraceptive advice from medical sources. A majority of Americans still learned about birth control from their relatives or friends.[54] The major movers in the campaign to spread contraceptive practice and to improve contraceptive technology during the 1950s were lay birth control advocates and social scientists.[55] Physicians reported that more married women complained of infertility than asked for contraceptive advice, and until the public demanded better contraceptive services, doctors were unlikely to take much more interest in providing them. A medical editor spoke for a good part of the general public as well as his profession when he declared, "Caustic self-analysis leads to only one honest conclusion: candid physicians are ashamed of these messy makeshifts . . . there is a sense of relative inadequacy . . . nourished by the contemplation of these disreputable paraphernalia." "The messy little gadgets, the pastes, and creams and jellies" were simply "an embarrassment to the scientific mind."[56]

The renewed "sex appeal" of condoms, diaphragms, jellies, and foams during the 1970s illustrated the point that social values played a significant part in the "embarrassment of the scientific mind" in the jelly/diaphragm/condom days of contraception. Christopher Tietze and Sarah Lewit, long-time research associates of the Population Council, recall that it was impossible to continue a large-scale study of the relative effectiveness of barrier methods of contraception once the public learned that an oral contraceptive was available. Hundreds of patients suddenly developed "the hurting diaphragm syndrome" and could be restored to health only with a pill.[57] The eagerness with which physicians embraced this new wonder of modern science reflected their common assumption with the lay public that many of life's most personal problems could be solved with a technological fix. Their patients could now have "spontaneous sex," and doctors had a birth control method which had the prestige of science and did not require them or their patients to touch genitalia, or to fumble with "messy little gadgets."

John Rock played an important role in the pill's development. The biologist Gregory Pincus chose Rock to test on women the synthetic hormone regimen that Pincus believed would work because of the animal studies conducted by his staff at the Worcester Foundation for Experimental Biology. Rock's odyssey, as he developed from a critic of birth control in the 1930s to an outspoken champion of population control in the 1960s, illustrates some of the forces that were reshaping medical attitudes toward contraception.[58]

Margaret Sanger originally opposed bringing Rock into the pill project, arguing that "he would not dare advance the cause of contraceptive research and remain a Catholic." Pincus insisted that Rock was the right man. He explained his view of Rock to his financial angel Katharine McCormick, and McCormick reported to Sanger that Rock was

a "reformed Catholic whose position is that religion has nothing to do with medicine or the practice of it and that if the Church does not interfere with him he will not interfere with it—whatever that may mean!" Sanger eventually changed her mind about Rock and marveled at his ability to win support for her cause. "Being a good R.C. and as handsome as a god, he can just get away with anything."[59]

Some Catholic officials were outraged by Rock's habit of proclaiming his faith while he was violating Catholic dogma in his medical practice. In telling the world that the Pope would surely accept a "natural" contraceptive of synthetic hormones as soon as he was able to review the facts, Rock provided a rationale for Catholic contraceptors. By the time Catholic authorities decided that the pill was no more natural than other contraceptives, many Catholic laymen had found the pill acceptable to them, regardless of the hierarchy's attitude. Rock sincerely believed himself a good Catholic, however, and his changing attitudes toward contraception were those of a conservative seeking to preserve stable family life.[60]

He first spoke out on the issue of contraception in a 1931 article criticizing the poor obstetrical training of Massachusetts physicians. The Harvard associate professor of obstetrics cited laws prohibiting contraceptive advice as a minor factor in the state's high maternal mortality rate, but he was quick to distinguish "medical contraception," prescribed only when a woman's life would be endangered by pregnancy, from "birth control." Indeed, all efforts to separate sex from procreation were fraught with social risk, he thought, since only child rearing provided the discipline and purpose essential to happy marriage.[61] As late as 1943, in an article advocating repeal of Massachusetts laws that restricted "medical birth control advice," Rock noted:

> I hold no brief for those young or even older husbands and wives who for no good reason refuse to bear as many children as they can properly rear and as society can properly engross. Ignorant of the fact that sustained happiness comes only from dutiful sacrifice, such deluded mates are perhaps doing society a backhanded favor. Whatever genetic trait may contribute to the intellectual deficiency which permits them selfishly to seek

more immediate comfort, is at least kept from the inheritable common pool, and in time their kind is thus bred out.[62]

Thirty years later Rock told a reporter, "I think it's shocking to see the big family glorified."[63] Despite the apparent contradiction in his views at different periods, Rock's attitudes toward the family and its place in society were consistent. He considered himself a humanist, in contrast to the contemplative "egoist" who saw man as part of a transcendental unit, or the hedonist-naturalist who believed that life had no spiritual purpose. In Rock's view, life's meaning derived from social interaction, and especially from service to others. Man was an animal, evolved from lower forms of life. Cultural values, derived from centuries of trial and error, made man human.

Sexuality was an immutable part of man's biological heritage. "Unprejudiced observation of so-called civilized man discloses that his fundamental coital pattern . . . is that of other primates, however his coital behavior may appear to be modified by social and spiritual factors." The family provided an essential social focus for sexual expression. For centuries society had needed all the young that women could bear. Thus, the immutable coital urge, when expressed in marriage, had been compatible with, if not essential to, social well-being.[64]

Rock, the father of five, shared the pronatalist values that were one of the givens of American culture during the first half of the twentieth century. By 1943, his experience as a gynecologist made it clear, however, that human fertility would have to be curbed in some situations if the family was to remain a strong institution in an industrial society. Rock did not believe that sexual repression was an acceptable solution for the great majority of Americans. Like the physicians who participated in the Physicians Club of Chicago symposium on "sexual hygiene" in 1898, he had learned that social order depended on satisfying sexual expression within marriage, but good sex without contraception would lead to more children than most American breadwinners could support. Gradually, Rock was coming to the view that physicians should provide the contraceptive advice necessary to protect the family from the economic burden of too many children.[65]

Rock associated his respect for the family with a Catholic heritage, but his views were widely shared by Protestants and Jews. Having gradually accepted contraception as an aid to marital sexual adjustment, while disapproving of those who were able to raise large families but refused to do so, Rock was ready to alter his position when his perception of social needs changed. As demographers like Princeton's Frank Notestein began after World War II to publicize their conviction that rapid population growth was a threat to social order in the Third World and ultimately in the West, social and professional leaders began to advocate population control and to treat the small family with more sympathy. Changes in Rock's views mirrored the redefinition of "the population problem" that was taking place among social scientists and the educated public. Rock was an invaluable ally for family planners because his background and competence gave him an aura of objectivity that they lacked. But his presence in their ranks in the 1960s was symbolic of a broad change in social attitudes, the decline of pronatalism as a more critical attitude toward population growth developed. Rock was no less a humanist in 1973 than he had been in 1931. His view of what mankind needed had simply changed.[66]

Medical attitudes toward contraception, in 1830 or in 1970, were primarily conditioned by the social values which physicians shared with other citizens, rather than by the state of contraceptive technology or by internal scientific standards for judging the usefulness of therapeutic procedures. One could hardly have expected the physicians to behave differently. They were chosen by a process that reflected ability to internalize the values of a professional culture which depended on public confidence and support. Their function was to comfort and to explain, and sometimes to cure—not to question the basic structure or justice of the social system. Contraceptives were not therapeutic means in a narrow sense, since they were usually sought by healthy women for social, as opposed to medical, reasons. From the era of James Marion Sims to the era of John Rock, physicians were increasingly confident, with good reason, of their ability to manage difficult pregnancies and to repair birth injuries. Healthy babies delivered of willing mothers represented a congenial challenge to their improving art. In contrast, birth control was, as Howard Taylor, Jr., complained more than once, a banal topic for the first-class clinician.[67] The medical profession would take an interest in contraceptive practice only when the fertility of healthy women began to seem a clear and present danger to the moral and economic order that it served.

NOTES

Most of the research upon which this paper is based was conducted in the Countway Library of Medicine, Boston, Mass. I am indebted to Richard Wolfe, the rare books librarian at Countway, for bringing a number of collections to my attention and for numerous professional favors that made working in the Countway a pleasure as well as a privilege.

1 There were some important changes in medical attitudes toward birth control between 1830 and 1960. One milestone was a 1937 AMA resolution which recognized contraception as a legitimate service to be provided to patients on request. This victory for birth control was the direct result of an intense lobbying effort by Dr. Robert L. Dickinson and a few allies. Their efforts are described in this paper. The 1937 resolution did not mark the end of medical reluctance to provide contraceptive services, however. Rather, it reversed a ludicrous 1936 report by the AMA Committee on Contraception which denied that safe and effective contraceptive means existed, and which denounced lay birth control supporters and their medical allies, who had been lobbying for recognition of contraception as a routine part of practice. For the 1937 resolution and the 1936 report, see *Journal of the American Medical Association*, 1936, *106:* 1910–11 and 1937, *108:* 2217–18. For a fuller discussion of American attitudes toward birth control, see James Reed, *From Private Vice to Public Virtue: The Birth Control Movement and American Society since 1830* (New York: Basic Books, 1978).

2 Early nineteenth-century birthrates must be constructed from inadequate sources, but the best projections available indicate that native-born white women averaged 7.04 children in 1800; 5.21 in 1860; 3.56 in 1900; 2.10 in 1936. The low fertility of the 1930s should not be viewed primarily as a result of the great depression, since fertility had been declining for 150 years. The rate of this long-term trend varied with geographical location and social class. The native-born white women of New England, for example, had ceased to reproduce themselves by the late nineteenth century. By the middle 1930s, however, the fertility of the whole population hovered around a level barely adequate to maintain the existing population, despite the dramatic declines in mortality during the preceding forty years. See Ansley Coale and Melvin Zelnik, *New Estimates of Fertility and Population in the United States* (Princeton: Princeton University Press, 1963), 33–37; Alan Sweezy, "The economic explanation of fertility changes in the United States," *Population Studies* 25 (July 1971): 255–67; Maris Vinovskis, "Demographic changes in America from the Revolution to the Civil War: an analysis of the socioeconomic determinants of fertility differentials and trends in Massachusetts," Ph.D. diss., Harvard, 1975.

3 Reed, "Birth control in American social science, 1870–1940," chap. 14 in *Birth Control Movement*, 197–210.

4 For a contrasting interpretation, see David M. Kennedy, *Birth Control in America: The Career of Margaret Sanger* (New Haven: Yale University Press, 1971), 176–79.

5 Reed, *Birth Control Movement*, 3–18. I concluded that these contraceptive practices worked for highly motivated users. The problem in assessing their impact on fertility is to determine their "psychological availability."

6 The substitution of latex, for rubber, in condoms during the 1930s was a significant advance in contraceptive technology, but, like the improvement of the spring-loaded diaphragm in the 1920s, the latex condom was simply a refinement of a contraceptive that had been available for some time. The development of plastic intrauterine devices followed the marketing of the birth control pill.

7 See "The search for professional order in 19th century American medicine," a working paper made available to me by Barbara Rosenkrantz of Harvard University; Charles E. Rosenberg, "The practice of medicine in New York a century ago," *Bulletin of the History of Medicine*, 1967, *41:* 223–53.

8 The use of disease sanctions to reinforce female sex roles is discussed by Carroll Smith-Rosenberg and Charles Rosenberg in "The female animal: medical and biological views of woman and her role in nineteenth-century America," in this volume. For a discussion of the attitudes of French doctors toward contraception which emphasizes the prescriptive nature of medical advice, see Angus McLaren, "Doctor in the house: medicine and private morality in France, 1800–1850," *Feminist Studies*, 1975, *2:* 39–54, and "Some secular attitudes toward sexual behavior in France, 1760–1860," *French Historical Studies* 8 (Fall 1974): 604–25.

9 The standard biography is Audrey Davis, *Dr. Kelly*

of Hopkins: Surgeon, Scientist, Christian (Baltimore: Johns Hopkins University Press, 1959). Donald Fleming provides a vivid portrait of Kelly in *William H. Welch and the Rise of Modern Medicine* (Boston: Little, Brown, 1954), 90–91. For an interesting exchange of views between Kelly and Robert Dickinson on the problem of genital changes related to masturbation, see Reed, *Birth Control Movement,* 160.

10 Seale Harris describes the development of the operation in *Woman's Surgeon: The Life Story of J. Marion Sims* (New York: Macmillan, 1950), chaps. 10–11. For the spring-loaded pessary, see James Marion Sims, *Clinical Notes* (New York: W. Wood and Co., 1871), 269, and fig. 11. On Foote, see Vincent J. Cirillo, "Edward Foote's *Medical Common Sense:* an early American comment on birth control," *Journal of the History of Medicine* 25 (July 1970): 341–45, and Cirillo, "Edward Bliss Foote: American advocate of birth control," *Bulletin of the History of Medicine* 47 (September–October 1973): 471–79.

11 On Comstock's arrest of physicians, see Heywood Broun and Margaret Leech, *Anthony Comstock: Roundsman of the Lord* (New York: A and C. Boni, 1927), 160, 167, and Comstock's reply to criticism of his activity in *Frauds Exposed* (New York: J.H. Brown, 1880), 542. Broad interpretations of the war on commercial vice are provided by David Pivar, *Purity Crusade: Sexual Morality and Social Control, 1868–1900* (Westport, Conn.: Greenwood, 1973), and R. Christian Johnson, "Anthony Comstock: reform, vice, and the American way," Ph.D. diss., University of Wisconsin, 1973.

12 Pivar, *Purity Crusade,* 88–99. See also the dissertation version of Pivar's work, "The new Abolitionists: the quest for social purity, 1876–1900" (University of Pennsylvania, 1965), 108, 267, 264, where the following source is quoted: Charles H. Kitchell, *The Social Evil* (New York: privately printed, 1886).

13 The 1937 resolution on birth control did follow the "One Package" federal court decision of 1936 which exempted physicians from the Comstock Act's ban on contraceptive information. In the 1950s, state and local Comstock laws were still having an effect on the prescription of diaphragms by physicians. On the decision, see C. Thomas Dienes, *Law, Politics, and Birth Control* (Urbana: University of Illinois Press, 1972), 112–13. Medical prescription of contraceptives in the 1950s is analyzed in Mary Jean Cornish et al., *Doctors and Family Planning* (New York: National Committee on Maternal Health, 1963), 56–58.

14 The Editorial Staff of the Alkalodia Clinic, eds. *Sexual Hygiene* (Chicago: privately printed, 1902), Preface, and 10–15. There are two copies of *Sexual Hygiene* in the Countway Library of Medicine.

15 Ibid., 95.

16 Ibid., 184.

17 Ibid., 188, 190.

18 Ibid., 186–87, 189–90.

19 The attitudes of many influential physicians toward higher education for women closely paralleled their stance on birth control. See, for example, Alexander J. C. Skene, *Education and Culture as Related to the Health and Diseases of Women* (Detroit: G. S. Davis, 1889), in which Skene denounces both higher education and attempts to avoid pregnancy as violations of the natural order. See my analysis of literature of this genre in "The suppression of contraceptive information," chap. 3, *Birth Control Movement.*

20 I provide a biography of Dickinson in *Birth Control Movement,* pt. 3. The Dickinson Papers (hereafter cited as RLD-CL), are in the Countway Library of Medicine, Boston, Mass.

21 J. Whitridge Williams, "Has the American Gynecological Society done its part in the advancement of obstetrical knowledge?" *Transactions of the American Gynecological Society,* 1914, *39:* 3–20.

22 Robert L. Dickinson and Lura Beam, *The Single Woman: A Study in Sex Education* (New York: Williams and Wilkins, 1934), 4; Dickinson, "Hypertrophies of the labia minora and their significance," *American Gynecology,* 1902, *1:* 225–54; "'Urethral labia' or 'urethral hymen': pathological structures due to repeated traction," *American Medicine,* 1904, *7:* 347–49, 347–49; "Marital maladjustment: the business of preventive gynecology," *Long Island Medical Journal,* 1908, *2:* 1–5; interview with Dorothy Dickinson Barbour, Cincinnati, Ohio, 2 June 1971.

23 Williams, "Has the American Gynecological Society."

24 Robert L. Dickinson, "Suggestions for a program for American gynecology," *Transactions of the American Gynecological Society,* 1920, *45:* 1–13.

25 *Surgery, Gynecology, and Obstetrics,* 1916, *23:* 185–90; Dickinson to Sanger, 7 November 1945, Margaret Sanger Papers, Sophia Smith Collection, Smith College, Northampton, Mass., (hereafter cited as MS-SS); Sanger to Dickinson, 9 November 1945, RLD-CL. These letters were exchanged when Dickinson was preparing an article on the early history of the birth control movement and wanted to check some of his dates with Sanger. For Dickinson's unsuccessful attempt to gain backing from the New York Obstetrical Society, and the early activities of the Committee on Maternal Health, see Reed, *Birth Control Movement,* chap. 21, "Clinical studies."

26 "Origins of National Committee on Maternal Health," undated, unsigned memo, RLD-CL.

27 Minutes of the Committee on Maternal Health, 28

November 1925; 28 May 1924; 13 June 1924; 1 February 1928; 12 March 1926, in RLD-CL (hereafter cited as CMH).

28 9 March 1923; 10 May 1923; 10 January 1924, CMH.

29 7 December 1923; 11 December 1924; 10 December 1925, CMH. On the history and influence of Sanger's Birth Control Clinical Research Bureau, see Reed, *Birth Control Movement*, chap. 9, "Providing clinics."

30 21 January and 10 December 1928, CMH; "Report of the Conference of the Maternal Health Committee and the Clinic Committee of the American Birth Control League, November 29, 1925"; "Minutes of the public hearing: January 15, 1926," Margaret Sanger Papers, Library of Congress (hereafter cited as MS-LC); Dickinson, "England and birth control," RLD-CL.

31 Sanger to Edward M. East, 28 May 1925, MS-LC; 17 January 1927, CMH; Clarence Little to Dickinson, 26 October 1925, MS-LC; Committee on Maternal Health, *Biennial Report: 1928*, 5–6, RLD-CL; Hannah Stone, "Therapeutic contraception," *Medical Journal and Record*, 1928, *127*: 9–17.

32 In 1956 the Clinical Research Bureau was still operating without a license, on advice of the Planned Parenthood Federation of America's counsel, Morris Ernst, in candid recognition of the fact that a dispensary license was unattainable. See Mary Calderone to Ethel Wortis, 25 October 1956, Mary Calderone Papers, Schlesinger Library, Radcliffe College, Cambridge, Mass., and the transcript of my interview with Dr. Calderone, Schlesinger-Rockefeller Oral History Project, Schlesinger Library, 9–10.

33 Morris Fisbein, *Medical Follies* (New York: Boni and Liveright, 1925), 125; Kennedy, *Birth Control in America*, 176–79; Reed, *Birth Control Movement*, 144–46.

34 Fishbein, *Medical Follies*, 56–58, 218–20, 142–49.

35 James F. Cooper, *Technique of Contraception* (New York: Day-Nichols, 1928), 23–24.

36 For discussion of a revealing attempt by Fishbein to impose his views on woman's proper social role on a woman author, see my interview with Emily H. Mudd, Ph.D., Schlesinger-Rockefeller Oral History Project, 124–27.

37 "Notes on the round table meeting of December 4, 1936," RLD-CL.

38 George Kosmak, "The broader aspects of the birth control propaganda," (discussion of paper) *American Journal of Obstetrics and Gynecology*, 1923, *6*: 351–53; George Kosmak, compiler, "Newspaper clippings on birth control, child birth deaths, etc.: 1917–1941" (hereafter cited as Kosmak Clippings), vol. 2, New York Academy of Medicine; Kosmak, "What

shall be the attitude toward the percent propaganda," *Medical Record*, *1917*, *91*: 268–73; Kosmak Clippings, 18 May 1939; Reed, *Birth Control Movement*, 168–71.

39 Kosmak, "The broader aspects."

40 Reed, *Birth Control Movement*, 181–90.

41 Ibid., 211–38.

42 "The accident of birth," *Fortune* (17 February 1938): 83–86, 108–14; "The lay press looks at birth control," *Journal of Contraception* 3 (March 1938): 60–61; Reed, *Birth Control Movement*, chap. 18, "Policing the market place," 239–46.

43 Reed, *Birth Control Movement*, 186–87; *Journal of the American Medical Association*, 1936, *106*: 1910–11.

44 Dienes, *Law, Politics, and Birth Control*, 112–113.

45 "Notes on informal meeting at Atlantic City . . . ," CMH; 24 Feburary 1937, CMH.

46 24 February 1937, CMH; "Notes on the round table meeting of December 4, 1936," RLD-CL.

47 "Notes on the round table meeting of December 4, 1936," RLD-CL.

48 "Report of the round table meeting, October 5, 1934," RLD-CL.

49 "Notes on the round table meeting of December 4, 1936," RLD-CL.

50 *Journal of the American Medical Association*, 1937, *108*: 2217–18.

51 Reed, *Birth Control Movement*, 5, "Birth control entrepreneur: the philanthropic pathfinding of Clarence J. Gamble."

52 14 June 1946, CMH; Reed, *Birth Control Movement*, 243.

53 George Corner, *The Hormones in Human Reproduction* (Princeton: Princeton University Press, 1947 [first edition, 1942]), 87; Reed, *Birth Control Movement*, 313–16.

54 Cornish et al., *Doctors and Family Planning*, passim.

55 Reed, *Birth Control Movement*, chaps. 21, 23, "The population explosion" and "The failure of simple methods: the IUD justified."

56 Editorial, *Western Journal of Surgery, Obstetrics, and Gynecology* 51 (September 1943): 381–83.

57 Interview with Sarah Lewit Tietze and Christopher Tietze, Schlesinger-Rockefeller Oral History Project, 10.

58 Reed, *Birth Control Movement*, 351–54.

59 Sanger to Marion Ingersoll, 18 February 1954; McCormick to Sanger, 19 July 1954; Sanger to Mrs. John D. Rockefeller, Jr., 19 February 1960, MS-SS.

60 Rock stated his views on oral contraception in *The Time Has Come: A Catholic Doctor's Proposals to End the Battle over Birth Control* (New York: 1963). For criticism of Rock by a Catholic spokesman, see remarks by Msgr. George Kelly. *New York Times*, 6 May 1963, 20. For criticism by a more liberal Catholic, see J.S.

Duhamel's review of *The Time Has Come* in *America* 108 (27 April 1963): 608. For criticism of Rock's rationalization of "the pill" by a fellow physician and birth control advocate, see Robert Hall's review in the *New York Times Review of Books* (12 May 1963), 30.

61 John Rock, "Maternal morality: what must be done about it," *New England Journal of Medicine*, 1931, *205:* 902.

62 "Medical and biological aspects of contraception," *Clinics* 1 (April 1943): 1601–2.

63 "Dr. John Rock at 83: an interview," *Boston Globe Sunday Magazine* (19 July 1973), 6–8.

64 "Medical and biological aspects," 1608–9.

65 Ibid., 1599–1601.

66 Ibid.

67 Interview with Howard Taylor, Jr., New York City, 27 April 1971; 24 September 1936; 2 April 1937; 27 April 1937; 6 October 1938, CMH.

CHILDBIRTH

Although American women and men became increasingly successful at limiting the size of their families in the nineteenth century—the number of children per married woman dropped from 7.04 in 1800 to 3.56 in 1900—childbirth remained a common female experience. When colonial women were "brought to bed," their women friends and relatives came to aid the midwife during labor and delivery and to help with domestic chores. This "social childbirth" continued to characterize American births throughout the nineteenth century even as male physicians increasingly replaced female midwives as attendants in the birthing rooms of the urban elite. The change to physician attendants at childbirth occurred for most nonelite women, especially the poor and immigrant women, during the first half of the twentieth century, although certain small segments of America's women continued to give birth with female midwife attendants throughout the twentieth century. Even with individual male attendants, however, birth remained predominantly a female affair and an important part of women's domestic culture until the twentieth century, when it moved away from women's homes and into the hospital.

In this section Catherine Scholten examines changes in childbirth attendant in the late-eighteenth- and early-nineteenth-century in the eastern seacoast cities, and Judith Leavitt and Whitney Walton explore women's perceptions of their birth experience as times of great physical danger when the presence of other women provided important psychological comforts. Virginia Drachman describes obstetrical training in the mid-nineteenth century, when male physicians' practical birth experience increased amidst a raging controversy. Finally, Judith Leavitt analyzes the paradoxical episode in the early twentieth century when feminist women sought to increase their control over the childbirth experience by taking drugs that allowed them to forget the whole thing.

In the twentieth century American childbirth moved to the hospital. While a small segment of women, usually the poorest and most alone, had delivered their babies in the hospital throughout the nineteenth century, the numbers of women going to the hospital, now predominantly those who had some degree of choice, exploded after 1920. By 1938 half of American babies first saw the world in hospital delivery rooms, and by 1955, 95 percent of women rushed to the hospital when their labors began. For a variety of reasons examined in this section, American women gave up their women-centered social childbirths for medicalized childbirths, during which women left their families at the labor room door and, in the words of one of them, delivered their babies "alone among strangers." Even though women participated in the transition from home to hospital, from the birthing women's point of view the changes have not all been positive.

10

"On the Importance of the Obstetrick Art": Changing Customs of Childbirth in America, 1760–1825

CATHERINE M. SCHOLTEN

In October 1799, as Sally Downing of Philadelphia labored to give birth to her sixth child, her mother, Elizabeth Drinker, watched her suffer "in great distress." Finally, on the third day of fruitless labor, Sally's physician, William Shippen, Jr., announced that "the child must be brought forward." Elizabeth Drinker wrote in her diary that, happily, Sally delivered naturally, although Dr. Shippen had said that "he thought he should have had occasion for instruments" and clapped his hand on his side, so that the forceps rattled in his pocket.[1]

Elizabeth Drinker's account of her daughter's delivery is one of the few descriptions by an eighteenth-century American woman of a commonplace aspect of women's lives—childbirth.[2] It is of special interest to social historians because it records the participation of a man in the capacity of physician. Shippen was a prominent member of the first generation of American doctors trained in obstetrics and, commencing in 1763, the first to maintain a regular practice attending women in childbirth.[3] Until that time midwives managed almost all deliveries, but with Shippen male physicians began to supplant the midwives.

The changing social customs and medical management of childbirth from 1760 to 1825 are the subjects of this article. By analyzing the rituals of childbirth it will describe the emergence of new patterns in private and professional life. It shows that, beginning among well-to-do women in Phila-

delphia, New York, and Boston, childbirth became less a communal experience and more a private event confined within the intimate family. In consequence of new perceptions of urban life and of women, as well as of the development of medical science, birth became increasingly regarded as a medical problem to be managed by physicians. For when Shippen, fresh from medical studies in London, announced his intention to practice midwifery in Philadelphia in 1763, he was proposing to enter a field considered the legitimate province of women.[4] Childbearing had been viewed as the inevitable, even the divinely ordained, occasion of suffering for women; childbirth was an event shared by the female community; and delivery was supervised by a midwife.

During the colonial period childbearing occupied a central portion of the lives of women between their twentieth and fortieth years. Six to eight pregnancies were typical, and pregnant women were commonly described as "breeding" and "teeming."[5] Such was women's natural lot; though theologians attributed dignity to carrying the "living soul" of a child and saluted mothers in their congregations with "Blessed are you among women," they also depicted the pains of childbirth as the appropriate special curse of "the Travailing Daughters of Eve."[6] Two American tracts written specifically for lying-in women dwelt on the divinely ordained hazards of childbirth and advised a hearty course of meditation on death, "such as their pregnant condition must reasonably awaken them to."[7]

Cotton Mather's pamphlet, *Elizabeth in Her Holy Retirement*, which he distributed to midwives to give

CATHERINE M. SCHOLTEN (1949–1981) was a doctoral candidate in American History at the University of California at Berkeley and a staff member of the regional Oral History Library, Bancroft Library.

Reprinted with permission from Pauline Scholten. This article originally appeared in *William and Mary Quarterly* 34 (1977): 426–445.

to the women they cared for, described pregnancy as a virtually lethal condition. "For ought you know," it warned, "your Death has entered into you, you may have conceived that which determines but about Nine Months more at the most, for you to live in the World." Pregnancy was thus intended to inspire piety.[8] John Oliver, author of *A Present for Teeming American Women,* similarly reminded expectant mothers that prayer was necessary because their dangers were many. He noted that women preparing for lying-in "get linnen and other necessaries for the child, a nurse, a midwife, entertainment for the women that are called to the labour, a warm convenient chamber, and etc." However, "all these may be miserable comforters," argued Oliver, for "they may perchance need no other linnen shortly than a Winding Sheet, and have no other chamber but a grave, no neighbors but worms."[9] Oliver counseled women to "arm themselves with patience" as well as prayer, and "abate somewhat those dreadful groans and cries which do so much to discourage their friends and relatives who hear them."[10]

Surely women did not need to be reminded of the risks of childbirth. The fears of Mary Clap, wife of Thomas Clap, president of Yale College, surface even through the ritual phrases of the elegy written by her husband after her death in childbirth at the age of twenty-four. Thomas remembered that before each of her six lyings-in his wife had asked him to pray with her that God would continue their lives together.[11] Elizabeth Drinker probably echoed the sentiments of most women when she reflected, "I have often thought that women who live to get over the time of Childbareing, if other things are favourable to them, experience more comfort and satisfaction than at any other period of their lives."[12]

Facing the hazards of childbirth, women depended on the community of their sex for companionship and medical assistance. Women who had moved away at marriage frequently returned to their parents' home for the delivery, either because they had no neighbors or because they preferred the care of their mothers to that of their in-laws. Other women summoned mothers, aunts, and sisters on both sides of the family, as well as female friends, when birth was imminent.[13] Above all, they relied on the experience of midwives to guide them through labor.

Women monopolized the practice of midwifery in America, as in Europe, through the middle of the eighteenth century. As the recognized experts in the conduct of childbirth, they advised the mother-to-be if troubles arose during pregnancy, supervised the activities of lying-in, and used their skills to assure safe delivery. Until educated male physicians began to practice obstetrics, midwives enjoyed some status in the medical profession, enhanced by their legal responsibilities in the communities they served.

English civil authorities required midwives to take oaths in order to be licensed but imposed no official test of their skills. The oaths indicate that midwives had responsibilities which were serious enough to warrant supervision. They swore not to allow any infant to be baptized outside the Church of England, and promised to help both rich and poor, to report the true parentage of a child, and to abstain from performing abortions. Oath-breaking midwives could be excommunicated or fined.[14]

Some American midwives learned their art in Europe, where midwifery was almost exclusively the professional province of women. Though barber surgeons and physicans increasingly asserted their interest in midwifery during the seventeenth century, midwives and patients resisted the intruders.[15] The midwives' levels of skill varied. Some acquired their medical education in the same way as many surgeons and physicians, by apprenticeship; some read manuals by more learned midwives and physicians; and after 1739, when the first British lying-in hospital was founded, a few were taught by the physicians who directed such hospitals.[16] But more often than not, women undertook midwifery equipped only with folk knowledge and the experience of their own pregnancies.[17]

Disparity of skills also existed among American midwives. Experienced midwives practiced alongside women who were, one physician observed, "as ignorant of their business as the women they deliver."[18] By the end of the eighteenth century physicians thought that the "greater part" of the midwives in America took up the occupation by accident, "having first been *catched,* as they express it, with a woman in labour."[19] The more diligent sought help from books, probably popular medical manuals such as *Aristotle's Masterpiece.*[20]

American midwives conducted their practice free,

on the whole, from governmental supervision and control. Only two colonies appear to have enacted regulatory statutes, and it does not seem that these were rigorously enforced. In the seventeenth century Massachusetts and New York required midwives, together with surgeons and physicians, not to act contrary to the accepted rules of their art. More specifically, in 1716 the common council of New York City prescribed a licensing oath for midwives, which was similar to the oaths of England, though without the provision on baptism. The oath included an injunction—significant for the theme of this article—that midwives not "open any matter Appertaining to your Office in the presence of any Man unless Necessity or Great Urgent Cause do Constrain you to do so."[21] This oath, which was regularly reenacted until 1763, suggests the common restriction of midwifery to women, excluding male physicians or barber surgeons, who, in any case, were few and usually ill trained. There are records of male midwives in New York, Philadelphia, Charleston, and Annapolis after 1740, but only one, a Dr. Spencer of Philadelphia, had London training in midwifery, and it was said of another that "he attended very few natural labors."[22]

Though their duties were not as well defined by law, American midwives served the community in ways similar to those of their British counterparts. In addition to assisting at childbed, they testified in court in cases of bastardy, verified birthdates, and examined female prisoners who pleaded pregnancy to escape punishment.[23] Some colonials also observed the English custom of having the midwife attend the baptism and burial of infants. Samuel Sewall reported that Elizabeth Weeden brought his son John to church for christening in 1677, and at the funeral of little Henry in 1685 "Midwife Weeden and Nurse Hill carried the Corps by turns."[24]

The inclusion of the midwife in these ceremonies of birth and death shows how women's relationships with their midwives went beyond mere respect for the latter's skill. Women with gynecologic problems would freely tell a midwife things "that they had rather die than discover to the Doctor."[25] Grateful patients eulogized midwives.[26] The acknowledgment of the services of one Boston midwife, recorded on her tombstone, has inspired comment since 1761. The stone informs the curious that Mrs. Phillips was " born in Westminster in

Great Britain, and Commission'd by John Laud, Bishop of London in ye Year 1718 to ye Office of a Midwife," came to "this Country" in 1719, and "by ye Blessing of God has brought into this world above 3000 Children."[27]

We may picture Mrs. Phillip's professional milieu as a small room, lit and warmed by a large fire, and crowded by a gathering of family and friends. In daytime, during the early stages of labor, children might be present, and while labor proceeded female friends dropped in to offer encouragement and help; securing refreshments for such visitors was a part of the preparation for childbirth, especially among the well-to-do families with which we are concerned. Men did not usually remain at the bedside. They might be summoned in to pray, but as delivery approached they waited elsewhere with the children and with women who were "not able to endure" the tension in the room.[28]

During the final stages of labor the midwife took full charge, assisted by other women. As much as possible, midwives managed deliveries by letting nature do the work; they caught the child, tied the umbilical cord, and if necessary fetched the afterbirth. In complicated cases they might turn the child and deliver it feet first, but if this failed, the fetus had to be destroyed. In all circumstances the midwife's chief duty was to comfort the woman in labor while they both waited on nature, and this task she could, as a woman, fulfill with social ease. Under the midwife's direction the woman in labor was liberally fortified with hard liquor or mulled wine. From time to time the midwife examined her cervix to gauge the progress of labor and encouraged her to walk about until the pains became too strong. There was no standard posture for giving birth, but apparently few women lay flat in bed. Some squatted on a midwife's stool, a low chair with an open seat. Others knelt on a pallet, sat on another woman's lap, or stood supported by two friends.[29]

Friends were "welcome companions," according to one manual for midwives, because they enabled the woman in labor "to bear her pains to more advantage," and "their cheerful conversation supports her spirits and inspires her with confidence."[30] Elizabeth Drinker endeavored to talk her daughter into better spirits by telling her that as she was thirty-nine "this might possibly be the last trial of this sort."[31] Some women attempted to cheer the mother-to-be by assuring her that her labor was easy compared to others they had seen, or provoked laughter by making bawdy jokes.[32]

For some attendants, a delivery could be a wrenching experience. Elizabeth Drinker relived her own difficult deliveries when her daughters suffered their labors, and on one such occasion she noted with irony, "This day is 38 years since I was in agonies bringing her into this world of troubles: she told me with tears that this was her birthday."[33] For others the experience of assisting the labors of friends was reminder of their sex. Sarah Eve, an unmarried twenty-two-year-old, attended the labor of a friend in 1772 and carried the tidings of birth to the waiting father. "None but those that were like anxious could be sensible of a joy like theirs," she wrote in her journal that night. "Oh! Adam's wife I mean—who could forget her today?"[34]

After delivery, the mother was covered up snugly and confined to her bed, ideally for three to four weeks. For fear of catching cold she was not allowed to put her feet on the floor and was constantly supplied with hot drinks. Family members relieved her of household duties. Restless women, and those who could not afford weeks of idleness, got up in a week or less, but not without occasioning censure.[35]

The social and medical hold of midwives on childbirth loosened during the half-century after 1770, as male physicians assumed the practice of midwifery among urban women of social rank. Initially, physicians entered the field as trained practitioners who could help women in difficult labors through the use of instruments, but ultimately they presided over normal deliveries as well. The presence of male physicians in the lying-in chamber signaled a general change in attitudes toward childbirth, including a modification of the dictum that women had to suffer. At the same time, because medical training was restricted to men, women lost their position as assistants at childbirth, and an event traditionally managed by a community of women became an experience shared primarily by a woman and her doctor.

William Shippen, the first American physician to establish a steady practice of midwifery, quietly overcame resistance to the presence of a man in the lying-in room. Casper Wistar's *Eulogies on Dr.*

Shippen, published in 1809, states that when Shippen began in 1763, male practitioners were resorted to only in a crisis. "This was altogether the effect of prejudice," Wistar remarked, adding that "by Shippen this prejudice was so done away, that in the course of ten years he became very fully employed."[36] A few figures testify to the trend. The Philadelphia city directory in 1815 listed twenty-one women as midwives, and twenty-three men as practitioners of midwifery. In 1819 it listed only thirteen female midwives, while the number of men had risen to forty-two; and by 1824 only six female midwives remained in the directory.[37] "Prejudice" similarly dissolved in Boston, where in 1781 the physicians advertised that they expected immediate payment for their services in midwifery; by 1820 midwifery in Boston was almost "entirely confined" to physicians.[38] By 1826 Dr. William Dewees, professor of midwifery at the University of Pennsylvania and the outstanding American obstetrician of the early nineteenth century, could preface his textbook on midwifery with an injunction to every American medical student to study the subject because "everyone almost" must practice it. He wrote that "a change of manners within a few years" had "resulted in almost exclusive employment of the male practitioner."[39]

Dewees's statement must be qualified because the "almost exclusive" use of men actually meant almost exclusive use among upper- and middle-class urban women. Female midwives continued throughout the nineteenth century to serve both the mass of women in cities and women in the country who were "without advantage of regular practitioners."[40] During the initial years of their practice physicians shared obstetrical cases with midwives. On occasion Philadelphia women summoned Shippen together with their midwives, and Dewees reports that when he began to practice in the 1790s he depended on midwives to call him when instruments were needed.[41] It is clear, however, that by the 1820s Dewees and his colleagues had established their own practice independent of midwives.

On one level the change was a direct consequence of the fact that after 1750 growing numbers of American men traveled to Europe for medical education. Young men with paternal means, like Shippen, spent three to four years studying medicine, including midwifery, with leading physicians in the hospitals of London and the class-rooms of Edinburgh. When they returned to the colonies they brought back not only a superior set of skills but also British ideas about hospitals, medical schools, and professional standards.[42]

In the latter part of the eighteenth century advanced medical training became available in North America. At the time of Shippen's return in 1762 there was only one hospital in the colonies, the Pennsylvania Hospital, built ten years earlier to care for the sick poor. Shippen and his London-educated colleagues saw that the hospital could be used for the clinical training of physicians, as in Europe. Within three years the Philadelphia doctors, led by John Morgan, established formal, systematic instruction at a school of medicine, supplemented by clinical work in the hospital.[43] Morgan maintained that the growth of the colonies "called aloud" for a medical school "to increase the number of those who exercise the profession of medicine and surgery."[44] Dr. Samuel Bard successfully addressed the same argument to the citizens of New York in 1768.[45]

In addition to promoting medical schools, Morgan and Bard defined the proper practitioner of medicine as a man learned in a science. To languages and liberal arts their ideal physician added anatomy, material medicine, botany, chemistry, and clinical experience. He was highly conscious not only of his duty to preserve "the life and health of mankind,"[46] but also of his professional status, and this new emphasis on professionalism extended to midwifery.

The trustees of the first American medical schools recognized midwifery as a branch of medical science. From its founding in 1768, Kings College in New York devoted one professorship solely to midwifery, and the University of Pennsylvania elected Shippen professor of anatomy, surgery, and midwifery in 1791. By 1807 five reputable American medical schools provided courses in midwifery.[47] In the early years of the nineteenth century some professors of midwifery began to call themselves obstetricians or professors of obstetrics, a scientific-sounding title free of the feminine connotations of the word midwife.[48] Though not compulsory for all medical students, the new field was considered worthy of detailed study along the paths pioneered by English physicians.

Dr. William Smellie contributed more to the development of obstetrics than any other eighteenth-century physician. His influence was established by his teaching career in London from 1741 to 1758, and by his treatise on midwifery, first published in 1752.[49] Through precise measurement and observation Smellie discovered the mechanics of parturition. He found that the child's head turned throughout delivery, adapting the widest part to the widest diameter of the pelvic canal. Accordingly, he defined maneuvers for manipulating an improperly presented child. He also recognized that obstetrical forceps, generally known for only twenty years when he wrote in 1754, should be used to rectify the position of an infant wedged in the mouth of the cervix, in preference to the "common method" of simply jerking the child out. He perfected the design of the forceps and taught its proper use, so that physicians could save both mother and child in difficult deliveries, instead of being forced to dismember the infant with hooks.[50]

To Smellie and the men who learned from him, the time seemed ripe to apply science to a field hitherto built on ignorance and supported by prejudice. Smellie commented on the novelty of scientific interest in midwifery. "We ought to be ashamed of ourselves," he admonished the readers of his *Treatise*, "for the little improvement we have made in so many centuries." Only recently have "we established a better method of delivering in laborious and preternatural cases."[51] Smellie's countryman Dr. Charles White reflected in his text on midwifery in 1793 that "the bringing of the art of midwifery to perfection upon scientific and medical principles seems to have been reserved for the present generation."[52]

Some American physicians shared this sense of the new "Importance of the Obstetrick Art." Midwifery was not a "trifling" matter to be left to the uneducated, Thomas Jones of the College of Medicine of Maryland wrote in 1812. Broadly defined as the care of "all the indispositions incident to women from the commencement of pregnancy to the termination of lactation," it ranked among the most important branches of medicine. "With the cultivation of this branch of science," women could now "reasonably look to men for safety in the perilous conditions" of childbirth.[53]

Jones maintained, as did other physicians, that the conditions of modern urban life produced a special need for scientific aid in childbirth. Both rich and poor women in large cities presented troublesome cases to the physican. Pelvic deformities, abortions, and tedious labors Jones considered common among wealthy urban women because of their indolent habits and confining fashionable dress, and among the poor because of inadequate diet and long hours of work indoors. There was, he believed, a greater need for "well informed obstetrick practitioners in large cities than in country places."[54]

Although it cannot be established that there was an increase in difficult parturitions among urban women, social as well as medical reasons account for the innovations in the practice of midwifery in such cities as Boston, Philadelphia, and New York. Physicians received their medical education in cities, and cities offered the best opportunities to acquire patients and live comfortably. Urban families of some means could afford the $12 to $15 minimum fee which Boston physicians demanded for midwife services in 1806.[55] Obstetrics was found to be a good way to establish a successful general practice. The man who conducted himself well in the lying-in room won the gratitude and confidence of his patient and her family, and they naturally called him to serve in other medical emergencies. It was midwifery, concluded Dr. Walter Channing of Boston, that ensured doctors "the permanency and security of all their other business."[56]

The possibility of summoning a physician, who could perhaps insure a safer and faster delivery, opened first to urban women. The dramatic rescue of one mother and child given up by a midwife could be enough to convince a neighborhood of women of a physician's value and secure him their practice.[57] Doctors asserted that women increasingly hired physicians because they became convinced "that the well instructed physician is best calculated to avert danger and surmount difficulties."[58] Certainly by 1795 the women of the Drinker family believed that none but a physician should order medicine for a woman in childbed, and had no doubts that Dr. Shippen or his colleague Dr. Nicholas Way was the best help that they could summon.[59]

Although she accepted a male physician as midwife, Elizabeth Drinker still had reservations about the use of instruments to facilitate childbirth and was relieved when Shippen did not have to use forceps on her daughter. Other women feared to call a physician because they assumed that any instruments he used would destroy the child.[60] However, once the capabilities of obstetrical forceps became known, some women may have turned to them by choice in hope of faster deliveries. Such hope stimulated a medical fashion. By about 1820 Dewees and Bard felt it necessary to condemn nervous young doctors for resorting unnecessarily to forceps.[61]

The formal education of American physicians and the development of midwifery as a science, the desire of women for the best help in childbirth, the utility of midwifery as a means of building a physician's practice, and, ultimately, the gigantic social changes labeled urbanization explain why physicians assumed the ordinary practice of midwifery among well-to-do urban women in the late eighteenth and early nineteenth centuries. This development provides insight into the changing condition of women in American society.

The development of obstetrics signified a partial rejection of the assumption that women had to suffer in childbirth and implied a new social appreciation of women, as admonitions to women for forbearance under the pain of labor turned to the desire to relieve their pain. Thus did Dr. Thomas Denman explain his life's work: "The law of a religion founded on principles of active benevolence, feelings of humanity, common interests of society, and special tenderness for women" demanded that men search for a method by which women might be conducted safely through childbirth.[62] In his doctoral dissertation in 1812 one American medical student drew a distinction between childbirth in primitive societies and his own. In the former, "women are generally looked on by their rugged lords as unworthy of any particular attention," and death or injury in childbirth is "not deemed a matter of any importance." Well-instructed assistants to women in childbirth were one sign of the value placed on women in civilized societies.[63]

The desire to relieve women in childbirth also signified a more liberal interpretation of scripture. At the University of Pennsylvania in 1804, Peter Miller, a medical student, modified the theological dictum that women must bear in sorrow. The anxieties of pregnancy and the anguish caused by the death of so many infants constituted sorrow enough for women, argued Miller. They did not need to be subjected to bodily pain as well.[64] Reiterating this argument, Dewees bluntly asked, "Why should the female alone incur the penalty of God?"[65] To relieve the pain of labor Dewees and his fellows analyzed the anatomy and physiology of childbirth and defined techniques for the use of instruments.

If the development of obstetrics suggests the rise of a "special tenderness for women" on the part of men, it also meant that women's participation in medical practice was diminished and disparaged. A few American physicians instructed midwives or wrote manuals for them, but these efforts were private and sporadic, and had ceased by 1820. The increasing professionalization of medicine, in the minds of the physicians who formed medical associations that set the standards of the field, left little room for female midwives, who lacked the prescribed measure of scientific training and professional identity.[66]

William Shippen initially invited midwives as well as medical students to attend his private courses in midwifery. His advertisement in the *Pennsylvania Gazette* in January 1765 related his experience assisting women in the country in difficult labors, "most of which was made so by the unskillful old women about them," and announced that he "thought it his duty to immediately begin" courses in midwifery "in order to instruct those women who have virtue enough to own their ignorance and apply for instructions, as well as those young gentlemen now engaged in the study of that useful and necessary branch of surgery." Shippen taught these private lessons until after the Revolution, when he lectured only to the students at the University of Pennsylvania, who, of course, were male.[67]

At the turn of the century Dr. Valentine Seaman conducted the only other known formal instruction of midwives. He was distressed by the ignorance of many midwives, yet convinced that midwives ought to manage childbirth because, unlike physicians, they had time to wait out lingering labors, and, as women, they could deal easily with female patients. Seaman offered his private lectures and demonstrations at the New York Almshouse lying-in ward, and in 1800 published them as the *Midwives Monitor and Mothers Mirror*.[68] A handful of other men wrote texts at least nominally directed to midwives between 1800 and 1810; some of these, like Seaman's, discussed the use of instruments.[69] In 1817 Dr. Thomas Ewell proposed that midwives be trained at a national school of midwifery in Washington, D.C., to be supported by a collection taken up by ministers. There is no evidence that Ewell's scheme, presented in his medical manual *Letters to Ladies*, ever gained a hearing.[70]

Seaman and Ewell, and other authors of midwives' manuals, presumed that if women mastered some of the fundamentals of obstetrics they would be desirable assistants in ordinary midwifery cases. In 1820 Dr. Channing of Boston went further in his pamphlet *Remarks on the Employment of Females as Practitioners of Midwifery*, in which he maintained that no one could thoroughly understand the management of labor who did not understand "thoroughly the profession of medicine as a whole." Channing's principle would have totally excluded women from midwifery, because no one favored professional medical education for women. It was generally assumed that they could not easily master the necessary languages, mathematics, and chemistry, or withstand the trials of dissecting room and hospital. Channing added that women's moral character disqualified them for medical practice: "Their feelings of sympathy are too powerful for the cool exercise of judgment" in medical emergencies, he wrote, "they do not have the power of action, nor the active power of mind which is essential to the practice of the surgeon."[71]

Denied formal medical training, midwives of the early nineteenth century could not claim any other professional or legal status. Unlike Great Britain, the United States had no extensive record of licensing laws or oaths defining the practice of midwifery. Nor were there any vocal groups of midwives who, conscious of their tradition of practice or associated with lying-in hospitals, were able to defend themselves against competition from physicians.[72] American midwives ceased practice among women of social rank with few words uttered in their defense.

The victory of the physicians produced its own problems. The doctor's sex affected the relationships between women and their attendants in childbirth, and transformed the atmosphere of the lying-in room. In his advice to his male students Dewees acknowledged that summoning a man to assist at childbed "cost females a severe struggle."[73]

Other doctors knew that even the ordinary gyne-cologic services of a physician occasioned embar-rassment and violated woman's "natural delicacy of feeling," and that every sensitive woman felt "deeply humilated" at the least bodily exposure.[74] Doctors recognized an almost universal repug-nance on the part of women to male assistance in time of labor.[75] Because of "whim or false delicacy" women often refused to call a man until their con-dition had become critical.[76] It is unlikely that phy-sicians exaggerated these observations, although there is little testimony from women themselves about their childbed experience in the early nine-teenth century.

The uneasiness of women who were treated by men was sometimes shared by their husbands. In 1722 the *Virginia Gazette* printed a denunciation of male midwifery as immoral. The author, probably an Englishman, attributed many cases of adultery in England to the custom of employing men at deliveries. Even in labor a woman had intervals of ease, and these, he thought, were the moments when the doctor infringed on the privileges of the husband. It would be a matter of utmost indiffer-ence to him "whether my wife had spent the night in a bagnio, or an hour of the forenoon locked up with a man midwife in her dressing room."[77] Such arguments were frequently and seriously raised in England during the eighteenth century.[78] They may seem ludicrous, but at least one American man of Dr. Ewell's acquaintance suffered emotional con-flict over hiring a male midwife. He sent for a phy-sician to help his wife in her labor, yet "very sol-emnly he declared to the doctor, he would demolish him if he touched or looked at his wife."[79]

Physicians dealt with the embarrassment of pa-tients and the suspicion of husbands by observing the drawing room behavior of "well-bred gentle-men." Dewees told his students to "endeavor, by well chosen conversation, to divert your patient's mind from the purpose of your visit."[80] All ques-tions of a delicate nature were to be communicated through a third party, perhaps the only other per-son in the room, either a nurse or an elderly friend or relative. The professional man was advised "never to seem to know anything about the parts of gen-eration, further than that there is an orifice near the rectum leading to an os."[81]

Physicians did not perform vaginal examina-tions unless it was absolutely important to do so,

and they often had to cajole women into permit-ting an examination at all. Nothing could be more shocking to a woman, Shippen lectured his stu-dents, "than for a young man the moment he en-ters the Chamber to ask for Pomatum and proceed to examine the uterus."[82] Doctors waited until a labor pain clutched their patients and then sug-gested an examination by calling it "taking a pain." During examination and delivery the patient lay completely covered in her bed, a posture more modest, if less comfortable, then squatting on a pallet or a birth stool. The light in the room was dimmed by closing the shutters during the day and covering the lamps at night. If a physician used forceps, he had to manipulate them under the cov-ers, using his free hand as a guide.[83] On this point doctors who read Thomas Denman's *Obstetrical Re-membrancer* were reminded that "Degorges, one of the best obstetricians of his time, was blind."[84]

The crowd of supportive friends and family dis-appeared with the arrival of the doctor. The phy-sician guarded against "too many attendants; where there are women, they must talk."[85] The presence of other women might increase the doctor's ner-vousness, and they certainly did not help the woman in labor. Medical men interpreted women's talk of other experiences with childbirth as mere gossip "of all the dangerous and difficult labours they ever heard any story about in their lives," which ought to be stopped lest it disturb the patient.[86] Especially distracting were the bawdy stories visitors told, ex-pecting the physician to laugh, too. Medical pro-fessors recommended "grave deportment," warn-ing that levity would "hurt your patient or yourself in her esteem."[87] Far from providing the consola-tion of a friend, the physician was often a stranger who needed to "get a little acquainted" with his patient. One medical text went so far as to coach him in a series of conversational icebreakers about children and the weather.[88]

Etiquette and prudery in the lying-in chamber affected medical care. Physicians were frustrated by their inability to examine their patients thor-oughly, for they knew full well that learning mid-wifery from a book was "like learning shipbuilding without touching timber."[89] Examinations were in-adequate, and the dangers of manipulating instru-ments without benefit of sight were tremendous. Dewees cautioned his students to take great care before pulling the forceps that "no part of the mother is included in the locking of the blades. This accident is frequent."[90] Accidental mutilation of infants was also reported, as the navel string had to be cut under the covers. Lecturers passed on the story of the incautious doctor who included the penis of an infant within the blades of his scissors.[91]

In view of such dangers, the conflict between social values and medical practice is striking. The expansion of medical knowledge brought men and women face to face with social taboos in family life. They had to ask themselves the question, Who should watch a woman give birth? For centuries the answer had unhesitatingly been female relatives and friends, and the midwife. The science of obstetrics, developing in the eighteenth century, changed the answer. Though women might socially be the most acceptable assistants at a delivery, men were potentially more useful.

In consequence of the attendance of male physicians, by 1825, for some American women, childbirth was ceasing to be an open ceremony. Though birth still took place at home, and though friends and relatives still lent a helping hand, visiting women no longer dominated the activities in the lying-in room. Birth became increasingly a private affair conducted in a quiet, darkened room. The physician limited visitors because they hindered proper medical care, but the process of birth was also concealed because it embarrassed both patient and physician.

Between 1760 and 1825 childbirth was thus transformed from an open affair to a restricted one. As one consequence of the development of obstetrics as a legitimate branch of medicine, male physicians began replacing midwives. They began to reduce childbirth to a scientifically managed event and deprived it of its folk aspects. Strengthened by the professionalization of their field, these physicians also responded to the hopes of women in Philadelphia, New York, and Boston for safe delivery. Although they helped some pregnant women, they hurt midwives, who were shut out of an area of medicine that had been traditionally their domain. All these innovations took place in the large urban centers in response to distinctly urban phenomena. They reflected the increasing privatization of family life, and they foreshadowed mid-nineteenth-century attitudes toward childbirth, mother, and woman.

NOTES

An earlier version of this article was read at the St. Louis meeting of the Organization of American Historians, April 1976. The author wishes to thank Gunther Barth, J. William T. Youngs, Jr., Regina Morantz, and Linda Auwers for comments on that draft.

1 Cecil K. Drinker, *Not So Long Ago: A Chronicle of Medicine and Doctors in Colonial Philadelphia* (New York, 1937), 59–61.

2 Although births are noted frequently in diaries and letters of the 17th, 18th, and early 19th centuries, the event itself is rarely described. For the most part, information on the medical procedures and social customs of birth analyzed in this article is derived from midwives' manuals, medical textbooks, and lecture notes of medical students. This literature mingles plain observation with partisan advocacy of medical reform. It seems reasonable to accept the physician's evaluations of midwifery as evidence of their desire for change, and their case histories as documents of the actual circumstances of birth. Despite ambiguities, the material provides a glimpse of social change not directly reflected in many conventional sources.

3 Betsy Copping Corner, *William Shippen, Jr.: Pioneer in American Medical Education* (Philadelphia, 1951), 103; Irving S. Cutter and Henry R. Viets, *A Short History of Midwifery* (Philadelphia, 1964), 150.

4 Cutter and Viets, *Short History,* 148–49.

5 For a discussion of childbearing patterns see Wilson H. Grabill, Clyde V. Kiser, and Pascal K. Whelpton, "A long view," in *The American Family in Social-Historical Perspective,* ed. Michael Gordon (New York, 1973), 392.; J. Potter, "The growth of population in America, 1700–1860," in *Population in History: Essays in Historical Demography,* ed. D.V. Glass, and D.E.C. Eversley (Chicago, 1965), 644, 647, 663, 679,; Robert V. Wells, "Demographic change and the life cycle of American families," in *The Family in History: Interdisciplinary Essays,* ed. Theodore K. Rabb and Robert I. Rotberg (New York, 1971), 85, 88.

When William Byrd II wrote in his diary in 1712, "my wife was often indisposed with breeding and very cross," he used a term common until the 19th century. Louis B. Wright and Marion Tinling, eds., *The Secret Diary of William Byrd of Westover, 1709–1712* (Richmond, Va., 1941), 548, "Breeding" was used colloquially and in popular medical literature.

The use of the term to describe the hatching or birth of animals parallels its application to humans. The word lingered longest in speech in the American south, where fertile or pregnant black slaves were called "breeding women," an indication of the animality implied in the word. *Oxford English Dictionary*, s.v. "breeding"; Mitford Mathews, ed., *A Dictionary of Americanisms on Historical Principles* (Chicago, 1951), s.v. "breeding." "Teeming," also considered archaic dialect by the *OED*, applied to women from the 16th through 18th century.

6 Benjamin Colman, *Some of the Honours that Religion Does unto the Fruitful Mothers in Israel* . . . (Boston, 1715), 8; Cotton Mather, *Elizabeth in Her Holy Retirement: An Essay to Prepare a Pious Woman for Her Lying-in; or, Maxims and Methods of Piety, to Direct and Support an Hand Maid of the Lord, Who Expects a Time of Travail* (Boston, 1710), 3; Cotton Mather, *Ornaments for the Daughters of Zion; or, The Character and Happiness of a Woman: in a Discourse*, 3d ed. (Boston, 1741), 2–3. Even a secular medical manual affirmed the curse of Eve: American edition of *Aristotle's Masterpiece*, 1766, discussed in Otho T. Beall, Jr., *"Aristotle's Master Piece in America*: a landmark in the folklore of medicine," *William and Mary Quarterly*, 1963, *3d ser. 20:* 216.

7 Mather, *Elizabeth in Her Retirement*, 1.

8 *The Diary of Cotton Mather* (Massachusetts Historical Society, *Collections*, 7th ser., pt. II [19121]), 8:618, 700; Mather, *Elizabeth in Her Retirement*, 2, 6, 7.

9 John Oliver, *A Present for Teeming American Women* (Boston, 1694), 3.

10 Ibid., 118.

11 [Thomas Clap], "Memoirs of a college president: womanhood in early America," ed. Edwin Stanley Wells, *Connecticut Magazine*, 1908, *12:* 233–239, esp. 235.

12 Drinker, *Not So Long Ago*, 48.

13 Stewart Mitchell, ed., *New Letters of Abigail Adams, 1788–1801* (Boston, 1947), 3–5, 56; Clayton Harding Chapman, "Benjamin Colman's daughters," *New England Quarterly*, 1953, *26:* 182; Malcolm R. Lovell, ed., *Two Quaker Sisters, from the Original Diaries of Elizabeth Buffam Chance and Lucy Buffam Lovell* (New York, 1937), 1, 12; Drinker, *Not So Long Ago, 51–60;* Mary Vial Holyoke's diary, in *The Holyoke Diaries, 1709–1856*, ed. George Francis Dow (Salem, Mass., 1911), 70, 73, 75, 83, 95, 100, 101, 107; *Diary of Samuel Sewall* (Massachusetts Historical Society, *Collections*, 5th ser., V–VII [1878–1882], 1: 11, 40, 110, 166, 222–223, 351, 394, 426; 2: 49, hereafter cited as *Diary of Sewall;* Ethel Armes, ed., *Nancy Shippen: Her Journal Book* (Philadelphia, 1935), 122–24.

14 James Hobson Aveling, *English Midwives: Their History and Prospects* (London, 1967 [orig. pub. 1872]), 3–4, 7, 10; E. H. Carter, *The Norwich Subscription Books: A Study of the Subscription Books of the Diocese of Norwich, 1637–1800* (London, 1937), 17–18, 134; facsimile oath of 1661, in Thomas Forbes, *The Midwife and the Witch* (New Haven, Conn., 1966), 145.

15 Cutter and Viets, *Short History*, 5–55; Isaac Flack, *Eternal Eve* (London, 1950), 218–19; Alfred McClintock, ed., *Smellie's Treatise on the Theory and Practice of Midwifery* (London, 1876–1878), 2: 248–50, 3: 26–27, 298, 317–19; Percival Willughby, *Observations in Midwifery*, ed. Henry Blenkinsop (Wakefield, Eng., 1972 [orig. pub. 1803]), 37, 155.

Save for midwifery, medical practice in England was divided among three guilds of physicians, surgeons, and apothecaries. Physicians, titled "doctor" and usually possessing university degrees, theoretically as gentlemen did not work with their hands. Surgeons, trained by apprenticeship and rarely holding degrees, dealt with structural emergencies. Apothecaries, also apprenticed, sold drugs. These distinctions disappeared in the rural areas and small towns of England, as well as in colonial America, where medical men, usually without formal training and indiscriminately called doctor, engaged in general practice. Even after 1765, the American men who were by strict definition physicians practiced general medicine. Richard Harrison Shryock, *Medicine and Society in America, 1660–1860* (Ithaca, N.Y., 1960), 2–3, 7, 10.

16 Aveling, *English Midwives*, 138–144; Alice Clark, *Working Life of Women in the Seventeenth Century* (London, 1919), 265, 269, 270–75; *The Compleat Midwifes Practice, in the Most Weighty and High Concernments of the Birth of Man* . . . (London 1656), 119–24; John Memis, *The Midwife's Pocket Companion; or, A Practical Treatise of Midwifery* (London, 1765), v–vii; Jane Sharp, *The Compleat Midwife's Companion; or, The Art of Midwifery Improved* . . . , 4th ed. (London, 1725), x–xii; Willughby, *Observations in Midwifery*, 73.

17 John Kobler, *The Reluctant Surgeon: A Biography of John Hunter* (New York, 1960), 31; Sharp, *Compleat Midwife's Companion, Introduction; Observations in Midwifery*, 102.

18 Valentine Seaman, *The Midwives Monitor, and Mothers Mirror: Being Three Concluding Lectures of a Course of Instruction of Midwifery* (New York, 1800), viii.

19 Ibid. See also Joseph Brevitt, *The Female Medical Repository* . . . (Baltimore, 1810), 6.

20 Beall, *"Aristotle's Master Piece," William and Mary Quarterly*, 1963, *3d ser. 20:* 209–10; Seaman, *Midwives Monitor*, ix. Beall's article is the best study of the popular manuals of "Aristotle." The *Masterpiece*, which was the creation of an English physi-

cian, "W. S.," and a succession of hack writers, first appeared in England in 1684. The numerous later editions were the only works on sex and gynecology widely available to 18th-century Americans.

21 Jane B. Donegan, "Midwifery in America, 1760–1860: a study in medicine and morality" (Ph.D. diss., Syracuse University, 1972), 9–10, 12; "A law for regulating mid wives within the city of New York," Minutes of the Common Council of New York, 1716, Appendix I, in Clarie E. Fox, "Pregnancy, childbirth and early infancy in Anglo-American culture, 1675–1830" (Ph.D. diss., University of Pennsylvania, 1966), 442–45; Richard Harrison Shryock, *Medical Licensing in America, 1650–1965* (Baltimore, 1967), 3, 16; James J. Walsh, *History of Medicine in New York: Three Centuries of Medical Progress* (New York, 1919), 2:22, 25.

22 Cutter and Viets, *Short History,* 145, 150; *Maryland Gazette* (Annapolis), Sept. 30, 1747; Francis R. Packard, *History of Medicine in the United States* (New York, 1931), 1: 52–53; Shryock, *Medicine and Society,* 11–12; J. Whitridge Williams, *A Sketch of the History of Obstetrics in the United States up to 1860* (Baltimore, 1903).

23 Wyndham B. Blanton, *Medicine in Virginia in the Seventeenth Century* (Richmond, 1930), 166; Packard, *History of Medicine,* 1: 52; Julia C. Spruill, *Women's Life and Work in the Southern Colonies* (Chapel Hill, N.C., 1938), 272; Herbert Thoms, *Chapters in American Obstetrics* (Springfield, Ill., 1961), 10.

24 *Diary of Sewall,* 1: 40, 114; Sharp, *Compleat Midwife's Companion,* frontispiece of midwife at christening.

25 Aristotle [pseud.], *Aristotle's Compleat and Experienc'd Midwife, in Two Parts. I. Guide for Childbearing Women. II. Proper and Safe Remedies for the Curing of All Those Distempers That Are Incident to the Female Sex . . . ,* 9th ed. (London [1700?]), iii.

26 Broadside of elegy to Mary Broadwell, in Francisco Guerra, *American Medical Bibliography, 1639–1783* (New York, 1962), 69.

27 Packard, *History of Medicine, 1:* 49.

28 Drinker, *Not So Long Ago,* 51, 52, 54; 59; Dow, ed. *Holyoke Diaries,* 70, 73, 75, 81, 83, 95, 101, 107; *Diary of Sewall,* 5: 40, 222–23, 394, 6: 49; Charles White, *A Treatise on the Management of Pregnant and Lying-in Women* (Worcester, Mass., 1793), 19–20.

29 Aristotle [pseud.], *Compleat and Experienc'd Midwife,* 50–51, 56, 57; Nicholas Culpepper, *A Directory for Midwives; or, A Guide for Women in Their Conception, Bearing, and Suckling Their Children* (London, 1651), 167; Drinker, *Not So Long Ago,* 60; *Diary of Sewall,* 5: 40; Sharp, *Compleat Midwife's Companion,* 81, 82, 124, 125, 128; White, *Treatise on Pregnant Women,* 20, 74; Willughby, *Observations in Midwifery,* 4, 11, 13, 19.

30 Seaman, *Midwives Monitor,* 90–91.

31 Drinker, *Not So Long Ago,* 59.

32 William Buchan, *Advice to Mothers on the Subject of Their Own Health* (Charleston, S.c., 1807), 28; *The London Practice of Midwifery by an American Practitioner* (Concord, N.H., 1826), 129; Thomas Chalkey James, "Notes from Drs. Osborne's and Clark's lectures on midwifery taken by T.C. James, London, 1790–1791," MS, Historical Collections, College of Physicians of Philadelphia.

33 Drinker, *Not So Long Ago,* 53, 59.

34 Mrs. Eva Eve Jones, ed., "Extracts from the journal of Miss Sarah Eve," *Pennsylvania Magazine of History and Biography,* 1881, 5: 195.

35 Mitchell, ed., *New Letters of Adams,* 4–5; Jack P. Greene, ed., *The Diary of Colonel Landon Carter of Sabine Hall, 1752–1788,* (Charlottesville, Va., 1965), 2: 86; Dow, ed., *Holyoke Diaries,* 49, 56, 58, 62, 63, 65, 67, 73, 77, 78, 82, 95, 100, 107; *Diary of Sewall,* 51; Sharp, *Compleat Midwife's Companion,* frontispiece drawing of lying-in; McClintock, ed., *Smellie's Treatise,* 1:380.

36 Corner, *Willilam Shippen,* 124; Cutter and Viets, *Short History,* 150.

37 *Kite's Philadelphia Directory for 1815* (Philadelphia, 1815), xi–xii; John Paxton. *The Philadelphia Directory and Register for 1819* (Philadelphia, 1819), n.p.; Robert Desilver, *The Philadelphia Directory and Register for 1824* (Philadelphia, 1824), n.p.

38 Walter Channing [John Ware?], *Remarks on the Employment of Females as Practitioners in Midwifery* (Boston, 1820), 1; *Independent Chronicle and the Universal Advertiser* (Boston), Nov. 8, 1781.

39 William Potts Dewees, *A Compendious System of Midwifery, Chiefly Designed to Facilitate the Inquiries of Those Who May Be Pursuing This Branch of Study* (Philadelphia, 1826), xiv.

40 William Buchan, *A Compend of Domestic Midwifery for the Use of Female Practitioners, Being an Appendix to Buchan's Domestic Medicine* (Charleston, S.C., 1815), 3; Frances E. Kobrin, "The American midwife controversy: a crisis of professionalization," in this volume; M. D. Learned and C. F. Brede, "An old German midwife's record, kept by Susanna Muller, of Providence Township, Lancaster County, Pennsylvania, during the years 1791–1815" (n.d.) Historical Collections, College of Physicians of Philadelphia; Mrs. Joseph Sarber, memorandum kept by Mrs. Joseph Sarber, midwife at the Falls of the Schuykill from 1814 to 1831, MS, Historical Society of Pennsylvania, Philadelphia,

41 Drinker, *Not So Long Ago,* 51–52; Dewees, *Compendious System of Midwifery,* 303.

42 Charles M. Andrews, *Colonial Folkways: A Chronicle of American Life in the Reign of the Georges* (New Ha-

ven, Conn., 1919), 147; Maurice Bear Gordon, *Aesculapius Comes to the Colonies: The Story of the Early Days of Medicine in the Thirteen Original Colonies* (Ventnor, N.J., 1949), 156–57, 460–65; Francis Packard, "How London and Edinburgh influenced medicine in Philadelphia in the eighteenth century," College of Physicians of Philadelphia, *Transactions*, 1931, *3d ser. 53:* 167.

43 Gordon, *Aesculapius*, 465; Packard, *History of Medicine*, 1: 181–230; Packard, "How London and Edinburgh influenced medicine," 163, 166.

44 John Morgan, *A Discourse upon the Institution of Medical Schools in America* (Baltimore, 1937 [orig. pub. 1765]), 33.

45 Samuel Bard, *Two Discourses Dealing with Medical Education in Early New York* (New York, 1921), 1.

46 Ibid., 10, 16, 19; Morgan, *Discourse upon the Institution of Medical Schools*, 14–17.

47 Packard, *History of Medicine*, 2: 1125–27; Williams, *Sketch of the History of Obstetrics*, 5–7.

48 OED, s.v. "obstetrics"; Packard, *History of Medicine*, 2: 1125–26.

49 Cutter and Viets, *Short History*, 26–28.

50 Ibid., 44–59; John Glaister, *Dr. William Smellie and His Contemporaries* (Glasgow, 1894), 170, 174, 178–179, 187; McClintock, ed., *Smellie's Treatise*, 2:250–51, 339.

51 McClintock, ed., *Smellie's Treatise*, 2: 339.

52 White, *Treatise on Pregnant Women*, viii, 70–71.

53 Thomas Dashiell Jones, *An Essay on the Importance of the Obstetrick Art; Submitted to the Examination of Charles Alexander Warfield, M.D., President of the Medical Faculty of the College of Medicine of Maryland . . .* (Baltimore, 1812), 5, 11, 21, 23.

54 Thomas Denman, *An Introduction to the Practice of Midwifery* (New York, 1802), 1:47; Jones, *Essay on Obstetrick Art*, 8, 17–19; Seaman, *Midwives Monitor*, x; White, *Treatise on Pregnant Women*, 79.

55 Boston Medical Association, *Rules and Regulations of the Boston Medical Association* (Boston, 1806), 4–5. The minimum fee escalated to $15/day case, $20/night by 1819, Boston Medical Association, *Rules and Regulations* (1819 ed).

56 Channing, *Remarks on Employment of Females*, 19; Edward Warren, *The Life of John Collins Warren, M.D., Compiled Chiefly from his Autobiography and Journals*, (Boston, 1860), 1: 219.

57 Dewees, *Compendious System of Midwifery* (Philadelphia, 1824), 307.

58 Ibid. (1826), xiv.

59 Drinker, *Not So Long Ago*, 51, 54–56, 59.

60 Dewees, *Compendious System of Midwifery* (1824), 307; Drinker, *Not So Long Ago*, 60.

61 Samuel Bard, *A Compendium of the Theory and Practice of Midwifery*, 5th ed. (New York, 1819), v, 176, 289;

Dewees, *Compendious System of Midwifery* (1826), xv.

62 Denman, *Introduction to Midwifery*, 235.

63 Jones, *Essay on Obstetrick Art*, 8.

64 Peter Miller, *An Essay on the Means of Lessening the Pains of Parturition* (Philadelphia, 1804), 340.

65 William Potts Dewees, *Essays on Various Subjects Connected with Midwifery* (Philadelphia, 1823), 24.

66 Channing, *Remarks on Employment of Females*, 6–12; Jones, *Essay on Obstetrick Art*, 20; Joseph Kett, *The Formation of the American Medical Profession: The Role of Institutions, 1780–1860* (New Haven, Conn., 1968), 10–30.

67 *Pennsylvania Gazette* (Philadelphia), Jan. 31, 1765.

68 Williams, *Sketch of the History of Obstetrics*, 13; Seaman, *Midwives Monitor*, iii–vii.

69 Bard, *Compendium of Theory and Practice of Midwifery*, iv, 289; Brevitt, *Female Medical Repository*, 149–155; Buchan, *Compend of Domestic Midwifery;* Samuel Jennings, *Married Lady's Companion, or Poor Man's Friend . . .* (NewYork, 1808), 135; Seaman, *Midwives Monitor*, 31–32. All of these works were directed entirely or in part to midwives.

70 Thomas Ewell, *Letters to Ladies, Detailing Important Information Concerning Themselves and Infants* (Philadelphia, 1817), vii–viii.

71 Channing, *Remarks on Employment of Females*, 4–7.

72 Aveling, *English Midwives*, 138–44, 153–59; Cutter and Viets, *Short History*, 43; Glaister, *William Smellie*, 32–36.

73 Dewees, *Compendious System of Midwifery* (1826), xv.

74 Channing, *Remarks on Employment of Females*, 16, 17; Ewell, *Letters to Ladies*, 27.

75 Jones, *Essay on Obstetrick Art*, 11.

76 Seaman, *Midwives Monitor*, iv.

77 *Virginia Gazette* (Purdie and Dixon), Oct. 1, 1772; reprinted in *New-London Gazette* (Conn.), Jan 29, 1773.

78 Elizabeth Nihell, *A Treatise on the Art of Midwifery, Setting Forth Various Abuses Therein, Especially as to the Practice with Instruments* (London, 1760), and S. W. Fores, *Man-Midwifery Dissected* (London, 1793), are outstanding examples of arguments made about the supposed immorality of man-midwives. Glaister, *William Smellie*, discusses other examples of such literature.

79 Ewell, *Letters to Ladies*, 27.

80 Dewees, *Compendious System of Midwifery* (1826), 189; Daniel B. Smith, "Notes on lectures of Thomas Chalkey James and William Potts Dewees, University of Pennsylvania, 1826," MS, Hist. Colls., College of Physicians of Philadelphia.

81 *London Practice of Midwifery*, 109.

82 Bard, *Compendium of Theory and Practice of Midwifery*, 181; lecture notes from lectures of William Shippen, Jr., University of Pennsylvania, n.d., MS,

Hist. Colls., College of Physicians of Philadelphia.

83 Bard, *Compendium of Theory and Practice of Midwifery*, 181; Dewees, *Compendious System of Midwifery* (1826), 189–90; *London Practice of Midwifery*, 108–109.

84 Thomas Denman, *The Obstetrical Remembrancer; or, Denman's Aphorisms on Natural and Difficult Parturition* (New York, 1848 [orig. U.S. publ, 1803]), 46.

85 *London Practice of Midwifery*, 129.

86 Ibid., 129–30.

87 James, "Notes from Osborne's and Clark's lectures," Hist. Colls., College of Physicians of Philadelphia; notes on Shippen lectures, ibid.

88 Notes on Shippen lectures, Hist. Colls., College of Physicians of Philadelphia; *London Practice of Midwifery*, 127.

89 Bard, *Compendium of Theory and Practice of Midwifery*, 220; Seaman, *Midwives Monitor*, ix.

90 Dewees, *Compendious System of Midwifery* (1826), 313.

91 Kobler, *Reluctant Surgeon*, 32; *London Practice of Midwifery*, 132–33.

11

"Down to Death's Door": Women's Perceptions of Childbirth in America

JUDITH WALZER LEAVITT AND WHITNEY WALTON

In the rugged lands of the Alaskan frontier in the early twentieth century an early winter avalanche pinned Martha Martin to a mountain ledge, isolating her from her family and breaking one of her arms and one of her legs.[1] Advanced in her pregnancy and struggling with severe weather conditions, she extracted herself and crawled home, where, during the next months, she managed to stay alive and prepare for her baby's arrival. Entirely alone, Martha Martin delivered her own baby and lived to be rescued during the spring thaw.

Martin had complete control over her birthing in the literal sense. No outside person and no set of institutional regulations determined how her childbirth occurred. Martin's experience is noteworthy, however, not because it exemplified the ultimate in potential control women can exercise over their birth experiences, but because it calls into question the very issue of what control in childbirth means. Rather than being able to dominate her own birth situation, in fact, Martin was at the mercy of her body. If any complications had occurred—a breech presentation, placenta previa, hemorrhage, or if her placenta had not come away entirely—Martin's control would have evaporated. She had no choice about how or where to have her baby, nor did she have the opportunity to be at-

tended by anyone who might have been able to help her through a difficult situation. This extreme circumstance highlights the three main components of the childbirth experience that have been important to American women since colonial times: assistance, choice, and safety. Although taking different forms over time and altered by socioeconomic and ethnic background, these three factors have shaped women's childbirth activity in the past, and they continue to be important issues for parturient women today.

Women's perceptions of childbirth and how they changed over time can best be revealed by reading women's own accounts of their birthing experiences. Because most historical analyses have been based on prescriptive advice literature or on the accounts of birth attendants, this essay relies heavily on personal and family accounts to provide a new perspective on one of women's most persistent and challenging experiences.[2]

Traditionally women attended other women in their confinements. Trained midwives or experienced friends and relatives came to help before or during labor, and many of them stayed for days or weeks afterward, participating in the transition to motherhood. The entrance of male physicians into normal obstetrics in the last third of the eighteenth century altered this traditional female event. Physicians provided the small group of urban women who wanted and could afford their services with additional options for their births, and the presence of men in the birthing rooms made the traditional women's event less exclusive. Recent social historians agree that the entrance of male physicians into normal childbirth and the subsequent growth of obstetric technology and drugs in the

JUDITH WALZER LEAVITT is Associate Professor of the History of Medicine and Women's Studies at the University of Wisconsin, Madison, Wisconsin.
WHITNEY WALTON is Assistant Professor of History at Hamline University, St. Paul, Minnesota.
Reprinted with permission from *Childbirth: The Beginning of Motherhood, Proceedings of the Second Motherhood Symposium,* April, 1981 (Madison: Women's Studies Research Center, 1982).

nineteenth century significantly altered the experiences of the birthing women. Men and intervention overturned centuries of female-directed noninterventionist childbirth.[3] But from parturient women's own perspective, neither the presence of men in the rooms usually reserved for women nor physicians' frequent use of drugs and instruments changed the basic structure of childbirth in America. Those women who were attended by male physicians—and they were less than half of all birthing women in America before 1900—continued to determine what happened behind the closed doors of their birthing rooms just as they had traditionally at midwife-attended births. Birthing women, accompanied by their friends and relatives, dominated home birthing rooms throughout the nineteenth century regardless of the sex or training of their birth attendants. Not until mid-twentieth-century women left their own homes and their supportive network of women and entered the birthing rooms of medicine did the power structure of American childbirth significantly change. In this transition to the hospital, which occurred for a majority of American women by 1940, women lost many of the controls over childbirth they had held for millennia.[4] This paper, in making the point that the twentieth-century move to the hospital was the most significant transition in childbirth history, explores why women and their birth attendants made choices that increasingly replaced the supportive aspects of traditional birthings—familiar home environments, the presence of friends and relatives, and the choice of attendants—with the sterile environment of a hospital, where in shining clean delivery rooms women found themselves "alone among strangers."[5]

Between the end of the eighteenth century and the beginning of the twentieth, two common themes emerge from American women's accounts of their childbirths. First, the company of other women before, during, and after the delivery was of paramount importance to birthing women. When other women, especially close friends and relatives, could be secured, parturients felt more relaxed and more in control of the situation. Second, the fear of pain, postpartum complications, and death equally pervaded women's consciousness. Women feared that the physical strain of childbirth would weaken them for long periods of time, make them lifelong invalids, or kill them. The importance of women companions helps explain why childbirth remained in women's domain as long as it did, and the importance of women's physical fears, as increasingly sophisticated obstetric techniques seemed to offer greater safety, helps explain why women ultimately agreed to go to the hospital to have their babies.

American women's perceptions of childbirth in the era of home deliveries were amazingly similar. Rich, poor, urban, and rural women all shared with each other, by virtue of their sex, an enormous bond of common experience. Circumstances obviously played their part, because money and access could broaden the number of birth options, but hundreds of women's accounts of their childbirths reveal that women's feelings about birth were not limited by particular circumstances. Women anticipated the event anxiously (and sometimes joyfully), suffered through the agonies and dangers, and sought each other's support, regardless of the details of their specific birth experiences. Childbirth was indeed, as Carroll Smith-Rosenberg has argued, one of the "functional bonds" that united women.[6] Owing to their common physical and social experience, women developed similar feelings, fears, and needs during pregnancy and delivery, despite their divergent life circumstances. Childbirth was a woman's event, and most women throughout American history consciously wanted it that way.

Women felt vulnerable when they discovered they were pregnant, and they hoped to prepare for their confinements by arming themselves with the strength of other women who had passed through the event successfully. Most crucial to the support networks women tried to establish were their own mothers. "If you could but be with me now, what wouldn't I give," wrote Anita McCormick Blaine to her mother, Nettie Fowler McCormick, in 1890 as she prepared for the birth of her first child. "Dearest mother mine—all would be complete if you were here."[7] Even though her mother was away, Anita Blaine moved into her childhood Chicago home to have her baby and arranged for her former governess to come from Virginia to be with her. Despite all Anita's preparations and the presence of an experienced doctor and nurse, Nettie McCormick yearned to be with her daughter. She wrote detailed instructions about her care, advising, for example, rubbing olive oil over the abdomen and perineal area to ease delivery. She worried that only a mother could rightfully do such an intimate job: "I don't know if you have a person you could let do it," she wrote, "but I wish I were there to do it."[8]

In the highly mobile nineteenth century, many American women shared Anita McCormick Blaine's predicament of finding themselves separated from their closest relatives during their pregnancies and confinements. Georgiana Bruce Kirby followed her husband to California in 1852 and found herself both pregnant and almost completely isolated. "I have seen the face of but one woman in four months," she lamented to her diary. Mother and other relatives totally beyond reach, Kirby was ready to settle for the company of any "congenial female companion." Her husband was attentive and kind, but, Kirby concluded, "Every good woman needs a companion of her own sex." She finally spent a few days and nights visiting another pregnant woman, who, Kirby wrote, "quite made me forget myself and my ailments."[9]

Letters formed a partial but usually frustrating substitute for many women whose marriages took them away from their childhood friends and relatives. Mary Hallock Foote prepared for her delivery by trying to follow the long-distance advice of her close friend Helena DeKay Gilder. "I have followed your advice in one of the two ways in which you recommended me to be anticipating the evil day that is coming—as to the hardening of the nipples—but I do not know how you mean about using oil," she wrote. "Is it the abdomen that is to be rubbed?"[10] Letters could never be as satisfying as the actual presence of the needed ones. "I thought of my mother," wrote Leah Morton about her pregnancy. "I wanted her, I needed her so that I could have cried, all the way over the long miles between us."[11]

Trying to overcome the problem of isolation, some women traveled long distances to be with their mothers at this most family-centered time. Dorothy Lawson McCall, the daughter of wealthy Massachusetts parents, went west to Oregon with her husband at the turn of the twentieth century, but returned to her parental home across the entire continent for each of her four childbirths.[12] Gladys

Brooks likewise returned to the family house to have her baby in the bed where her husband had been born.[13] Despite the difficulty of travel during their advanced pregnancies, many women who could not find appropriate women to attend them went home to mother.[14]

Emily McCorkee Fitzgerald, an army doctor's wife on the Alaskan frontier in the 1870s, could not travel home to mother, and so she made elaborate plans for neighboring women to attend her during and after her delivery. She had the additional security that most women did not share of having her physician-husband at hand. Even so, after her terrible ordeal of childbirth and the difficulty of scheduling her women-helpers, she wrote to her mother, "I hope I will never have any more babies where I can't have some of my relatives with me."[15]

Frequently even the best plans for gathering women together went astray in the haste of an early labor or in the midst of the proverbial snowstorm. Quite often when rural women went into labor, husbands hastened to summon the nearest neighbor or to send for the midwife or doctor and returned to find the babe already born. Countless women found themselves unexpectedly and totally alone during their deliveries. "When mother went into labor," wrote one daughter, "she called father from the field by waving a dishtowel. He had to unhitch the team, unharness one of them, harness him again, and then drive off to fetch the woman who served as mid-wife. She lived two miles down the road from our house. But, just as father drove out of the yard, a son, large and husky, was born."[16] Another woman, finding herself in active labor three weeks before expected, quickly turned to the chapter in her baby book "What to do before the doctor comes." While her husband raced for the doctor, her baby was born.[17] A logger's wife recounted how her husband barely rescued her 1908 breech delivery:

> When Bill was gone once . . . I broke water and was having too much pain. Feeling that baby with my hands I knew for certain it was going to breech. I put the kids to bed to keep warm and told the older ones to keep that fire going no matter what. . . . I got . . . on a pallet under my quilts and Lordy did I pray for Bill to come back. He came blowing in

that night. Said he just had a feeling. I was never so glad to see anyone. He pulled that baby out [feet first.][18]

Whether women chose midwives or doctors or experienced neighbors to attend them, whether they lived in cities or in the hinterlands, whether they lived at the beginning of the nineteenth century or the beginning of the twentieth century, they sought the company of women friends and relatives to be with them through their ordeals. Scarcely any family accounts of women in childbirth fail to mention this important element of the experience. From the South, Laura Norwood wrote to her mother, "It would be a great comfort to me to have Sarah [her sister?] or some of you with me."[19] From the Wisconsin frontier in 1851, Elizabeth Atkinson Richmond wrote her mother about the gracious neighbors who came to help her, concluding, "I can't tell you, dear Mother, how many times I have wished *you* near me to advise me."[20] From Boston, Mrs. A. Graves pitied her friend who delivered when "deprived of all intercourse with her kindred or friends" at a time when "the presence of a mother is so anxiously longed for and so much needed."[21] Grace Lumpkin's fictional account of a poor woman in South Carolina in the first decade of the twentieth century, who delivered her child with the sole assistance of her own father, captures the common feelings:

> As she gulped down the warm coffee she wished in herself there was a woman who would know what to do without telling. And she wished the men were where they belonged when a woman was in travail—somewhere out on the mountains or at a neighbor's. . . . [her father] must see her as he had not seen her since she was a naked baby in her mother's arms. Soon, maybe, it would be over.[22]

If mothers, relatives, and friends were the preferred companions of childbirths, women settled for any women who happened to be nearby. The presence of even strange women to share the pain and the fears and the joys of childbirth could provide comfort. Men could not know the women's experience; as one woman recorded, "His life has not been in jeopardy. Except in sympathy his nerves have not been racked, his muscles strained, his joints wrenched, his fibers torn, his blood spilled."[23] More simply another woman wrote: "Only a woman can know what a woman has suffered or is suffering."[24]

Women found other women necessary in part because of society's separation of the sexes into sex-determined roles and spheres. Nineteenth-century women were accustomed to sharing certain of their experiences and feelings only with other women, just as men cordoned off parts of their lives as men's business. The fears and joys of childbirth could be best understood by other women, especially those who had themselves had babies. Women who had not had children could still be more empathetic than men because childbirth was part of a whole network of experiences from menstruation to menopause that women shared with one another. Even when women invited male physicians to attend them in childbirth, they continued to yearn for and need comforting women around them.[25]

Although some women gave birth alone and others could not find female companions, most parturients throughout the home birth period delivered with the assistance of other women. Whether attended by midwives or male physicians, women continued to have women friends and relatives with them through their labors and deliveries. The presence of women in the birthing room where they traditionally determined events fostered the continuation of women's dominance of childbirth. Physicians realized that they needed to get approval from the attending women to use the forceps or administer anesthesia. In the beginning of the nineteenth century, for example, one physician found that "the women in attendance put their veto" upon a procedure of which they did not approve. Almost one hundred years later a doctor noted that he "cannot be too insistent with his patients over whom, usually, he has no control."[26] With birth in the woman's home domain, and with the presence of experienced women, childbirth remained a woman's event until the twentieth century.

Women's companionship was important because women perceived birth as part of woman's sphere, but also because women so commonly feared their birthings. Women were afraid of the pain and suffering of birth, afraid of developing agonizing gynecologic problems that would be with them the rest of their lives, and afraid of death. The possibility of this ultimate loss of control made women gather to themselves all the strengths they could muster. The familiar walls and sounds of their homes and the reassurances of trusted women relatives and friends thus served as important bulwarks against the uncontrollable.

Death fears remained central to women's perceptions of their births throughout the nineteenth and early twentieth centuries. Georgiana Kirby began to keep a journal when she learned she was pregnant in 1852 because, she wrote, "I think that perhaps I may die and my babe live."[27] Bessie Rudd, just a few years later, wrote to her husband that preparatory to her confinement she was arranging her household accounts so that he could understand them. "I have everything in order & fixed to my mind, should any unforeseen sorrow come to me. You know we must think of all things, Edward & have everything in readiness . . . I sometimes think I am ready to [die]. . . . though Life was never dearer to me than now."[28]

"As the time draws near I fear & tremble," wrote Persis Sibley Andrews to her diary in 1847, "I have suffered much in the last four weeks & often find myself indulging in forbodings of evil—of years of ill health as was the case before & all & the worst ills to be feared in the case. God help me."[29] Andrews feared childbirth the more because of the invalidism that followed her first birth, and her perceptions were shared by many other women who had survived their first births only to find themselves again pregnant. Agnes Reid's second pregnancy evoked this letter: "I confess I dreaded it with a dread that every mother must feel in repeating the experience of childbearing. I could only think that another birth would mean another pitiful struggle of days' duration, followed by months of weakness, as it had been before."[30] Another mid-nineteenth-century woman found herself "walking under the shadow of maternity. . . . Then came the week when there seemed no hope from day to day that even one life could be given for the other, but that both would perish together."[31] "Between oceans of pain," wrote one woman of her third birth in 1885, "there stretched continents of fear; fear of death and dread of suffering beyond bearing."[32]

Surviving a childbirth did not allow women to forget its horrors. Lillie M. Jackson, recalling her 1905 confinement, wrote "While carrying my baby, I was so miserable. . . . I went down to death's door to bring my son into the world, and I've never

forgotten. Some folks say one forgets, and can have them right over again, but today I've not forgotten, and that baby is 36 years old."[33] Too many women shared with Hallie Nelson her feelings upon her first birth: "I began to look forward to the event with dread—if not actual horror." Even after Nelson's successful birth, she "did not forget those awful hours spent in labor."[34]

Women recounted their trials with wrenching repetitiveness. One wrote: "[My child] nearly killed me as he tore his way into life." Another: "My body and spirits were so extremely weak, I could only just bear to look at those I loved." Another: "The two of us were close to death. . . . The strain of having him had exhausted me." Another: "The angels of life and death wrestled over my baby's life and over mine in that little pioneer fort." Another: "I lay at the point of death. And out of that hour in which I touched the hand of death, two months before her time, came my daughter."[35] Women suffered in the anticipation and in the reality of childbirth.

Many women managed to find joy or purpose despite their hard experiences. Mary Foote recounted her 1877 childbirth as a "long dreadful day and night . . . a dim bewildering Hall of pain all day—growing worse & worse and then came Heaven at last. . . . I am weak and happy." In another letter to her friend she admitted that motherhood was "a sort of pendulum . . . between joy & dread."[36] Josephine Peabody agreed that her childbirth in 1908 was "the most terrible day" of her life, but concluded to her diary, "Now that it is over—I would not for anything . . . give up the awfulness of it. For I am wiser in the height and the depth, for this knowledge of the almost inconceivable agony . . . I can never forget—or explain—that apocalyptic hugeness of the thing. . . . I have crossed the abyss now. . . . That anything so wonder-small and wonder-soft and helpless and exquisite should come of anything so cruel and unimaginable as Birth," she marveled.[37] Another new mother rejoiced that out of her "time of great difficulty and distress" she emerged "the living mother of a living and perfect child."[38]

Death remained a persistent threat and a too-common reality in the years before the 1930s and 1940s, when America's maternal mortality rates finally began to fall. Statistics before the twentieth century are unreliable and sketchy, but early-twentieth-century mortality figures were high, indicating that in the years before germ theory rates may have been considerably higher. Between 1900 and 1935 approximately sixty white women and over a hundred nonwhite women died for every ten thousand live births.[39] Certainly the perception of childbirth's dangers was a constant in the minds of pregnant women. A daughter wrote: "My mother died suddenly, giving premature birth, when I was seventeen (in 1879). She herself was only thirty-eight." A husband wrote: "In June [1875] my wife gave birth to my youngest daughter. From this sickness she never recovered. She suffered terribly . . . and finally died . . . leaving three boys and two girls to mourn her loss." A neighbor wrote of a mission wife in Oregon who, while her husband was away, "went down into the valley of the shadow of death" after delivering her first baby. A New England woman wrote: "My friend, Mrs. John Howard, of Springfield, has died as she has expected to,—under the most aggravated circumstances that a woman can leave the world. She never gave birth to her child; but died in the effort. In this dreadful manner have six of my youthful contemporaries departed this life." A desolate husband turned from his wife's death in childbirth in 1830: "I am undone forever." These are not isolated incidents. The U.S. Children's Bureau studies in the early twentieth century catalogued the intimate knowledge of death that pregnant women, especially in rural isolated areas, carried with them along with their swollen bellies.[40]

Women's fears of death and the persistent examples that their fears were not unfounded eroded the comfortable feelings that women received from their companions during traditional births. The threat of death and physical debility led women to search for safer and less painful childbirths. Because of the dangers, women tried to modify traditional births by incorporating new possibilities as they became available. Thus some eighteenth-century women readily invited physicians to attend them, despite their worries about the propriety of having strange men participate in intimate events, in the hope that the man-midwives could provide easier and safer births. As modesty faded, increasing numbers of women in the nineteenth century followed the example of seeking "expert" attendance.[41] Women, desiring relief from their misery, welcomed physicians' forceps and drugs, and anes-

thesia quickly became, in the words of Fanny Appleton Longfellow, the first American woman to receive ether in childbirth in 1847, "the greatest blessing of this age."[42]

Most of the middle-class women who formed the vanguard of Americans to be attended by physicians continued traditional practices at the same time as they incorporated the newest techniques. Anita McCormick Blaine, for example, in 1890 sequestered herself in her childhood home where "every chair and table speaks to me of dear familiar times," surrounded herself with loving female helpers, and then allowed a physician to deliver her baby while she was under the influence of chloroform. She united the old benefits of traditional female-home-centered birth with the new obstetric technologies. The doctor managed her birth in the context that she created.[43]

The twentieth-century move to the hospital extended earlier attempts to subdue the dangerous forces of childbirth. Obstetricians who could use the newest technology and take advantage of the expanding hospital services seemed to offer women an opportunity to survive their pregnancies in good health. The move of general obstetrics to the hospital in the twentieth century was influenced by the developing specialty of obstetrics, drug and technological advances, the expansion of hospitals themselves, immigration patterns, and the automobile, among other factors. Perceptions of childbirth as a time when death threatened contributed to women's willingness to make the move to the hospital. Their extreme worries explain why they gave up the consolatory company of close women friends and relations within the familiar walls of their own homes. Women allowed the increasing medicalization of childbirth out of their fears of losing their lives or their babies' lives, out of their will to survive and alleviate suffering. However, in gaining what they thought would be life itself, women lost for future generations what had been traditionally very common—the strength that comes from being surrounded by familiar and loving people during times of stress.

The move to the hospital was qualitatively different from previous changes in childbirth procedures. During the nineteenth century women had maintained their own environment for their births and their own selection of company and attendants. Women still controlled their births in the sense that they invited attendants into their homes knowing what interventions those attendants could use. Snug in their own homes, women made all the domestic arrangements. Regardless of the actual birth techniques used by the attendants, women found solace in the familiar—the ancestral bed, the wallpaper, the smells and noises of home. Even Martha Martin alone in her Alaska cabin felt good about arranging her room to make it suitable for birth. If they could not control the physical birth itself, women at home could determine the birth environment and company. Some women chose all available attendants to be with them at one time; women friends and relatives, midwives, and doctors frequently found themselves gathered around the same childbirth bed.[44] Throughout the home-birth period women incorporated whatever new ideas they had access to or wanted into the traditional experience of birth. The comforts of home and the ability to have the company of their choice were central to women's perceptions of what they needed during the difficult times; but women who went to the hospital gave up these choices and opted instead for safety, which they thought more important.

Women delivering their babies in the nineteenth century felt that they had little control over their physical fate; their birth attendants also felt powerless before raging puerperal infections and other complications that overcame women so forcefully. Trying to control the risks of death and of fallen wombs, vesicovaginal and rectovaginal fistulas, perineal tears, and a host of undefined "female complaints" that resulted from childbirths, women sought birth methods that could guarantee them physical security. When hospital births seemed to promise the long-awaited relief, women who suffered and watched their friends die in childbirth eagerly tried the new opportunity. They had their lives to gain if the new obstetrics succeeded in reducing childbirth mortality and postbirth complications.[45]

In hospital deliveries women left their family and friends at the door of the labor room and faced their birthings alone, as did this unnamed woman who delivered her baby in the 1930s:

> Arriving [at the hospital] . . . she is immediately given benefit of one of the modern analgesics or pain-killers. Soon she is in a dreamy, half-conscious state. . . . She knows nothing about being taken to the spotlessly clean delivery room, placed on a sterile table, draped with sterile sheets; neither does she see her attendants, the doctor and nurses, garbed for her protection in sterile white gowns and gloves; nor the shiny boiled instruments and antiseptic solutions. She does not hear the cry of her baby when first he feels the chill of this cold world, or see the care with which the doctor repairs such lacerations as may have occurred. . . . Finally she awakes in smiles, a mother with no recollection of having become one.[46]

This woman clearly had a very different childbirth experience from the women who delivered at home. She was separated from the people she loved, she was in an unfamiliar environment controlled by others, and she was unconscious for her childbirth. Women did not view the transition to the hospital as a time when they lost important parts of traditional birth experiences, but rather as a time when they gained life and health, aspects of birth that had been elusive and uncertain in the past. Whether or not women were correct in their assumption that hospital births would be safer for them (and the evidence based on physicians' own assessments in the 1930s indicates that they were wrong), they *thought* specialists' attendance in hospitals and the use of the newest technology would be safer.[47] "I have placed myself in the hands of . . . a specialist in obstetrics," wrote Lella Secor to her mother in 1918. "I have every confidence in him and it is a great relief."[48] The hospital appealed to women because it was modern, well equipped, and staffed by experts: it represented the newest medical advance. "I have nothing to worry about . . . and have only to concentrate on giving birth," wrote a mid-twentieth-century mother about going to the hospital: "All this peace of mind, plus expert medical attention, makes me wonder why anybody would consider it a 'privilege' to have a baby at home." Another woman agreed: the "hospital is equipped with every modern device for the safe delivery of babies, nursing and medical attention is available at any hour of the day or night. How much simpler—and more restful—to be in a hospital where babies are an accepted business."[49] Women gave up some aspects of control for others, because on balance the new benefits seemed more important. Since they could not control all the major aspects of birth—the environment, the people with them, the pain, and the dangers—at the same time, women seeking control over birth's pains and dangers gave up control over the environment and companionship. In seeking life and health, women relinquished consciousness and self-determination.

Some of the women who went to the hospital to deliver their babies—and this number increased to 95 percent of American women by 1955—missed features of home births and found hospital births lacking in the human dimension. Continuing to appreciate the safety factors they believed existed in hospitals, many women in the 1950s attacked the "cruelty in the maternity wards." "My first two deliveries were pure torture," wrote one woman from Jeffersonville, New York, to the *Ladies' Home Journal*, which exposed these conditions. "So many women," agreed a new mother from Elkhart, Indiana, "receive such brutal inconsiderate treatment that the whole thing is a horrible nightmare." Another woman concurred that she had been "foiled in every attempt to follow her own wishes."[50] These women noticed that the physical removal of childbirth from a woman's home to the physicians' institution shifted the balance of power with it. Birth was no longer part of the woman's domain, as it had been during all the years it remained in the home. Women who in their own homes could be attended by physicians and still determine what would happen—could demand ether, or refuse specific procedures—still controlled much of their own births. But women who entered the birthing rooms of medicine were captured by institutional routine and could not determine what kinds of birth they would have. An Ohio woman observed that "many normal deliveries are turned into nightmares for the mothers by 'routine' obstetrical practices." Women drew the analogy to the assembly line when they described their hospital births and agreed with the mother from Bozeman, Montana, who wrote, "The cruelest part of [hospital] childbirth is being alone among strangers."[51] By the middle of the twentieth century, women had not achieved childbirth experiences that were safe, comfortable, and psychologically satisfying, components they had been seeking throughout American history.

By listening to women who went down to death's door to bring their babies into this world we begin to understand that childbirth, a persistent event in women's lives, is a historical raw nerve that exposes and reveals important elements in women's lives in the past. Women who feared childbirth and yet found themselves repeatedly pregnant experienced significant physical pressures and conflicts for much of their adult lives. Their efforts to relieve their afflictions led them to make choices—circumscribed as they were—that aided physicians in medicalizing childbirth. Women participated in leaving us a legacy of impersonal and institutional birth, which we can accept only through understanding the pervasiveness of suffering in their lives.

NOTES

This paper is a revised version of a paper delivered at the symposium "Childbirth, The Beginning of Motherhood," sponsored by the Department of the History of Medicine and the Women's Studies Program, University of Wisconsin, April, 1981. We gratefully acknowledge the research assistance of Elizabeth Black, Eve Fine and Calvin Dexter, and we would like to thank Susan Friedman, Gerda Lerner, and Ronald L. Numbers for their comments on the earlier draft.

1 Martha Martin [pseud.], *O Rugged Land of Gold* (New York: Macmillan, 1953). See also the shortened version of this edited diary in the *Ladies' Home Journal*, 1952, *69:* 35, 87–121.

2 Evidence for this paper was gathered from women and other family members who participated in various ways in childbirths. Many of them are memory accounts written years later. Over two hundred accounts form the base for the conclusions drawn here. We have not tried in any way to make this a quantitative study. Most women left no written records of their births, and any attempt to generalize from our small group to women in general would be problematic. Yet we have been struck at how similar the accounts we used have been, and we do believe that the quality of the feelings expressed as we describe them in this paper give a legitimate reflection of women's childbirth experiences.

3 See for example, Catherine M. Scholten, "'On the importance of the obstetrick art': changing customs

of childbirth in America, 1760 to 1825," in this volume; and Richard W. Wertz and Dorothy C. Wertz, *Lying-In: A History of Childbirth in America* (New York: Free Press, 1977); and Janet Bogdan, "Care or cure? childbirth practices in nineteenth-century America," *Feminist Studies*, 1978, *4:* 92–99. For an overview of recent literature on the history of childbirth, see Nancy Schrom Dye, "The history of childbirth in America," *Signs*, 1980, *6:* 97–108.

4 In 1940, 55.8 percent of American women delivered their babies in hospitals. See Neal Devitt, "The transition from home to hospital birth in the United States, 1930–1960," *Birth and the Family Journal*, 1977, *4:* 47–58.

5 Woman from Bozeman, Montana, quoted in Gladys Denny Shultz, "Cruelty in maternity wards," *Ladies' Home Journal*, May 1958, 45.

6 Carroll Smith-Rosenberg, "The female world of love and ritual: relations between women in nineteenth-century America," in this volume.

7 Anita McCormick Blaine to Nettie Fowler McCormick, August 1890, McCormick Papers, Wisconsin State Historical Society Archives.

8 Nettie McCormick to Anita McCormick Blaine, August 1890, McCormick Papers.

9 Georgiana Bruce Kirby journal, in Erna Olafson Hellerstein, Leslie Parker Hume, and Karen Offen, eds., *Victorian Women: A Documentary Account of Women's Lives in Nineteenth-Century England, France, and the United States* (Stanford: Stanford University Press, 1981), 211–13.

10 Mary Hallock Foote Letters, Stanford University Library, transcripts of letters to Helena DeKay Gilder 1874–86, Department of Special Collections, M115, M305. Quoted with permission.

11 Elizabeth G. Stern [Leah Morton, pseud.], *I Am a Woman—and a Jew* (New York: Arno, 1969; orig. pub. 1926), 87.

12 Dorothy Lawson McCall, *The Copper King's Daughter: From Cape Cod to Crooked River* (Portland, Ore: Binfords & Mort, 1972).

13 Gladys Brooks, *Boston and Return* (New York: Atheneum, 1962).

14 See, for example, Forest W. McNeir, *Forest McNeir of Texas* (San Antonio: Naylor Company, 1956); Elsa Maxwell, *R.S.V.P. Elsa Maxwell's Own Story* (Boston: Little, Brown, 1954); Malcolm R. Lovell, *Two Quaker Sisters: From the Original Diaries of Elizabeth Buffum Chase and Lucy Buffum Lovell* (New York: Liveright, 1937); Mattie White Briscoe, *Dun-Movin: The Memoirs of a Minister's Wife* (New York: Exposition Press, 1963); and Susan Allison, *A Pioneer Gentlewoman in British Columbia: The Recollections of Susan Allison*, ed. Margaret A. Ormsby (Vancouver: University of British Columbia Press, 1976).

15 Emily McCorkee Fitzgerald, *Army Doctor's Wife on the Frontier: Letters from Alaska and the Far West 1874–1878*, ed. Abe Laufe (Pittsburgh: University of Pittsburgh Press, 1962).

16 Frances Jacobs Alberts, ed., *Sod House Memories* (Hastings, Neb.: Sod House Society, 1972), memoir of C. O. and Ann Almquist of Nebraska, 7.

17 Marguerite Wallace Kennedy, *My Home on the Range* (Boston: Little, Brown, 1951), 274–75.

18 Patricia Cooper and Norma Bradley Buferd, *The Quilters: Women and Domestic Art* (Garden City, N.Y.: Doubleday, 1977) (oral history interviews with women in the Southwest), 154.

19 Laura Lenoir Norwood letter, in Hellerstein et al., *Victorian Women*, 218.

20 Elizabeth Y. Atkinson Richmond, Papers 1851–1898, Wisconsin State Historical Society Archives (emphasis added). See also, Stella B. Gowan, *Wildwood: A Story of Pioneer Life* (New York: Vantage Press, 1959).

21 Mrs. A. Graves, *Girlhood and Womanhood . . . Sketches of My Schoolmates* (Boston: Carier 1844), History of Women collection.

22 Grace Lumpkin, *To Make My Bread* (New York: Macaulay Co., 1932). My thanks to Mari Jo Buhle for calling this reference to my attention.

23 See for example, Susan Allison, *A Pioneer Gentlewoman*, 28; Elizabeth Avery Meriwether, *Recollections of Ninety-two Years, 1824–1916* (Nashville, Tenn.: Tennessee Historical Commission, 1958), 109–10. Quote is from Mrs. Carrie W. Keeley correspondence, 1905–11, Wisconsin State Historical Society Archives, letter dated 1910.

24 Mrs. W. H. Maxwell, *A Female Physician to the Ladies of the United States, Being a Familiar and Practical Treatise on Matters of Utmost Importance Peculiar to Women; Adapted for Every Woman's Own Private Use* (New York: Pub. by Mrs. W. H. Maxwell, M.D., 1860), 3.

25 On the importance of the female sphere, see Rosenberg, "Female World"; Sheila Rothman, *Woman's Proper Place: A History of Changing Ideals and Practices, 1870 to the Present* (New York: Basic Books, 1978), and Nancy F. Cott and Elizabeth H. Pleck, eds., *A Heritage of Her Own: Toward a New Social History of American Woman* (New York: Simon and Schuster, 1979).

26 Robert P. Harris, "History of a pair of obstetrical forceps sixty years old," *American Journal of Obstetrics and Diseases of Women and Children*, 1871, *4:* 55–59; J. H. Mackay, Letter to the Editor, *Journal of the American Medical Association*, 1912, *58:* 720. These reactions were fairly typical. See Judith Walzer Leavitt, " 'Science' enters the birthing room: obstetrics in America since the eighteenth century," paper

presented to the Seventh Annual International Symposium on the Comparative History of Medicine East and West, Japan, September 1982.

27 Georgiana Kirby, in Hellerstein et al., *Victorian Women*, 211.

28 Bessie Hunting Rudd to her husband, Edward Payson Rudd, dated [Sag] Harbor, May 27, 1860, Schlesinger Library, Radcliffe College, Cambridge, Mass. Quoted with permission.

29 Persis Sibley Andrews diary, in Hellerstein et al., *Victorian Women*, 218–19.

30 Agnes Just Reid, *Letters of Long Ago* (Caldwell, Idaho: Coston Printers, 1936), 25. Daughter wrote these letters based on mother's actual experiences and mother edited them, 1871 birth.

31 Augustin Caldwell, *The Rich Legacy: Memories of Hannah Tobey Farmer, Wife of Moses Gerrish Farmer* (Boston: Privately printed, 1892), 97.

32 Elizabeth H. Emerson; *Glimpses of a Life* (Burlington, N.C.: J. S. Sargent & Co., 1960), 4–5.

33 Lillie M. Jackson, *Fanning the Embers* (Boston: Christopher Publishing House, 1966), 90–91.

34 Hallie F. Nelson, *South of the Cottonwood Tree* (Broken Bow, Neb.: Purcells, 1977), 173.

35 Harriet Connor Brown, *Grandmother Brown's Hundred Years, 1827–1927* (Boston: Little, Brown, 1929), 158; Susanna Corder, *Life of Elizabeth Fry, Comp. from her Journal* (Philadelphia: H. Longstreth, 1855), 109–10 (History of Women Collection); Evalyn Walsh McLean, *Father Struck It Rich* (Boston: Little, Brown, 1936), 161; Mrs. Hal Russell, "Memoirs of Marian Russell," *Colorado Magazine*, 1944, *21*: 35–36; Stern, *I Am a Woman*, 90.

36 Mary Hallock Foote letter of May 1877 to Helena DeKay Gilder.

37 Josephine Preston Peabody, *Diary and Letters of Josephine Preston Peabody*, ed. Christina Hopkinson Baker (Boston: Houghton Mifflin, 1925), 229.

38 Caroline Gardner Cary Curtis, ed., *The Cary Letters* (Cambridge: Riverside Press, 1891), 60.

39 Sam Shapiro, Edward R. Schlesinger, and Robert E. L. Nesbitt, Jr., *Infant, Perinatal, Maternal and Childhood Mortality in the United States* (Cambridge: Harvard University Press, 1968), 143–58.

40 Ella Reeve Bloor, *We Are Many* (New York: International Publications, 1940), 33; *Memoirs of Paul Henry Kendricksen* (Boston: Privately printed, 1910), 302; Theressa Gay, *Life and Letters of Mrs. Jason Lee* (Portland, Ore.: Metropolitan Press, 1936), 84; Anne Lesley, in Susan Inches Lesley, *Recollections of My Mother* (Boston: Press of George H. Ellis, 1889), 306. Ebenezer Pettigrew journal entry, in Hellerstein et al., *Victorian Women*, 220; U.S. Children's Bureau.

41 Numerous women in this study sought doctors when they anticipated or faced trouble, indicating the belief that doctors were more skilled than midwives and friends. Part of the decision depended on cost, and women early learned that if they were going to call a physician at all, they should call right away. Typically, physicians charged the same amount for a full delivery or a placenta delivery (if called late) or sometimes just being called if a midwife was already there. See for example, Kershaw County, S.C., 1891 fee bill, in George Rosen, *Fees and Fee Bills: Some Economic Aspects of Medical Practice in Nineteenth-Century America* (Baltimore: Johns Hopkins Press, 1946), 80, and the Waukesha County (Wis.) Physicians Fee Bill of 1846, which charged $5.00 for obstetrical attendance and $10–$30 if the physician was called after a midwife. Fee bill in University of Wisconsin History of Medicine Department, reproduced in *Wisconsin Medicine: Historical Perspectives*, ed. Ronald L. Numbers and Judith Walzer Leavitt (Madison: University of Wisconsin Press, 1981). The question of whether doctors actually were experts in obstetrics in the nineteenth century does not concern us here, where we are following women's perceptions. Some interesting recent work on physicians' obstetric education sheds light on this issue. See for example, Lawrence D. Longo, "Obstetrics and gynecology," in *The Education of American Physicians: Historical Essays*, ed. Ronald L. Numbers (Berkeley: University of California Press, 1980), 205–25; Virginia G. Drachman, "The Loomis trial: social mores and obstetrics in the mid-nineteenth century," in this volume. See also Judy Barrett Litoff, *American Midwives* (Westport, Conn.: Greenwood Press, 1978); Jane B. Donegan, *Women and Men Midwives: Medicine, Morality, and Misogyny in Early America* (Westport, Conn.: Greenwood Press, 1978); and Leavitt, "Science enters the birthing room."

42 *Mrs. Longfellow: Selected Letters and Journals of Fanny Appleton Longfellow (1817–1861)*, ed. Edward Wagenknecht (New York: Longmans, Green, 1956), 130. Twilight sleep in the early twentieth century similarly looked enticing to women who sought greater control over the risks of childbirth. Judith Walzer Leavitt, "Birthing and anesthesia: the debate over twilight sleep," in this volume.

43 McCormick Papers, Wisconsin State Historical Society Archives.

44 See, for example, *Incidents in the Life of a Pioneer Woman: True Stories by the Daughters of the Pioneers of Washington* (State Association of the Daughters of Pioneers of Washington, 1975), 19–20, 29, 65, 71, 86; Gertrude DeWeiser Bricker, *Preacher's Girl* (Philadelphia: Dorrance and Co., 1957); Mrs. Hal Russell, "Memoirs of Marian Russell."

45 Many factors not discussed in this paper also influenced the move of normal obstetrics into the hos-

pital in the twentieth century. The development of the specialty of obstetrics, drug and technological advances that could be monitored best in the hospital, the expansion of hospitals themselves, and transportation improvements with the automobile are some of the factors that would have to be analyzed to make this analysis complete. In this paper we have discussed only women's perceptions of their own physical dangers to see how those perceptions helped change birth procedures.

46 R. P. Finney, *The Story of Motherhood* (New York: Liveright, 1937), 6–7.

47 Neil Devitt, "The transition," argues that the hospital was not the only factor in declining childbirth mortality and morbidity. See also Leavitt, "Science enters the birthing room."

48 Lella Secor, *Lella Secor: A Diary in Letters, 1915–1922,* ed. Barbara Moeuch Florence (New York: Burt Franklin, 1978), letter to mother, April 4, 1918.

49 Women quoted in M. F. Ashley Montagu, "Babies should be born at home!" *Ladies' Home Journal* 72 (August 1955): 52–53.

50 Women quoted in Shultz, "Cruelty in maternity wards," 45.

51 Ibid.

12

The Loomis Trial:
Social Mores and Obstetrics
in the Mid-Nineteenth Century

VIRGINIA G. DRACHMAN

Throughout the nineteenth century changes in medical science, professional status, and medical education were central to the concerns of American physicians. The shift from lay midwifery to male-dominated obstetrics, the faltering professional status of doctors, and the need for reform in the organization, content, and method of medical education often engendered heated, acrimonious debates among practitioners. Sometimes these debates overflowed into the public arena, through newspaper articles or other means, and became intertwined with public attitudes toward health, disease, and even female modesty. The libel trial in 1850 of Dr. Horatio N. Loomis, a private practitioner in Buffalo, was one such event that attracted widespread public attention.[1] In this trial physicians were called upon to debate the value of a controversial pedagogical innovation—demonstrative midwifery, the practice of allowing medical students to observe women in labor as part of their training. But, through their testimony, doctors' concerns over much larger health-related issues surfaced quickly: the demise of midwifery and the establishment of obstetrics as a legitimate field of medicine for male physicians, the relationship of doctors to the larger community, and the relationship of private practice to medical education and hospital practice. "As connected with the introduction of a mode of teaching," noted the *Buffalo Medical Journal* at the time, and "as involving medical ethics, and affording indications of medical sentiment of the present time, the trial will rank among

VIRGINIA DRACHMAN is Assistant Professor of History at Tufts University, Boston, Massachusetts.

Reprinted with permission from *Health Care in America*, ed. by Susan Reverby and David Rosner (Philadelphia: Temple University Press, 1979), pp. 67–83.

the events which make up the history of medicine."[2] This chapter examines the trial within the general context of the history of nineteenth-century American medicine.[3]

The events leading up to the trial began in January 1850, when Dr. James Platt White, professor of obstetrics at Buffalo Medical College, allowed his students to observe while he attended a woman in labor. As the fetal head emerged from the pubic arch, approximately twenty students watched him remove some of the patient's clothing to demonstrate the proper technique for supporting the perineum. This was the first time in the United States that medical students had been permitted to observe a delivery. White's students were aware of the importance of this first incidence of demonstrative midwifery, and they publically praised their instructor in a written statement sent to the *Buffalo Medical Journal*.[4] Subsequently, one of the city's general newspapers, the *Buffalo Commercial Advertiser*, published an editorial in support of demonstrative midwifery.[5] Shortly thereafter, an article critical of demonstrative midwifery appeared in another newspaper, the *Buffalo Courier*. The author, a Buffalo physician who identified himself merely as "L.," charged White with offending the modesty of the female patient by exposing her to the "meretricious curiosity" and "salacious stare" of his students and thereby committing a "gross outrage upon public decency" for the purpose of furthering his own professional reputation.[6] In response, Professor White's students issued another statement in his support.[7] To quiet the mounting controversy, the faculty of the college published their own statement of support, claiming that

White's clinical instruction furthered "the interests of the students in their acquisition of useful knowledge, and, thereby, the interests of medical science and of humanity."[8] Meanwhile, Dr. Horatio Loomis, a private practitioner suspected of being "L.," purchased additional copies of the critical letter that had appeared in the *Courier* and distributed them to citizens of Buffalo. To save his reputation, White brought Loomis to trial for libel, ultimately losing the case because he could not prove that Loomis was the author of the newspaper article.

Although White lost the case, this single incident of demonstrative midwifery signaled a major medical advance, for it set the stage for the routine practice of ocular deliveries in medical schools, a necessary precondition for the development of modern obstetrics. But there were many doctors who denounced demonstrative midwifery, defining it as medically unethical, pedagogically unnecessary, and professionally unsound.[9] In the mid-nineteenth century, after all, obstetrics as a legitimate area of medical practice for male physicians was not universally accepted among either lay people or doctors themselves. Until the mid-eighteenth century childbirth was understood to be a uniquely female experience that took place amidst female friends and relatives under the direction of the female midwife. Toward the end of the eighteenth century male physicians began to gain access to the delivery room. Some returning from Europe with new medical skills, and others having attended lectures in cities such as Boston and New York on the subject of midwifery, made themselves available as accoucheurs in complicated or dangerous cases. The presence of the skilled male accoucheur implied a changing attitude toward childbirth. No longer was it seen simply as an event of nature. Instead, it began to be understood as a complex physiological process that often required the medical expertise of a trained physician. The implication that scientific knowledge and skill were now deemed necessary to avoid the dangers of childbirth set the stage for the eventual discrediting of midwives and for the legitimization of the skilled obstetrician.[10]

By the time of the Loomis trial it was not so unusual for male physicians, particularly in the urban centers of Boston, New York, and Philadelphia, to attend women in labor. Nevertheless, the male physician's position as accoucheur was far from secure. The midwife still presented formidable competition for him, for many women continued to prefer to deliver surrounded by female relatives, friends, and the midwife. Male physicians seeking access to the delivery room were haunted by this tradition. "It is indeed, in our remembrance," explained one doctor, "that the very presence of a male practitioner in the house was scarce endured."[11] In addition to the persistence of the tradition of midwifery, women were beginning to break into the medical profession by 1850, competing with male physicians for access to the delivery room. Two women's medical colleges had already been founded, the New England Female Medical College and the Woman's Medical College of Pennsylvania, and Elizabeth Blackwell had completed her instruction at Geneva Medical College and become the first woman to graduate from a regular medical school in the United States. The takeover of the delivery room by the male obstetrician was a process that took almost two centuries to complete.[12]

While by midcentury most male physicians seemed to agree on the validity of the male accoucheur, they disagreed over how he should behave in the delivery room. The male physician was expected to act simultaneously as both doctor and gentleman. As a doctor, his duty was to provide the best medical service possible to his patient. As a gentleman, however, he was expected to preserve the dignity and modesty of the woman. Dr. D. Humphreys Storer, professor of midwifery at Harvard, explained in his introductory lecture to the medical class of 1855–56 that the female patient "does expect that uniformly gentlemanly deportment, that constant kindness, that fidelity, which ever characterize the true physician."[13] These dual responsibilities often placed the physician in a difficult dilemma of conflicting professional and social roles.

This problem was not new to male physicians. They had been facing it throughout the nineteenth century as they increasingly sought female patients. It manifested itself, for example, as doctors began to rely on the new instruments of medical technology in treating women. When some physicians began to use the vaginal speculum, for instance, many others resisted the innovation. By the time of the Loomis trial this controversy was in full swing. Routine use of the speculum was denounced by many because it involved an ocular examination of the female genitalia, a radical deviation from the traditional mode of examining female patients. Throughout the first half of the nineteenth century physicians had relied primarily on their sense of touch when they gave an internal examination; some looked at the female genitals in an emergency. Yet most generally agreed that to both look at and touch the female genitals unnecessarily, as in the case of a routine examination, was to sacrifice female delicacy and ignore medical ethics. The influential Dr. Charles D. Meigs, professor of medicine and diseases of women and children at Jefferson Medical College in Philadelphia, was one doctor who urged restraint in the use of the speculum and reliance on it only when absolutely necessary. To Meigs, indiscriminate use of the speculum was an affront to female modesty and virtue. In fact, he explained that the doctor's primary obligation was not to fulfill his professional responsibility to heal the sick but to fulfill his social responsibility to preserve the moral fabric of society. Meigs explained this to his medical students:

It is perhaps best, upon the whole, that this great degree of modesty should exist even to the extent of putting a bar to researches, without which no very clear and understandable notions can be obtained of the sexual disorders. I confess I am proud to say that in this country generally, certainly in many parts of it, there are women who prefer to suffer the extremity of danger and pain rather than wave those scruples of delicacy which prevent their maladies from being explored. I say it is fully an evidence of the dominion of a fine morality in our society.[14]

Demonstrative midwifery met similar resistance because, like the speculum, it involved exposing the female genitalia to the male eye. Previously medical students had learned about the birth process from pictures in books. Unless they had received some practical training as an apprentice, they usually would not have observed a delivery until they were practicing on their own. Most physicians and medical educators of the day considered this an adequate system of training. They believed that to allow students to observe a woman in labor for the purpose of instruction was unneces-

sary and therefore offensive to the modesty and virtue of the expectant mother. Loomis's attorney expressed these sentiments in his opening statement to the jury. "The exposure of this woman in labor," he charged, "was . . . a startling and bestial innovation. . . . Against the exposure of this woman," he continued, "we do protest. And we expect that you will by your verdict vindicate the delicacy of the sex."[15]

Even those doctors who championed demonstrative midwifery understood the importance of respecting the modesty of their female patients. White himself had heeded traditional medical etiquette and taken special precautions to protect his patient from the indiscriminate stares of his students. When the fetal head presented itself, he had covered the perineum with napkins while he demonstrated the proper method of supporting the perineum. From the testimony of the students it appears that their view of the patient's genitals had been effectively obscured. One student stated that "her genitals were not exposed."[16] Another testified:

I didn't see any of the front part of her body. As the clothes were raised, I saw something in the form of flesh and blood; what it was I couldn't say. . . . I don't recall whether one or both hands supported the perineum. Professor White had a napkin in his hand. The woman was covered when the placenta was delivered.[17]

The students also testified that proper decorum had been preserved. In response to the charge in the letter by L. that the patient had been subjected to the "meretricious curiosity" and "salacious stare" of "a score of scarcely adolescent youth," one student explained that "the best of order was preserved in the room. I don't recollect any talking except between Professor White and the nurse."[18] Another student described the atmosphere in the room in more detail:

There was no talk, unless the woman wanted something. There was no talk among the students.—There was no laughing or jesting. I saw one smile. Dr. White talked about the labor, for the purpose of instructing the class, his talk had no other tendency than to instruct the class. Professor White enjoined decorum and order. The house, as I said before, was still.[19]

White and his students clearly believed that demonstrative midwifery could take place without violation of female modesty and virtue.

Despite the differences of opinion expressed at the trial, there seems to have been an underlying consensus among the doctors there regarding the importance of preserving female delicacy and virtue. Yet the doctors also seemed to share the understanding that one could modify this principle of preserving female virtue. While they spoke about respecting the virtues of womanhood in general, it appears that they were most concerned about upholding the virtues of middle-class and upper-class women. They loosened their rigid standards when the woman in question was poor. White's patient, Mary Watson, for example, was a recent immigrant from Ireland, an unmarried woman living in the Erie County poorhouse. From the testimony of the physicians at the trial one sees hints of a double standard of medical practice whereby such women because of their ethnicity, economic condition, and marital status were treated differently from more well-to-do female patients. One physician testified, for example, that he would "be fearful of introducing [demonstrative midwifery] into a private institution" and that in his "private practice he never expose[d] the female."[20] Another stated that "there ought to be a difference made between medical instructions to a class and private practice," that he "considered them entirely different," and that he "would not pretend to make the ladies in private practice the means of instruction to classes."[21]

We may better appreciate this way of thinking if we examine the response of physicians to demonstrative midwifery within the context of their relationship to the community. Because their access to the delivery room was far from absolute, doctors understood that what went on behind its door was by no means a purely private matter. They realized that the community at large was watching closely as they attended women in childbirth. Each uneventful, successful delivery they attended could heighten their reputations as respectable accoucheurs and further justify their presence in the delivery room. Similarly, any type of complication or event of note, such as demonstrative midwifery,

could damage their reputation and destroy the uneasy alliance they were building with female patients. Hence, physicians resisted demonstrative midwifery in part because they feared that it would attract unfavorable attention and engender public controversy that would keep women away from them.

Throughout the trial doctors revealed their concern about the response of the community at large to the practice of demonstrative midwifery. They continually echoed the theme that demonstrative midwifery was "prejudicing the moral sense of the community against doctors."[22] One physician, a graduate of the University of Pennsylvania and a practicing physician for twenty-two years, explained:

> I disapprove of [demonstrative midwifery]...
> for the same general reason that has been
> stated here—it is contrary to the moral sense
> of the community. It is a principle in Medical
> Ethics, not to do anything to excite the public against the Medical Profession. Gregarious teaching in midwifery is improper.[23]

Another practicing physician of twenty-seven years echoed that "according to Medical Ethics, all unnecessary acts are to be avoided which are calculated to excite the public or create a prejudice against the profession."[24]

In seeking to maintain the favor of the community, physicians were particularly concerned about their relationship with female members of well-to-do families, who held the key to male physicians' entrance into obstetrics. Their allegiance and support could guarantee lucrative private obstetric practices and at the same time lend legitimacy and respectability to the major shift from midwifery to obstetrics.[25] For these reasons male doctors were careful not to offend well-to-do women as they sought to woo them into becoming their obstetric patients. Thus they adapted their medical behavior to conform to social etiquette.

Five years before the Loomis trial, this same fear of alienating the women of well-to-do families had prompted Boston physicians to reject a proposal to provide clinical instruction in midwifery for medical students at the Massachusetts General Hospital. The committee reviewing the proposal concluded that wealthy women, as well as self-respecting poor women, would refuse to tolerate such exposure. They argued that if the hospital lost the patronage of its respectable female patients, it would also lose the philanthropic support of the wealthy members of the Boston community. Like physicians in Boston, those at the Loomis trial feared demonstrative midwifery would destroy their delicate alliance with the community as they sought to strengthen their hold on the field of obstetrics.

The concern expressed by the physicians who testified at the Loomis trial should also be seen within the context of the public's general dissatisfaction with regular doctors. Physicians at midcentury were attempting to establish a strong professional identity and a comfortable relationship with the lay public. Their efforts were complicated, however, by the public's growing disenchantment with doctors' ineffective and often harmful therapeutics. By the end of the first third of the nineteenth century, this disenchantment had mushroomed into the rejection of regular medicine by large portions of the public, the growth of numerous medical sects offering alternatives to regular medicine, and a willingness among lay people to rely on these medical alternatives.[26] Though the challenge to regular medicine had peaked before midcentury, public disrespect for it and enchantment with medical sectarianism were still riding the crest of that peak at the time of the Loomis trial. Regular doctors, who deemed themselves the only respectable medical representatives, were in a quandary as to how best to cope with this assault. One response was the establishment of the American Medical Association in 1848. Among its initial tasks, the AMA sought to improve medical education, standardize medical practices, and regulate the numbers of regular physicians. In so doing, the American Medical Association sought to upgrade the public image of regular physicians and to strengthen their defense against medical sectarians. We may, therefore, understand the uproar among doctors over demonstrative midwifery as growing in part out of these attempts by regular physicians to monitor and to regulate their own medical practices.

We may also appreciate it if we place it within the context of regular doctors' attempts to distance themselves from the public at large. As part of their attempt to gain greater respect from the community and improve their professional image, they sought to distinguish themselves as different from lay people. In so doing, they increasingly came to see medical issues as their concern alone. Public input was deemed inappropriate. Thus, for some of the doctors at the Loomis trial, the significant issue was not so much White's demonstration of delivery to his students as the public discussion of it. "I do not think the transaction at the College as objectionable as the publication of it," explained one physician.[27] A colleague of White's explained that, while he had assented to White's demonstrating a delivery to his students, he had "not advise[d] the publication of the Demonstration."[28] Similarly, another of White's colleagues testified, "[I] don't so much object to its publication in a medical journal as in a secular newspaper, which I condemn *in toto*."[29] It was the article in the *Buffalo Commercial Advertiser* in defense of demonstrative midwifery that he thought was "injudicious." The American Medical Association echoed these sentiments in its report on demonstrative midwifery:

> It is to be regretted that this subject has been brought at all upon the popular arena. It is wholly a professional question, and should be discussed by the profession in a calm, considerate and dignified manner. It is no subject for newspaper warfare, nor for a warfare in medical journals in newspaper style.[30]

A single physician at the trial voiced a minority opinion. He explained that generally he would "disapprove of a publication in a secular newspaper, like that in the *Commercial*. But in this case it was different—the public mind had become excited on this subject, and that article was published for the purpose of allaying the excitement."[31]

The controversy over demonstrative midwifery was also a response to the changing standards of medical education. In the first half of the century most physicians were trained by apprenticing themselves to practicing doctors. Despite its popularity, this system of apprenticeship presented a variety of problems. There was, for example, no adequate way of regulating standards of medical education. Instead, the training of each individual medical student varied, depending on the knowledge and skill of his particular preceptor. In addition, as medical science progressed, the preceptor grew increasingly less competent to provide sufficient medical training.[32]

While most physicians in the first half of the nineteenth century had been trained by means of the apprenticeship system, some went to medical schools. The wealthier students went either to schools in Europe or to American medical schools such as the Philadelphia Medical College, Kings College in New York City, and Harvard, all of which had been founded during the last third of the eighteenth century and modeled after the schools in Europe. Other students attended any of the more local and less prestigious medical schools that had been growing in numbers throughout the nineteenth century. Not surprisingly, the quality of education varied greatly from school to school, and the lack of a standard program of medical education was one of the major problems of medical school training in the early nineteenth century. Another serious problem was that medical schools omitted what the apprenticeship stressed, practical training. The students' learning experience in medical school was confined almost solely to lectures; clinical and laboratory instruction were rare. Unless a student went to medical school and apprenticed himself to a physician as well, there was no way for him to get both theoretical knowledge and practical experience. The debate over demonstrative midwifery was part of the midcentury reevaluation among doctors of medical school education and particularly of the value of clinical training.

While this atmosphere of self-improvement had opened the door for reforms in medical education, we should not be surprised that physicians resisted introducing demonstrative midwifery into medical schools. Historically, resistance had been a predictable response to innovation among doctors. In the seventeenth century, for example, they had greeted the theory of circulation of the blood with much skepticism; in the eighteenth century they responded similarly to the practice of inoculation; and at the same time that Dr. White was trying to bring changes to the teaching of obstetrics, physicians were adamantly resisting new ideas regarding the contagious nature of puerperal infection.[33]

The resistance of physicians to demonstrate midwifery also was a defensive response in part for they realized that to acknowledge its pedagogical value was to concede the inadequacy of their own training experience. Thus physicians at the Loomis trial insisted that the traditional mode of learning obstetrics, by studying plates of the female anatomy and by tactile internal examination, was entirely sufficient. One physician, for example, explained that "the student can learn the distention of the perineum properly only by the sense of touch. The external parts can as well be seen upon plates as by ocular demonstration."[34] With plates, explained another physician, "the student can have all the parts before him at once, both of the internal and external organs; while he cannot have the living subject before him, except at long intervals. . . . The plates are almost perfect, exhibiting all the stages of labor during parturition."[35]

Those supporting the innovation of demonstrative midwifery responded quite differently. White's students were overwhelmingly in its favor, testifying that their instructor had given them a valuable learning experience that greatly enhanced their understanding of the birth process. "In my opinion," one explained, "demonstrative midwifery is important and useful as a means of imparting valuable instruction."[36] Another testified that he had "derived such confidence as to enable [him] to proceed better when called to attend a sick bed,"[37] while another explained that the ocular demonstration had "impressed upon his mind the *practical* part of what he only knew before by theory."[38]

White's graduates were not the only witnesses to speak in favor of the pedagogical benefits of demonstrative midwifery. Practicing doctors also testified as to its value. Several of this latter group were men whose training had taken them to European cities such as Edinburgh, Paris, and Amsterdam, where demonstrative midwifery was an integral part of medical education. Their testimony in favor of the practice may have been particularly significant because many American doctors then believed European medicine was superior to American medicine and wished to use it as a model for American medical practice.[39]

The debate over demonstrative midwifery was not contained within the walls of the Erie County courtroom; doctors throughout the country participated in the controversy, carrying on the debate in their numerous medical journals, echoing the same themes of concern as those expressed by the doctors at the trial. Addressing the need for reform in medical education, for example, a letter from a physician to the *Boston Medical and Surgical Journal* praised White for "his endeavors to make the instruction in his department as practicable as possible."[40] Similarly, another doctor explained in the *New Orleans Medical Journal* that "our teachers of medicine have heretofore, devoted too much of their lectures to theoretical medicine to turn out competent graduates; practical *clinical* teaching will ultimately triumph."[41] In chiding the profession for resisting reform in medical education, one doctor surmised that the Buffalo physicians opposing demonstrative midwifery were members of the "opposition factions, so commonly found surrounding and impeding medical schools."[42] Another doctor, in a letter of support to the *New York Journal of Medicine*, reminded his colleagues that "novelty in practice . . . always meets with opposition" and asked, as an illustration that reminds us of the insecurity male doctors felt regarding their relationship to female patients, "who does not recollect the bitter persecution which attended the introduction of the stethoscope (not to mention the speculum) into general practice, and the more than bitter persecution which was encountered by the early male-practitioners of obstetrics?"[43]

A letter to the *Charleston Medical Journal and Review* addressed this issue of reform of medical education as well as the issue of the autonomy of the medical profession from the public:

> If an attempt to do in this country, what has been quite common in Europe for years past, is to be frowned down by the mischievous uprising of the ignorant and uneducated, merely because it seems repugnant to their sense of what is fit—if the laity are to determine the *quid deciat* for the Medical Profession, then we had better content ourselves with lying down supinely, and waiting for their sanction, before attempting any improvements, however recommended by the progress of science, the advance of an enlightened civilization, or even the long experience of others.[44]

In a letter to the *Louisville Medical Journal* a doctor addressed both of these concerns as well as the question of the responsibility of physicians to uphold female virtue. He labeled the opposing physicians the "prudish Miss Nancies of Buffalo" and chided them for "their excessive modesty and shamefacedness."[45]

With demonstrative midwifery evoking such a nationwide controversy, it is interesting to look at the reaction of the newly formed American Medical Association. At its third annual meeting in 1850, the association decided to undertake an investigation of "whether any practicable scheme can be devised to render instruction in Midwifery more practical than it has hitherto been in the medical schools of the United States."[46] Curiously, the Committee on Education was assigned the task of investigation rather than the Committee on Obstetrics, even though both committees agreed that the latter would have been the more appropriate investigating group. Unfortunately, the transactions of the meeting do not indicate the motives behind this decision. However, the very fact that this task fell to the Committee on Education suggests that the AMA preferred to define demonstrative midwifery primarily as an educational issue rather than as one of obstetric practice. In its report the following year, the Committee on Education rejected demonstrative midwifery first and foremost as an unnecessary and inadequate form of instruction. "We not only object to the mode of instruction, adopted in the plan at Buffalo, as unnecessary," the committee explained, "but we object to it, also, as being utterly *incompetent to give the student* that knowledge which he needs in the practice of obstetrics."[47] In addition, it was sensitive to the obstetric issues as well and expressed deep concern about the impact of demonstrative midwifery on the relationship between male doctors and female patients:

> The confidential relation existing between women and our profession, so essential to the full and proper treatment of her diseases, may be impaired either by the practices of individuals, or by those which may prevail very generally in the profession. Great carefulness, therefore, is needed on this point. The object, both of the individual practitioner and of the profession, should be to meet most fully the demands of science and humanity, and yet not offend a sensitive, but rational delicacy, nor give countenance to an unblushing shamelessness.
>
> It is principally the prejudice which indelicate practices among medical men have engendered in the public mind, that has given

rise to the project for training female practitioners of medicine.[48]

In effect, the medical profession's major vehicle for promoting medical policy in the nation had rejected an innovation that many physicians throughout the country had greeted with great acclamation. The voice of caution in the face of change, the American Medical Association thus revealed the tenuous position of the medical profession as it sought to treat women. Its conservatism, however, was contrary to the winds of progress. The editor of the *New Orleans Medical Journal* correctly forecast the future when he wrote about demonstrative midwifery: "Practical clinical teaching will ultimately triumph over those who oppose it as alike grossly offensive to morality and common decency."[49]

In the post–Civil War period doctors evolved a working, though unspoken, agreement with the growing population of poor urban women, not unlike Mary Watson. They gave them medical attention, and, in return, used them as a resource for medical instruction. Within a relatively short period of time after the Loomis trial, demonstrative midwifery became an acceptable mode of medical instruction among doctors as well as the public. Within this context, the Loomis trial gives us a snapshot of physicians during a period of transition as they struggled to come to grips with issues that would shape medicine for generations to come: establishing a female clientele, improving their professional relationship with the public, and reforming medical education.

NOTES

I would like to thank Douglas Jones for his thoughtful criticism and advice.

1 Frederick T. Parsons, *Report of the Trial, The People versus Dr. Horatio N. Loomis, for Libel* (Buffalo: Jewett, Thomas and Co., 1850); also reprinted in Charles Rosenberg and Carroll Smith-Rosenberg, eds., *The Male-Midwife and the Female Doctor* (New York: Arno Press, 1974). An original publication of the report is in the archives at SUNY, Buffalo. The best copy of the report is the Arno Press reprinted edition, from which all quotes in this paper are taken.

2 *Buffalo Medical Journal and Monthly Review of Medical and Surgical Science* 6 (July 1850): 115.

3 Other historians have recognized the significance of the Loomis trial in the history of American obstetrics: Jane Donegan, "Midwifery in America, 1760–1860: A Study in Medicine and Morality" (Ph.D. diss., Syracuse University, 1972); Herbert Thoms, *Chapters in American Obstetrics* (Springfield: Charles C. Thomas, 1961); and Richard Wertz and Dorothy C. Wertz, *Lying-In: A History of Childbirth in America* (New York: Free Press, 1977), 85–89.

4 *Buffalo Medical Journal* 5 (February 1850): 565, reprinted in *Report of the Trial*, appendix, 42.

5 *Buffalo Commercial Advertiser*, 19 February 1850, reprinted in *Report of the Trial*, appendix, 43.

6 *Buffalo Courier*, 27 February 1850, reprinted in *Report of the Trial*, appendix, 44–45.

7 Written statement by graduates of Buffalo Medical College session of 1849–50, 15 February 1850, *Report of the Trial*, appendix, 43–44.

8 Resolutions of the Faculty of the Medical Department of the University of Buffalo, 26 February 1850, *Report of the Trial*, appendix, 44.

9 Seventeen Buffalo physicians publicly denounced demonstrative midwifery in a letter to Dr. Austin Flint, dean of the Buffalo Medical College and editor of the *Buffalo Medical Journal*. The letter appeared in *Buffalo Medical Journal* 5 (March 1850): 621 and in *Boston Medical and Surgical Journal* 42 (29 May 1850): 349, reprinted in *Report of the Trial*, appendix, 44.

10 For a discussion of midwifery in early America and the changing attitudes toward childbirth, see Catherine M. Scholten, "'On the importance of the obstetric art': changing customs of childbirth in America, 1760 to 1825," in this volume.

11 *American Journal of the Medical Sciences* 20 (October 1850): 449.

12 For evidence of the resistance to the move toward obstetrics, see Samuel Gregory, *Letters to Ladies, in Favor of Female Physicians* (New York: Fowlers and Wells, 1850), reprinted in Rosenberg and Smith-Rosenberg, *The Male-Midwife and the Female Doctor*; Samuel Gregory, *Man-Midwifery Exposed and Corrected; or, The Employment of Men to Attend Women in Childbirth, and in Other Delicate Circumstances Shown to Be a Modern Innovation* (Boston: G. Gregory, 1848), reprinted in *The Male-Midwife and Female Doctor*; and George Gregory, *Medical Morals: Illustrated with Plates and Extracts from Medical Works; Designed to Show the Pernicious Social and Moral Influence of the Present System of Medical Practice, and the Importance of Establishing Female Medical Colleges, and Educating and Em-*

ploying Female Physicians for Their Own Sex (Boston: 1853), reprinted in *The Male-Midwife and Female Doctor*.

13   David Humphreys Storer, *An Introductory Lecture before the Medical Class of 1855/56 of Harvard University* (Boston: David Clapp, 1855), 11.

14   Charles D. Meigs, *Females and Their Diseases* (Philadelphia: Lea and Blanchard, 1848), cited in James V. Ricci, *The Development of Gynaecological Surgery and Instruments* (Philadelphia: Blakiston Co., 1949), 313.

15   *Report of the Trial*, p. 9.

16   Ibid., 9.

17   Ibid., 10.

18   Ibid., 10.

19   Ibid., 9.

20   Ibid., 27.

21   Ibid., 29.

22   Ibid., 14.

23   Ibid., 15.

24   Ibid., 16.

25   A physician, D. W. Cathell, expressed this understanding in a book on how to establish a successful medical practice that was widely read by doctors toward the end of the nineteenth century. D. W. Cathell, *The Physician Himself and What He Should Add to the Scientific Acquirements*, ed. Charles E. Rosenberg (New York: Arno Press, 1972).

26   For a discussion of the low esteem of the medical profession and the use of sectarian medicine, see, for example: William Rothstein, *American Physicians in the Nineteenth Century: From Sects to Science* (Baltimore: Johns Hopkins University Press, 1972); Richard Harrison Shryock, *Medicine and Society in America, 1660–1860* (Ithaca, N.Y.: Cornell University Press, 1960); Richard Harrison Shryock, "The American physician in 1846 and in 1946: a study in professional contrasts," *Medicine in America* (Baltimore: Johns Hopkins Press, 1966); and Richard Harrison Shryock, "Sylvester Graham and the Popular Health Movement, 1830–1870," *Medicine in America* (Baltimore: Johns Hopkins Press, 1966).

27   *Report of the Trial*, 15.

28   Ibid., 26.

29   Ibid., 27.

30   "Report of the Committee on Education in relation to 'Demonstrative midwifery,'" submitted at the fourth annual meeting of the American Medical Association, in *Transactions of the American Medical Association*, 1851, *4:* 436–37.

31   *Report of the Trial*, 29.

32   On medical education, see, for example, William Rothstein, *American Physicians in the Nineteenth Century: From Sects to Science;* and Shryock, *Medicine and Society in America, 1660–1860*.

33   *Report of the Trial*, p. 6.

34   Ibid., 13.

35   Ibid., 12–13.

36   Ibid., 19.

37   Ibid., 20.

38   Ibid., 20.

39   See Shryock, *Medicine and Society in America, 1660– 1860*.

40   *Boston Medical and Surgical Journal* 42 (29 May 1850): 258.

41   Editorial, *New Orleans Medical Journal* 6 (May 1850): 809.

42   *Cincinnati Medical Journal*, May 1850, reprinted in *Report of the Trial*, appendix, 48.

43   *New York Journal of Medicine and the Collateral Sciences* 4 (May 1850): 395.

44   *Charleston Medical Journal and Review* 5 (September 1850): 672.

45   *Louisville Medical Journal*, June 1850, quoted in Thomas, *Our Obstetrical Heritage*, 108.

46   *Minutes of the Third Annual Meeting of the American Medical Association, Transactions of the American Medical Association*, 1850, *3:* 42.

47   "Report of the Committee on Medical Education in relation to 'Demonstrative midwifery,'" submitted at the fourth annual meeting of the American Medical Association, *Transactions of the American Medical Association*, 1851, *4:* 440.

48   Ibid., 440.

49   Editorial, *New Orleans Medical Journal* 6 (May 1850): 809.

13

Birthing and Anesthesia:
The Debate over Twilight Sleep

JUDITH WALZER LEAVITT

"At midnight I was awakened by a very sharp pain," wrote Mrs. Cecil Stewart, describing the birth of her child in 1914. "The head nurse . . . gave me an injection of scopolamin-morphin. . . . I woke up the next morning about half-past seven . . . the door opened, and the head nurse brought in my baby. . . . I was so happy."[1] Mrs. Stewart had delivered her baby under the influence of scopolamine, a narcotic and amnesiac that, together with morphine, produced a state popularly known as "twilight sleep." She did not remember anything of the experience when she woke up after giving birth. This 1914 ideal contrasts with today's feminist stress on being awake, aware, and in control during the birthing experience. In 1914 and 1915, thousands of American women testified to the marvels of having babies without the trauma of childbirth. As one of them gratefully put it, "The night of my confinement will always be a night dropped out of my life."[2]

From the perspective of today's ideology of woman-controlled births, it may appear that women who want anesthesia sought to cede control of their births to their doctors. I will argue however, that the twilight sleep movement led by women in 1914 and 1915 was not a relinquishing of control. Rather, it was an attempt to gain control over the birthing process. Feminist women wanted the parturient, not the doctor or attendant, to choose the kind of delivery she would have. This essay examines the apparent contradiction in the women's demand to control their births by going to sleep.

JUDITH WALZER LEAVITT is Associate Professor of the History of Medicine and Women's Studies at the University of Wisconsin, Madison, Wisconsin.

Reprinted with permission from *Signs* 6 (1980): 147–164. © 1980 by The University of Chicago Press.

THE PROCESS

The attendants, location, and drugs or instruments used in American women's birthing experiences varied in the early decades of the twentieth century. America's poorer and immigrant women delivered their babies predominantly at home, attended by midwives who seldom administered drugs and who called physicians only in difficult cases. A small number of poor women gave birth in charity or public hospitals where physicians attended them. Most upper- and middle-class women, who had more choice, elected to be attended by a physician, usually a general practitioner but increasingly a specially trained obstetrician, rather than a midwife. At the turn of the twentieth century, these births, too, typically took place in the woman's home; however, by the second decade of the century, specialists, aided partly by the twilight sleep movement, were moving childbirth from the home to the hospital.[3]

Physicians used drugs and techniques of physical intervention in many cases, although the extent cannot be quantified accurately. In addition to forceps, physicians relied on opium, chloroform, chloral, cocaine, quinine, nitrous oxide, ergot, and ether to relieve pain, expedite labor, prevent injury in precipitous labors, control hemorrhage, and prevent sepsis.[4] In one study of 972 consecutive births in Wisconsin, physicians used chloroform during the second stage of labor in half of their cases and forceps in 12 percent.[5] The reports indicate that drugs and instruments may have made labors shorter but not necessarily more enjoyable. Because most drugs could not be used safely throughout the labor and delivery, either because they affected muscle function or because they were dangerous for the baby, women still experienced pain. The use of forceps frequently added to discomfort and caused perineal tears, complicating postdelivery recovery. Maternal mortality remained high in the early decades of the twentieth century, and childbirth, whether attended by physicians or midwives, continued to be risky.[6]

Most women described their physician-attended childbirths as unpleasant at best. Observers of the declining birthrates among America's "better" classes worried that the "fear of childbirth has poisoned the happiness of many women"[7] and caused them to want fewer children. One woman told her doctor that her childbirth had been "hell.... It bursts your brain, and tears out your heart, and crashes your nerves to bits. It's just like hell, and I won't stand it again. Never."[8] In scopolamine deliveries, the women went to sleep, delivered their babies, and woke up feeling vigorous. The drug altered their consciousness so that they did not remember painful labors, and their bodies did not feel exhausted by their efforts.[9] Both the women who demanded scopolamine and the doctors who agreed to use it perceived it as far superior to other anesthesia because it did not inhibit muscle function and could be administered throughout the birthing process. It was the newest and finest technique available—"the greatest boon the Twentieth Century could give to women," in the words of Dr. Bertha Van Hoosen, one of its foremost medical advocates.[10]

However, women's bodies experienced their labors, even if their minds did not remember them. Thus observers witnessed women screaming in pain during contractions, thrashing about, and giving all the outward signs of "acute suffering." Residents of Riverside Drive in New York City testified that women in Dr. William H. W. Knipe's twilight sleep hospital sent forth "objectionable" noises in the middle of the night.[11]

A successful twilight sleep delivery, as practiced by Dr. Van Hoosen at the Mary Thompson Hospital in Chicago, required elaborate facilities and careful supervision. Attending physicians and nurses gave the first injection of scopolamine as soon as a woman appeared to be in active labor and continued the injections at carefully determined intervals throughout her labor and delivery. They periodically administered two tests to determine the effectiveness of the anesthesia: the "call-

ing test," which the parturient passed if the doctor could not arouse her even by addressing her in a loud voice, and the "incoordination test," which she passed if her movements were uncoordinated. Once the laboring woman was under the effects of scopolamine, the doctors put her into a specially designed crib-bed to contain her sometimes violent movements. Van Hoosen described the need for the bed screens: "As the pains increase in frequency and strength, the patient tosses or throws herself about, but without injury to herself, and may be left without fear that she will roll onto the floor or be found wandering aimlessly in the corridors. In rare cases, where the patient is very excitable and insists on getting out of bed.... I prefer to fasten a canvas cover over the tops of the screens, thereby shutting out light, noise and possibility of leaving the bed."[12] When delivery began, attendants took down the canvas crib and positioned the patient in stirrups, familiar in modern obstetrical services. Van Hoosen advised the use of a continuous sleeve to ensure that patients did not interfere with the sterile field. The canvas crib and the continuous sleeve were Van Hoosen's response to a common need in twilight sleep deliveries: a secure, darkened, quiet, contained environment.

THE EVENTS

Twilight sleep became a controversial issue in American obstetrics in June 1914, when *McClure's Magazine* published an article by two laywomen describing this newly popular German method of painless childbirth.[13] In the article, Marguerite Tracy and Constance Leupp, both visitors at the Freiburg women's clinic, criticized high-forceps deliveries (which they called the common American technique) as dangerous and conducive to infection. They contrasted these imperfect births to the safety and comfort of twilight sleep. The new method was so wonderful that women, having once experienced it, would "walk all the way [to Germany] from California" to have their subsequent births under twilight sleep. The physicians at the Freiburg clinic thought the method was best suited for the upper-class "modern woman ... [who] responds to the stimulus of severe pain ... with nervous exhaustion and paralysis of the will to carry labor to conclusion." They were less certain about its usefulness for women who "earn their living by manual labor" and could tolerate more pain.[14]

The women who took up the cause of twilight sleep concluded that it was not in general use in this country because doctors were consciously withholding this panacea. Physicians have "held back" on developing painless childbirth, accused Mary Boyd and Marguerite Tracy, two of the most active proponents, because it "takes too much time." "Women alone," they asserted, "can bring Freiburg methods into American obstetrical practice."[15] Others echoed the call to arms: journalist Hanna Rion urged her readers to "take up the battle for painless childbirth.... Fight not only for yourselves, but fight for your ... sex."[16] Newspapers and popular magazines joined the chorus, advocating a widespread use of scopolamine in childbirth.[17]

The lay public's anger at the medical profession's apparent refusal to adopt a technique beneficial to women erupted into a national movement. The National Twilight Sleep Association, formed by upper-middle-class clubwomen,[18] was best epitomized by its leaders. They included women such as Mrs. Jesse F. Attwater, editor of *Femina* in Boston; Dr. Eliza Taylor Ransom, active women's rights advocate and physician in Boston; Mrs. Julian Heath of the National Housewife's League; author Rheta Childe Dorr of the Committee on the Industrial Conditions of Women and Children; Mary Ware Dennett of the National Suffrage Association (and later the National Birth Control League); and Dr. Bertha Van Hoosen, outspoken women's leader in medical circles in Chicago.[19] Many of these leaders saw the horrors of childbirth as an experience that united all women: "Childbirth has for every woman through all time been potentially her great emergency."[20] Dr. Ransom thought that the use of twilight sleep would "create a more perfect motherhood" and urged others to work "for the betterment of womankind."[21] Because they saw it as an issue for their sex, not just their class, and because many of the twilight sleep leaders were active feminists, they spoke in the idiom of the woman movement.[22]

The association sponsored rallies in major cities to acquaint women with the issue of painless childbirth and to pressure the medical profession into adopting the new method. In order to broaden their appeal, the association staged meetings "between the marked-down suits and the table linen" of department stores where "the ordinary woman" as well as the activist clubwoman could be found.[23] At these rallies, women who had traveled to Freiburg testified to the wonders of twilight sleep "I experienced absolutely no pain," claimed Mrs. Francis X. Carmody of Brooklyn, displaying her healthy baby at Gimbels. "An hour after my child was born I ate a hearty breakfast. ... The third day I went for an automobile ride. ... The Twilight Sleep is wonderful." Mrs. Carmody ended with the familiar rallying cry: "If you women want it you will have to fight for it, for the mass of doctors are opposed to it."[24]

Department store rallies and extensive press coverage brought the movement to the attention of a broad segment of American women. Movement leaders rejoiced over episodes such as the one in which a "tenement house mother ... collected a crowd" on a street corner where she joyfully told of her twilight sleep experience.[25] Many working-class women were attracted to twilight sleep not only because it made childbirth "pleasanter" but because they saw its use as "an important cause of decreased mortality and increased health and vitality among the mothers of children."[26] Some feared, however, that twilight sleep would remain a "superadded luxury of the wealthy mother" because it involved so much physician time and hospital expense.[27] Although different motivations propelled the physician-advocates who believed twilight sleep was safe, middle- and upper-class women who wanted the newest thing medicine had to offer, and working-class women who wanted simple relief from childbed suffering, they were all united by their common desire to make childbirth safer and easier for women.

Van Hoosen emerged as the most avid advocate of twilight sleep in the Midwest. She received her M.D. from the University of Michigan Medical School and worked at the New England Hospital for Women and Children in Boston before setting up practice in Chicago in 1892. Her enthusiasm for the method came from two sources: her strong commitment to the best in obstetrical care and her equally strong commitment to women's rights. Through her use of scopolamine in surgery and obstetrics, she became convinced that twilight sleep offered women a "return of more physiological births" at the same time that it increased the efficiency of physicians, giving them "complete control of everything."[28] She guided many other physicians to the twilight sleep method.[29] In terms of safety and comfort, she could not imagine a better method of birthing.

Increasingly, doctors began to deliver twilight sleep babies. Some traveled to Germany to learn the Freiburg technique and subsequently offered it to both private and charity patients.[30] A few physicians even became enthusiastic about the possibilities of twilight sleep. "If the male had to endure this suffering," said Dr. James Harrar of New York, "I think he would resort very precipitously to something that might relieve the ... pain."[31] Dr. W. Francis B. Wakefield of California went even further, declaring, "I would just as soon consider performing a surgical operation without an anesthetic as conducting a labor without scopolamin amnesia. Skillfully administered the best interest of both the mother and the child are advanced by its use."[32] Another physician listed its advantages: painless labor, reduction of subsequent "nerve exhaustion that comes after a prolonged hard labor," better milk secretion, fewer cervical and perineal lacerations, fewer forceps deliveries, less strain on the heart, and a "better race for future generations" since upper-class women would be more likely to have babies if they could have them painlessly.[33] There was also, it was claimed, an "advantage to the child: To give it a better chance for life at the time of delivery; a better chance to have breastfeeding; a better chance to have a strong, normal mother."[34]

Despite the energy and enthusiasm of the twilight sleep advocates, many American doctors resisted the technique. They lashed out against the "pseudo-scientific rubbish" and the "quackish hocuspocus" published in *McClure's*[35] and simply refused to be "stampeded by these misguided ladies."[36] These physicians did not believe that nonmedical people should determine therapeutic methods; it was a "question of medical ethics."[37] Other physicians refused to use scopolamine because they feared its dangers either to the mother or the child. The *Journal of the American Medical Association* concluded that "this method has been thoroughly investigated, tried, and found wanting, because of the danger connected with it."[38]

Because the evidence about safety was mixed, many doctors were frustrated in their attempts to find out whether scopolamine was harmful or safe

for use in obstetrics. Earlier experience with the unstable form of the drug led some to refuse to try scopolamine again, although at least one pharmaceutical company had solved the problem of drug stability by 1914. "The bad and indifferent results which were at first obtained by the use of these drugs we now know to have been due entirely to overdosage and the use of impure and unstable preparations," concluded one physician in a report on his successful results with 1,000 twilight sleep mothers in 1915.[39] Dr. Van Hoosen had successfully performed surgery on 2,000 patients with the help of scopolamine by 1908[40] and began using the drug routinely in deliveries in 1914. She concluded after 100 consecutive cases that scopolamine, properly administered, "solves the problems of child-bearing" and is safe for mother and child.[41] But the medical literature continued to express concern about the possible ill effects of a breathing irregularity in babies whose mothers had been given scopolamine and morphine late in labor.[42] Doctors trying to understand the evaluation of twilight sleep must have been confused. In one journal, they read that the procedure was "too dangerous to be pursued," while another journal assured them that scopolamine, when properly used during labor, "has no danger for either mother or child."[43] Increasingly, by 1915, medical journals published studies that at least cautiously favored twilight sleep (the January 1915 issue of *American Medicine* published nine such articles),[44] although they frequently ran editorials warning of the drug's potential dangers and stressing the need for caution. Practicing physicians faced a dilemma when pregnant women demanded painless childbirth with scopolamine.[45]

While physicians debated the desirability of using scopolamine in 1914 and 1915, the public, surer of its position, demanded that twilight sleep be routinely available to women who wanted it. Hospitals in the major cities responded to these demands and to physicians' growing interest in the method by allowing deliveries of babies the Freiburg way.[46] In order to gain additional clinical experience, and possibly in response to some women's requests, some doctors used twilight sleep in hospital charity wards. But the technique was most successful in the specialty wards where upper- and middle-class patients increasingly gave birth and hospital attendants and facilities were available. By May 1915, *McClure's Magazine*'s national survey reported that the use of twilight sleep, although still battling for acceptance, "gains steadily" around the country.[47]

Because of the need for expertise and extra care in administration of scopolamine, the twilight sleep movement easily fed into widespread efforts in the second decade of the twentieth century to upgrade obstetrical practice and eliminate midwives.[48] Both the women who demanded the technique and the doctors who adopted it applauded the new specialty of obstetrics. Mary Boyd desired to put an end to home deliveries when she advocated twilight sleep for charity patients: "Just as the village barber no longer performs operations, the untrained midwife of the neighborhood will pass out of existence under the effective competition of free painless wards."[49] Not only did scopolamine advocates try to displace midwives, but they also regarded general practitioners as unqualified to deliver twilight sleep babies. "The twentieth century woman will no more think of having an ordinary practitioner attend her in childbed at her own home," said two supporters; "she will go to a [twilight sleep] hospital as a matter of course."[50] Specialists agreed that "the method is not adapted for the general practitioner, but should be practiced only by those who devote themselves to obstetrics."[51] Eliza Taylor Ransom went so far as to recommend the passage of a federal law forbidding "anyone administering scopolamine without a course of instruction and a special license."[52]

Some obstetricians used this issue to discredit their general practitioner colleagues and the midwives who still delivered large numbers of America's babies. Another factor that might have pushed obstetricians to support twilight sleep was that births under scopolamine could be managed more completely by the physician. As one succinctly put it, anesthesia gave "absolute control over your patient at all stages of the game. . . . You are 'boss.'"[53] Physicians' time at the bedside could even be used for other pursuits. "I catch up on my reading and writing," testified one practitioner, "I am never harassed by relatives who want me to tell them things."[54]

THE ISSUE OF CONTROL

How do we explain the seeming contradictions in this episode in medical history? Why did women demand to undergo a process which many physi-

cians deemed risky and in which parturients lost self-control? Why did some physicians resist a process that would have given women an easier birthing experience and would have reinforced physicians' control over childbirth in a hospital environment?

Several factors contributed to the open tensions about the use of twilight sleep. One was safety. Many physicians rejected scopolamine because they did not have access to facilities like those at the Mary Thompson Hospital or because they believed the drug too risky under any circumstances. Because of the variability among physicians' use of scopolamine and the contradictory evidence in the professional journals, we know that safety was a guiding motivation of many physicians. However, this is not enough to explain physician reluctance since so many doctors administered other drugs during labor despite questionable safety reports.[55] Differing perceptions about pain during childbirth also contributed to the intensity of feeling about twilight sleep in 1914 and 1915. Although many physicians believed that women's "extremely delicate nervous sensibilities" needed relief, others were reluctant to interfere with the natural process of childbirth. One anti-twilight-sleep physician argued, "when we reflect that we are dealing with a perfectly healthy individual, and an organ engaged in a purely physiological function . . . I fail to see the necessity of instituting such a measure in a normal labor and attempt[ing] to bridge the parturient woman over this physiological process in a semi-conscious condition."[56] Women perceived, too, that some physicians used anesthesia only for "suffering when it becomes a serious impediment to the birth process."[57] However, women who had suffered greatly, or whose friends had suffered greatly, actively sought relief from their "physiological" births: They thought pain in itself a hindrance to a successful childbirth experience and "demanded" that their physicians provide them with more positive, less painful experiences in the future.[58]

Both sides in the twilight sleep debate grappled with a third important question: whether the women or the attendants should determine and control the birthing process.[59] The women who demanded that doctors put them to sleep were partially blind to the safety issue because the issue of control (over pain, bodily function, decision making) was so important to them. Control became important when doctors refused to allow women "to receive the same benefits from this great discovery that their sisters abroad are getting."[60] Twilight sleep advocates demanded their right to decide how they would have their children. Tracy and Boyd articulated this issue: "Women took their doctor's word before. They are now beginning to believe . . . that the use of painlessness should be at *their* discretion."[61] Although women were out of control during twilight sleep births—unconscious and needing crib-beds or constant attention to restrain their wild movements—this loss of control was less important to them than their determination to control the decision about what kind of labor and delivery they would have. Hanna Rion, whose influential book and articles had garnered support for the method, wrote:

> In the old-fashioned days when women were merely the blindfolded guardians of the power of child-bearing, they had no choice but to trust themselves without question in the hands of the all-wise physician, but that day is past and will return no more. Women have torn away the bandages of false modesty; they are no longer ashamed of their bodies; they want to know all the wondrous workings of nature, and they demand that they be taught how best to safeguard themselves as wives and mothers. When it comes to the supreme function of childbearing every woman should certainly have the choice of saying *how* she will have her child.[62]

Twilight sleep women wanted to control their own births by choosing to go to sleep. They were not succumbing to physicians or technology but were, they thought, demanding the right to control their own birthing experiences.

This feminist emphasis on control over decision making appears in the writings and lectures of the leaders of the twilight sleep movement; its followers sought simple relief from pain.[63] Many leaders were active suffragists whose commitment to twilight sleep was rooted in their belief in women's rights.[64] Although these activists agreed with most physicians that birth should increasingly be the domain of the obstetricians and that women should not suffer unnecessarily, they disagreed vehemently about who should decide what the birthing woman's experience would be. They clearly and

adamantly wanted women to have the right to decide their own method of birthing.[65]

In the face of advancing obstetrical technology, many physicians wanted to retain their traditional professional right and duty to decide therapy on the basis of their judgment about the medical indications. They refused to be "dragooned" into "indiscriminate adoption" of a procedure that they themselves did not choose.[66] Even the doctors who supported twilight sleep believed that in the final analysis, the method of childbirth was "a question for the attending man and not the patient to decide."[67] It was principally this question of power over decision making that separated the movement's proponents from its opponents.

THE DECLINE

In the very successes of the twilight sleep movement lay the seeds for its demise. Pressured by the clubwomen's associations and their own pregnant patients, doctors who had not been trained in the Freiburg method delivered babies with scopolamine. There was an enormous variation in the use of the drug, its timing through labor, the conditions in which the woman labored, and the watchfulness of attendants. As its advocates had feared, problems emerged when scopolamine was not properly monitored in a hospital setting. Following reports of adverse effects on the newborn, the drug fell into ill repute, and some hospitals that had been among the first to use it stopped administering it routinely.[68]

Those physicians who continued to advocate twilight sleep believed that accidents were due to misuse of the Freiburg method and not to the drug itself. Commenting on its discontinuation at Michael Reese Hospital in Chicago, Dr. Bertha Van Hoosen noted that "it is . . . probable that this adverse report demonstrates nothing more than the inexperience of the people using this anesthetic."[69] Dr. Ralph Beach agreed that "there is no doubt that all of the bad results which have been reported due to this method, are due to an improper technic, or the administration of unstable preparations."[70] Simultaneously, in 1915, some hospitals expanded their obstetric services to offer twilight sleep, and others began cutting back its use. Either because they judged the drug dangerous or because they did not use it correctly, some hospitals found the method too troublesome to administer on a routine basis to all patients. Most reached a compromise and continued to use scopolamine during labor's first stage (when it was deemed safe), thus preempting their patients' protests without compromising their medical beliefs. A second inhibitory factor appeared in August 1915 when Mrs. Francis X. Carmody, one of the country's leading exponents of twilight sleep, died during childbirth at Long Island College Hospital in New York. Although doctors and her husband insisted that her death was unrelated to scopolamine, it nonetheless harmed the movement.[71] Mrs. Carmody's neighbor started a new movement to oppose twilight sleep, and women became more alert to the question of safety than they had been.[72] Doctors and some former twilight sleep advocates, emphasizing the issues of safety and difficulty of administration, began exploring other methods of achieving painless childbirth.[73]

The obstetric literature after 1915 indicates that twilight sleep did not die in that year. The women's movement may have failed to make scopolamine routinely available to all laboring women, but it succeeded in making the concept of painless childbirth more acceptable and in adding scopolamine to the obstetric pharmacopoeia. In fact, obstetricians continued to use scopolamine into the 1960s during the first stage of hospital births.[74] The use

of anesthesia (including scopolamine) in childbirth grew in the years after 1915, since women, aware of the possibility of painlessness, continued to want "shorter and less painful parturition" and since physicians felt they could disregard these desires "only at great risk to [their] own practice."[75]

The attempt by a group of women, including some feminists, to control their birthing experiences backfired. The medical profession retained the choice of birth procedures and perhaps gained additional control as a result of this episode. Partial acceptance by the profession quieted the lay revolt, and women lost the power they had sought. Ironically, by encouraging women to go to sleep during their deliveries, the twilight sleep movement helped to distance women from their bodies. Put to sleep with a variety of drugs, most parturient women from the 1920s to the 1960s did not experience one of their bodies' most powerful actions and thus lost touch with their own physical potential.[76] The twilight sleep movement helped change the definition of birthing from a natural home event, as it was in the nineteenth century, to an illness requiring hospitalization and physician attendance. Parturient feminists today, seeking fully to experience childbirth, paradoxically must fight a tradition of drugged, hospital-controlled births, itself the partial result of a struggle to increase women's control over their bodies.

NOTES

I am grateful to William J. Orr, Jr., and Susan Duke for their assistance in the preparation of this study. I would also like to thank Mari Jo Buhle, Norman Fost, Susan Friedman, Lewis Leavitt, Elaine Marks, Regina Morantz, and Ronald Numbers for their comments on earlier drafts of this paper.

1 Testimony quoted in Marguerite Tracy and Mary Boyd, *Painless Childbirth* (New York: Frederick A. Stokes Co., 1915), 188–89. For a thorough account of the twilight sleep controversy in America, see Lawrence G. Miller, "Pain, parturition, and the profession: twilight sleep in America," in *Health Care in America: Essays in Social History*, ed. Susan Reverby and David Rosner (Philadelphia: Temple University Press, 1979). 19–44.

2 Tracy and Boyd, *Painless Childbirth*, 198.

3 For more information on childbirth practices in this period, see Judy Barrett Litoff, *American Midwives: 1860 to the Present* (Westport, Conn.: Greenwood Press, 1978).

4 J. F. Ford, "Use of drugs in labor," *Wisconsin Medical Journal*, 1904–5, *3*:257–65.

5 Ibid.

6 See, e.g., Dorothy Reed Mendenhall ("Prenatal and natal conditions in Wisconsin," *Wisconsin Medical Journal*, 1917, *15*:353–69), who reported, "The death rate from maternity is gradually increasing in Wisconsin, as it is throughout the United States" (364). Dr. Mendenhall also noted that death rates for physician-attended births were higher than for midwife-attended births in Wisconsin (353). I would like to thank Dale Treleven for calling this article to my attention.

7 Mary Boyd, "The story of Dammerschlaf: an American woman's personal experience and study at Freiburg," *Survey*, 1915, *33*:129.

8 Quoted in Russell Kelso Carter, *The Sleeping Car "Twilight," or Motherhood without Pain* (Boston: Chapple Publishing Co., 1915), 10–11.

9 Scopolamine is an alkaloid found in the leaves and

seeds of solanaceous plants. It is a sedative and a mild analgesic as well as an amnesiac, causing forgetfulness of pain rather than blocking the pain sensation. For obstetrical twilight sleep, scopolamine was administered with morphine—the most active alkaloid of opium—in the first dose and alone for subsequent doses.

10   Bertha Van Hoosen, *Scopolamine-Morphine Anaesthesia* (Chicago: House of Manz, 1915), 101.

11   *New York Times*, June 9, 1917, 13.

12   Van Hoosen, *Scopolamine-Morphine*, 42.

13   Marguerite Tracy and Constance Leupp, "Painless childbirth," *McClure's Magazine*, 1914, *43*:37–51.

14   Ibid., 43. For the same sentiment among American physicians, see e.g., John O. Polak, "A study of scopolamin and morphine amnesia as employed at Long Island College Hospital," *American Journal of Obstetrics*, 1915, *71*:722; and Henry Smith Williams, *Painless Childbirth* (New York: Goodhue Co., 1914), 90–91. The classic descriptions of the ideal scopolamine delivery are Bernhard Kronig, "Painless delivery in Dammerschlaf" (1908); and Carl J. Gauss, "Births in artificial Dammerschlaf" (1906) and "Further experiments in Dammerschlaf" (1911), all translated and reprinted in Tracy and Boyd, *Painless Childbirth*, 205–308.

15   Mary Boyd and Marguerite Tracy, "More about painless childbirth," *McClure's Magazine*, 1914, *43*:57–58.

16   Hanna Rion, *Painless Childbirth in Twilight Sleep* (London: T. Werner Laurie, 1915), 239; see also her "The painless childbirth," *Ladies' Home Journal*, 1914, *31*:9–10.

17   See, e.g., "Is the twilight sleep safe—for me?" *Woman's Home Companion*, 1915, *42*:10, 43; William Armstrong, "The 'twilight sleep' of Freiburg: a visit to the much talked of Women's Clinic," *Woman's Home Companion*, 1914, *41*:4, 69; *New York Times*, September 17, 1914, 8; November 28, 1914, 2.

18   On women's clubs and clubwomen, see Mary P. Ryan, *Womanhood in America: From Colonial Times to the Present* (New York: New Viewpoints, 1975), 227–32; Edith Hoshino Altbach, *Women in America* (Lexington, Mass.: D. C. Heath & Co., 1974), 114–21; William L. O'Neill, *Everyone Was Brave: A History of Feminism in America* (Chicago: Quadrangle Books, 1969), 107–68; Sheila M. Rothman, *Woman's Proper Place: A History of Changing Ideals and Practices, 1870 to the Present* (New York: Basic Books, 1978), 63–93.

19   Carter, *Sleeping Car "Twilight,"* 174–75.

20   Tracy and Boyd, *Painless Childbirth*, 145.

21   Eliza Taylor Ransom, "Twilight sleep," *Massachusetts Club Women*, 1917, *1*:5. I am grateful to Regina Markell Morantz for this reference.

22   The connections between clubwomen and suffrage or other women's issues are explored in Altbach, *Women in America*, 114–15; O'Neill, *Everyone Was Brave*, 49–76, 146–68; Ryan, *Womanhood in America*, 230–49; and Eleanor Flexner, *Century of Struggle: The Woman's Rights Movement in the United States* (New York: Atheneum Publishers, 1970), 172–92. The term "woman movement," in the nineteenth and early twentieth centuries, described the movement to better women's condition, including, but not limited to, the drive for suffrage.

23   Tracy and Boyd, *Painless Childbirth*, 145.

24   Quoted in *New York Times*, November 18, 1914, 18.

25   Tracy and Boyd, *Painless Childbirth*, 145.

26   Clara G. Stillman, "Painless childbirth," *New York Call*, July 12, 1914, 15.

27   Sam Schmalhauser, "The twilight sleep for women," *International Socialist Review*, 1914, *15*:234–35. I am grateful to Mari Jo Buhle for this and the previous reference.

28   Bertha Van Hoosen, *Petticoat Surgeon* (Chicago: Pellegrini & Cudahy, 1947), 282–83.

29   See, e.g., Bertha Van Hoosen, "A fixed dosage in scopolamine-morphine anaesthesia," *Woman's Medical Journal*, 1916, *26*:57–58; and "Twilight sleep in the home," ibid., 132.

30   For early American trials, see William H. Wellington Knipe, "'Twilight sleep' from the hospital viewpoint," *Modern Hospital*, 1914, *2*:250–51; A. M. Hilkowich, "Further observations on scopolamine-narcophin anesthesia during labor with report of two hundred (200) cases," *American Medicine*, 1914, *20*:786–94; William H. Wellington Knipe, "The Freiburg method of Dammerschlaf or twilight sleep," *American Journal of Obstetrics*, 1914 *70*:364–71; and James A. Harrar and Ross McPherson, "Scopolamine-narcophin seminarcosis in labor," *Transactions of the American Association of Obstetricians and Gynecologists*, 1914, *27*: 372–89.

31   Quoted during discussion of Rongy, Harrar, and McPherson papers, *Transactions of the American Association of Obstetricians and Gynecologists*, 1914, *27*:389.

32   W. Francis B. Wakefield, "Scopolamine amnesia in labor," *American Journal of Obstetrics*, 1915, *71*:428. For more of this kind of enthusiasm, see also Elizabeth R. Miner, "Letter and report of nineteen cases in which 'twilight' was used," *Woman's Medical Journal*, 1916, *26*:131.

33   Ralph M. Beach, "Twilight sleep," *American Medicine*, 1915, *21*:40–41.

34   Bertha Van Hoosen, *Scopolamine-Morphine Anaesthesia*, 101. Some physicians reported success using twilight sleep at home, but most thought the method best suited to hospital deliveries.

35   Quoted from the *Journal of the American Medical Association* in "Another 'twilight sleep,'" *Literary Digest*,

1915, *50:*187; W. Gillespie, "Analgesics and anesthetics in labor, their indication and contraindications," *Ohio Medical Journal*, 1915, *11:*611.

36 "Twilight sleep again," *American Medicine*, 1915, *21:*149.

37 "'Twilight sleep' in the light of day," *Scientific American*, 1915, *79 supp. 2041:*112. See also *New York Times*, October 20, 1914, 12; November 28, 1914, 12; February 5, 1915, 10; February 11, 1915, 8.

38 *Journal of the American Medical Association* (June 6, 1914), quoted in "'Twilight sleeps' and medical publicity," *Literary Digest*, 1914, *49:*60.

39 Ralph M. Beach, "Twilight sleep: report of one thousand cases," *American Journal of Obstetrics*, 1915, *71:*728.

40 Frederick A. Stratton, "Scopolamine anesthesia," *Wisconsin Medical Journal*, 1908–9, *8:*27.

41 Van Hoosen, *Scopolamine-Morphine Anaesthesia*, 101.

42 This condition, called "oligopnea," usually resolved after a few hours, but it was frightening to observe, especially for attendants who had no experience with it (Gauss, "Further experiments in Dammerschlaf," 302).

43 See discussion of the Polak paper (n. 14 above) in *American Journal of Obstetrics*, 1915, *7:* 798; and Hilkowich, "Further observations," 793.

44 *American Medicine*, 1915, *21:*24–70.

45 See, e.g., the discussion following Knipe's paper (n. 30 above) in the *American Journal of Obstetrics*, 1914, *70:*1025. For articles with positive conclusions, see John Osburn Polock, "A study of twilight sleep," *New York Medical Journal*, 1915, *101:* 293; Robert T. Gillmore, "Scopolamine and morphine in obstetrics and surgery," *New York Medical Journal*, 1915, *102:* 298; William H. Wellington Knipe, "'Twilight sleep' from the hospital viewpoint," 250; W. Francis B. Wakefield, "Scopolamin-amnesia in labor," *American Journal of Obstetrics*, 1915, *71:* 428; Samuel J. Druskin and Nathan Ratnoff, "Twilight sleep in obstetrics—with a report of 200 cases," *New York State Journal of Medicine*, 1915, *15:* 152; Charles B. Reed, "A contribution to the study of 'twilight sleep,'" *Surgery, Gynecology and Obstetrics*, 1916, *22:* 656. For a negative conclusion, see Joseph Louis Baer, "Scopolamin-morphin treatment in labor," *Journal of the American Medical Association*, 1915, *64:* 1723–28. The actual dangers of the drug varied according to dosage and timing, and it is impossible for the historian to assess the events accurately without individual case records. Any drug can be dangerous if misused, and the variability in advice about scopolamine suggests that some disasters occurred with it.

46 E.g., see *New York Times*, August 22, 1914, 9; and September 10, 1914; and the American hospitals mentioned in Tracy and Boyd, *Painless Childbirth*.

47 Anna Steele Richardson's survey was reported in the *New York Times*, May 10, 1915, 24.

48 Litoff, *American Midwives*, 69–70.

49 Mary Boyd, "The story of Dammerschlaf," *Survey*, 1914, *33:* 129. See the same statement in Tracy and Boyd, *Painless Childbirth*, 69.

50 Constance Leupp and Burton J. Hendrick, "Twilight sleep in America," *McClure's Magazine*, 1915, *44:* 172–73. The argument about expertise appeared repeatedly (see e.g., William H. W. Knipe, "The truth about twilight sleep," *Delineator*, 1914, *85:* 4. Twilight sleep women were aware that theirs was an expensive demand. They expected the cost of physician-attended childbirth to jump from twenty-five to eighty-five dollars (Tracy and Boyd, *Painless Childbirth*, 180).

51 Druskin and Ratnoff, "Twilight sleep in obstetrics," 152.

52 *New York Times*, April 30, 1915, 8.

53 Quoted from the *New Orleans Medical and Surgical Journal* in Miller, "Pain, parturition," 24.

54 Van Hoosen, *Petticoat Surgeon*, 282.

55 Fifty percent of 100 general practitioners surveyed in rural districts and small towns in Wisconsin indicated that they used ergot during labor, although its use was blamed for "a very large per cent of necessary operations for repair of injuries to the floor and pelvic organs of the female patient" (Ford, "Use of drugs," 257).

56 Dr. Francis Reder, during a discussion of Rongy, Harrar, and McPherson papers, *Transactions of the American Association of Obstetricians and Gynecologists*, 1914, *27:*386.

57 Tracy and Boyd, *Painless Childbirth*, 149.

58 For physicians' perceptions of "demanding" women, see e.g., the discussion following the Rongy and Harrar papers, *Transactions of the American Association of Obstetricians and Gynecologists*, 1914, *27:*382–83.

59 Other contributing factors cannot be developed here. Growing professionalization and specialization with medicine produced tensions among groups of doctors that surfaced during this debate. The method's German "origins" invalidated it with many Americans during the war years. My emphasis here on the issue of control is not meant to minimize these and other factors. However, because others, especially Lawrence Miller (n. 1 above), have explored the general outlines, I have focused on the previously unanalyzed question of decision-making power. Its importance, I think, is indicated by the intensity in the women's arguments on this issue.

60 Letter from "Ex-Medicus" in *New York Times*, November 28, 1914, 12.

61 Tracy and Boyd, *Painless Childbirth*, 147, (emphasis in original).

62 Rion, *Painless Childbirth*, 47.

63 Tracy and Boyd claimed "four to five million" twilight sleep followers, obviously an exaggeration (*Painless Childbirth*, 144).

64 See, e.g, *New York Times*, November 28, 1914, 12.

65 See esp. Tracy and Boyd, *Painless Childbirth*; Rion, *Painless Childbirth*; Ransom, "Twilight sleep"; and Van Hoosen, *Scopolamine-Morphine*.

66 *New York Times*, September 26, 1914, 10.

67 Dr. Arthur J. Booker in his remarks defending Van Hoosen's use of scopolamine, quoted in Van Hoosen, *Scopolamine-Morphine*, 12.

68 *New York Times*, April 24, 1915, 10; April 30, 1915, 8; May 29, 1915, 20; August 25, 1915, 10; August 16, 1916, 7.

69 Van Hoosen, "A fixed dosage," 57.

70 Beach, "Twilight sleep," 43.

71 *New York Times*, August 24, 1915, 7.

72 Ibid., August 31, 1915, 5.

73 See, e.g., Frank W. Lynch, "Nitrous oxide gas analgesia in obstetrics," *Journal of the American Medical Association*, 1915, *64*:813.

74 See, e.g., Henry Schwartz, "Painless Childbirth and the safe conduct of labor," *American Journal of Obstetrics and Diseases of Women and Children*, 1919, *79*:46–63; and W. C. Danforth and C. Henry Davis, "Obstetric analgesia and anesthesia," *Journal of the American Medical Association*, 1923, *81*:1090–96.

75 See the assessment of anesthesia used in childbirth in New York Academy of Medicine Committee on Public Health Relations, *Maternal Mortality in New York City: A Study of all Puerperal Deaths, 1930–1932* (New York: Commonwealth Fund, 1933), 113; see also Joyce Antler and Daniel M. Fox, "Movement toward a safe maternity: physician accountability in New York City, 1915–1940," *Bulletin of the History of Medicine*, 1976, *50*:569–95.

76 The legacy for the parent-infant bond and for subsequent child development is explored in M. H. Klaus and J. H. Kennell, *Maternal Infant Bonding: The Impact of Early Separation or Loss on Family Development* (St. Louis: C. V. Mosby Co., 1976). For a feminist perspective on women's missing their deliveries, see Adrienne Rich, *Of Woman Born: Motherhood as Experience and Institution* (New York: W. W. Norton & Co., 1976).

WOMEN'S DISEASES AND TREATMENTS

Many nineteenth-century observers noted that America seemed to be breeding physically inferior women. One of Catharine Beecher's friends wrote her at midcentury that among all her woman acquaintances in the city of Milwaukee she did "not know one perfectly healthy woman in the place." We have already noted that physicians believed that women's reproductive organs governed their lives and put them repeatedly at great physical risk. This section of the book addresses the general question of women's health and analyzes the extent to which illnesses were sex-specific and whether treatments of diseases were determined by the gender of the patient and the healer.

Joan Jacobs Brumberg explores the relationship between culture- and gender-specific diseases in her article on chlorosis among female adolescents in the late nineteenth and early twentieth centuries. In the next article, Mark Connelly argues that gender also helped determine the progressive response to gonorrhea and syphilis, especially in the social prescriptions for eliminating venereal diseases. Ann Douglas Wood, using literary sources in addition to more traditional ones, analyzes the popular idea that nineteenth-century American women were sickly and posits that nineteenth-century misogynist attitudes in part created the problem. Regina Morantz counters Wood's inter-

pretation, which she believes is too strongly based on the idea of woman as victim, by emphasizing the complexity of the analyses needed to understand women's health.

The last articles in this section examine three very different nineteenth-century therapeutic modes. Kathryn Kish Sklar describes hydropathy—which served men as well as women—and the psychologically supportive environments of the popular water cures. Sarah Stage, in a chapter from her book on Lydia Pinkham's wide-selling cure for women's complaints, addresses questions of self-help and domestic medicine. Lawrence Longo, in describing the development of gynecological surgery, examines one important episode in the relationship between women and the medical profession.

The existence of specific women's health problems, only some of which were directly related to reproduction, and the possibility of unequal treatment based on sex raise difficult and controversial questions about the history of women and health. This section of the book, perhaps more than any other, forces us to analyze a woman's relationships to her own body, to her healers, and to society's views of femaleness. Ideology and physicality, mind and body considerations, form the basis of the historical analysis of this topic.

14

Chlorotic Girls, 1870–1920:
A Historical Perspective on Female Adolescence

JOAN JACOBS BRUMBERG

Students of human development generally fail to appreciate the relevance of historical study to understanding biomedical phenomena, particularly those that relate to specific stages of the life course. Our identification of contemporary female adolescence with both anorexia nervosa and bulimarexia raises larger questions about the evolution of gender- and age-specific symptomatologies, questions that may be answered in part by reference to the history of American women. Consequently, this essay poses a deceptively simple but nevertheless important question: What can we learn from the historical study of a particular disease?

The complete answer is part of a more extensive investigation of the changing symptomatology of American girlhood from 1850 to the present.[1] What you will read here is not a biomedical diagnosis or an epidemiological explanation but a historical description and analysis of chlorosis, a disease which was linked solely to female adolescence in the period 1870–1920. While there was neither a precise constellation of symptoms nor a medical consensus as to its cause, there was agreement about the constituency for this popular form of anemia. Chlorotic girls, not boys, were the focus of attention from medical men, parents, and educators. In fact, chlorosis represented an entire conception of the female adolescent rather than a simple anemia.

This analysis is guided by a set of assumptions drawn from the fields of anthropology, history, the sociology of medicine, and human development. First, since the contexts for human development

JOAN JACOBS BRUMBERG is Assistant Professor in the Department of Human Development and Family Studies and in the Women's Studies Program at Cornell University, Ithaca, New York.

Reprinted with permission from *Child Development* 53 (1982): 1468–1477.

invariably shape physiological, cognitive, and behavioral growth processes,[2] historical study can and should be enlisted in the effort to define the relationship between structural and cultural changes and the evolving psychological orientations of young women. Second, modern anthropological studies, particularly Margaret Mead's (1928) pioneering description of adolescence as a biocultural transition,[3] clearly demonstrate that what is pathological within one cultural setting may be modal in another or vice versa. It is a logical corollary that variations with respect to what is atypical or modal can also occur over time within a single culture as well as cross-culturally. A striking case in point is the changing age of menarche in the United States; in 1833, the normative age for the onset of the menses may have been as high as 17; in 1972, it was 13 years of age.[4] Third, historical and sociological study reveals that in addition to the systematic study of the physical world and its phenomena, science is also an expression of our culture and our social relations.[5]

Thus, the clinical object—disease—must be regarded as both cultural artifact and somatic phenomenon. Consequently, a single disease may have a biography or life history all its own, responsive to social as well as medical cure. Previous studies point to the limited duration of chlorosis[6] without providing adequate cultural explanations for why it was that chlorosis was so prevalent among a single age and sex group. Hudson relates the rise of the disease to advances in laboratory medicine (particularly in the field of hematology) and the demise of the disease to a generalized improvement in nutrition (which he does not document). Siddall links the declining frequency of the disease to change in prenatal care, that is, the elimination of "bloodletting" in the care of expectant mothers.[7] Huang, the most extensive scholarly investigation to date, attributes the decline in incidence by 1900 to increased medical acceptance of the "iron deficiency hypothesis" and the parallel development of a successful treatment, namely, iron therapy in correct dosages. In this scenario, medical men, not patients, play a primary role in the cure. Figlio attributes the origin of chlorosis and other chronic diseases in late-nineteenth-century Britain to the exigencies of class. In England, chlorosis was linked to the idle daughters of the aristocracy and the bourgeoisie; yet their physicians, according to Figlio, were only "marginal members" of the middle class. As a result, both the cure and the explanatory etiology of chlorosis were shaped by class tensions. And as a cure, British doctors promoted a "medicalized condemnation" of the luxurious habits associated with the leisure of girls in the privileged classes.

In the American case, the diverse social settings in which chlorosis developed undercut a strictly class explanation. This article argues that medical pathlogies linked to adolescent girls may emerge at particular moments in time, their appearance and disappearance not entirely explained by empirical factors. Moreover, adolescent girls are more directly implicated in the cure for chlorosis than either the Hudson or Huang studies allow. Certainly chlorosis cannot be understood fully without exploring its meaning for the patient. What you will read here is a rather straightforward exposition of the relationship between the biomedical diagnosis of the disease, medical conceptions of the female adolescent, and the changing social experience of girls. This essay places chlorosis in the context of its "life and times" in order to suggest the complex interplay of adolescent physiology, medicine, and social and family life.

Writing in the fifth volume of his massive medical compendium, *A System of Medicine*, T. Clifford Allbutt (1905) set forth the distinguishing characteristics of chlorosis, a form of anemia named for the greenish tinge that allegedly marked the skin of the patient. Allbutt reported that chlorosis was a "malady of women, and primarily of young women at or about the age of puberty . . . consisting in defect of the red corpuscles of the blood, a defect partly of numbers, chiefly of hemoglobin; the plasma being constant, or even enriched."[8] The term chlorosis had been in use throughout the

nineteenth century. In *Females and Their Diseases,* Charles Meigs referred to a "puberic condition" that "the French call *pâles couleurs,* and which we term green sickness or chlorosis."[9] In *The Lady's Manual of Homeopathic Medicine,* written some twenty years later, E. H. Ruddock defined chlorosis as "a condition of general debility affecting young women" caused by a "deficiency" in the red corpuscles.[10] To the modern eye, chlorosis appears to be merely a curious, archaic name for iron deficiency anemia, yet Allbutt's comprehensive medical discussion of the etiology and symptoms of the disease suggests no easy one-to-one equivalent.

Allbutt distinguished chlorosis from other anemias by its constituency (girls between fourteen and twenty-five) and on the basis of patient reports of difficult respiration or dyspnea. "The heart is irritable," he wrote; "it often palpitates to the great distress of the patient. The palpitation makes itself felt . . . on the least exertion."[11] In addition to shortness of breath and energy, chlorotic girls were said to experience a wide variety of symptoms, including "caprices and perversions" of the appetite, amenorrhea, inertia and melancholy, headaches, "mental disposition," and a "desire for sleep and repose."[12] The patients' complexions, however, were not always pale or conspicuously tinted, as the name of the disease suggested. "Chlorotic girls still blush readily enough," wrote Allbutt, "and even in the height of an attack of their malady some of them never lose a vivid carmine on the malar eminences."[13]

Allbutt's synthesis of the medical literature on chlorosis suggests how popular a malady it had become during the nineteenth century. Among female adolescents, chlorosis existed on a number of different diagnostic levels that are easy enough to hypothesize but almost impossible to quantify. After about 1870, some young women, probably those of the middle and upper classes living in urban or commercial centers with a well-educated professional class, were clinically diagnosed as chlorotics on the basis of actual analysis of their blood. In these cases, hemoglobin deficiencies did exist. Many other patients, however, were called chlorotic by less careful and less knowledgeable doctors simply on the basis of symptoms described to them in a medical interview. No blood tests were made on this group of patients; rather, the age and gender of the patients triggered the diagnosis. Since the disease conveyed no particular status liabilities, it was easy enough to assign, particularly to those girls who may have used being "sickly" as a means of securing special attentions within the family or among friends. Still other girls, generally those without access to a physician or without the means to pay one, used the term chlorosis to describe their debilities and followed self-diagnosis with a home cure, that is, patent medicine designed to improve and strengthen the female constitution.[14]

Because chlorosis existed on both the clinical and popular levels, it was regarded as altogether commonplace and democratic. "The chlorotic girl," Allbutt wrote, "is known in every consulting-room, public or private. The disease is no respecter of rank or fortune."[15] Maintaining that chlorotic girls came from farms as well as urban centers, from all walks and stations of life, Allbutt claimed the broadest constituency for the disease despite evidence, drawn from his own clinical practice, that might point to a hereditary propensity for the condition. For example, Allbutt reported that he had treated at least two, and possibly three, generations of chlorotic daughters in a single family. When another doctor associated the disease with blondes, suggesting a possible link to race, Allbutt dismissed the claim with the remark that the disease was simply "more conspicuous" in fair people. A 1915 analysis of the disease by physician Richard C. Cabot, later the founder of the Department of Social Ethics at Harvard, pointed to the large number of Irish domestics in Boston who, apparently, reported the disease. Yet, Cabot could not find much additional evidence for an Irish propensity for chlorosis since factory girls of the same ethnic background seemed not to be affected. Among the Germans, Cabot noted, girls who "have moved to the city, from the country" were likely to develop chlorosis.[16]

Rather than scientifically refine the constituency for chlorosis by establishing its connection to specific racial or social variables, Allbutt and others advanced the notion that all adolescent girls were potentially chlorotic: "Perhaps, every girl passes as it were, through the outer court of chlorosis in her progress from youth to maturity." In fact, Allbutt suggested that even those who appeared well might be suffering from the disease: "It is a common experience that many girls otherwise healthy and living under the best conditions of life become chlo-

rotic; perhaps, no girl escapes it altogether; some, however, show it but little and recover rapidly." Finally, Allbutt posited that the physician was needed to distinguish between the healthy and the diseased girl. If, as Allbutt maintained, "every girl may be regarded as potentially chlorotic," then the boundary between the normal and the pathological was, in his own words, an "arbitrary one."[17] Every female adolescent raised the specter of chlorosis.

The actual cause of chlorosis was the subject of much debate. According to Huang, nineteenth-century etiologies focused on three major causes: environmental, moral, and constitutional.[18] Typical of the first is an 1869 medical guide that linked chlorosis to "confinement" in badly ventilated or poorly lighted rooms.[19] In the United States these environmental causes were present in all classes. Among factory girls, chlorosis was linked to poor diet and "bad living"; among college girls, the disease was linked to excessive study and lack of outdoor exercise. Different doctors had their own favorite constitutional and moral interpretations, ranging from "derangement of the menstrual function," to "impoverished blood," to a "disease of the nervous system," to "a morbid condition of the organs of generation." Allegedly, the last of these was the result of masturbation. One medical adviser, urging mothers "to find out whether the disease may not be induced by secret habits," suggested that girls be watched "unobtrusively" and allowed "as little as possible to remain alone."[20] Although masturbation was not widely hypothesized as a direct cause of chlorosis, doctors like Allbutt were unwilling to disassociate the "master vice" completely. Allbutt advised his fellow physicians that in looking for the cause of chlorosis "if epithelial debris be found repeatedly in the urine, masturbation must not be forgotten, and corroborative evidence of the habit . . . detected."[21]

Menstruation, however, was almost always implicated in the etiology of chlorosis because the disease was associated with puberty in girls, not boys. In *Modern Medicine* readers found the following tentative analysis: "Judging from the fact that chlorosis is confined to the female, and that it occurs in the period immediately after the establishment of the function of menstruation, we can hardly help suggesting that there is some immediate relation between menstruation and chlorosis, but we can go no further. We have nothing to say as to what that relation is, or whether we are right in supposing any such relation exists. The figures suggest it; that is all we can say."[22] Medical men were obviously confused by the fact that some girls developed chlorosis even before the onset of the menses, making a direct causal relationship unlikely. Consequently, popular medical tracts, such as Lucien Warner's *A Treatise on the Functions and Diseases of Women* (1875), glossed the issue of the premenstrual chlorotic girl, offering this common interpretation of the origins of the pathology: "the real seat of the disease is in the nervous system, although it manifests itself chiefly in impoverishment of the blood. It occurs most frequently at the time of puberty, because the system is then in such a transition, that it requires slighter disturbing causes for its development."[23]

Clearly, in the transitionary period from childhood to adulthood girls were "at risk" for disease. In women, puberty and the onset of the menses marked the beginning of a period of psychological as well as physiological crisis that would continue until menstruation was regularized or "firmly established." Medical tracts urged both girls and their parents to consider the need for a special "hygiene of puberty."[24] Because of "large demands upon the resource of the female adolescent system," Lucien Warner advised close parental supervision of the diet, clothing, exercise, sleep, and mental and moral training of girls. In the 1870s, Dr. Edward Clarke, professor of medicine in Harvard College, argued against higher education for young women precisely because he believed that the "complicated apparatus peculiar to the female" needed time and ease to develop, free from the drain of intellectual activity. Clarke's influential but controversial book, *Sex in Education* (1873), presented case studies, allegedly drawn from clinical practice, of girls whose "catamenial function," ovarian development, and general health were ruined by inattention to the special demands of their new "periodicity."[25] In the view of many, female adolescence was especially dangerous because menstruation raised the specter of multiple crises of a social as well as a medical nature. Only marriage insured a formal, guaranteed, and effective resolution of the difficult transition period. As a result, marriage was sometimes

suggested as a cure for chlorosis.[26] Warner wrote of this kind of therapy: "It should in no case be resorted to except upon the recommendation of some responsible physician."[27]

While most medical men implicated menstruation in the etiology of chlorosis, some did not. For example, in *Chlorosis: The Special Anemia of Young Women* (1897), E. Lloyd Jones, an instructor in pathology at Cambridge and a research scholar for the British Medical Association, reported that there simply was "not sufficient evidence to show that chlorosis is due to menstrual loss." Rather, Jones proposed an interpretation of the causes of the disease that reflected new research techniques and insights derived from the science of hematology. Chlorosis, Jones argued, was best understood in relation to the blood changes that occurred at puberty, particularly a drop in specific blood gravity among females. Using the centrifugal method (whirling tubes of blood at a speed of 1,000 rpm), Jones discovered that the average ratio between serum and corpuscles could be differentiated by gender and age. This disparity in female and male blood was presented in a number of charts and tables, which gave the treatise an empirical aura and in turn documented in chlorotic girls a reduction in the amount of hemoglobin, a diminution of the number of red corpuscles, and an increase in the proportion of serum to corpuscles. Yet, like Allbutt, Jones had difficulty distinguishing the normal from the pathological: "the blood of the chlorotic subject exhibits an exaggeration of the fall in specific gravity which occurs in healthy young women about the age of puberty; and, indeed, it is likely that I included among my healthy women some who were in reality chlorotic."[28]

If hematology failed to establish absolute distinctions between the blood of healthy and diseased girls, diagnosis was confused even further by the fact that the pathological was also regarded as the ideal type. That is to say that girls with the disease were also the most attractive and, possibly, the best potential mothers. In fact, Jones claimed that chlorosis in adolescence was positively correlated with high fertility. "Those women who have the lowest specific gravity of the blood, and the largest number of brothers and sisters," Jones wrote, "are generally fair, with pretty pink and white complexions, blue or light eyes, fine hair, with a goodly amount of subcutaneous fat. Such women are, I believe, unusually prolific."[29] Jones's attention to the looks of the chlorotic girl was not unusual. According to one medical report, chlorosis was "the anemia of good looking girls."[30] Medical men generally agreed with Allbutt's statement of their physiological normality: "chlorotic girls do not lack size, nor do they fall away from the main lines of development."[31] Jones, however, took the association between chlorosis and good looks a step further, claiming that while the "lips and ears" of a chlorotic girl might be "pallid," her cheeks certainly were not. Jones asserted that the face of the chlorotic girl remained a "pretty pink and white color" precisely because her blood vessels were so "well-filled."

The medical notion of the chlorotic girl as simultaneously diseased, fertile, and attractive fit within the framework of the Victorians' sentimentalization of sickly women.[32] In the nineteenth century, adult women in the United States were prone to a generalized invalidism as well as both hysteria and neurasthenia, the latter a polite but "profound physical and mental exhaustion."[33] Neurasthenia, like chlorosis, had an imprecise constellation of symptoms including sick headaches, palpitations, and nervous dyspepsia. (In his classic work, *American Nervousness* [1881], George Beard called neurasthenia "slippery, fleeting, and vague.")[34] For the study of female adolescence the crucial point is that invalidism and neurasthenia were not uncommon pathologies among mothers, aunts, teachers, and family friends who conditioned the psychological orientation and experiences of younger women. Chlorotic girls and sickly mothers did share some common symptoms and probably legitimated each other's complaints. It is also important to understand that among nineteenth-century physicians the same cluster of symptoms (e.g., exhaustion, headaches, heart palpitations, and indigestion) could result in different diagnoses depending on the age and gender of the patient. In this way, the labeling of medical conditions by nineteenth-century doctors reinforced the gender and age categories that were the basis of the Victorian social order.

The coexistence of both disease and physical attractiveness among chlorotics was also a telling reflection of the state of medical and scientific knowledge, particularly with respect to ovarian function. For example, Jones, who was typical of many late-nineteenth-century physicians, attributed the chlorotic girl's good looks, that is, her rosy glow, to the fact that her vessels were "well-filled." Moreover, he maintained that girls bled from the finger more easily than boys. These claims were based on the belief that in chlorotic women there was an absolute increase in the total volume of blood. Jones and others attributed the alleged increase in blood volume to the tendency to "store up blood during the intermenstrual periods"; at each menstrual period, girls would receive "blood changes" or experience "fresh additions to the reserve laid aside." Allbutt's experience confirmed Jones's view; he posited that chlorosis was "the exaggeration of the fertile blood, of blood, that is, which has for its end the storage of nutritive materials for the foetus during pregnancy."[35]

The clinical portrait of the chlorotic girl was obviously confused by a lack of understanding of menstrual physiology. Until the work of Westphalen in 1896, prevailing theory held that menstruation was set in motion by the "tubal nerve," that is, a "nerve irritation" produced by the ovary caused the blood vessels to dilate just prior to ovulation; if unfertilized, the ovum was swept away by the flow. Westphalen first described the cyclical changes in the uterine lining and the continual process of building up and breaking down of that lining.[36] Jones, however, who had only a rudimentary understanding of what took place in the uterus during menstruation, was able to associate chlorosis with greater blood volume and fecundity at the same time that he reported amenorrhea in his chlorotic patients. Ultimately, Jones revealed his ambivalence about the simple hematological calculus he had proposed, calling chlorosis "a chronic autointoxication brought about by some substances which are probably the products of uterine, fallopian or ovarian metabolism, and producing effects on the blood by inducing changes in the gastrointestinal canal by the medium of the nervous system."[37]

In calling chlorosis an "autointoxication," Jones raised the issue of the involvement of adolescent girls in the creation of their own disease. As already noted, chlorosis was the kind of condition that depended in large measure on self-reporting or reports from parents. According to clinical observations, many adolescents presented themselves at the office of the family doctor with a diagnosis in hand. "I think my blood must be out of order," was the characteristic analysis in the experience of an Erie, Pennsylvania, practitioner. Still other patients reported what their peers had said: "friends . . . commented on the lack of color in my face."[38] According to Lucien Warner, concerned parents recited the sad case histories of daughters who were "unusually dull and listless," whose "fits of sadness and weeping" appeared to be without cause. Ruddock reported that his chlorotic patients were "sombre and taciturn, weeping without cause; and sighing involuntarily."[39] Generally, however, the symptoms described by late-nineteenth-century physicians were physiological rather than psychological, although the doctors never promoted the notion of a happy chlorotic or discredited the idea that the ultimate cause might be emotional (e.g., lovesickness, homesickness, shock). The most commonly reported symptoms were progressive loss of strength, difficulty in respiration, and loss of appetite.

Lethargy and shortness of breath received mention but little elaboration; Allbutt noted that girls who once could "trip upstairs" easily were reduced to a state of inactivity by chlorosis. More interesting, however, were the eating disorders associated with chlorosis, all of which acted to confirm what the 1897 *American Journal of Medical Science* called the "capricious appetite" of young women. Nearly thirty years before, a homeopathic medical guide for women noted that in the chlorotic girl the appetite was "lost or so perverted that substances such as chalk, cinders, etc. are desired."[40] In 1875, Lucien Warner's popular medical compendium associated chlorosis with "loss of appetite, loathing of food, and often a desire which almost amounts to a passion, for such indigestible and repulsive articles as charcoal, slate-stones, chalk, plaster, flies, bugs, and other similar substances."[41] Another report stated that the commonest dietary abnormality among chlorotics was "a special fondness for pickles and sour things."[42]

In 1897, E. Lloyd Jones linked chlorosis to a less bizarre diet, but to an eating "disorder" nonetheless. Chlorotic girls, he observed, were not simply prone to the excessive consumption of carbohydrates; they eschewed an important nutritive source: "Almost all chlorotic girls are fond of biscuits, potatoes, etc. while they avoid meat on most occasions, and when they do eat meat, they prefer the burnt outside portion."[43] Meigs confirmed the same problem in a dialogue between a physician and an adolescent girl. "'Oh, I like pies and preserves but I can't bear meat,' the young woman reportedly told her family doctor."[44] Apparently, while many chlorotic patients assured their doctors that they ate meat, physicians regularly found that their meat eating actually involved only the scantiest quantities of burnt, overcooked parts. J. H. Montgomery, a Pennsylvania physician, observed this "disgust for meat in any form"; a medical guide reported that among chlorotics "the appetite for animal food completely ceases."[45] In articulating his cure for chlorosis, Allbutt wrote: "it is of the first importance to overcome the common distaste for meat. Girls will say that the entry of a dish of hot meat into the room makes them feel sick."[46]

The repugnance for animal flesh among Victorian adolescents clearly had a larger cultural significance. In fact, meat eating was tied to female physiology, sexuality, and, consequently, behavior as an adult woman. In negotiating the difficult biological transition to adulthood, Warner suggested that meat eating could actually accelerate sexual development; at the same time, a restriction on the carnivorous aspect of the diet could tame premature or rampant sexuality as well as overabundant menstrual flow: "If there is any tendency to precocity in menstruation, or if the system is very robust and plethoric, the supply of meat should be quite limited. If, on the other hand, the girl is of sluggish temperament and the menses are tardy in their appearance, the supply of meat should be especially generous."[47] In excess, meat eating was popularly linked to nymphomania.[48] A stimulative diet of meat and condiments was recommended only for those girls whose development of the passions seemed, somehow, "deficient."

If a meatless diet could insure their sexual morality, it is no wonder that so many middle-class girls, aspiring to be good, evidenced distaste for a food that, allegedly, increased the menstrual flow and made them more passionate. In making the refusal of meat a positive social virtue, middle- and upper-class girls increased the likelihood of their incurring iron deficits of exactly the kind that led to iron deficiency anemia. Moreover, Allbutt's important synthesis of the medical literature on chlorosis reveals that even as early as 1905, American girls had fallen victims to the grand obsession:

slimness. "Many young women, as their frames develop, fall into a panic fear of obesity," Allbutt wrote, "and they not only cut down on their food, but swallow vinegar and other alleged antidotes to fatness."[49] Consequently, voluntary restrictions on diet were part of female adolescent life in the United States before the twentieth century. Whether a girl chose to avoid meat because she found its associations "disgusting" or she ate less for fear of expanding her waistline, the fact of the matter is that these cultural attitudes were in place, tying feminine goodness and attractiveness to an ideal body type. Thus, there were cultural sources as well as organic reasons for the "loss of appetite" and the "peculiarities of diet" associated with chlorotic girls.

As therapy for these patients, physicians debated the effectiveness of rest versus outdoor exercise. However, most doctors prescribed daily supplements of iron salts even though there was little consensus on how organic and inorganic iron actually affected the blood and few studies of the iron intake of chlorotics.[50] Blaud's Pills, a well-known patent medicine that combined iron and potassium carbonate, were frequently cited by doctors writing about the clinical treatment of chlorotic girls. Iron supplements from drug manufacturers were praised by professional medical men; Allbutt, in fact, called the patent medical business "our excellent allies." Popular advertising in newspapers and magazines promoted "blood and nerve remedies" by the score, keeping pace with both the physicians' clinical diagnosis of chlorosis and the girls' self-reporting and self-diagnosis of their weak condition. E. Lloyd Jones typically prescribed Blaud's Pills after each meal along with small doses of bismuth salicylate with morphine (to relax the stomach before eating) and a diet of underdone meat, no potatoes, and little bread. J. H. Montgomery, who also ordered sulphate of iron in doses of 6– 12 grains daily, was careful to point out that the iron supplements should not be prematurely discontinued as soon as the hemoglobin reached normal. Rather, Montgomery, warning of relapse, encouraged continuation of the supplements for at least two months and the cultivation of "better habits." Another source estimated that "under treatment" the disease was usually relieved "well within six months" and recommended that the patient go from one 0.3-gram pill after each meal in the first week to three pills after each meal, or 2.7 grams

per day, in the third week.[51] Despite medical faith in the efficacy of supplementary iron, doctors were willing to concede that "it is also true that patients will improve without the administration of iron, provided we correct their constipation and improve their general hygiene."[52] Generally, however, a regimen of Blaud's Pills accomplished a satisfactory "cure." Once past the age of twenty-five, or at such time as they married, the risk of developing chlorosis was drastically reduced.

By 1900, chlorosis was already on the decline; by the 1930s the disease was moribund. Statistical evidence from both the wards and the dispensary at Massachusetts General Hospital indicates that between 1898 and 1907 the number of cases declined by nearly 90 percent.[53] Practicing physicians confirmed the same trend. In 1915, Dr. Richard C. Cabot reported: "We do not see chlorosis now as we used to ten years ago." Cabot carefully described how this decline in cases could not be explained away by "supposing that we now call the same cases by another name."[54] In other words, chlorosis was not simply a diagnostic entity that was subsumed into a different category. By 1936, an Iowa physician, W. M. Fowler, was moved to eulogize the disease in an article entitled "Chlorosis—an Obituary," published in the *Annals of Medical History*. "What disease," Fowler asked, "can compare with chlorosis in having occupied such a prominent place in medical practice only to disappear spontaneously while we are still speculating as to its etiology?"[55] Thus, the chlorotic era, which reached its peak in the last three decades of the nineteenth century, came to be regarded as something of a medical curiosity at the very time when massive economic deprivation, in the form of the great depression, should have increased the constituency for anemias of all kinds.

"Very little of the decrease in chlorosis can be attributed to direct medical intervention," writes Robert P. Hudson, a contemporary medical historian.[56] If the demise of chlorosis is not the self-conscious accomplishment of American medicine, how then did it occur? Hudson claims that certain changes in the day-to-day life of Americans in the first few decades of this century had consequences for the future of chlorosis, specifically, a general improvement in nutrition, diminishing prejudice against the eating of meat,[57] the abandonment of corsets or "tight lacing," and a related increase in physical activity among women. While all of these changes are relevant, they fail to capture the essential dynamic of the chlorotic era. That is to say, neither more effective iron therapy, improved nutritional levels, nor increased physical activity, each a legitimate biomedical factor, provides the essential cipher for decoding the social construction of chlorosis.

At a basic level, chlorosis depended for its existence on the popular notion that adolescence, marked by the onset of the menses, made a girl ripe for disease. So long as medical men misunderstood the true nature of the ovulatory cycle and the menstrual flow, women did, in fact, appear to be strangely afflicted. Important discoveries that marked the beginning of the modern endocrine perspective on menstrual physiology came only after 1900; in particular, the 1908 description of the cycle of changes in the endometrium, by Hitschmann and Adler, paved the way for a more accurate understanding of the significance of menstruation. Between 1903 and 1928, the role of ovarian hormones in triggering the cycle was established through animal experimentation.[58] Taken together, these and other developments in the history of gynecology finally condemned the notion of menstruation as a "crisis." Once it was discovered that the menstrual cycle actually lasted for twenty-eight days and then routinely began again, it became difficult to argue that the process itself made adolescent girls susceptible to disease. In effect, the rise of endocrinology in the early twentieth century undercut the medical diagnosis of chlorosis. Informed and better-educated doctors were simply less likely to assume that adolescent girls were either "at risk" or sick.

Finally, the patients and their families must be implicated in the demise of chlorosis. However iatrogenic medical practice may be,[59] the prevalence of chlorosis depended both on young female patients' presenting a certain set of complaints and the biomedical diagnosis and labeling by medical men. Girls who were told that they had chlorosis learned how to have it from family, friends, and the popular press as well as from their doctors; their behavior as "sick" persons was surely affected by the expectations of the people and the institutions with whom they interacted. The fact that neurasthenic conditions were fashionable among the adult women who superintended their school,

church, and family life is essential to understanding the psychology of chlorotic girls. It may well be that nineteenth-century mothers and daughters, particularly among the middle and upper classes, were bonded together by their common ill health rather than their vigor.

As social and cultural values changed, American girls began to choose activity over inactivity, the meeting place over the malaise. Chlorotic girls, with their problems of respiration and limited energy, were aptly suited to a domesticated nineteenth-century environment where they could conscientiously take their iron pills and their requisite afternoon naps. As the lives of girls became more public and standardized, chlorosis became a problem. Geared increasingly to attendance in public high schools, programs of physical activity, peer-group associations beyond the home and family, as well as the "dating system"[60] and the media of romance (film, radio, and popular press), girls replaced concern about their blood with a different set of anxieties about face and figure.

So, too, parents and parental expectations changed. For American mothers, the years between 1900 and 1920 were significant for the emphasis put in the popular women's press on the idea that there was a "scientific nutrition" with application to the home. Dieticians such as Sarah Tyson Rorer, domestic editor of the *Ladies' Home Journal* from 1897 to 1911, charged American mothers with "building and repairing the human body" through right diet.[61] Other pioneers in applied nutrition addressed the general public through bulletins issued by the U.S. Department of Agriculture. In the 1890s, W. O. Atwater developed dietary guides which Ellen Swallow Richards, founder of the home economics movement, translated into family menu planning. Between 1916 and 1923, the USDA popularized the concept of five basic food groups, adapting it for kitchen use.[62] Once this information was available and incorporated into the day-to-day domestic routines of American women of the middle class, mothers were simply less likely to tolerate having a nutritional disease in the home.

In effect, both mothers and daughters had moved beyond invalidism and chlorosis. Complaints of weakness and loss of appetite, as well as the notion of "rest cures," simply did not "fit" with the plethora of institutions and programs servicing American girlhood by World War I. By 1920, a girl with chlorosis was not only a social "drag" but a liability with respect to her own mother's perception of herself as a competent domestic manager and nurturer. If, as the contemporary Geritol commercials

repeatedly remind us, iron deficiency anemia never disappeared, chlorosis surely did precisely because the cultural and familial context that stimulated its construction changed dramatically.

NOTES

Earlier versions of this paper were presented to the Department of Human Development and Family Studies and the Women's Studies Sex and Gender Study Group, both at Cornell. The author has profited from her colleagues' critical comments and from perceptive readings by Nancy Tomes and Will Provine.

1 Female adolescence is a largely neglected area of psychological, sociological, and historical study. See G. H. Elder, Jr., "Adolescence in historical perspective," in *Handbook of Adolescent Psychology*, ed. J. Adelson (New York: Wiley, 1980), for commentary on this lacuna in the developmental literature. Among historians, important studies of adolescence and youth in Europe and the United States by John Gillis (*Youth and History: Tradition and Change in European Age Relation, 1770–Present* [New York: Academic Press, 1974]), and Joseph Kett (*Rites of Passage: Adolescence in America, 1790 to the Present* [New York: Basic, 1977]), focus primarily on the patterns and behaviors of males. Carol Dyhouse's *Girls Growing Up in Victorian and Edwardian England* (London: Routledge & Kegan Paul, 1981) is essentially a study of the socialization of girls in English schools.

2 U. Bronfenbrenner, *The Ecology of Human Development* (Cambridge, Mass.: Harvard University Press, 1979).

3 M. Mead, *Coming of Age in Samoa* (New York: Morrow, 1928).

4 V. Bullough, "Age at menarche: a misunderstanding," *Science*, 1981, *213*:365–66; P. Laslett, "Age of menarche in Europe since the eighteenth century," in *The Family in History*, ed. T. Rabb and R. Rotberg (New York: Harper and Row, 1971); J. Money and A. E. Ehrhardt, *Man and Woman, Boy and Girl: The Differentiation and Dimorphism of Gender Identity from Conception to Maturity* (Baltimore: Johns Hopkins, 1972), 197–98.

5 E. Mishler et al., *Social Contexts of Health, Illness, and Patient Care* (New York: Cambridge University Press, 1981); E. D. Pellegrino, "Medicine, history, and the idea of man," *Annals of the American Academy of Political and Social Science*, 1963, *346*:9–20.

6 K. Figlio, "Chlorosis and chronic disease in nineteenth-century Britain: the social constitution of so-

matic illness in a capitalist society," *Social History*, 1978, *3*:167–97; R. P. Hudson, "The biography of disease: lessons from chlorosis," *Bulletin of the History of Medicine*, 1977, *51*:448–63; S.-R. Huang, "Chlorosis and the iron controversy: an aspect of nineteenth-century medicine," Ph.D. diss., Harvard University, 1978.

7 A. C. Siddall, "Chlorosis: etiology reconsidered," *Bulletin of the History of Medicine*, 1982, *56*:254–60.

8 T. Clifford Allbutt, "Chlorosis," in *A System of Medicine*, ed. T. C. Allbutt (New York: Macmillan, 1905).

9 C. Meigs, *Females and Their Diseases* (Philadelphia: Lea and Blanchard, 1848), 344.

10 E. H. Ruddock, *The Lady's Manual of Homeopathic Medicine* (New York: Smith, 1869), 31–32.

11 Allbutt, "Chlorosis," 501.

12 Ibid.; E. L. Jones, *Chlorosis: The Special Anemia of Young Women* (London: Balliere, Tindall, and Cox, 1897); Ruddock, *Lady's Manual*; R. L. Tait, *Diseases of Women* (Philadelphia: Lea, 1889).

13 Allbutt, "Chlorosis," 499.

14 S. Stage, *Female Complaints: Lydia Pinkham and the Business of Women's Medicine* (New York: Norton, 1979).

15 Allbutt, "Chlorosis," 497.

16 R. C. Cabot, "Chlorosis," in *Modern Medicine*, ed. W. Osler and T. McCrae (New York: Lea and Febinger, 1915), 647.

17 Allbutt, "Chlorosis," 484, 486, 492.

18 Huang, "Chlorosis and the iron controversy."

19 Ruddock, *Lady's Manual*, 32.

20 Ibid., 35.

21 Allbutt, "Chlorosis," 487.

22 Cabot, "Chlorosis," 648.

23 L. Warner, *A Treatise on the Functions and Diseases of Women* (New York: Manhattan, 1875), 68–69.

24 A. Howard, *Medical Gynecology* (New York: Appleton, 1908), 67.

25 E. H. Clarke, *Sex in Education; or, A Fair Chance for Girls* (Boston: Osgood, 1873). G. Stanley Hall (*Adolescence*, 2 vols. [New York: Appleton, 1904]) built a psychology of adolescent development based on the law "that there is a trophic or nutritive background to everything" and that the "profound metamorphoses of puberty involve adjustments far more radical than are usually imagined" (1:252). In a

chapter entitled "Diseases of body and mind," Hall detailed various nosological peculiarities of adolescence including chlorosis (1:260). Hall's conception of "periodicity" and the consequent crisis of female adolescence was expressed in romantic metaphors: "Puberty for a girl is like floating down a broadening river into an open sea. Landmarks recede, the water deepens and changes in its nature, there are new and strange forms of life, the currents are more complex, and the phenomena of tides make new conditions and new dangers. The bark is frail, liable to be tossed by storms of feeling, at the mercy of wind and wave, and if without chart and compass and simple rules of navigation, aimless drifting in the darkness of ignorance, amidst both rocks and shoals, may make of the weak or unadvised wrecks or castaways" (1:507–8).

26 Huang, "Chlorosis and the iron controversy."
27 Warner, *Treatise*, 74.
28 Jones, *Chlorosis*, 20.
29 Ibid., 15–17.
30 Tait, *Diseases of Women*, 282–83.
31 Allbutt, "Chlorosis," 497.
32 V. Bullough and M. Voght, "Women, menstruation, and nineteenth-century medicine," in this volume; B. Ehrenreich and D. English, *Complaints and Disorders: The Sexual Politics of Sickness* (Old Westbury, N.Y.: Feminist Press, 1973); J. Haller and R. Haller, *The Physician and Sexuality in Victorian America* (Urbana: University of Illinois Press, 1974); R. Morantz, "The lady and her physician," in *Clio's Consciousness Raised: New Perspectives on the History of Women*, ed. M. S. Hartman and L. Banner (New York: Harper and Row, 1974); C. Rosenberg and C. Smith-Rosenberg, "The female animal: medical and biological views of woman and her role in nineteenth-century America," in this volume; A. D. Wood, "'The fashionable diseases': women's complaints and their treatment in nineteenth-century America," in this volume.
33 B. Sicherman, "The uses of a diagnosis: doctors, patients, and neurasthenia," *Journal of the History of Medicine and Allied Sciences*, 1977, *32*:33–54; I. Veith, *Hysteria: The History of a Disease* (Chicago: University of Chicago Press, 1965).
34 G. Beard, *American Nervousness* (New York: Putnam's, 1881).
35 Allbutt, "Chlorosis," 483–84.
36 R. Leonardo, *History of Gynecology* (New York: Froben, 1944).
37 Jones, *Chlorosis*, 67.
38 J. H. Montgomery, *Clinical Observations on Cases of Simple Anemia or Chlorosis Occurring in Young Women in the Decade Following Puberty* (Erie, Pa.: Author, 1919).
39 Ruddock, *Lady's Manual*, 32.
40 Ibid., 32.
41 Warner, *Treatise*, 70.
42 Cabot, "Chlorosis," 649.
43 Jones, *Chlorosis*, 39.
44 Meigs, *Females and Their Diseases*, 361.
45 Montgomery, *Clinical Observations;* Ruddock, *Lady's Manual*, 34.
46 Allbutt, "Chlorosis," 517.
47 Warner, *Treatise*, 54.
48 Bullough and Voght, "Women, menstruation."
49 Allbutt, "Chlorosis," 485.
50 Huang, "Chlorosis and the iron controversy."
51 Jones, *Chlorosis*, 57–60.
52 Allbutt, "Chlorosis," 515.
53 Cabot, "Chlorosis," 646–47.
54 Ibid., 646.
55 W. M. Fowler, "Chlorosis—an obituary," *Annals of Medical History*, 1936, *8*:168.
56 Hudson, "Biography of disease," 459.
57 The last decades of the nineteenth century may be an important transitional period in the history of nutrition throughout the Western world. For example, research by J. C. Toutain (*La Consommation alimentaire en France de 1789 à 1964* [Geneva: Droz, 1971]) suggests that in France animal proteins accounted for only about 25 percent of the total protein intake until after 1880–90.
58 Leonardo, *History of Gynecology*, 255–58.
59 I. Illich, *Medical Nemesis* (New York: Bantam, 1977).
60 J. Modell, "Pre–World War II courtship patterns in the United States," unpublished paper, Cornell University, March 1982.
61 L. Boyd, "Sarah Tyson Rorer," in *Notable American Women*, ed. E. T. James (Cambridge, Mass.: Harvard University Press, 1971), vol. 3.
62 A. Hertzler and H. L. Anderson, "Food guides in the United States," *Journal of the American Dietetic Association*, 1974, *64*:18–28; I. Leitch, "The evolution of dietary standards," *Nutrition Abstracts and Reviews*, 1942, *2*:509–21.

15

Prostitution, Veneral Disease, and American Medicine

MARK THOMAS CONNELLY

The American medical profession's concern about the physical and social consequences of venereal disease infused antiprostitution in the progressive years with a particular urgency. Physicians and laymen, to be sure, had pointed much earlier to the relationship between prostitution and venereal disease. Dr. William Sanger, for instance, in his 1858 investigation of prostitution in New York City, argued that uncontrolled prostitution made the city a "hotbed where . . . syphilis may be cultivated and disseminated." During the late decades of the nineteenth century, however, important advances in venereology, which were part of the great efflorescence of medical research accompanying the rise of bacteriology, gave venereal disease and, by implication, prostitution a new and more serious dimension.[1]

After 1838, the year in which Philippe Ricord demonstrated that syphilis and gonorrhea were distinctly different diseases, progress in the understanding of venereal disease came rapidly.[2] In 1854, Pierre Diday published his account of the symptoms of congenital syphilis. In the late 1860s, Jean Alfred Fournier stressed the fact of latency in syphilis and traced a variety of serious physical and mental problems to syphilitic infection. Albert Neisser isolated and identified the gonococcus, the gonorrhea bacterium, in 1879. In 1903, Elie Metchnikoff and Emile Roux transmitted the syphilis organism to monkeys, thus making possible the experimental study of the disease. Two years later, Fritz Schaudinn and Erich Hoffman discovered and isolated the syphilis bacterium,

Treponema pallidum. The next year, Karl Landsteiner perfected the dark-field microscopic technique, which allowed researchers to see *Treponema pallidum* clearly and alive.

The advances in the control and treatment of venereal disease were equally impressive. In 1884 the German obstetrician Karl Siegmund Crede discovered that a solution of silver nitrate put into the eyes of newborn babies prevented gonorrheal ophthalmia, a condition often resulting in total blindness in children born of mothers infected with gonorrhea. Working with the principles of the newly discovered complement fixation tests, August von Wassermann and his colleagues in 1906 developed a serological test for determining the presence of the syphilis bacterium in human blood. And in 1910, Paul Ehrlich and Sahachiro Hata discovered that an arsenical compound, later named Salvarsan, could be used to kill the syphilis bacterium. These developments were well known to informed American physicians and stimulated an intense appreciation of both the possibility and the necessity of controlling venereal contagion.

For the American medical community, the prophylaxis of venereal disease became inextricably tied to the issue of prostitution by virtue of the fundamental assumption that prostitution was the major, and to some the only, source of venereal contagion. During the progressive years, any analysis of the issue of venereal disease invariably stressed its relationship to prostitution.[3] The case was succinctly stated by Lavinia L. Dock, a member of the Nurses' Settlement in New York City, who maintained in her 1910 nursing manual for venereal disease that prostitution "is now as certainly the abiding place and inexhaustible source of . . . venereal disease, as the marshy swamp is the abode of the malaria-carrying mosquito, or the polluted water supply of the typhoid bacillus."[4] By the sec-

MARK THOMAS CONNELLY is a Research Associate in the Office of Legislative Services in Trenton, New Jersey.

Originally published in *The Response to Prostitution in the Progressive Era*, by Mark Thomas Connelly. Copyright 1980 The University of North Carolina Press. Reprinted by permission of the publisher.

ond decade of the century, this belief rested on two seemingly unassailable bodies of evidence. The first of these, drawn from group studies of prostitutes conducted after 1914, indicated that a large percentage of prostitutes—between 28 and 100 percent—were infected with venereal disease, which they communicated to their patrons.[5] The second body of data, contained in the records of hospitals, clinics, and private practitioners, suggested that most cases of venereal infection in men could be traced to contact with prostitutes.[6]

Whether prostitution actually was responsible for most of the contagion of venereal disease in the progressive years is not easily determined.[7] In recent times, when the venereal disease rate in some areas has been at extremely high levels, only 5 percent of all reported venereal disease cases can be traced to prostitution.[8] This figure contrasts strikingly with the statistics from the progressive years. The low contemporary figure certainly reflects, however, two important changes in sexual behavior that have occurred in the last half-century: the decrease in the number of contacts of American men with prostitutes and the concurrent increase in sexual activity not related to prostitution.[9] The continuing progress in the medical control of venereal disease is also an important consideration. During the early decades of the twentieth century, both the etiology and the treatment of venereal disease were in a state of flux. Furthermore, even after Salvarsan and fairly reliable serological tests became available in the teens, it cannot be assumed that prostitutes immediately made use of them. Since 1943, however, when penicillin was first used in the treatment of syphilis, the effectiveness of both personal and professional prophylaxis has improved to a point where a knowledgeable prostitute can achieve a control over venereal infection far superior to that of her counterpart in the early decades of the century.

It was probably the case, therefore, that prostitution played a significant role in the spread of venereal disease during the progressive era; at least it played a more important role then than it does today. But what is finally important about the belief that prostitution was the major source of venereal disease was its implication that venereal disease was a "result" of prostitution and that therefore, by a logical deduction, all the pernicious social and physical effects of venereal disease were also "re-

sults" of prostitution. Given these convictions, any attempt to ameliorate the consequences of venereal disease would have to focus on prostitution.[10] This is the point at which the medical community's concern over venereal disease most perfectly dovetailed with antiprostitution.

Though physicians agreed that prostitution was the source of venereal disease, they could not cite any authoritative statistics indicating the extent of venereal infection on a national level. To be sure, data on most diseases in the early twentieth century were incomplete or sketchy, but reliable statistics on venereal disease were virtually nonexistent.[11] There were at least three reasons for this state of affairs: the prudery and conspiracy of silence surrounding discussion of venereal disease, which enlightened elements within the medical profession were only beginning to challenge effectively in these years; the fact that the venereal diseases had not been included in the late-nineteenth-century public health regulations requiring the reporting of other infectious diseases; and the practice by both physicians and hospitals of recording cases of venereal disease under more socially acceptable medical classifications. By 1910, then, there existed a rather ironic situation: although knowledge of the medical and social aspects of venereal disease was steadily progressing, physicians, in the absence of reliable official figures, did not know exactly how extensive venereal infection was.

Physicians were unanimous in bemoaning the lack of official vital statistics on venereal disease, but the dearth of such material did not prevent many practitioners from compiling and publicizing what unofficial figures were available.[12] In 1901, a committee of seven physicians of the Medical Society of the County of New York circulated a questionnaire to 4,750 physicians in the New York City area asking each practitioner to state the number of venereal disease cases he was treating. On the basis of 678 replies, the Committee of Seven estimated there to be 200,000 syphilitics in New York City.[13] Several years later, in 1904, Prince Morrow, the chairman of the Committee of Seven, estimated that 60 percent of the adult male population in the United States contracted either gonorrhea or syphilis at some time in their lives; his figure translated into about 450,000 new infections per year.[14] The next year another physician cited evidence of 50,000 new cases of syphilis in New York City each year.[15] In 1909 still another practitioner calculated that the national rate of venereal infection in the 1860s, 85.11 per 1,000, had grown by 1908 to 194.5 per 1,000.[16] In 1910 it was reported that 80 percent of urban males, and 60 to 75 percent of "marriageable age" men, had gonorrhea.[17] And by the teens there was an extensive medical literature of estimates of venereal infection, all of which pointed to an enormous amount of venereal disease in the United States.[18]

The sources and basis for these high figures were, however, sometimes sharply questioned. For instance, in 1911 the distinguished Massachusetts physician Richard C. Cabot, in delivering the Shattuck lecture before the Massachusetts Medical Society, questioned Prince Morrow's estimate of the extent of gonorrhea in the United States. Morrow had maintained in his book *Social Diseases and Marriage* (1904) that 75 percent of American men contracted gonorrhea, so that it was in his opinion the most widespread disease in the adult male population. Cabot doubted that this was the case. "Many wild guesses about the proportion of adult males afflicted with venereal disease have . . . been published for campaign purposes," he claimed. But he argued that there was "no solid basis" for such estimates and further asserted that "gonorrheal infection ranks very far below . . . tubercular infection in the numbers of persons attacked each year." Hospital records, Cabot insisted, contained the only reliable data on venereal disease, and, on the basis of an examination of the records of 8,031 adult males admitted to the Massachusetts General Hospital over eighteen years, he found that 35 percent had contracted gonorrhea sometime in their lives. The discrepancy between this figure and Morrow's was the result, Cabot felt, of Morrow's wild guessing.[19]

Morrow quickly registered a brief in his own defense: "It may be laid down as a general proposition that the statistics of general hospitals as to the actual or relative frequency of venereal morbidity are absolutely worthless. It would be just as absurd to compute the proportion of prostitutes or drunkards in a community from the census of a church congregation." Most cases of venereal disease, Morrow argued, never reached a hospital, and the ones that did were often admitted under a "re-spectable pseudonym." A much more accurate body of data, he pointed out, was the statistics on venereal infection in military posts, because they were based on a more representative cross section of the population than were hospital statistics. But no matter how many sets of data were used, he concluded, "It is only by reading between the lines that we can arrive at any adequate conception of the extent of venereal morbidity."[20]

Who was right? There is no way of knowing for sure, but both estimates were probably higher than the actual incidence of the disease among the general population. Yet, with due regard to Cabot's criticism of inflammatory figures, Morrow better understood the social context of venereal disease in 1910 and was absolutely correct in seeing the essential uselessness of hospital records for determining the extent of venereal disease. Morrow was convinced—and rightly so—that any one set of figures on venereal disease would be inaccurate and misleading; an accurate computation of venereal infection could be achieved only by "reading between the lines" of many sets of data in an attempt to account for such irrational factors as fear, shame, ignorance, and deception. This was hardly an exact procedure, and in our own age of labyrinthine data banks and imposing computer technology, it at first appears utterly primitive. But even today, in fact, most countries in the world do not have reliable statistics on venereal disease. In the United States, the Public Health Service concedes that because only a small percentage of venereal disease cases are reported (8 to 12 percent for infectious syphilis and 7 to 11 percent for gonorrhea), it must employ extrapolation techniques, a sophisticated form of reading between the lines, to arrive at a reliable estimate of the national rate.[21]

In 1917 one physician wrote that "the actual number of cases of gonorrhea and syphilis contracted and treated in a large city is a hundred fold greater than is indicated by the official reports."[22] This was undoubtedly an overstatement, but given the low percentage of venereal disease that is reported even today, it was not as irrational as it might first appear. More importantly, it manifestly articulated the contemporary belief that venereal disease was rampant and out of control, a belief just as vital in focusing medical and public attention on the problem of prostitution and venereal disease as the concurrent explosion of new medical knowledge of the nature and consequences of venereal infection.

Even though American physicians believed that the incidence of venereal infection was very high, there was no immediate agreement on how to approach the problem. By the late teens, an influential wing of the medical profession was loosely united in an attitude toward venereal disease that was fundamentally scientific and secular, but this unity was achieved only after more than a decade of conflict of opinion.

The most formidable obstacle to a rational approach was the traditional cultural censorship imposed on any frank discussion of the subject. Medical history is replete with instances where an atmosphere of fear and shame hindered a reasoned approach to certain diseases. The problems surrounding the treatment of cholera and tuberculosis in the nineteenth century are salient examples. But because the venereal diseases were associated in both an actual and an emotional sense with illicit sexual behavior (itself a tabooed subject), any forthright discussion of syphilis and gonorrhea had to confront a conspiracy of polite silence more tenaciously maintained than was the case with other diseases. Thus, around the turn of the century, Howard Kelly, an eminent gynecologist and professor at the Johns Hopkins Medical School, asserted at a meeting of the American Medical Association that the discussion of venereal disease was "attendant with filth and we besmirch ourselves by discussing it in public."[23] And throughout the progressive years, many physicians who supported an open discussion of venereal disease also supported the belief that fear of infection acted as a deterrent to illicit intercourse and that infection, if contracted, constituted the just wages of sin.[24] The American Society of Sanitary and Moral Prophylaxis, although in some respects marking a new departure in the approach to venereal disease, also incorporated much of the older legacy of fear. "The only way to make these diseases effective guardians of virtue," Prince Morrow argued, "is to expose their true significance and real danger, to substitute a wholesome fear, for the ignorant contempt in which they are now held, the fear of infection, the fear of microbes, to appeal to enlightened self interest. After all, fear is the protective genius of the human body, and the basis upon which all hygienic precepts are inculcated."[25]

During these same early years of the century, however, there emerged an increasingly scientific and more socially responsible attitude.[26] There was, to begin with, a growing belief among physicians that the atmosphere of ignorance and misinformation surrounding the venereal diseases could be effectively countered by a program of education in sex hygiene.[27] There was also slow but encouraging growth in the number of clinics, and in particular evening clinics, for the treatment of venereal patients.[28] In 1903 the American Medical Association established a standing committee on venereal disease, and the annual meeting of that association in 1906 held two important symposia. One, on the "Duty of the Profession to Womankind," considered the dire effects of ignorance of the consequences of venereal disease on married women, marriage, and the family. The other, on the venereal diseases in general, centered on the need for the medical profession to take an active role in educating the public on the seriousness of unchecked venereal infection.[29] In 1913 there were three signs of progress: the French playwright Eugene Brieux's *Les Avaries* (translated as *Damaged Goods*), a drama dealing with the marital and social consequences of syphilis, was produced with commercial success in New York, Washington, and Chicago;[30] the morally oriented purity forces merged with the medically oriented groups to form the American Social Hygiene Association;[31] and the Rockefeller-financed Bureau of Social Hygiene formally opened. And in 1914 the first number of the *Journal of Social Hygiene*, a publication devoted to the discussion of venereal disease, prostitution, and related issues, appeared.

All of these developments clearly signaled the emergence of a recognizably modern trend in both attitude and therapy, but the contest with prudery, ignorance, and superstition was not resolved by 1915. Much of the enlightenment that took place within the medical profession never extended beyond it. Throughout the period, physicians complained that quack remedies for venereal infection, sold at drugstores or from the back of a wagon, were still popular and frequently resorted to by the general public.[32] Even the enlightenment within the profession was not complete. For instance, well into the teens, concerned physicians were declaring the state of instruction in venereology in most medical schools to be inadequate and thus productive of practitioners unqualified to diagnose and treat venereal diseases adequately.[33]

There was also the problem of inadequate facilities for the treatment of patients. In New York City in 1905, there were only 96 hospital beds available for venereal patients (this in comparison to 960 beds in Paris, a city with only two-thirds the population of New York). In New York City in 1916, only ten of the thirty general hospitals would admit cases of active syphilis, and in Pennsylvania in 1912, a survey revealed that of fourteen major hospitals none would accept venereal disease cases.[34] Throughout the progressive years there were demands that hospital authorities change these restrictive admission policies and enlarge the facilities available for treatment of venereal disease.[35] In some cases it was common practice, again well into the teens, to list admitted patients as having more socially acceptable diseases—an approach that, in addition to reflecting a moralistic attitude, hindered the compilation of accurate statistics on the incidence of venereal infection.[36]

There was, then, tension between old and new modes of thought and attitudes. On the one hand, an older legacy of fear and shame was manifest in a variety of forms. On the other hand, many physicians were beginning to separate the patient from the illness and to treat the venereal diseases without regard to the moral or social character of either the patient or the disease. Because of the unique nature of venereal disease and because it was so closely associated with the emotionally volatile issue of prostitution, this was no easy task.

Most physicians found the venereal infection statistics compelling. Even more alarming, however, were the catastrophic physical and societal consequences of the unchecked spread of syphilis and gonorrhea. By the onset of the twentieth century, medical research had conclusively demonstrated the relationships between syphilis and certain birth deformities (congenital syphilis, commonly called "syphilis of the innocent") and between gonorrhea and infant blindness.[37] At a symposium on venereal disease held in Rhode Island in 1905, for instance, specialists estimated that between 25 and 40 percent of blindness in infants was the result of gonorrheal conjunctivitis. An estimate a decade later was even higher.[38]

Perhaps most horrifying was the relationship between syphilis and general paresis (paralysis and insanity, the final form of tertiary syphilis). Early in his career, Prince Morrow had translated into English the French venereologist Jean Alfred Fournier's work on the correlation between syphilis and paresis; and by the opening decade of the twentieth century, American physicians—at least those who kept up with the medical journals—were well aware of the widespread incidence of syphilis-induced insanity.[39] Some physicians and public health officers estimated that between 8 and 20 percent of insanity cases under treatment could be linked to a syphilitic infection in the patient's past.[40] These were staggering figures, both for the toll in human suffering they represented and for the cost to the public of institutional care, and they were among the most important facts marshalled by physicians concerned with the consequences of venereal disease for American life.[41]

It is important to understand, however, that physicians and laymen perceived the venereal diseases as clearly distinct from other infectious diseases of similar medical seriousness. The venereal diseases were more than an ordinary health problem: they had, and still have today, although to a diminished degree, an emotional dimension that other diseases did not. The spread of syphilis and gonorrhea posed serious threats not only to the public health but also to the integrity of certain conceptualizations of great cultural and psychological value: the "race," marriage, the family, motherhood, womanhood, and manhood. These concepts were key components of civilized morality. The reproductive act, in its proper setting, marriage, was central to the fate of these ideals and values. The venereal diseases, because they were transmitted in this most sacred of acts and because they were so closely associated with prostitution and illicit sexuality, blighted and corrupted the meaning of those ideals and the moral system they represented. The idea of marriage, and particularly of the middle-class married woman, stood at the focal point of these ideals, and it was the fate of the married woman that became a master symbol of the disastrous consequences of venereal disease, its transmitters—profligate men—and its source—prostitution.

Physicians argued, albeit with little hard evidence, that venereal disease was responsible for most of the sterility in marriages that many middle-class Americans were finding so alarming. When President Roosevelt introduced the phrase "race suicide" into the public parlance (in reference to the fact that the birthrate of patrician Anglo-Saxon Americans was declining), it was widely assumed that he was referring to the result of voluntary birth control.[42] Physicians disagreed and argued instead that barren marriages, and what Prince Morrow called "one child sterility," were rather the result of the physiological effects of gonorrheal infection in either the husband or, more often, the wife.[43] One physician, writing in 1910, argued that prior to 1850, just 2 percent of "our native born white women" were sterile, whereas by 1900 the ratio had increased to one in five. Venereal disease, he asserted, was behind this disconcerting increase. Other physicians presented figures purporting to show that from 20 to 75 percent of childless marriages were the result of venereal-disease-induced sterility.[44] It requires only a sympathetic sensibility to appreciate the emotional impact of such figures on an age and culture in which parenthood and especially motherhood were envisioned as almost sacred roles.

Physicians also pointed to an alarming connection between venereal disease and divorce, namely, the instances in which marriages collapsed after the wife was infected with venereal disease by her husband, who had contracted it from a prostitute. Prince Morrow bemoaned these calamities in his *Social Diseases and Marriage* and, as president of the American Society of Sanitary and Moral Prophylaxis, continued to warn against the "morbid irradiations [of venereal disease] when introduced into married life." "Notwithstanding the conspiracy of concealment between the husband and physician," he asserted, "women often learn the name and nature of their trouble, which not infrequently leads to the breaking-up of the family. The number of applications for divorce from this cause, especially in the middle and upper classes of society is much larger than is commonly supposed. In divorce proceedings, the cause of action usually appears under some non-compromising name, such as 'cruelty,' 'non-support,' 'desertion,' while the true cause is never made public."[45] The same argument, put forth in 1910 by a prominent physician in the widely circulated *Pearson's Magazine*, simply read: "Divorce increasing? Of course; cannot you all see why? Divorce increases in direct ratio to the increase in venereal diseases. We cannot stop the effect until we stop the cause."[46] Here prostitution, venereal disease, and divorce seemed locked in a vicious triangle. The belief that prostitution was the main source of venereal disease, along with the belief that a substantial percentage of the men frequenting prostitutes were married (a fact that most investigations of prostitution regretfully verified), made the connection among prostitution, venereal disease, and divorce a logical, if not irrefutable, proposition.

Another serious result of venereal contagion, related to the issues of sterility and divorce, involved women, invariably depicted as innocent wives, constrained to undergo serious gynecological surgery after being infected with gonorrhea by their husbands. At a meeting of the American Gynecological Society in 1879, the eminent German physician Emil Noeggerath proposed to his American audience that most serious diseases of the female reproductive organs were related to gonorrheal infection. At the time, American physicians were not willing to accept the implications of such a theory.[47] By the opening decades of the twentieth century, however, many of them conceded Noeggerath's case.

Prince Morrow, not known for the flippancy of his remarks, asserted in 1904 that "there is more venereal disease among virtuous wives than among professional prostitutes in this country," a proposition that, although questionable in a purely statistical sense, nonetheless pointed to a most distressing problem.[48] Indeed, numerous physicians argued that gonorrheal infection by husbands stood in the shadows in between 10 and 75 percent of cases of women requiring major gynecological surgery (including hysterectomies or removal of the fallopian tubes because of acute salpingitis).[49] Katharine Houghton Hepburn (mother of the actress), a Hartford, Connecticut, suffragist active in the anti-prostitution activities in that city, wrote in 1910 that "Seventy-five per cent of all operations peculiar to women are necessary because the husband has infected the wife with one of the diseases which are spread through all ranks of society by means of the social evil."[50] This matter had an emotional as well as a medical impact, for what was at stake was the very sanctity of marriage. "What more distressing picture can be portrayed," asked one physician, "than that of a young wife of but a few weeks, one who, in her youthful innocence of venery and its subsequent possibilities, is looking forward to a future containing all the blessings of married life, being forced to consult her physician, who finds in her a new victim of the insatiable appetite of the venereal spectre."[51]

This was a most serious situation in itself, and was treated as such, but it was also an indication of another less readily verifiable but equally serious problem: the existence of a secret collusion between physicians and male patients, either husbands or prospective husbands, which resulted in unsuspecting women being infected with venereal disease.[52] The "medical secret," as this was called, operated in either of two ways: a physician might treat a male patient for venereal disease without insisting that the patient inform his wife or fiancée; or, if the wife should subsequently be infected and seek medical aid, the physician might attempt to treat her without her learning of the nature or the source of her disease. It is next to impossible to calculate how pervasive was the practice of the "medical secret" within the profession, short of examining the records or the diaries of thousands of general practitioners and specialists. One point, however, merits notice here. The "medical secret," when it was operative, was deeply entangled in the psychology of male power and loyalty, and recent studies have shown that a similar situation prevailed in other areas of medical diagnosis, therapy, and ethics.[53] But whatever the actual extent of this complicity between physician and patient, the medical profession's concern for venereal-disease-related surgery for women speaks for itself and for the mental and physical suffering inflicted on untold numbers of women.

The situation was not, however, one of unrelieved gloom, and many physicians pointed to several ways of avoiding these marital disasters. Almost all physicians concerned with the consequences of prostitution and venereal disease felt that some kind of a national or local program of sex hygiene education—especially for adolescents—was an immediate desideratum. The main emphasis of these programs was not, however, on prophylactic techniques—the use of condoms, for example—but rather on the practice of sexual continence for males, or what was often referred to as the single

standard of morals. Much of this educational propaganda was aimed at the doctrine of "male sexual necessity," the traditional belief that sexual intercourse was necessary for male physical and psychological health.[54] Social hygienists argued that this belief had no medical basis, that it was one of the root causes of prostitution, that it was the foundation of the double standard of morals, and that it resulted in the spread of venereal disease. Some physicians in the early decades of the century, however, continued to support the doctrine of male necessity or at least to express misgivings about the gospel of continence. One physician, for instance, remarked: "Now, if men could be continent or chaste without women they would not need to marry. It may be inquired if any officer of this model society [the Philadelphia Society for the Study and Prevention of Social Diseases] has not found it more comfortable to cohabit with a wife than to live in absolute chastity as a celibate."[55] To counterbalance this kind of thinking, other social hygienists and physicians loudly proclaimed that sexual continence was absolutely compatible with perfect health.[56]

The repressive nature of the gospel of continence is obvious. So too is the emphasis on male sexuality to the almost total exclusion of female sexuality. And the phrase "sex-hygiene education" is somewhat misleading, because what was advocated was not an open knowledge of sexuality and sexual behavior but rather an enlightened indoctrination in proper and safe sex roles. But, given the belief that prostitution, via the uncontrolled male sex drive, was the main course of venereal infection, the idea of male continence, notwithstanding the psychological problems that can be seen in it today, seemed a logical solution to a serious problem.

Other physicians, particularly those allied with the public health movement, pointed to two other ways to avoid or check the ravages of prostitution and venereal disease: the mandatory reporting of cases of venereal disease, and legislation making an examination for venereal disease a prerequisite for marriage. Although in the nineteenth century numerous states enacted legislation mandating the reporting of cases of various communicable and infectious diseases, venereal disease had not come under the purview of such legislation.[57] Throughout the first decade of the twentieth century, however, more and more physicians argued that compulsory reporting was as necessary for venereal disease as for any other disease. Some physicians were quick to voice their opposition, usually on the grounds that reporting venereal disease would violate the confidentiality of the doctor-patient relationship (which was especially important given the social taboo on venereal disease), that reporting was unworkable because many doctors would refuse, and that many individuals would not seek a physician's aid and might have recourse instead to a quack if they knew that their malady would be reported to public health authorities.[58]

The forces that supported the reporting of venereal disease were, however, clearly dominant.[59] There was, to be sure, disagreement about exactly how such a system should work—for instance, whether cases should be reported by full name or, instead, by a numbered code. But reporting by one method or another was, by the teens, clearly the trend of the future. By 1922 all forty-eight states had enacted some kind of legislation requiring the reporting of venereal disease.[60]

The proposal that freedom from venereal disease be a state-enforced prerequisite for marriage was also widely supported by physicians and public health authorities as a way to safeguard marriage and the family from some of the consequences of prostitution and venereal disease. As with the issue of reporting venereal disease cases, there was some opposition. Prince Morrow, curiously enough, felt that such a measure would not work. "So far as the woman is concerned such examination is entirely unnecessary," he asserted, "as women almost never introduce these infections into marriage; besides, many sensitive, refined women would rather forego marriage than be subjected to a physical examination which they would regard as an outrage upon their modesty, and an indignity to their persons."[61] Other physicians articulated reservations similar to Morrow's, but by the teens, when fairly accurate serological tests for syphilis were available, the medical profession in general was favorable to what one physician termed the "guarantee of safety in the marriage contract."[62]

In 1910, Evangeline Young, a Boston physician, put the matter in clear and certain terms: "The young woman should know the actual conditions in society. . . . It is a crime to marry a clean woman to a diseased man, for her to find out when it is too late that she is sharing the disease of the women of the street; that almost to a certainty she will become sterile, or an invalid, or suffer death itself, an innocent victim to the double standard of morals. At the very least, she should have a choice in the matter." Laws requiring a premarriage examination, in addition to "educating young women to realize the dangers of marrying young men who cannot meet these requirements," would also serve "as a warning to the young men, who will realize as in no other way that venereal disease will disqualify him for honorable marriage."[63] Support for mandatory examinations grew steadily in the following years. Washington passed such legislation in 1909 and Wisconsin in 1913, and by 1921 twenty states had enacted statutes of various kinds declaring freedom from venereal disease a prerequisite for marriage.[64] Sometimes the efforts of physicians and public health authorities to promote these laws received the support of local eugenics groups, which saw such provisions as "eugenical marriage laws." But actually the two movements were quite distinct in orientation and objective; as an authority on the eugenics movement has succinctly observed, "eugenics was concerned with genes, not germs."[65]

One characteristic of many of the early laws requiring premarriage examinations merits special notice: the stipulation that only the prospective husband, not the wife, demonstrate freedom from infection.[66] Though there may have been a medical rationale for this rather peculiar exemption, what seems to have been equally at work was a recrudescence of the Victorian penchant for envisioning women as suffering victims. This was a dominant theme in antiprostitution in general; it was especially visible when the focus was on venereal disease, because it was always an innocent bride or wife who suffered from a male's contaminating association with a prostitute. There was hardly a single reference in the medical literature on prostitution and venereal disease to an innocent husband's being infected by his wife.

This point is interesting for the illumination it sheds on the medical profession's perception of women, but it is also important to note that the depiction of brides and wives as innocent victims of venereal infection ran counter to the logic of a key component of antiprostitution: the belief in widespread clandestine prostitution. Because "clandestine prostitution" referred to such a broad range of female sexual activity, there were poten- tially thousands of women in America in 1915 who were involved in clandestine sexual behavior and were, therefore, possibly infected with venereal disease if and when they married. Thus, according to a basic assumption of antiprostitution and to the reasoning used to support premarriage exams, women should have been covered in the legislation requiring such exams. This situation stands in cu- rious tension with the willingness of medical and nonmedical groups and individuals to support leg- islation requiring prenuptial examinations only for males. Much of the explanation for this inconsist- ency lies in the powerful cultural commitment to the idea that, as Morrow put it, "men are the re- sponsible authors of these social crimes—women the victims," and to the vision of married and mar- riageable women as pure and ethereal mothers, wives, and helpmates who could never transmit the most morally reprehensible diseases into the fun- damental relationship of family life.[67]

The advocacy of premarriage examinations is thus a complex matter for interpretation. For, on the one hand, the belief in the efficacy of such exams was forward looking and educational; as Evangeline Young pointed out, it encouraged young women to "know the actual conditions in society," to be conscious of and exercise some control over an important aspect of their lives. On the other hand, the argument behind the early premarriage exams, in emphasizing only the role of the male in spreading venereal disease, depicted women in the orthodox nineteenth-century manner: as passive victims. This is not to say that women did not suf- fer under the moral, sexual, and medical conven- tions of the society in which they lived. They did. And it would be similarly inaccurate to argue that women (excepting prostitutes) were as central to the spread of venereal disease in the early years of the twentieth century as were men, although there is much more work to be done on this subject. But to insist that women could not spread venereal dis- ease simply because they were women embodied an attitude that, even by 1915, was becoming in- creasingly absurd.

The mandatory reporting of venereal disease and the premarriage exam, topics of sharp disagree- ment in the progressive era, are now established practices. Another heatedly debated issue pertain- ing to the control of venereal disease, however, is only vaguely remembered today. This was the question whether the spread of venereal disease could be most effectively and efficiently controlled by the medical inspection and regulation of segre- gated prostitution districts. Such regulation was the subject of great controversy in both England and America in the nineteenth century, and it is some- times assumed that the conflict of opinion substan- tially died out by the end of the century. In part it did. In England the Contagious Diseases Acts (which instituted medical inspection of prostitutes in cer- tain cities) were eventually repealed, and in the United States, after the demise of the 1870 St. Louis experiment in medical inspection, there were only sporadic attempts to repeat it.[68] But on an intellec- tual and emotional level, the medical regulation of prostitution remained well into the twentieth cen- tury an issue which those concerned about pros- titution and venereal disease felt constrained to address. Indeed, one of the achievements of anti- prostitution in the progressive era was the final resolution of this question.

The controversy stemmed from the medical profession's belief that prostitution was the main source of venereal disease. Given this assumption, there was a certain logic to medical inspection: if prostitution was the principal agent in the spread of venereal disease, one could propose that con- trolling that agent was a practical objective. Many voices, however, were raised in opposition to this way of thinking, and the cacophonous debate con- tinued throughout the progressive years. It was an exceedingly complicated controversy, and many participants, both physicians and laymen, ap- proached it from points of view that can only be described as perversely idiosyncratic. Then, too, there were some physicians who framed their ar- guments in such careful wording that it is impos- sible to place them on one side or the other. Never- theless, two distinctly opposing positions can be discerned.

Those who supported the medical control of prostitution were usually called regulationists. The regulationists, most of whom were male physi- cians, argued that the only way to curb the ravages of venereal disease was to confine the practice of prostitution to a certain section of a city (this was already the existing situation in most cities) and to subject it to rigorous medical supervision.[69] The regulationists insisted that the medical profession take a strictly pragmatic attitude toward the problem of prostitution and venereal disease. "As far as the prevention of disease is concerned," one physician wrote, "the physician should be the chaperon of the house of ill fame."[70] Supporters of regulation, conceding that no system could completely control the spread of venereal disease, nonetheless maintained that in American cities where regulation was in de facto operation—in Cincinnati, for example—the spread of venereal disease had been curtailed.[71]

The regulationists allowed that earlier European experiments in medical inspection had not proven very effective but argued that the fault lay not in the concept of regulation itself but in the primitive medical knowledge that prevailed in the nineteenth century. The ever-increasing progress in the diagnosis and treatment of venereal diseases, the regulationists argued, would constantly improve the effectiveness of a system of medical inspection. This view found impressive endorsement in 1916 by Albert Neisser, the German researcher who had first identified the gonococcus in 1879.[72] Many regulationists also pointed to programs in European cities and in the U.S. military as examples of how medical inspection worked to control venereal disease.[73] The regulationists also held that the medical inspection of prostitutes would help to prevent prostitution from spreading throughout the urban community, and, as prostitution would no longer be illegal, the widespread network of corruption involving police and public officials would disappear. In fact, under most proposed systems of medical inspection, implementation would be carried out by professional and disinterested public health officials, rather than the police.[74]

Opposition to the regulation of prostitution came from a broad and disparate collection of groups, interests, and individuals.[75] The Women's Christian Temperance Union and the purity groups held to the antiregulation position they had espoused since the latter decades of the nineteenth century. The social hygiene forces—most notably the American Society of Sanitary and Moral Prophylaxis and later the American Social Hygiene Association—also opposed a system of regulation.[76] So did numerous physicians, both male and female.[77] The vice commission reports and the white slave narratives declared against regulation in the strongest language, even though these documents were quite different in other respects.[78] Feminists were appalled at the idea of regulation, and local women's clubs and groups also took a rigorous stand against it. Jane Addams, the muckraking journalist George Kibbe Turner, and social worker Maude E. Miner lent their voices to the opposition.[79] Theodore Roosevelt, who had had some experience in dealing with prostitution as police commissioner of New York City, wrote, in characteristic style, that "there should be no toleration of any 'tenderloin' or 'red light' district, and that above all there should be the most relentless war on commercialized vice." In 1912 the *American City*, in an editorial entitled "Shall Chicago Legalize Hell?" answered a resounding "no" to regulation. The following year, in a consideration of the issue of regulation, the *Independent* declared that "Mormon Polygamy is better."[80]

The antiregulationists agreed with the regulationists that prostitution was the source of venereal disease.[81] They argued, however, that the remedy was, not the regulation of prostitution, but rather its repression. The antiregulationists argued that although a system of regulation might control prostitution, it would also centralize and advertise it. In addition, a segregated district would invariably become a magnet for all kinds of criminal elements and could only foster a disrespect for law and order. Even more importantly, the medical inspection of prostitutes would not accomplish its object: the control of venereal disease. Systems of medical inspection had not reduced the incidence of venereal disease in the past and would not do so in the future, not because of any medical technique that was or was not used, but because of a basic flaw in the philosophy of regulation itself, namely, that only the prostitute would be treated, and the "masculine spreader of disease" (in Prince Morrow's words) would be ignored.[82] What would be the good, antiregulationists asked, of a medical document certifying a prostitute's freedom from venereal disease, renewed weekly, when she might be infected by a patron immediately after her examination? Indeed, the false sense of security that such an official certificate would promote would actually lead to an increase in the incidence of venereal disease.[83]

The antiregulationists also insisted that the military example used by the regulationists was inappropriate, because a fluid and mobile group of prostitutes could not be controlled like a military post.[84] In addition, the antiregulationists, especially the feminists and women among their number, warned that any system of regulation and inspection could potentially abuse the rights and personal freedom of many women, prostitute and nonprostitute alike. Lastly, antiregulationist physicians contended that any complicity with a system of medical inspection could only discredit and disgrace the medical profession. Howard Kelly of Johns Hopkins, in a talk given at a 1904 meeting of the American Medical Association, addressed exactly this point. "Consider for a moment, gentlemen," he warned, "what effect the legalization of vice will have on the medical profession. The necessity for examining women licensed to carry on their business will create in our midst a vile and odious specialty, akin and closely allied to the professional abortionist, degrading to our profession and justly bringing it into contempt by making it thus pander to vice. . . . What a lowering of our standards when we come to that!"[85]

Until 1914, the antiregulation position was for the most part diffuse and unintegrated, lacking a central, all-encompassing statement of purpose and philosophy. In that year, however, this problem was remedied by the publication of Abraham Flexner's *Prostitution in Europe.* Indeed, Flexner's book gave the antiregulationist position an authority never to be seriously challenged.

Flexner's career and achievements constitute one of the more impressive twentieth-century American biographies. The son of German-Jewish immigrants, Flexner grew up in Louisville, Kentucky, and graduated from Johns Hopkins University in 1886. He gained national prominence in 1910 with the publication of his *Medical Education in the United States,* the result of an investigation of medical schools conducted under the auspices of the Carnegie Foundation for the Advancement of Teaching. Flexner's detailed description of the appalling state of medical instruction was so compelling, and so damning, that it forced many American "medical schools" out of existence. In 1912, just as he was completing a study of medical education in Europe, Flexner was asked by John D. Rockefeller, Jr., who just recently had financed the founding of the Bureau of Social Hygiene, to conduct an inves-

tigation of prostitution in Europe. The bureau had recently commissioned its first study of prostitution, George Jackson Kneeland's *Commercialized Prostitution in New York City,* and, as Flexner later in life recalled, "there were those who believed that America had much to learn from European experience." Flexner accepted the assignment and spent the next two years surveying the sexual underworld of twenty-eight cities in the British Isles, the Continent, and Scandinavia.[86]

Flexner approached his task with characteristic thoroughness. He toured the brothels, bordellos, and shady haunts of the European cities (Theodore Dreiser accompanied him in Paris); conversed with prostitutes, police, and public officials; and watched hundreds of women being examined for venereal disease in those cities where regulation existed. Flexner recounted all of these experiences, including a brief but frank discussion of homosexual prostitution, in sober and clear prose. In addition to his own investigations, he used and indeed seems to have mastered the forbidding body of German, French, and British scholarship on prostitution, including the bewildering and constantly proliferating statistical material on the subject. But *Prostitution in Europe* was much more than a collection of copious citations. It was the high-water mark in the flood tide of progressive fact-finding investigations, even though it was, at least nominally, about Europe.

Its title was, however, somewhat imprecise. For what Flexner set out to investigate, and what he wrote of, was not prostitution in Europe but the various European policies concerning prostitution. It is this overarching emphasis which makes *Prostitution in Europe* a central document in the American controversy over medical inspection. Before leaving for Europe, Flexner remembered some years later, he talked with physicians and social workers who indicated that "on the Continent at least, prostitution was so regulated that the dangers to health were minimized." His experience in Europe did not bear out this claim. In fact, he found that on matters of European regulation, Americans were "completely ignorant."[87]

The major thrust of Flexner's argument was that European systems of medical examination of prostitutes were worthless. He argued that those who held up European systems as models for the United States were in error and that, indeed, the regulation of prostitution did not help maintain public order or control the spread of venereal disease. He was particularly adamant on the latter point. In many of the cities he visited, the prostitutes who were enrolled on the official rosters were compelled to appear at municipal centers, sometimes the police headquarters, where they were examined for venereal infection. This had been the prevailing situation in numerous Continental cities for several decades, and regulationists argued that it effectively controlled venereal contagion. Flexner asserted that this claim was nonsensical. His arguments, all of which were accompanied with appropriate statistical evidence, were many. The regulated prostitutes comprised only a small fraction—perhaps just one-quarter—of the total number of professional and clandestine prostitutes in any city. The actual medical inspection was usually hurried and careless and seldom included microscopic examinations of smears. Accordingly, syphilis in its most infectious forms was usually detected, but chronic gonorrhea was not. Also, experienced prostitutes were able to disguise certain kinds of symptoms of infection and thus escape detection. "The clinical method," Flexner argued, "is utterly incompetent to detect any considerable portion of infectious disease." In fact, he produced figures showing that regulation, by making prostitution seem "safe," actually led to an increase in venereal disease.[88]

Flexner presented evidence showing that cities in which prostitution was not regulated had a lower rate of venereal infection than did regulated cities. European authorities, he reported, were finally understanding this variation, for the number of regulated cities was steadily declining. Flexner admitted that prostitution was "by far the main factor in the spread of venereal disease," but he argued that the proper remedy was the rational and intelligent repression of prostitution and the provision of clinical treatment for all venereal sufferers, not just prostitutes.[89]

Flexner's study offered the most thorough understanding of European dealings with prostitution available to Americans in the progressive years. But *Prostitution in Europe*, despite its title, was also a book about the United States. For just as Tocqueville analyzed democracy in America with one eye looking back to Europe, Flexner studied prostitution in Europe with one eye focused on his

native land. He produced not only a scholarly and informative study but also a treatise on comparative morality. The driving force of *Prostitution in Europe* was a commitment to the belief that America must remain above the moral and political corruption that European systems of regulation both symbolized and embodied. Flexner devoted an entire chapter, "The Real Inwardness of Regulation," to showing that the regulation of prostitution in Europe was a product of social and political conservatism, class distinctions, militarist values, and the vested interests of corrupt police systems.[90] The message to antiprostitution forces in the United States was clear: there was nothing in Europe for a young and virtuous democratic nation to emulate.

What emerges in *Prostitution in Europe* is a familiar picture: a democratic and optimistic American exploring the dark and twisted streets of thousand-year-old European cities—ancient or medieval cities burdened with a history of corruption, superstition, and moral compromise and chained to the atavistic social arrangements and attitudes of a dark and repressive past. Considering the purpose of his journey, Flexner cannot be said to have been an innocent abroad, but, nonetheless, the clash between American innocence and European corruption is the sotto voce theme of his book. European regulation of prostitution was to Flexner what European imperialism was to Woodrow Wilson: an irrational expression of decadent European culture, with which American civilization must have no alliance.[91]

Flexner's work touched a nerve in the United States: it was reviewed and synopsized widely and at length and was seen as a document just as relevant and important to American concern with prostitution as were the vice commission reports, which dealt with the subject on native grounds. Indeed, *Prostitution in Europe* was the last major prewar expression of antiprostitution and seemed to be the definitive resolution to the controversy over regulation.[92]

Because regulationists and antiregulationists often used the same studies and statistics to support their opposite conclusions, the controversy over regulation might at first appear to be only a matter of different interpretations of the same facts. This was not, however, the case, for the two positions were based on fundamentally different social and moral assumptions. The regulationists clearly did not "approve" of prostitution, but they saw prostitution and venereal disease as serious problems that, although insoluble in any total sense, could be rationally and scientifically *managed.* They were aware that the solution they advocated was at profound variance with some of the dominant beliefs of their age, but they felt that the seriousness of the problem made such an accommodation imperative.

There is a quiet irony here. In effect, the regulationists were proposing to deal with prostitution and venereal disease in a fashion well within the parameters of the liberal gradualism that so permeated the progressive political outlook in general. The key goal of the regulationists' program of medical inspection was the imposition of order, stability, control, and predictability on a potential source of irrationality and conflict. Many of the antiregulationists supported this approach when applied to other social problems. For instance, progressive reformers did not often propose that the solution to the problem of poverty was the annihilation of the economic order itself. Quite the contrary, it was the dominant progressive approach that social and economic problems could be gradually controlled and rationalized. Yet many who endorsed this basically meliorist approach concerning a broad range of social issues—Theodore Roosevelt, for instance—did not apply it to the problem of prostitution but instead called for a total solution: absolute repression and annihilation.

Why such a position? An immediate explanation for the antiregulationists' position lies in the fact that the issues of prostitution and venereal disease, because of their association with illicit sexuality, were so anxiety producing that a "conventional" or "rational" response was simply impossible. But there were deeper and more specific reasons. The antiregulationists saw quite clearly that the idea of the medical inspection of prostitutes, of setting apart a group of women for the sole purpose of sexual service, outrageously violated the vision of the ideal woman as reserved, reticent, and rather asexual. The very thought of lines of outcast women waiting their turn to be probed, inspected, and graded as so many heads of cattle, like the thought of a sanitary, antiseptic, efficiently run, and openly, administered medical bureaucracy that would certify women as medically safe for sexual use, was a spec-

ter to which the antiregulationists could respond only with shock and moral indignation.

But even more fundamentally, the antiregulationists deplored the medical inspection of prostitutes because it would publicly contravene the basic canons of civilized morality, especially those decreeing that sex was meant to serve only the purposes of reproduction, that all sexual activity must take place within the context of marriage, and that male continence prior to marriage was the truest sign of manhood.[93] Abraham Flexner commented, "Regulation implies the absence of any expectation of male self-restraint; it is society's tacit assent to laxity." The feminist Anna Garlin Spencer went even further. "Do we accept monogamic marriage as the only right and wise arrangement for the union of the sexes?" she asked. If so, "then we can no longer tolerate the brothel, with all its vulgar concerns turned over to the police force, while the rest of us shut our eyes." Regulation, she went on, would be "a tacit admission that we do not mean what we say by the marriage laws."[94]

The antiregulationists clearly understood that at the heart of the regulationists' position was the assumption that prostitution was "necessary"—that it was a phenomenon which, no matter how onerous, seemed to be deeply rooted in biological reality and the very structure of social and moral relationships. The medical examination of prostitutes would be a public and symbolic declaration that this assumption was correct. Therefore, those who were fully committed to the ideals of civilized morality had to oppose regulation, for to do otherwise would be tantamount to an admission that civilized morality was not working.

By 1914, however, antiregulation was more than an affirmation of a moral system; it was an affirmation of a moral system in the process of collapse. There was an additional irony here. By 1914 the segregated prostitution districts, which would have been a key component of most systems of medical inspection, were also in a state of decline. This decline was attributable in part to the increase of sexual activity unrelated to prostitution, which was one of the results of the demise of civilized morality. Thus, the crisis in civilized morality, while on the one hand providing much of the fuel for antiregulation, was on the other hand rendering it, willy-nilly, a superfluous position.

This analysis, it should be emphasized, is intended only to put the antiregulationist position in its complete cultural context; it does not invalidate the humanitarian concerns of the antiregulationists. To the contrary: many of the concerns of the opponents of regulation—most importantly their recognition that, as dehumanizing as prostitution was, an official complicity in that dehumanization could only be worse—still have relevance and meaning today.

In the postpenicillin era, much of the progressive concern about venereal disease might at first seem exotic and strangely removed from contemporary experience. Surely we would wince today to hear a physician say, as one did in 1910: "The cough spray of a syphilitic may be more dangerous than the discharge of a gun into a person's face." Today most cases of both syphilis and gonorrhea can be completely cured with a single massive dose of penicillin, and this simple fact has profoundly influenced the general view of venereal disease.[95]

In 1900 the death rate for syphilis was 13 per 100,000; in 1970 it stood at .03 per 100,000.[96] Sir Alexander Fleming's discovery of penicillin was mainly responsible for this extraordinary change, but it has created a problem of historical interpretation. Venereal disease is still a matter of concern, but because of the existence of penicillin and other antibiotics, the problem is no longer primarily one of curing the disease but rather one of reaching the infected person. Physicians in the prepenicillin era, and particularly in the early decades of the twentieth century, were working under very different circumstances. The fact of this historical divide must be kept in mind in evaluating their performance. The penicillin era is about the length of the atomic age; in contrast, physicians in the progressive years were working at the end of a period that stretched back at least as far as the Renaissance.

The differences between the two eras appear quite clearly. There was not, for all practical purposes, any completely effective cure for syphilis and gonorrhea in the early twentieth century. Salvarsan and the arsphenamines raised hope in this direction (regarding syphilis), but treatment with Salvarsan was an expensive and lengthy procedure. Most could not afford it, and those who could often did not go through with the whole program. During World War I, rigidly enforced programs of prophylaxis were surprisingly effective, but it was

widely recognized that such a policy could not work with a civilian population.

This lack of an effective cure had many effects. It can account in part for two of the policies advocated to halt the spread of venereal disease: sexual continence and the repression of prostitution. Notwithstanding the fact that they were related to issues other than venereal disease, they had a certain logic as a prophylactic against venereal disease in the prepenicillin age. The absence of a completely effective cure also made prostitution much more than morally obnoxious: it was, in fact, a locus of a disease for which there was no sure cure. This factor, in turn, points to another difference between the progressive concern over prostitution and venereal disease and our own. Now, although prostitution is still seen by many as morally reprehensible, it is seldom seen as a serious health problem—largely because of the existence of penicillin.[97]

As striking as these differences are, they ought not to obscure the similarities and common problems regarding venereal disease that span the first three-quarters of this century. Although penicillin is a very effective cure for venereal disease, many of the problems surrounding the control of venereal disease that plagued progressive era physicians persist today. Some physicians in the progressive years understood an important component of this problem: the unique nature of venereal disease. Whereas other infectious and communicable diseases were related to such agents as mosquitoes and impure water sources, or such habits as spitting, venereal disease was connected with something of far greater complexity: human sexual behavior. The streets might be swept, the common drinking cup abolished, spitting educated out of existence, and the pools of stagnant water irrigated away, but the sex instinct, as many psychologists were coming to understand, was not susceptible to such rational approaches. Physicians like Prince Morrow argued that the irrational aspects of sexual behavior might be counterbalanced by education and sexual continence. In this attitude he exhibited the general nineteenth-century belief in reason and education, but in his understanding that individuals might irrationally *choose* to expose themselves to venereal disease, he pointed to a basic conundrum of venereal disease control.[98] And, just as individuals might choose to take a chance on contracting venereal disease, they might also, if infected, choose to stay away from a physician because of the shame associated with illicit sex and venereal disease. For the same reasons, a physician might not report a case of venereal disease under his care. These factors were important in the progressive years, and they still are today.

These considerations should help to put the progressive effort to deal with prostitution and venereal disease in a contemporary and sympathetic perspective. Progressive physicians certainly threw a beam of light on what had been a dark corner of medicine and social policy, and they made an important start in framing a rational approach to venereal disease control. But their attempt was only partially successful, both because of the limitations of their own cultural commitments and, even more importantly, because of the social and cultural dynamics of venereal disease. Unfortunately, the latter still plague us today.

NOTES

1 William W. Sanger, *The History of Prostitution: Its Extent, Causes, and Effects throughout the World* (1858; rpt. New York: Eugenics, 1937), 633.

2 For a general overview of the history of medical research on venereal disease, see Owsei Temkin, "Therapeutic trends and the treatment of syphilis before 1900," *Bulletin of the History of Medicine*, 1955, *29:* 309–16; Kenneth M. Flegel, "Changing concepts of the nosography of gonorrhea and syphilis," *Bulletin of the History of Medicine*, 1974, *48:* 571–88; Theodor Rosebury, *Microbes and Morals: The Strange Story of Venereal Disease* (New York: Viking, 1971); R. S. Morton, *Venereal Diseases* (Baltimore: Penguin, 1974), 21–34; William Allen Pusey, *The History and Epidemiology of Syphilis* (Springfield, Ill.: Charles C. Thomas, 1931); H. Goodman, *Notable Contributors to the Knowledge of Syphilis* (New York: Froben, 1943), Stewart M. Brooks, *The V.D. Story* (New York: A. S. Barnes, 1971), and Harry F. Dowling, *Fighting Infection: Conquests of the Twentieth Century* (Cambridge, Mass.: Harvard University Press, 1977), 82–104. The factual material in this and following paragraphs is drawn from these works.

3 Today, in direct contrast, one can pick up any recent textbook on venereal disease and find at most only a passing reference to prostitution. For instance, in his *Textbook of Venereal Diseases and Treponematoses* (2d ed. [Springfield, Ill.: Charles C. Thomas, 1964]), R. R. Wilcox devotes several pages (423–25) to the relationship between prostitution and venereal disease and concludes that prostitution is not an important factor in the spread of venereal disease. The U.S. Public Health Service, in its 1968 *Syphilis: A Synopsis*, does not mention prostitution at all.

4 Lavinia L. Dock, *Hygiene and Morality* (New York: G. P. Putnam, 1910), 35. See also Prince Morrow, "A plea for the organization of a 'Society of Sanitary and Moral Prophylaxis,'" *Medical News*, 1904, *84:* 1073; Prince Morrow, "The Society of Sanitary and Moral Prophylaxis," *American Medicine*, 1905, *9:* 320; Abraham L. Wolbarst, "The problem of venereal prophylaxis," *Boston Medical and Surgical Journal*, 1906, *155:* 280; V. G. Vecki, "Can we abolish, shall we ignore, or must we regulate prostitution?" *American Journal of Dermatology and Genito-Urinary Diseases*, 1910, *14:* 215; J. Rosenstirn, "Should the sanitary control of prostitution be abandoned?" *Medical Record*, 1914, *85:* 1070; A. J. McLaughlin, "Pioneering in venereal disease control," *American Journal of Obstetrics and Diseases of Women and Children*, 1919, *80:* 639; George Jackson Kneeland, *Commercialized Prostitution in New York City* (1913; rpt. Montclair, N.J.: Patterson Smith, 1969), 134–35; Minneapolis, *Report of the Vice Commission of Minneapolis* (1911), 45–46; Anna Garlin Spencer, "Social nemesis and social salvation," *Forum*, 1913, *50:* 433; and Massachusetts, *Report of the Commission for the Investigation of the White Slave Traffic, So Called* (1914), 45.

5 See Jau Don Ball and Hayward G. Thomas, "A sociological, neurological, serological and psychiatrical study of a group of prostitutes," *American Journal of Insanity*, 1918, *74:* 647–65 (of 320 prostitutes, 74 percent had a positive Wassermann reaction, and 23 percent admitted having had syphilis or were under treatment for it); Jane Deeter Rippin, "Municipal detention of women," *Proceedings of the National Conference of Social Work*, 1918, *45:* 132–40 (of a group of 750 women detained at the Court and House of Detention for Girls and Women in Philadelphia, 259—34 percent—had either syphilis or gonorrhea or both); W. R. Jones, "Prostitution in Seattle," *Northwest Medicine*, 1918, *17:* 239–42 (of 384 prostitutes examined by the Seattle Health Department, 60 percent had syphilis, 37 percent had gonorrhea, and 17 percent had both); W. F. Draper, "The detention and treatment of infected women as a measure of control of venereal diseases in extra-cantonment zones," *American Journal of Obstetrics*

and Diseases of Women and Children, 1919, *80:* 642–46 (of a group of 208 prostitutes, all had gonorrhea, and 40 had both syphilis and gonorrhea); Edith L. Spaulding, "Mental and physical factors in prostitution," *Woman's Medical Journal,* 1914, *24:* 133–36 (of a group of 243 prostitutes studied, 99.5 percent had either gonorrhea or syphilis, and 55.8 percent had both); and Massachusetts, *Report of the Commission for the Investigation of the White Slave Traffic, So Called* (1914), 45–46 (of 80 prostitutes examined at the Suffolk County House of Correction in Boston, 87.5 percent had either syphilis or gonorrhea). Although all these studies were conducted after 1914, there is no evidence to indicate that the incidence of venereal infection among prostitutes would have been much different if such studies had been made, say, in 1905.

6   Figures from a New York City venereal disease clinic (given in William F. Snow, "Occupations and the venereal diseases," *Journal of the American Medical Association,* 1915, *65:* 2055) revealed the following:

Source of Infection	Percentage of Patients
Street prostitutes	36.3
House prostitutes	18.9
Domestic servants	10.0
Friends	10.0
Working women	7.7
Wives	1.5
Unknown	14.7

These figures show that some 55 percent of the venereal disease cases could be linked with prostitution. In 1910, Frederick Bierhoff, a New York City physician, presented figures from his private practice and from three hospital dispensaries in New York City, dealing with male patients who were infected with gonorrhea. Of a group of 1,429 such patients, 1,056, or 74 percent, traced the origin of their infection to public prostitutes. See Bierhoff, "Concerning the sources of infection in cases of venereal diseases in the city of New York," *New York Medical Journal,* 1910, *92:* 949–51. These figures—and any like them from other studies—are not absolutely conclusive. One would have to know, for instance, the economic class of the patients, their age spread, and approximately what percentage, of the estimated total number of venereal disease cases in New York City, these *reported* cases of venereal disease constituted.

7   Some physicians, however, argued that the public and professional full-time prostitute was *not* the main source of venereal contagion and that ordinary promiscuous sexual intercourse was the real problem. Professional prostitutes, the argument went, were sufficiently experienced and well informed to

avoid venereal disease or to seek a cure for it. See A. H. Powers, "Prostitution and venereal disease," *New England Medical Gazette,* 1905, *40:* 559–61.

8   See Charles Winick and Paul M. Kinsie, *The Lively Commerce: Prostitution in the United States* (Chicago: Quadrangle Books, 1971), 64; Harry Benjamin and R. E. L. Masters, *Prostitution and Morality* (London: Souvenir Press, 1965), 406; and "Is prostitution still a significant health problem?" *Medical Aspects of Human Sexuality,* 1968, *2:* 42.

9   This point was made in both of the Kinsey reports. The studies indicated that for the post–World War I generation (men born after 1900), the percentage of males who had experiences with prostitutes was roughly the same as for the pre-1900 generation, but the *frequency* with which American males went to prostitutes was, for the postwar generation, about half of that for the pre-1900 generation. Kinsey argued that the frequency of intercourse with non-prostitute women increased markedly for the younger generation. See Alfred B. Kinsey et al., *Sexual Behavior in the Human Female* (Philadelphia: W. B. Saunders, 1953), 300; and Alfred B. Kinsey et al., *Sexual Behavior in the Human Male* (Philadelphia: W. B. Saunders, 1948), 411. The problems with the Kinsey data are well known; here the difficulty is the bias in the sample of males.

10   By 1920 a change in emphasis was appearing. Discussions of venereal disease were focusing almost exclusively on the disease itself, with little consideration of prostitution. This attitude would have been highly exceptional just a decade earlier. See, for instance, Jules Schevitz, "Are we controlling venereal disease?" *Modern Medicine,* 1920, *2:* 507–9. See in general Odin W. Anderson, *Syphilis and Society: Problems of Control in the United States, 1912–1964* (Chicago: University of Chicago Press, 1965).

11   See, on this subject, James H. Cassedy, "The registration area and American vital statistics," *Bulletin of the History of Medicine,* 1965, *39:* 221–31.

12   For complaints about the lack of statistics, see Prince Morrow, "Prophylaxis of social diseases," *American Journal of Sociology,* 1907, *13:* 22; L. Chargin, "The reporting and control of venereal diseases," *American Journal of Public Health,* 1915, *5:* 298; F. H. Baker, "The control of venereal diseases by health departments," *American Journal of Public Health,* 1915, *5:* 293; and Henry D. Holton, "The duty of the state toward venereal diseases," *Journal of the American Medical Association,* 1906, *47:* 1249.

13   For the Committee of Seven see James F. Gardner, Jr., "Microbes and morality: the social hygiene crusade in New York City, 1892–1917," Ph.D. diss., Indiana University, 1973, 85–91. Gardner sees the activities of the committee as the beginning of social

hygiene agitation in New York State and argues, persuasively, that the high figures on venereal infection were used, at least in one sense, to scare other physicians and the general public into action. The 200,000 figure for New York City was stated again in 1913 by Hermann M. Biggs, an eminent public health authority. See Biggs, "Venereal diseases: the attitude of the Department of Health in relation thereto," *New York Medical Journal*, 1913, *97*: 1011.

14   Morrow, "A plea for the organization of a 'Society of Sanitary and Moral Prophylaxis,'" 1904. For similar figures see R. N. Wilson, "The relation of the medical profession to the social evil," *Journal of the American Medical Association*, 1906, *47*: 29; and Dock, *Hygiene and Morality*, 49.

15   Duncan Bulkley, "Syphilis as a disease innocently acquired," *Journal of the American Medical Association*, 1905, *44*: 682.

16   J. Van R. Hoff, "Is there a venereal peril for us?" *Medical Record*, 1909, *76*: 897. For other statements on an increase in venereal disease, see L. T. Wilson," A few remarks on the prevalence of venereal disease," *American Journal of Public Hygiene*, 1907–8, *4*: 39; and McLaughlin, "Pioneering in venereal disease control," 638.

17   J. H. Hager, "Cost of venereal infection," *Kentucky Medical Journal*, 1910, *8*: 1172; Evangeline W. Young, "The conservation of manhood and womanhood," *Woman's Medical Journal*, 1910, *20*: 52. See also Wilson, "A few remarks on the prevalence of venereal disease," 39.

18   For two general summaries of the statistical information on venereal disease, each of them based on more than twenty sources, see J. Patterson, "An economic view of venereal infections," *Journal of the American Medical Association*, 1914, *62*: 668–71; and G. V. R. Merrill, "Supervision of the venereally diseased," *New York State Journal of Medicine*, 1911, *11*: 136–38.

19   Richard C. Cabot, "Observations regarding the relative frequency of the different diseases prevalent in Boston and its vicinity," *Boston Medical and Surgical Journal*, 1911, *165*: 155–57. Cabot's findings on the incidence of syphilis were close to Morrow's: Morrow believed that from 5 to 18 percent of males suffered from the disease; Cabot placed the figure at either 11 or 14.8 percent.

20   Morrow, "The frequency of venereal diseases," *Boston Medical and Surgical Journal*, 1911, *165*: 521, 522–25.

21   Rosebury, *Microbes and Morals*, 208. The actual number of Americans infected with venereal disease in the progressive years is still not known. The U.S. Public Health Service estimates that 10 percent of the population had syphilis. However, during World War I, about 5.6 percent of the draftees had either syphilis or gonorrhea. Both of these figures, needless to say, could be very inaccurate. See U.S. Public Health Service, *Syphilis: A Synopsis*, 13; and Fred Davis Baldwin, "The American enlisted man in World War I," Ph.D. diss., Princeton University, 1964, 66.

22   M. Scholtz, "The problem of social evil in a large municipality," *Journal of Sociological Medicine*, 1917, *18*: 104.

23   Kelly is quoted in Denslow Lewis, "The need of publicity in venereal prophylaxis," *Medical Record*, 1906, *69*: 863. Kelly's attitude became more tolerant during the first decade of the century. See his "The protection of the innocent," *American Journal of Obstetrics and Diseases of Women and Children*, 1907, *55*: 447–81; "The best way to treat the social evil," *Medical News*, 1905, *86*: 1157–63; "The regulation of prostitution," *Journal of the American Medical Association*, 1906, *46*: 397–401; and "What is the right attitude of the medical profession toward the social evil?" *Journal of the American Medical Association*, 1905, *44*: 679–81.

24   See, for instance, J. N. Upshur, "Venereal diseases as a social menace," *Virginia Medical Semi-Monthly*, 1904–5, *9*: 294; H. J. Scherck, "Venereal disease and the social evil," *St. Louis Medical Review*, 1910, *4*: 39–41; M. L. Heidingsfeld, "The control of prostitution and the prevention of the spread of venereal diseases," *Journal of the American Medical Association*, 1904, *42*: 306; A. L. Wolbarst, "The venereal diseases," *American Journal of Dermatology and Genito-Urinary Diseases*, 1910, *14*: 268; H. A. Brann, "Social prophylaxis and the Church," *Medical News*, 1905, *87*: 74–75; E. W. Ruggles, "The physician's relation to the social evil," *New York Medical Journal*, 1907, *85*: 159–60; A. Williams, "The anti-venereal campaign," *Detroit Medical Journal*, 1909, *9*: 40; and T. D. Crothers, "Some scientific conclusions concerning the vice problem," *Texas Medical Journal*, 1913–14, *29*: 386.

25   Morrow, "The Society of Sanitary and Moral Prophylaxis," 320.

26   This point is also made in John C. Burnham, "The Progressive Era revolution in American attitudes toward sex," *Journal of American History*, 1973, *59*: 885–908.

27   A. Vanderveer, "In the relation we bear to the public, what use shall we make of our knowledge of the evil effects of venereal disease?" *American Journal of Obstetrics and Diseases of Women and Children*, 1911, *64*: 1033–42; R. H. Everett, "Publicity and the campaign against venereal disease," *American Journal of Public Health*, 1919, *9*: 854–58; Lewis, "The need of publicity in venereal prophylaxis," 863–65;

F. W. Tomkins, "Sanitary science and the social evil," *Pennsylvania Medical Journal*, 1909–10, *13:* 172–74; L. D. Bulkley, "Should education in sexual matters be given to young men of the working classes?" *Interstate Medical Journal*, 1906, *13:* 300–304; George R. Dodson, "The Black Plague and the educational remedy," *Bulletin of the American Academy of Medicine*, 1910, *11:* 490–95; M. Call, "A plan for the prevention of venereal disease," *Virginia Medical Semi-Monthly*, 1904, *9:* 295.

28   W. R. Jones, "Seattle prostitution from inside the quarantine," *Northwest Medicine*, 1919, *18:* 237; W. R. Jones, "A successful venereal prevention campaign," *Journal of the American Medical Association*, 1918, *71:* 1297; A. N. Thomson, "Attacking the venereal peril," *Long Island Medical Journal*, 1916, *10:* 144; Michael M. Davis, Jr., "Evening clinics for syphilis and gonorrhea," *American Journal of Public Health*, 1915, *5:* 310–11; M. M. Davis, "Efficient dispensary clinics a requisite for adequate coping with venereal diseases," *Journal of the American Medical Association*, 1915, *65:* 1983–86; M. F. Gates, "The prophylaxis of venereal disease," *Pennsylvania Medical Journal*, 1910–11, *14:* 258; W. Bieberbach, "Venereal disease and prostitution," *Boston Medical and Surgical Journal*, 1915, *172:* 208; J. Rosenstirn, "The Municipal Clinic of San Francisco," *Medical Record*, 1913, *83:* 467–76; Scholtz, "The problem of social evil in a large municipality," 109–10.

29   See "Duty of the profession to womankind," *Journal of the American Medical Association*, 1906, *47:* 1886–96, 1947–49; and "Symposium on venereal diseases," *Journal of the American Medical Association*, 1906, *47:* 1244–58. There were no women physicians at either of these symposiums. See also "Symposium on the venereal peril," *Providence Medical Journal*, 1905, *6:* 59–78; and "Symposium on the social evil," *Kentucky Medical Journal*, 1910, *8:* 1163–78.

30   See Burnham, "The Progressive Era revolution in American attitudes toward sex," 905–7. For a typical medical endorsement of the play see "Damaged goods," *Lancet-Clinic*, 1913, *110:* 450.

31   The American Purity Alliance (1895) and the National Vigilance Committee (1906) merged in 1912 to form the American Vigilance Association. The American Society of Sanitary and Moral Prophylaxis (1905) merged with other social hygiene groups to form the American Federation for Sex Hygiene in 1910, which merged with the American Vigilance Association to form the American Social Hygiene Association in 1913.

32   See Wilson, "A few remarks on the prevalence of venereal disease," 41, 45; C. F. Bolduan, "Venereal diseases," *American Journal of Public Health*, 1913, *3:* 1087–93; Chargin, "The reporting and control of venereal diseases," 297–304; M. M. Davis, "Efficient dispensary clinics a requisite for adequate coping with venereal diseases," 1983–86; A. N. Thomson, "Methods of controlling venereal disease," *American Journal of Nursing*, 1916–17, *17:* 1069–70; Thompson, "Attacking the Venereal Peril," 141–46; Scholtz, "The problem of social evil in a large municipality," 110–11; and H. G. Giddings, "The evils of drug store prescribing in venereal diseases," *Rhode Island Medical Journal*, 1917, *1:* 154–58.

33   This finding is not really surprising, given the conclusions of the famous Flexner Report (1910), which documented the inadequate training and preparation offered in most medical schools at the time. For comments on the sorry state of instruction in venereal disease, see D. E. Gardner, "The relation of the general practitioner to the treatment of venereal diseases," *American Journal of Dermatology and Genito-Urinary Diseases*, 1910, *14:* 263; C. L. Demeritt, "Venereal prophylaxis from a practical standpoint," *American Journal of Dermatology and Genito-Urinary Diseases*, 1910, *14:* 425; Abner Post, "What should be the attitude of boards of health toward venereal diseases?" *American Journal of Public Hygiene*, 1907–8, *9:* 48; Prince Morrow, "Education within the medical profession," *Medical News*, 1905, *86:* 1153–56; J. M. Anders, "The role of the medical profession in combatting the social evil," *Medicine*, 1906, *12:* 824–25; and T. N. Hepburn, "Demand for an open change of attitude toward the social evil," *Yale Medical Journal*, 1907–8, *14:* 167.

34   Prince Morrow, "The sanitary and moral prophylaxis of venereal diseases," *Journal of the American Medical Association*, 1905, *44:* 675–79; J. H. Stokes, "Hospital problems of gonorrhea and syphilis," *Journal of the American Medical Association*, 1916, *67:* 1960; H. M. Christian, "The social evil from a rational standpoint," *Pennsylvania Medical Journal*, 1912, *15:* 790.

35   J. M. Baldy, "The most effective methods of control of venereal diseases," *Transactions of the American Gynecological Society*, 1918, *43:* 198; G. M. Muren, "A contribution to the prophylaxis of venereal diseases," *American Medicine*, 1903, *6:* 481; Merrill, "Supervision of the venereally diseased," *New York State Journal of Medicine*, 1911, *11:* 138; Scholtz, "The problem of social evil in a large municipality," 106–8; Morrow, "The frequency of venereal diseases," 525; Spaulding, "Mental and physical factors in prostitution," 133–36; S. A. Knopf, "Some thoughts on the etiology, prophylaxis, and treatment of the social ill," *New York Medical Journal*, 1908, *87:* 825; Bolduan, "Venereal diseases," 1091. By the end of the teens, some progress had been made, according to one physician, in changing the admission policies

of hospitals. See E. R. Kelley, "The state clinics for the treatment of venereal diseases," *Boston Medical and Surgical Journal*, 1919, *181:* 311.

36 Williams, "The anti-venereal campaign," 41; Prince Morrow, "Health department control of venereal diseases," *New York Medical Journal*, 1911, *94:* 131; Prince Morrow, "Publicity as a factor in venereal prophylaxis," *Journal of the American Medical Association,*, 1906, *47:* 1244–45; D. T. Atkinson, *Social Travesties and What They Cost* (New York: Vail-Ballou, 1916), 33–34; G. Frank Lydston, *The Diseases of Society* (Philadelphia: Lippincott, 1904), 311.

37 See Pusey, *The History and Epidemiology of Syphilis*, 59–64; and William Trufant Foster, ed., *The Social Emergency* (Boston: Houghton Mifflin, 1914), 32–44.

38 "Symposium on the venereal peril," 71–72. The later estimate (60–80 percent) is in Atkinson, *Social Travesties and What They Cost*, 41. Atkinson noted that only an estimate could be given because of the lack of accurate records in the United States. There is some evidence to indicate that these estimates were probably too high. For example, in 1914 the Massachusetts Commission for the Blind informed a Massachusetts state commission investigating prostitution that 10 percent of the cases of blindness treated at three Boston hospitals were the result of venereal disease. See Massachusetts, *Report of the Commission for the Investigation of the White Slave Traffic, So Called*, 47.

In the white slave narratives, gonorrheal blindness in babies took on the emotional and melodramatic tone that permeated these documents as a whole. See Ernest Bell, ed., *War on the White Slave Trade* (Chicago: Charles C. Thompson, 1909), 283–85, where it is claimed that there are *"half a million blind"* in the world (ten to twelve thousand in the United States) from venereal disease. The text is accompanied by a pathetic picture of a "blind baby in a poor house."

39 John C. Burnham, "Medical inspection of prostitutes in America in the nineteenth century," *Bulletin of the History of Medicine*, 1971, *45:* 212, especially n. 31; Burnham, "The Progressive Era revolution in American attitudes toward sex," 890–94.

40 The 8 percent figure is from a study of 1,698 cases admitted to the psychopathic department of the Boston State Hospital. See B. H. Mason, "Compulsory reporting and compulsory treatment of venereal diseases," *Boston Medical and Surgical Journal*, 1919, *181:* 36. The 20 percent figure was supported by F. T. Simpson, neurologist to the Hartford Hospital, Hartford, Conn. See his "The extent and importance of the venereal diseases in the social body," *Virginia Medical Semi-Monthly*, 1909–10,

14: 128. A Massachusetts commission investigating prostitution in 1914 reported similar figures: for the first 2,600 admissions to all insane hospitals in the state in 1912, 8.65 percent; for Boston Psychopathic Hospital, 6.8 percent; for Danvers State Hospital for the Insane, 20 percent; for the State Hospital for Epileptics, 10.63 percent. See Massachusetts, *Report of the Commission for the Investigation of the White Slave Traffic, So Called*, 47. For similar statements on the prevalence of insanity owing to syphilis, see Walter T. Sumner, "General considerations on the vice problem," *Chicago Medical Recorder*, 1913, *35:* 103; N. E. Aronstam, "The prevention of the venereal peril," *Indianapolis Medical Journal*, 1912, *15:* 190; Hepburn, "Demand for an open change of attitude toward the social evil," 172; G. H. Bogart, "The menace of clandestine prostitution," *Medical Herald*, 1911, *30:* 495; E. G. Ballenger, "The social evil," *Atlanta Journal-Record of Medicine*, 1907, *9:* 8; William Lee Howard, "The havoc of prudery," *Pearson's Magazine*, 1910, *24:* 591; Chicago Vice Commission, *The Social Evil in Chicago* (1911), 25; and Syracuse Morals Survey Committee, *The Social Evil in Syracuse* (1913), 82.

The white slave narratives presented the relationship between syphilis and insanity in statements such as *"The red mills grind out men's brains,"* or *"The red mill destroys the spinal cord,"* giving testimonies from physicians that 75 percent of insanity was the result of syphilitic infection. See Clifford G. Roe, *The Great War on White Slavery* (n.p.: Clifford G. Roe and B. S. Steadwell, 1911), 310–12.

41 See, for instance, the figures for the state of Massachusetts, in J. H. Cunningham, "The importance of venereal disease," *Boston Medical and Surgical Journal*, 1913, *168:* 80. Cunningham estimated that the cost for institutional care in state institutions for the unquestionably syphilitic insane was just under $110,000 per year. Counting inmates in institutions for remote effects of syphilis, the figure was $300,000.

42 The "race suicide" alarm is discussed, from different points of view, in David M. Kennedy, *Birth Control in America: The Career of Margaret Sanger* (New Haven: Yale University Press, 1970), 42–44; Mark H. Haller, *Eugenics: Hereditarian Attitudes in American Thought* (New Brunswick, N.J.: Rutgers University Press, 1963), 79–81; Peter Gabriel Filene, *Him-Her Self: Sex Roles in Modern America* (New York: New American Library, 1975), 36–38; and Linda Gordon, *Woman's Body, Woman's Right: A Social History of Birth Control in America* (New York: Grossman, 1976), 136–58. Physicians concerned with the problem saw "race suicide" in a much broader context than that of the birth control controversy and related it not

only to the birthrate (which could be consciously controlled) but to the ravages of various diseases on the population. Two of these were, of course, hereditary syphilis and gonorrhea. See D. Clinton Guthrie, "Race suicide," *Pennsylvania Medical Journal*, 1911–12, *15:* 855–59; Emory Lanphear, "Gonorrhea and race suicide," *Medico-Pharmaceutical Critic and Guide*, 1907, *8:* 7–8; Simpson, "The extent and importance of the venereal diseases in the social body," 126, 129; Upshur, "Venereal diseases as a social menace," 293; C. F. Hodge, "Instruction in social hygiene in the public schools," *Bulletin of the American Academy of Medicine*, 1910, *11:* 515; Hager, "Cost of venereal infection," 1175; Bieberbach, "Venereal disease and prostitution," 202–3; Ballenger, "The social evil," 8; Merrill, "Supervision of the venereally diseased," 137; D. E. Stannard, "The crime of sexual ignorance, showing why the doctor is to blame," *American Journal of Clinical Medicine*, 1910, *17:* 1172; A. L. Wolbarst, "The venereal diseases," *Medical Review*, 1913, *62:* 269, 271; "The deeper reason," *Texas Medical Journal*, 1913–14, *29:* 394; and Prince Morrow, "Venereal diseases and their relation to infant mortality and race deterioration," *New York Medical Journal*, 1911, *94:* 1315–17.

43 Morrow, "Venereal diseases and their relation to infant mortality and race deterioration," 1317. Morrow was referring to instances where a woman gave birth to one child but a subsequent venereal infection rendered her sterile.

44 F. C. Walsh, "Venereal diseases and marriage," *American Journal of Dermatology and Genito-Urinary Diseases*, 1910, *14:* 225. See also the following statements on the percentage of childless marriages caused by venereal infection: Upshur, "Venereal diseases as a social menace," 292 (70 percent); Cunningham, "The importance of venereal disease," 79–80 (67 percent); Albert Burr, "The guarantee of safety in the marriage contract," *Journal of the American Medical Association*, 1906, *47:* 1887 (75 percent); Prince Morrow, "Eugenics and Venereal Diseases," and *Dietetic and Hygiene Gazette*, 1911, *27:* 15 (17–25 percent).

45 Prince Morrow, "Social prophylaxis and the medical profession," *American Journal of Dermatology and Genito-Urinary Diseases*, 1905, *9:* 269; Prince Morrow, "The relations of social diseases to the family," *American Journal of Sociology*, 1909, *14:* 629.

46 Howard, "The havoc of prudery," 591. For similar sentiments see Wilson, "The relation of the medical profession to the social evil," 30; J. C. Irons, "The social evil," *West Virginia Medical Journal*, 1907–8, *2:* 347; Ballenger, "The social evil," 8; Upshur, "Venereal diseases as a social menace," 292–94; Call,

"A plan for the prevention of venereal disease," 294; and Young, "The conservation of manhood and womanhood," 51.

47 See the recollection by G. W. Potter, in "Symposium on the Venereal Peril," 66.

48 Morrow, "A plea for the organization of a 'Society of Sanitary and Moral Prophylaxis,'" 1075. Morrow at another time pointed out the irony that prostitutes, who were usually experienced in matters of venereal disease, normally got swifter and better treatment for venereal diseases than did a middle-class wife. Here it seems that prostitutes were far more advanced in knowledge of their own physiology than were most other women in early twentieth-century American society.

49 See the obstetricians' and gynecologists' figures cited in Wilson, "The relation of the medical profession to the social evil," 31; and Bierberbach, "Venereal disease and prostitution," 204. Prince Morrow cited a statement of the president of the American Gynecological Society in 1907 to the effect that "70 per cent of all the work done by specialists in diseases of women in this country was the result of gonococcus infection" (Morrow, "The relations of social diseases to the family," 626). These statements also asserted that from 30 to 70 percent of married women seeking medical treatment for venereal disease had been infected by their husbands. For general statements on the plight of "innocent wives," see W. A. Newman Dorland, "The social aspect of gonoccocal infection of the innocent," *Bulletin of the American Academy of Medicine*, 1910, *11:* 469; Walsh, "Venereal diseases and marriage," 225; Stannard, "The crime of sexual ignorance, showing why the doctor is to blame," 1167–68; Bransford Lewis, "What shall we teach the public regarding venereal diseases?" *Journal of the American Medical Association*, 1906, *47:* 1255; Hepburn, "Demand for an open change of attitude toward the social evil," 172; D. C. Brockman, "What can we do to prevent the sacrifice of the innocents?" *Iowa Medical Journal*, 1904, *10:* 431–36; A. Ravogli, "Education and instruction in sexual relations as a prophylaxis against venereal diseases," *New York Medical Journal*, 1910, *91:* 1221; G. Frank Lydston, "The social evil and its remedies," *American Journal of Clinical Medicine*, 1909, *16:* 156–57; Robert N. Wilson, *The American Boy and the Social Evil* (Philadelphia: J. C. Winston, 1905), 106; and Atkinson, *Social Travesties and What They Cost*, 19, 20.

50 See Katharine Houghton Hepburn, "Communications," *Survey*, 1910, *24:* 637–38.

51 Walsh, "Venereal diseases and marriage," 225.

52 Morrow mentioned this collusion in his comment on venereal disease and divorce, quoted above (n. 49), although he did not elaborate on it elsewhere.

One can find condemnations of the "medical secret," implying that it was a widespread phenomenon, in Edmund Alden Burnham, "Abatement of the social evil," in *Recent Christian Progress: Studies in Christian Thought and Work during the Last Seventy-five Years*, ed. Lewis Bayles Paton (New York: Macmillan, 1909), 480; and Dock, *Hygiene and Morality* (1910), 145–46.

53 See Ann Douglas Wood, "The Fashionable Diseases," in this volume; and, in general, John S. Haller, Jr., and Robin M. Haller, *The Physician and Sexuality in Victorian America* (Urbana: University of Illinois Press, 1974); and G. J. Barker-Benfield, *The Horrors of the Half-Known Life: Male Attitudes toward Women and Sexuality in Nineteenth Century America* (New York: Harper & Row, 1976).

54 For an overview of the general subject of sex education, see Bryan Strong, "Ideas of the early sex education movement in America, 1890–1920," *History of Education Quarterly*, 1972, *12:* 129–61. The doctrine of male sexual necessity is discussed in James L. Wunsch, "Prostitution and public policy: from regulation to suppression," Ph.D. diss., University of Chicago, 1976, 101–21.

55 G. B. H. Swayze, "Social evil dilemma," *Medical Times*, 1906, *34:* 228. For similar attitudes, see C. E. Lack, "The physician's duty regarding the prophylaxis of venereal diseases," *Medical Times*, 1909, *37:* 47; Wolbarst, "The problem of venereal prophylaxis," 285; F. Bierhoff, "Venereal diseases," *New York Medical Journal*, 1912, *96:* 1012; and E H. Williams and J. S. Brown, "Venereal diseases and practical eugenics in small communities," *Medical Record*, 1913, *84:* 1020.

56 The belief in the value of sexual continence permeated the medical literature on prostitution and venereal disease. For some examples, see F. H. Gerrish, "A crusade against syphilis and gonorrhea," *Boston Medical and Surgical Journal*, 1910, *163:* 5–6; J. N. Upshur, "The limitation and prevention of venereal disease," *American Journal of Dermatology and Genito-Urinary Diseases*, 1910, *14:* 349; Demeritt, "Venereal prophylaxis from a practical standpoint," 424; Lydston, "The social evil and its remedies," 158–59; Ravogli, "Education and instruction in sexual relations as a prophylaxis against venereal disease," 1219; E. L. Keyes, "The sexual necessity," *Medical News*, 1905, *87:* 73, 74; J. H. Landis, "The social evil in relation to the health problem," *American Journal of Public Health*, 1913, *3:* 1076; Lewis, "What shall we teach the public regarding venereal diseases?" 1253; W. F. Snow, "Public health measures in relation to venereal diseases," *Journal of the American Medical Association*, 1916, *66:* 1006; William Cullen Bryant, "The social evil," *Pittsburgh Medical Journal*, 1913–14, *1:* 37–40; Hepburn, "Demand for an open

change of attitude toward the social evil," 170–71; Young, "The conservation of manhood and womanhood," 52; Ballenger, "The social evil," 11–12; Sprague Carleton, "The prostitute," *Hahnemannian Monthly*, 1908, *43:* 825; Maude Glasgow, "On the regulation of prostitution with special reference to paragraph 79 of the Page Bill," *New York Medical Journal*, 1910, *92:* 1321–22; Ruggles, "The physician's relation to the social evil," 159; P. B. Brooks, "The relation of the general practitioner to prevention of venereal diseases," *New York State Journal of Medicine*, 1913, *13:* 102; Call, "A plan for the prevention of venereal disease," 296; "Sowing wild oats," *Texas Medical Journal*, 1913–14, *24:* 410–11; C. E. Smith, Jr., "Some observations on public health and morality," *St. Paul Medical Journal*, 1912, *14:* 201; W. J. Herdman, "The duty of the medical profession to the public in the matter of venereal diseases, and how to discharge it," *Journal of the American Medical Association*, 1906, *47:* 1247; Foster, *The Social Emergency*, 28–31, 98, 130, 142, 145; Dock, *Hygiene and Morality*, 60–62; Rabbi Rudolph I. Coffee, "Pittsburgh clergy and social evil," *Survey*, 1913, *29:* 815; "Is it crime as well as sin?" *Independent*, 1913, *74:*176; Clara E. Laughlin, "A single standard," *Pearson's Magazine*, 1914, *31:* 737–38; Howard, "The havoc of prudery," 597; Minneapolis, *Report of the Minneapolis Vice Commission* (1911), 9; and Newark Citizen's Committee on Social Evil, *Report of the Social Evil Conditions of Newark* (1914), 133.

57 See Barbara Gutmann Rosenkrantz, *Public Health and the State: Changing Views in Massachusetts, 1842–1936* (Cambridge, Mass.: Harvard University Press, 1972), 110–12.

58 N. P. Rathbun, "The control of social disease," *Long Island Medical Journal*, 1908, *2:* 22; Baldy, "The most effective methods of control of venereal disease," 196–97; E. L. Keys, "The prenuptial sanitary guarantee," *New York Medical Journal*, 1907, *85:* 1203; W. M. L. Coplin, "Departmental influence in the suppression of social disease," *New York Medical Journal*, 1907, *85:* 1206; Demeritt, "Venereal prophylaxis from a practical standpoint," 424, 424. The heavy opposition of New York physicians to a New York reporting regulation is discussed in Gardner, "Microbes and morality," 307–8.

59 This proreporting sentiment was widespread in the medical literature, and, although journal opinion cannot be taken as an absolute indication of physicians' opinions, it clearly indicated an atmosphere, or a set of attitudes, that looked to the future. See, for some examples, Smith, "Some observations on public health and morality," 200; "Symposium on the venereal peril," 65–66; Lack, "The physician's duty regarding the prophylaxis of venereal dis-

ease," 48; Young, "The conservation of manhood and womanhood," 53; Ballenger, "The social evil," 10; Merrill, "Supervision of the venereally diseased," 138–39; C. C. Pierce, "Progress of venereal disease control," *Journal of the American Medical Association,* 1919, *73:* 421; W. Elder, "The reporting of venereal diseases by physicians," *Journal of the American Medical Association,* 1920, *74:* 1764; Brooks, "The relation of the general practitioner to prevention of venereal diseases," 103; J. Rosenstirn, "The notification of venereal disease," *Medical Record,* 1914, *86:* 343; Bolduan, "Venereal diseases," 1088; Gerrish, "A crusade against syphilis and gonorrhea," *Boston Medical and Surgical Journal,* 1910, *163:* 10–12; Post, "What should be the attitude of boards of health toward venereal diseases?" 47; and W. A. Purrington, "Professional secrecy and the obligatory notification of venereal diseases," *New York Medical Journal,* 1907, *85:* 1209.

60 See, in general, Biggs, "Venereal diseases," 1009–12; S. L. Strong, "A symposium on the reportability and control of venereal diseases," *Boston Medical and Surgical Journal,* 1913, *169:* 903–7; Kelley, "The state clinics for the treatment of venereal diseases," 310; Mason, "Compulsory reporting and compulsory treatment of venereal diseases," 37–38; H. G. Irvine, "The venereal disease campaign in retrospect," *Journal of Cutaneous Diseases including Syphilis,* 1919, *37:* 750; and Joseph Mayer, *The Regulation of Commercialized Vice* (New York: n.p., 1922), 31–32. The anti-venereal-disease campaign during World War I gave an important boost to the demand for reporting laws. See Thomas Parran, *Shadow on the Land: Syphilis* (New York: Raynal and Hitchcock, 1937), 80–88; Baldwin, "The American enlisted man in World War I," 31–49; 111–15; and Mark Thomas Connelly, *The Response to Prostitution in the Progressive Era* (Chapel Hill: University of North Carolina Press, 1980), chap. 7.

61 Morrow, "The relations of social diseases to the family," 632. It is interesting here to compare Morrow's conception of feminine modesty in 1909 with the sensibility of Mencken's 1915 essay "The flapper," a famous sentence of which reads: "She has been converted, by Edward W. Bok, to the gospel of sex hygiene. She knows exactly what the Wassermann reaction is, and has made up her mind that she will never marry a man who can't show an unmistakable negative" ("The flapper," *Smart Set,* 1915, *45:* 1).

62 For positive attitudes, see Burr, "The guarantee of safety in the marriage contract," 1888; "Marriage laws and Wisconsin's experience," *Texas Medical Journal,* 1913–14, *29:* 395–96; Patterson, "An economic view of venereal infections," 671; G. G. H.

Swayze, "Shall social evil infections be legally repressed?" *Medical Times,* 1906, *34:* 257; Smith, "Some observations on public health and morality," 201; M. Lederer, "The value of the gonorrheal complement fixation test and the Wassermann reaction in determining the fitness of a person to marry," *Long Island Medical Journal,* 1913, 7: 102–4; Williams, "The anti-venereal campaign," 45; C. D. Lockwood, "Venereal diseases in children," *Bulletin of the American Academy of Medicine,* 1910, *11:* 482; W. F. Snow, "The preventive medicine campaign against venereal diseases," *American Medical Association Bulletin,* 1914, *9:* 193; Mason, "Compulsory reporting and compulsory treatment of venereal diseases," 38; Sumner, "General considerations on the vice problem," 103; Aronstam, "The prevention of the venereal peril," 196; Irons, "The social evil," 348; Knopf, "Some thoughts on the etiology, prophylaxis, and treatment of social ill," 822; Gardner, "The relation of the general practitioner to the treatment of venereal diseases," 265; F. H. Gerrish, "A crusade against syphilis and gonorrhea," *Medical Communications of the Massachusetts Medical Society,* 1910, *21:* 723–60; and Wolbarst, "The problem of venereal prophylaxis," 280–86.

The vice commission reports also supported premarriage medical tests. See, for example, Newark, *Report of the Social Evil Conditions of Newark* (1914), 134; Minneapolis, *Report of the Vice Commission of Minneapolis* (1911), 2; Chicago, *The Social Evil in Chicago* (1911), 56, 68, 292; and Syracuse, *The Social Evil in Syracuse* (1913), 64, 82.

63 Young, "The conservation of manhood and womanhood," 53.

64 This matter deserves some elaboration. By 1914 seven states had passed legislation dealing with venereal disease and marriage. The Michigan (1899) and Utah (1909) laws declared it unlawful for infected men to marry but provided for no means of enforcement. The Pennsylvania (1913) statute required males applying for marriage licenses to sign affidavits indicating freedom from venereal disease. The Washington (1909), North Dakota (1913), Wisconsin (1913), and Oregon (1913) legislation required males to present physicians' certificates (but *not* the results of serological tests) certifying the absence of venereal infection. In 1914, Edward L. Keyes, a leading physician in the social hygiene movement, commented: "No state requires the physical examination of the prospective bride. We may admit the impracticality of requiring such an examination. Yet its omission nullifies the intent of the law" (Keyes, "Can the law protect matrimony from disease?" *Journal of Social Hygiene,* 1914–15, *1:* 10). In 1917, New York State stipulated that both

applicants for a marriage license must sign affidavits; and in 1919, Alabama called for males to present physicians' certificates. By 1922 twenty states had provisions concerning venereal disease and marriage on the books, but none of them required serological tests. See Michael F. Guyer, "Review of Wisconsin's 'Eugenics Legislation,'" *American Journal of Obstetrics and Diseases of Women and Children*, 1918, *77:* 485–92; J. S. Lawrence, "Recent legislation in New York State, relating to the control of venereal disease," *Medical Record*, 1919, *95:* 669–70; "Antenuptial examination of males for venereal infection," *Public Health Reports*, 1920, *35:*1401; Hugh Cabot, "Syphilis and society," *Journal of Social Hygiene*, 1915–16, *2:* 347–51; Bernal C. Roloff, "The eugenics marriage laws of Wisconsin, Michigan, and Indiana," *Journal of Social Hygiene*, 1920, *6:* 227–54; Mayer, *The Regulation of Commercialized Vice*, 31; and Fred S. Hall and Elizabeth Brooke, *American Marriage Laws in Their Social Aspects* (New York: Russell Sage Foundation, 1919).

By 1936 the situation was only somewhat improved. Twenty-eight states had passed legislation, but ten states still required only affidavits from males, and four states (Del., N.Y., Nebr., and Pa.) required affidavits from both parties. Only Connecticut required the results (from both male and female) of serological tests. See Parran, *Shadow on the Land*, 251–52.

By 1939 some progress had been made. Sixteen states (Calif., Colo., Conn., Wash., W.Va., Ill., Ind., Ky., Mich., N.H., N.J., N.Y., Pa., R.I., S.Dak., Tenn.) required male and female to present the results of serological tests. But nineteen states (Ariz., Ark., Fla., Ga., Idaho, Iowa, Kans., Maine, Md., Mass., Minn., Miss., Mo., Mont., Nev., N.Mex., Ohio, Okla., S.C.) had no legislation dealing with venereal disease and marriage. Seven states (Ala., La., N.C., Oreg., Tex., Wis., Wyo.) still required only physicians' certificates from both parties, and three (Utah, Vt., Va.) stated that persons with venereal disease could not marry but set up no means of enforcement. Figures from Bascom Johnson, ed., *Digest of Laws and Regulations Relating to the Prevention and Control of Syphilis and Gonorrhea in the Forty-eight States and the District of Columbia* (New York: American Social Hygiene Association, 1940).

65   Haller, *Eugenics*, 142. A distinction between the eugenics orientation and the campaign against venereal disease is made in Snow, "Public health measures in relation to venereal diseases," 1008.

66   See note 64.

67   Morrow, "The relations of social diseases to the family," 633.

68   For the nineteenth-century controversy over regu-

lation, see Wunsch, "Prostitution and public policy," 38–100; Burnham, "Medical inspection of prostitutes in America in the nineteenth century," 203–18; and David J. Pivar, *Purity Crusade: Sexual Morality and Social Control, 1868–1900* (Westport, Conn.: Greenwood Press, 1973), 50–77.

69   See W. E. Harwood, "A Practical Lesson in Reglementation," *Journal of the American Medical Association*, 1906, *47:* 2076–78; Frederic Bierhoff, "The Page Bill and regulation of prostitution," *Medico-Pharmaceutical Critic and Guide*, 1910, *13:* 437–42; F. Bierhoff, "The problem of prostitution and venereal diseases in New York City," *New York Medical Journal*, 1911, *93:* 557–61, 618–22; Vecki, "Can we abolish, shall we ignore, or must we regulate prostitution?" 213–20; F. H. Hancock, "Regulation of prostitution in the city of Norfolk, Virginia," *Virginia Medical Semi-Monthly*, 1912–13, *17:* 559–61; Landis, "The social evil in relation to the health problem," 1073–86; Bryant, "The social evil," 42, 45–48; J. Huici, "The necessity of isolating prostitutes who suffer from syphilis," *American Journal of Public Hygiene*, 1909–10, *6:* 523–30; Christian, "The social evil from a rational standpoint," 789–90; Bieberbach, "Venereal disease and prostitution," 206; A. W. Herzog, "A plan to regulate prostitution," *Medical Brief*, 1905, *33:* 381–83; Denslow Lewis, "What shall we do with the prostitute?" *American Journal of Dermatology and Genito-Urinary Diseases*, 1907, *11:* 485–93; Aronstam, "The prevention of the venereal peril," 192–93, 196; J. C. Wood, "The social evil," 573; and Swayze, "Shall Social Evil Infections Be Legally Repressed?" 257.

70   Lewis, "What shall we do with the prostitute?" 491.

71   For Cincinnati see D. E. Robinson and J. G. Wilson, "Tuberculosis among prostitutes," *American Journal of Public Health*, 1916, *6:* 1164–65, 1171–72; and J. H. Landis (Cincinnati health officer), "What health departments can do to solve the venereal problem under existing conditions," *Medical Review of Reviews*, 1915, *21:* 535–38. For some brief comments on the system of medical regulation in Cincinnati, See Zane L. Miller, *Boss Cox's Cincinnati* (New York: Oxford University Press, 1968), 98, 177–78, 218. For Cleveland and Toledo see Theodore A. Bingham, "The girl that disappears," *Hampton's Magazine*, 1910, *25:* 570.

72   A. Neisser, "Is it really impossible to make prostitution harmless as far as infection is concerned?" 289–99.

73   For European cities, see F. Griffith, "Observations upon the protective value of the inspection of public women as carried out in Paris," *Medical Record*, 1904, *65:* 651–52; Frederic Bierhoff, "Police methods for the sanitary control of prostitution in some

of the cities of Germany," *New York Medical Journal,* 1907, *86:* 298–305, 354–59, 400–406, 451–56 (Bierhoff admitted that the German system, for a number of reasons, was not effective, but argued that the faults could be remedied); H. P. deForest, "Prostitution: police methods of sanitary supervision," *New York State Journal of Medicine,* 1908, *8:* 516–35 (deForest, a police surgeon in the New York City police department and a professor of obstetrics, was somewhat unique among regulationists in that he advocated, along with the inspection of prostitutes, the inspection of their male customers); and Wilhelm Dreuw, "The modern examination of prostitutes," *Urologic and Cutaneous Review,* 1914, *18:* 182–91 (this is a detailed and illustrated article describing the procedure, instruments, and techniques used in examining prostitutes in Berlin, Germany; it was, in short, a specific model for U.S. physicians to follow).

The military analogy was two-sided. First, it was contended that military programs which required prophylaxis for men after sexual contact (shore leave, etc.) reduced the rate of venereal disease and thus showed that similar programs applied to prostitutes would also work. See E. O. J. Eytinge, "A system of venereal prophylaxis and its results," *Military Surgeon,* 1909, *25:* 170–71; Gates, "The prophylaxis of venereal disease," 255–59; and Robert A. Bachman, "Venereal prophylaxis: past and present," *Providence Medical Journal,* 1913, *14:* 231–44. It was also argued that in military areas where prostitution was under medical supervision, the rate of venereal infection for military personnel was decreased. See H. Goodman, "Prostitution and community syphilis," *American Journal of Public Health,* 1919, *9:* 515–20.

74 An exception was the program advocated by Theodore A. Bingham, former chief of the New York City police, who argued that a system of medical inspection should be run by the police, in cooperation with the public health authorities. See Bingham, "The girl that disappears," 572–73.

75 The opposition to the regulation of prostitution was not organized in the progressive years, and it cannot be assumed that the individuals and groups mentioned in this paragraph worked together or even were entirely aware of what the others were doing. Their activities are presented simply as expressions of a particular pattern of response to the idea of regulation. It should also be emphasized that these groups did not share the same outlook on many other social issues and, indeed, were many times on opposite sides of particular questions.

76 For a typical statement by Prince Morrow opposing the regulation of prostitution, see his "The sanitary and moral prophylaxis of venereal diseases," 675. In its first major publication, George Jackson Kneeland's *Commercialized Prostitution in New York City* (1913), the Bureau of Social Hygiene concluded that a policy of regulation was useless (9).

77 Glasgow, "On the regulation of prostitution with special reference to paragraph 79 of the Page Bill," 1320–23; Maude Glasgow, "Side lights on the social peril," *New York Medical Journal,* 1911, *93:* 1186–90; Kelly, "The regulation of prostitution," 398; Lydston, "The social evil and its remedies," 279; Call, "A plan for the prevention of venereal disease," 295; Crothers, "Some scientific conclusions concerning the vice problem," 391; Gerrish, "A crusade against syphilis and gonorrhea," *Medical Communications of the Massachusetts Medical Society,* 1910, *21:* 732–36; Post, "What should be the attitude of boards of health toward venereal diseases?" 47–48; Chargin, "The reporting and control of venereal diseases," 298; Ballenger, "The social evil," 9; P. F. Rogers, "The sociologic aspect of the venereal diseases," *Wisconsin Medical Journal,* 1909–10, *8:* 256; George W. Goler, "The municipality and the venereal disease problem," *American Journal of Public Health,* 1916, *6:* 357; J. M. Mabbott, "The duties of the gynecologist in relation to the state control of vice," *American Journal of Obstetrics and Diseases of Women and Children,* 1911, *64:* 227–37; Heidingsfeld, "The control of prostitution and the prevention of the spread of venereal diseases," 308; Hepburn, "Demand for an open change of attitude toward the social evil," 167–73; "Symposium on the venereal peril," 64; Ruggles, "The physician's relation to the social evil," 160.

78 See Chicago, *The Social Evil in Chicago* (1911), 26; Syracuse, *The Social Evil in Syracuse* (1913), 87–88; Minneapolis, *Report of the Vice Commission of Minneapolis* (1911), 34–36, 37, 52, 53; Massachusetts, *Report of the Commission for the Investigation of the White Slave Traffic, So Called* (1914), 45; and Illinois, *Report of the Senate Vice Committee* (1916), 42–45.

For the white slave narratives see Bell, *War on the White Slave Trade,* 257–60; Roe, *The Great War on White Slavery,* 362; E. Norine Law, *The Shame of a Great Nation: The Story of the "White Slave Trade"* (Harrisburg, Pa.: United Evangelical Publishing House, 1909), 183; and Clifford G. Roe, *The Girl Who Disappeared* (Chicago: American Bureau of Moral Education, 1919), 302, 306–11.

79 See the statements written by Anna Garlin Spencer: "State regulation of vice and its meaning," *Forum,* 1913, *49:* 587–601; "The scarlet woman," *Forum,* 1913, *49:* 276–89; and "A world crusade," *Forum,* 1913, *50:* 182–95. See also Jane Addams, *A New Conscience and an Ancient Evil* (New York: Macmillan, 1912), 45–49; Jane Addams, "A challenge

to the contemporary church," *Survey*, 1912, *28:* 195–98; George Kibbe Turner, "The strange woman," *McClure's Magazine*, 1913, *41:* 33; and Maude E. Miner, *Slavery of Prostitution* (New York: Macmillan, 1916), 138–42, 155–61. Much of the opposition to regulation drew inspiration from the efforts of Josephine Butler in opposing the medical inspection of prostitutes in England in the nineteenth century. See Anna Garlin Spencer, "Josephine Butler and the English crusade," *Forum*, 1913, *49:* 703–16.

80 Theodore Roosevelt, *Autobiography* (New York: Scribner, 1925), 237; "Shall Chicago legalize hell?" *American City*, 1912, *7:* 405–6; "California dux," *Independent*, 1913, *74:* 1064–65.

81 This acceptance of the same basic assumption sometimes took amusing forms. For instance, the Minneapolis Vice Commission was at pains to show that prostitution was the major source of venereal disease and that therefore prostitution ought to be repressed and not regulated. The commission used some figures gathered by Frederick Bierhoff, a New York City physician, which showed that three-quarters of venereal disease cases could be traced to prostitution. What is interesting is that Bierhoff had presented these figures in the course of an article in support of a policy of medical regulation. See Minneapolis, *Report of the Vice Commission of Minneapolis* (1911), 46, for the citation of Bierhoff's figures. For Bierhoff's presentation, see his "Concerning the sources of infection in cases of venereal diseases in the city of New York," 949–51.

82 Morrow, "The sanitary and moral prophylaxis of venereal diseases," 675.

83 M. L. Heidingsfeld, a private practitioner in Cincinnati, argued that during the years 1900–1903, when Cincinnati had a system of medical inspection, his volume of venereal disease cases *increased,* and that a high percentage of these cases could be traced to "inspected prostitutes." See Heidingsfeld, "The control of prostitution and the prevention of the spread of venereal diseases," 305–9. (Other Cincinnati officials came to the opposite conclusion. See the citations in note 71 above.) A Cleveland physician, a superintendent of a community dispensary, also presented figures showing that regulation did not work. He argued that during the eight months before the closing of the segregated district in Cleveland, the dispensary handled 112 cases of venereal disease, whereas in the first eight months *after* the closing of the district, there were only 53 cases. See A. R. Warner, "The result of closing the segregated vice district upon the public health of Cleveland," *Cleveland Medical Journal*, 1916, *15:* 171–73.

84 See Demeritt, "Venereal prophylaxis from a prac-

tical standpoint," 422–23; Lydston, *The Diseases of Society*, 407; and Dock, *Hygiene and Morality*, 131–32. Pivar, *Purity Crusade*, discusses earlier nineteenth-century American opposition from purity reformers to military programs for the regulation of prostitution (218–24).

85 Kelly, "What is the right attitude of the medical profession toward the social evil?" 681.

86 Abraham Flexner, *I Remember* (New York: Simon & Schuster, 1940), 186. Flexner's early life, see 3–184. There is some material on Flexner's relationship with Rockefeller and the Bureau of Social Hygiene in Gardner, "Microbes and morality," 248–49.

87 Flexner, *I Remember*, 188.

88 Abraham Flexner, *Prostitution in Europe* (1914; rpt. Montclair, N.J.: Patterson Smith, 1969), 231.

89 Ibid., 12, 286–394.

90 Ibid., 265–85.

91 For this interpretation of Wilson's approach to European imperialism, see N. Gordon Levin, Jr., *Woodrow Wilson and World Politics*, (New York: Oxford University Press, 1968), 1–10.

92 For reviews, see "A hopeful book on the social evil," *Outlook*, 1914, *106:* 293–94; James Bronson Reynolds, "Prostitution in Europe," *American City*, 1914, *10:* 155–56; "A real social evil treatise," *Nation*, 1914, *19:* 75–76; "Prostitution in Europe," *Survey*, 1914, *31:* 471–73; and C. V. Carrington, "An analysis of the report of Abraham Flexner on the regulation of prostitution in Europe," *Virginia Medical Semi-Monthly*, 1916–17, *21:* 11–16. These were all laudatory reviews, but for one that questioned Flexner's interpretation, see D. C. McMurtrie, "A study of prostitution in Europe," *Medical Record*, 1914, *85:* 325–28.

93 Although most physicians subscribed to civilized morality, its rhetoric, especially the belief in sexual continence, was most strenuously espoused by the physicians and others who were against regulation. Those who supported regulation were not, usually, proselytizers for the gospel of continence. And those who supported the belief in continence usually were strongly against the regulation of prostitution. One can see this breakdown in a crude sense by noting that the physicians listed in note 69 above as regulationists do not appear in note 56, with the proponents of continence. And, the physicians listed in note 55 as critics of the gospel of continence do not appear in note 77, with the antiregulationists. There were, of course, some exceptions. For instance, J. H. Landis supported both the regulation of prostitution and the theory of continence (see "The social evil in relation to the health problem," 1073–86).

94 Flexner, *Prostitution in Europe*, 219; Spencer, "State regulation of vice and its meaning," 600. Spencer's

article is one of the fullest analyses of the significance of the regulation of prostitution to be found in the progressive years.

95 Hodge, "Instruction in social hygiene in the public schools," 515.

96 Brooks, *The V.D. Story*, 22.

97 The physicians interviewed in "Is prostitution still a significant health problem?" basically agreed that prostitution is no longer as important a factor in venereal disease control as it once was but argued that it is a problem in terms of drug abuse and diseases such as hepatitis.

98 Morrow, "The sanitary and moral prophylaxis of venereal diseases," 677.

16

"The Fashionable Diseases": Women's Complaints and Their Treatment in Nineteenth-Century America

ANN DOUGLAS WOOD

Historians of nineteenth-century American culture and society have become increasingly aware that many of the medical theories and practices of the period fall within their province rather than within that of the scientist. Furthermore, the historical consensus seems to be that nineteenth-century treatments of mental illness, "nervous" conditions, and sexual difficulties, although telling little about scientific advancement, are particularly sensitive indicators of cultural attitudes. Historians Huber and Meyer, for example, have considered the "mind cure" movement of the late nineteenth and early twentieth centuries not as incipient psychoanalysis, but as an expression of contemporary conflict-laden ideas of success and achievement. Rothman has based his recent study of development of the asylum in the Jacksonian period on the stated assumption that "the march of science cannot by itself explain the transformation in the American treatment of the insane." He proceeds to analyze the asylum and the methods it adopted as the result of the tensions and ideas of Jacksonian society.[1]

Such an approach is clearly dictated in the consideration of nineteenth-century diagnosis and treatment of American women's nervous and sexual diseases.[2] The historian reading through the health books and medical manuals of the day dealing with the topic is confronted at once with a combination of scientific imprecision and emotionally charged conviction which demands interpretation.

Books written in the period between 1840 and 1900 consistently, if questionably, assert that a large number, even the majority, of middle-class American women were in some sense ill. Catharine Esther Beecher, daughter of the famous minister Lyman Beecher and a pioneer in women's education and hygiene, took as her chief concern in later life "the *health of women and children*" which, she wrote in 1866, had become "a matter of alarming interest" to all. In *Physiology and Calisthenics* she had already warned her readers that "there is a delicacy of constitution and an increase of disease, both among mature women and young girls, that is most alarming, and such as was never known in any former period." In *Letters to the People on Health and Happiness* she attempted to back up her apocalyptic rumblings with statistics. She had asked all of the numerous women she knew in cities and towns across the United States to make a list of the ten women each knew best, and rate their health as "perfectly healthy," "well," "delicate," "sick," "invalid," and so on. Her report, which covered hundreds of middle-class women, was as "alarming" as Beecher could have desired. Milwaukee, Wisconsin, provides a typical example:

> Milwaukee, Wisc. Mrs. A. frequent sick headaches. Mrs. B. very feeble. Mrs. S. well, except chills. Mrs. L. poor health constantly. Mrs. D. subject to frequent headaches. Mrs. B. very poor health. Mrs. C. consumption. Mrs. A. pelvic displacements and weakness. Mrs. H. pelvic disorders and a cough. Mrs.

ANN DOUGLAS is Professor of English at Columbia University, New York, New York.

Reprinted from *The Journal of Interdisciplinary History*, IV (1973), 25–52, by permission of *The Journal of Interdisciplinary History* and The M.I.T. Press, Cambridge, Massachusetts. Copyright © 1973, by the Massachusetts Institute of Technology and the editors of *The Journal of Interdisciplinary History*.

B. always sick. Do not know one healthy woman in the place.[3]

The accuracy of Beecher's findings is clearly open to question. How representative of other American women were her friends? How bad did a headache have to be to qualify a woman for ill health? And what woman in 1855 wanted to admit to so crude a state as robust vitality? Heroines of the sentimental fiction so popular with the women in the middle ranks of society whose health concerned Beecher were more often than not bearing up under a burden of sickness that would have incapacitated any less noble being. Indeed, as commentators on American society at the time emphasized, ill health in women had become positively fashionable and was exploited by its victims and practitioners as an advertisement of genteel sensibility and an escape from the too pressing demands of bedroom and kitchen.[4]

If the reliability of Beecher's statistics is shaky, their significance, on which this essay will focus, is not. Although American women of the eighteenth century may have been more sickly than their supposedly frail nineteenth-century descendants, they did not talk of themselves as sick; they did not define themselves through sickness, and their society apparently minimized rather than maximized their ill health, whatever its actual extent. As Meyer has argued, "attention" to a problem in a given period is as telling to the cultural historian as its actual "incidence," which may be almost impossible to determine.[5] Beecher's statistics at least reveal that a sizable number of American women wanted or needed to consider themselves ill.

Equally important, the self-diagnosis of these women was confirmed, even encouraged, by their society. Literary observers of the American scene like Cooper and Hawthorne were appalled at the delicate health of American women.[6] The doctors who specialized in women's diseases were equally gloomy and a good deal more verbose on the subject. Alcott, a noted Boston physician and author of several books on women's health, had estimated that one half of American women suffered from the "real disease" of nervousness. When Clarke of the Harvard Medical School published his controversial *Sex in Education,* he saw the ill health of middle- and upper-class American women as so

pervasive that he pessimistically concluded they would soon be unable to reproduce at all. "It requires no prophet to foretell that the wives who are to be mothers in our republic must be drawn from trans-Atlantic homes," he announced.[7]

Beecher not only emphasized that many American women in the middle and upper ranks of society were sick, but also implied that they were ill precisely *because they were women.* Most of the ailments that she records—pelvic disorders, sick headaches, general nervousness—were regarded as symptoms of "female complaints," nervous disorders thought to be linked with the malfunctioning of the feminine sexual organs.

This is not to imply that men could not and did not display similar symptoms. Napheys, for example, in 1878, noted peevishness, listlessness, pallor, and headaches in men and boys who practiced the "secret vice" of masturbation. Beard found men and women suffering from what he termed "American nervousness."[8] No doctor implied that signs of nervous disorder were apparent only in women in nineteenth-century America, and the historian should not overlook this evidence. The fact remains, nonetheless, that to some extent the *diagnosis,* and to a greater extent the *treatment* by doctors of these symptoms in women, were different from their interpretation of the same signs in men. This difference was inevitable, because medical analysis of a woman began and ended with consideration of an organ unique to her, namely her uterus. Here, supposedly, lay the cause and the cure of many of her physical ailments. As a result of this special focus, medical reactions to female nervous complaints are indicative of nineteenth-century American attitudes not only toward disease and sexuality in general but, more significantly, toward feminine sexual identity in particular.

Doctors in America throughout the nineteenth century directed their attention to the womb in a way that seems decidedly unscientific and even obsessive to a modern observer. Popular manuals on women's health neglected discussion of widespread and fatal diseases like breast cancer and consumption and concentrated on every type of menstrual and uterine disorder conceivable.[9] Hubbard, a professor from New Haven, addressing a medical society in 1870, explained that it seemed "as if the Almighty, in creating the female sex, *had taken the uterus and built up a woman around it.*"[10] And the uterus, so essential to womankind, was apparently a highly perilous possession. Dewees, professor of midwifery at the University of Pennsylvania in the early part of the nineteenth century, stated in his standard work on the diseases of females that woman was subject to twice the sicknesses that affected man just because she has a womb. Her uterus exercises a "paramount power" over her physical and moral system, and its sway is "no less whimsical than potent." Furthermore, "she is constantly liable to irregularities in her menstrua, and menaced severely by their consequences."[11] It was these highly contagious irregularities in her womb's workings which were thought to produce the headaches, nervousness, and feebleness detailed by Beecher. Byford, professor of gynecology in the 1860s at the University of Chicago, was moved to exclaim in his monograph on the uterus, "It is almost a pity that a woman has a womb."

Rather complacently viewing the havoc that their natural biological disadvantages wreaked on women, these doctors detailed the symptoms of a typical case of (uterine-caused) nervous prostration. Its victims, like the women on whose health Beecher reported, according to Byford, would usually lose weight: They would frequently show a peevish irritability and suffer every kind of nervous disorder ranging from hysterical fits of crying and insomnia to constipation, indigestion, headaches, and backaches.[12] Since many of the practitioners of the first half of the nineteenth century traced all of these problems to disorders of the uterus, they consequently tried to cure them through what came to be called "local treatment," remedies specifically directed at the womb. This meant that not only the woman suffering from *prolapsus uteri* as the result of childbearing or the lady with cancer of the uterus or any menstrual difficulty, but also the girl suffering from backache and an irritable disposition with no discernible problem in her uterus might well be subjected to local treatment in the period 1830–1860.

"Local treatment" could mean manual adjustment by a doctor of a slipped uterus, a problem all too current in an age of poor midwifery, and the insertion of various pessaries for its support. It was more frequently used to designate a course of local medication for everything from cancer to cantan-

kerousness. This treatment had four stages, although not every case went through all four: a manual investigation, "leeching," "injections," and "cauterization." Dewees and Bennet, a famous English gynecologist widely read in America, both advocated placing the leeches right on the vulva or the neck of the uterus, although Bennet cautioned the doctor to count them as they dropped off when satiated, lest he "lose" some. Bennet had known adventurous leeches to advance into the cervical cavity of the uterus itself, and he noted: "I think I have scarcely ever seen more acute pain than that experienced by several of my patients under these circumstances."[13] Less distressing to a twentieth-century mind, but perhaps even more senseless, were the "injections" into the uterus advocated by these doctors. The uterus became a kind of catchall, or what one exasperated doctor referred to as a "Chinese toy shop": Water, milk and water, linseed tea, and "decoction of marshmellow . . . tepid or cold" found their way inside nervous women patients.[14] The final step, performed at this time, one must remember, with no anesthetic but a little opium or alcohol, was cauterization, either through the application of nitrate of silver, or, in cases of more severe infection, through the use of the much stronger hydrate of potassa, or even the "actual cautery," a "white-hot iron" instrument.[15] The principle here is medically understandable and even sound: to drive out one infection by creating a greater inflammation, and thus provoking the blood cells to activity great enough to heal both irritations. But the treatment was used, it must be remembered, even when there was no uterine infection, and it was subject to great abuses in itself as its best practitioners realized. "It is an easy matter," Byford noted, "to do violence to the mucous membrane by a very little rudeness of management." In a successful case, the uterus was left "raw and bleeding" and the patient in severe pain for several days; in an unsuccessful one, severe hemorrhage and terrible pain might result.[16] It should be noted that the cauterization process, whether by chemicals or by the iron, had to be repeated several times at intervals of a few days.[17]

In the 1870s and 1880s, this form of treatment was largely dropped. Austin, in his book *Perils of American Women,* came out against local treatment and dismissed cauterization as a relic of the barbaric past of a decade ago:

Thus it happened that thousands of women have been doomed to undergo the nitrate-of-silver treatment—their mental agony and physical torture were accounted nothing—in cases where soap and water and a gentle placebo would have been amply sufficient.[18]

Austin had his own panacea for women's nervous diseases, however. He was a devoted believer in the Philadelphia doctor S. Weir Mitchell and his famous "rest cure."

Firmly opposed to the cauterization school, Mitchell evolved a method of his own, which, in his own words, was "a combination of entire rest and of excessive feeding, made possible by passive exercise obtained through steady use of massage and electricity."[19] When he said "entire rest," he meant it. For some six weeks, the patient was removed from her home, and allowed to see no one except the doctor and a hired nurse. Confined to her bed flat on her back, she was permitted neither to read, nor, in some cases, even to rise to urinate. The massage treatment which covered the whole body lasted an hour daily. Becoming progressively more vigorous, it was designed to counteract the debilitating effects of such a prolonged stay in bed. Meanwhile the patient was expected to eat steadily, and gain weight daily. Mitchell's claims to have cured menstrual disorders and every kind of "nervous" ailment met with widespread acceptance. He was the best known and most successful woman's doctor of his generation.

Both the local treatment and the rest cure look to a modern viewer at best like very imperfect forms of medical treatment for complex problems. The first was always painful and often fruitless; the second was frequently tedious and occasionally irrelevant. Both, as we will see, could exacerbate rather than diminish the nervous state they were designed to cure. One's first temptation is to dismiss them as the products of an unscientific age, and there is ample evidence to support such an attitude.

Before the Civil War the American doctor was quite simply ignorant, and even his post–Civil War successor did not receive the training expected of a doctor today. Few medical schools before 1860 required more than two years of attendance; almost none provided clinical experience for their fledgling physicians.[20] Furthermore, gynecology at this period was perhaps the weakest link in the already weak armor of the nineteenth-century doctor's medical knowledge. Lectures on "midwifery" and the sexual organs, as Elizabeth Blackwell was to learn, usually provided a professor more opportunity for dirty jokes than for the dissemination of knowledge.[21] J. Marion Sims, a pioneer in gynecological surgery, frequently lamented the frightening ignorance which seemed especially to attend doctors on the subject of women's ailments. He wrote feelingly about one lady who had long suffered from internal problems and from the cures designed to relieve them:

> The leeching, the physicking, the blistering, the anodynes, the baths, the mountain excursions, the sea-bathing and sea voyages that this poor patient suffered and endured for years are almost incredible![22]

He restored her to health by a simple operation.

Doctors had some excuse for their ignorance of woman's internal organs, although little for their pretended knowledge. Ladies were expected, even by their doctors, to object to "local examination," to prefer modesty to health, and many of them did.[23] The French physician Médéric Louis Elie Moreau de St. Méry had commented on the unwillingness of Philadelphia women in the late eighteenth century to undergo even crucially necessary medical scrutiny, and Dewees, in the same city at the start of the next century, recounted several tales of women who put themselves in the hands of quacks rather than endure this ordeal. Bennet, the London authority, crusaded against the "absolutely criminal" delicacy of doctors who respected such fears in female patients.[24] He rightly attributed the birth of gynecology as a science to the increased possibility of uterine examination because of the use of the speculum and gradually changing attitudes.

Yet the ignorance of American doctors and the difficulties in the way of overcoming it certainly cannot explain the *forms* of the treatments they devised for nervous women. To understand these, one must cease to regard these fledgling gynecological techniques as part of a developing science and scrutinize them as part and parcel of a fully formed culture, and, as such, sharing in all the biases and assumptions about women which that culture possessed. This in no way suggests a failure of concern or goodwill on the part of nineteenth-century American doctors. Undeniably, the majority of these physicians were anxious to aid their female patients. J. Marion Sims, who devoted his life to the intelligent relief of woman's diseases, is only an illustrious example of what was surely a numerous class. Yet it seems equally undeniable that a complicated if unacknowledged psychological warfare was being waged between the doctors and their patients. Even the best-intentioned practitioner was forced into a role in part hostile to his woman patients simply by the misconceptions he was trained to hold. Until well after the Civil War, for example, physicians in America, as in Europe, arguing by analogy with the animal world, maintained that woman's fertile period was right before and after menstruation.[25] Hence the nineteenth-century American woman, perhaps in ill health and eager to practice a semirespectable form of birth control, conscientiously slept with her spouse squarely in the middle of her menstrual cycle.

Given the presumably disastrous results action on this belief must have produced, one must turn from the world of science to the realm of culture to explain its surprising tenacity, and the equal persistence with which treatments like cauterization and the rest cure kept their hold in the medical world. Physicians both of the cauterist school and of the rest cure school brought certain unexplored but pervasive presuppositions to their work. They assumed, as already mentioned, that women were physically dominated by their wombs. They held, moreover, even less carefully scrutinized beliefs about the social and psychological nature of femininity and its role and responsibilities in their society, beliefs which colored their attitude toward the illness of their female patients.

The first point to be noted is the element of distrust, even of condemnation, lurking behind their diagnoses. Physicians tended to stress a certain moral depravity inherent in feminine nervous disorders and to waver significantly between labeling it a result and analyzing it as the cause of the physical symptoms involved. The patient, according to Byford's experience, may become "a changed woman"—irritable, indecisive, lacking in willpower, morose, jealous. She is likely to show "a guarded cunning, a deceitful and perverted consciousness"; indeed, she may commit "acts of a de-

praved and indecent nature," and neglect her "duty in all the relations of life."[26]

In part, Byford was indirectly expressing his doubts as to whether or not his patients were truly sick. Such doubts were widely shared. Dixon, in *Woman and Her Diseases,* cautioned the physician always to pay "profound attention" to what he delicately called "moral circumstances." These moral causes were often, he warned, not of a nature "calculated to move our sympathy," and he was all too aware that women were cunning enough to "pretend hysteric attacks, in order to excite sympathy and obtain some desired end."[27] Even more important, of course, was the doctor's unspoken guess at the *reason* behind this calculated exploitation of illness. Who can doubt that, in an age when sex and childbirth involved very real threats to the health and life of women, some women would use the pretext of being "delicate" as a way not only of escaping household labor but also of closing the bedroom door while avoiding the guilt consequent upon a more flagrant defiance of their "duties"? Harriet Beecher Stowe understood the process and dramatized it at its worst in her portrait of Mrs. St. Clair (in *Uncle Tom's Cabin*) lying on her sofa, shirking responsibility and demanding attention. And Stowe herself, who suffered the burden of relative poverty and of a weak and dependent but potent husband, took periodic refuge from him and their numerous offspring in those havens of escape, the health establishments.[28]

Clearly, in the case of a woman like Stowe, however, we do not have the simple problem of a woman failing to live up to her sexual and domestic responsibilities as we do in the case of her own fictional creation, Mrs. St. Clair. It is rather that her responsibilities, despite all her histrionic and martyred posturings about them, were genuinely more than she could handle: They were almost killing her. Doctors of the period were intermittently and partially aware of the frustrations inherent in the middle-class woman's lot. Alexander Combe, the Scottish phrenologist so influential in America, attributed the high level of insanity in women of this class to the monotony of their lives.[29] In 1834, Dr. Alcott of Boston advocated that ladies be trained as nurses because "these are individuals who need some employment, for the sake even of the emolument; but more especially to save them from ennui, and disgust, and misery—sometimes from speedy or more protracted suicide."[30] Professional work, however, was hardly a socially acceptable escape from a lady's situation, but sickness, that very nervous condition brought on by the frustrations of her life, was.

Yet, many doctors, despite the apparent conscious understanding shown in the analysis of Combe and Alcott, in practice tended unconsciously to see the neuralgic ailments of their female patients as a threatening and culpable shirking of their duties as wives and mothers, and to look upon those duties as the cure, not the cause, of the illness. Self-sacrifice and altruism on a spiritual level, and childbearing and housework on a more practical one, constituted healthy femininity in the eyes of most nineteenth-century Americans. Dr. Clarke of Harvard, who believed that girls of the 1870s were ill because they were quite literally destroying their wombs and their childbearing potential by presuming to pursue a course of higher education intended by nature only for the male sex, was very much a spokesman for the doctors of his generation.

One finds an underlying logic running through popular books by physicians on women's diseases to the effect that ladies get sick *because* they are unfeminine—in other words, sexually aggressive, intellectually ambitious, and defective in proper womanly submission and selflessness. Bad health habits were often put forth by doctors and others as causes of nervous complaints. But these, consisting as they did of improper diet, light reading, late hours, tight lacing, and inadequate clothing, were in themselves a badge of the "fashionable" and flirtatious female, only a step removed in popular imagination from the infamous one. Byford believed that "the influence of lascivious books" and frequent "indulgence" in intercourse would precipitate neuralgia.[31] Significantly, in Mitchell's fiction, the sick woman is almost invariably the closest thing he has to a villainess and she is often intelligent and usually predatory to an extreme. In *Roland Blake*, published in 1886, Octapia Darnell, an invalid, is branded by her name. Octopuslike, she uses her sickness like tentacles to try to squeeze the life out of her innocent young cousin, Olivia Wynne. Although we see her in genuine nervous spasms, Mitchell never shows her seized by a convulsion

where it would be inconvenient to her purposes, nor does he let us forget that when she needs physical strength to accomplish her will, she always summons it. Again, the heroine of *Constance Trescott* (1905), his last and best novel, is driven by a demonic will to possess utterly where she loves and to revenge totally where she hates. Rather predictably she turns to invalidism at the book's close to gain her ends.

It is not that Mitchell totally condemns these women. Instead, he understands them, and adopts a tone of pitying patronage toward them. He thinks they are genuinely sick, but he believes, as did Clarke, that the root of their sickness was their failure to be women, to sacrifice themselves for others, and to perform their feminine duties. Typically, Octapia Darnell has a brief period of improvement when a "recent need to think of others had beneficently taken her outside of the slowly narrowing circle of self-care and self-contemplation, and, by relieving her of some of the morbid habits of disease, had greatly bettered her physical condition."[32] The truth is that Mitchell does not even need to blame or punish her: In his view, nature has conveniently done that job for him.

Mitchell's analysis, then, one standard with doctors in the nineteenth century, served an important psychological purpose, whatever its medical validity. The doctor, on some unacknowledged level, feared his female patient. Could he so emphasize the diseased potency of woman's unique and mysterious organ, the womb, if he did not worry that his sex, the constant companion of hers, was in some way menaced? How comfortable Mitchell must have felt, when, addressing a graduating Radcliffe class, he expressed his clearly faint hope "that no wreck from these shores will be drifted into my dockyard."[33] They might begin as his competitors, but, despite it—in fact, because of it—they would end as his patients.

Mitchell and his peers could indeed afford to pity the fair sex, even perhaps to "cure" them. Yet the consequent "cures" bore unmistakable signs of their culturally determined origin, for they made a woman's womb very much a liability. Since her disease was unconsciously viewed as a symptom of a failure in femininity, its remedy was designed both as a punishment and an agent of regeneration, for it forced her to acknowledge her womanhood and made her totally dependent on the professional prowess of her male doctor. The cauterizer, with his injections, leeches, and hot irons, seems suggestive of a veiled but aggressively hostile male sexuality and superiority, and the rest cure expert carried this spirit to a sophisticated culmination.

Mitchell's treatment depended in actuality not so much on the techniques of rest and overfeeding, as on the commanding personality and charismatic will of the physician. "A slight, pale lad of no physical strength" by his own description, he moved as a young man in the shadow of his dominating, joyous, strong doctor-father.[34] To be the strong, healing male in a world of ailing, dependent women had obvious charms for him. "Electric with fascination" for women as his granddaughter saw him, he acknowledged that he played the "despot" in the sickroom, and boasted of reducing patients to the docility of children.[35] Doctors had always preferred to keep women in ignorance, and Mitchell was no exception. In a characteristically urbane and aphoristic remark, he said, "Wise women choose their doctors and trust them. The wisest ask the fewest questions."[36] But he wanted to be more than trusted: He wished to be revered, even adored, and he succeeded. The totality of the power he could acquire is revealed in a letter he received from a sick woman who positively grovels before him as she rhapsodizes on his potency:

> Whilst laid by the heels in a country-house with an attack of grippe, also an invalid from gastric affection, the weary eyes of a sick woman fall upon your face in the *Century* of this month—a thrill passed through me—at last I saw the true physician![37]

It is clear, moreover, that Mitchell encouraged this worshiping attitude as an important element in his "cure." A doctor, in his view, if he had the proper mesmeric powers of will, could become almost godlike.[38] Women doctors would always be inferior to male physicians, he believed, precisely because they could not exercise such tyranny: They were unable to "obtain the needed control over those of their own sex."[39] Mitchell here skated on the edge of a theory of primitive healing through mesmeric sexual powers.[40] Furthermore, his treatment was designed to make his female patients take his view of the doctor's role. They were allowed to

see no one but him, and to talk of their ills and problems to no one else. As doctor he became the only spot of energy, the only source of *life*, during the enforced repose of a cure process.

Undoubtedly, if Mitchell were aware of what he was doing, he would have felt it justifiable and even merciful. He was curing his patients—by restoring them to their femininity or, in other words, by subordinating them to an enlightened but dictatorial male will. His admirers delighted to tell how, when a strangely recalcitrant patient refused to rise from bed after Mitchell had decreed that her rest cure was over, Mitchell threatened to move into bed with her if she did not get up, and even started to undress. When he got to his pants, she got up. Although the story may well be apocryphal, its spirit is not. Not surprisingly, the lady in question was fleeing the fact where she embraced the shadow, for symbolically, Mitchell, like his cauterizing predecessor, played the role of possessor, even impregnator, in the cure process. Dominated, overfed often to the point of obesity, caressed and (quite literally) vibrating, were not his patients being returned to health—to womanhood?[41] The only other time that the Victorian lady took to her bed and got fat was, in fact, before delivery. J. Marion Sims had noted that his colleagues were erroneously wont to lament about a sick woman: "If she could only have a child, it would cure her."[42] Although he was a generation later, Mitchell was not so different from the doctors Sims opposed who looked to pregnancy for the cure of all feminine ills.

Here one senses a clue to the pertinacity with which doctors told women anxious to avoid pregnancy that they should sleep with their husbands only during what we now know as their most fertile period. In a sense, the practices and writings of the medical profession provide the other half of the picture of ideal womanhood presented in the sentimental literature of the day. Woman was at her holiest, according to the genteel novels and poetry of Victorian America, as a mother. Pregnancy itself, however, was avoided by the authors of such works as completely as the act of impregnation. The medical manual took on the role of frankness disowned by its more discreet companion. All the logic of contemporary medical lore adds up to the lesson that women were at their most feminine when they were pregnant. Pregnant, they were visible emblems of masculine potency.

It is impossible to determine how many nine-teenth-century middle-class American women went to doctors, just as it is difficult to tell how real their much-advertised ailments were. Reluctant as American women apparently were to undergo local examination, many of them presumably stayed home and suffered with no medical aid except that provided by earlier versions of Lydia Pinkham's patent medicine. Others trusted to the hydropathic remedies provided at numerous water cures or used homeopathic drugs, both of which represented forms of protest against current medical practices.[43] Furthermore, the majority of women suffering from uterine and/or nervous disorders who underwent a form of local treatment or, later, the rest cure were presumably in real distress and glad of whatever help their physician could offer.[44] Some, however, were undoubtedly using prescribed treatments for their own purposes. According to numerous masculine and feminine observers, many women grew positively addicted to local treatment as others did later to the rest cure, but, not surprisingly, these women have not left any direct confessions to posterity.[45]

What we do have record of is a masked but almost hysterical paranoia among a small group of feminist hygiene experts and lady doctors, a paranoia stemming from their exaggerated but astute perception of the unconscious purposes underlying the attitudes and practices of doctors with women patients. In their excited view, current medical treatment was patently not science, for which they professed respect, but a part of their male-dominated culture, for which they had both fear and contempt. They saw it as a form of rape, designed to keep woman prostrate, a perpetual patient dependent on a doctor's supposed professional expertise.

No one expressed this attitude better than did two Beecher women, Catharine Esther Beecher, who crusaded against local treatment, and her grandniece Charlotte Perkins Gilman, who protested against Mitchell's rest cure a generation later. Each of them wrote a work dedicated to exposing what they felt were the unstated motives of physicians treating women patients. In *Letters to the People on Health and Happiness,* Beecher described with heavy-handed irony the ineffectuality of the string of "talented, highly-educated and celebrated" doctors who had tried to cure her own severe nervous

ailments (115).[46] She consumed sulphur and iron, she let one doctor sever the "wounded nerves from their centres," she let another cover her spine with "tartar emetic pustules," she subjected herself to "animal magnetism" and the water cure, but all to no purpose.

Beecher does not admit to having personally undergone local treatment, but when she discusses it, her tone changes from the condescending playfulness she uses to devastate such methods as the "tartar emetic pustules" to one of outraged horror. Doctors playing professional games with pustules had kept her sick perhaps, but they had left her with her honor. Local treatment, roughly equivalent to rape according to Beecher, seldom allowed a lady to retain that valuable possession. It is "performed," she explains, "with bolted doors and curtained windows, and with no one present but patient and operator," by doctors who have all too often "freely advocated the doctrine that there was no true marriage but the union of persons who were in love." Predictably, these immoral practitioners were said to have "lost all reverence for the Bible." With his "interesting" female patients, such a physician "naturally," in Beecher's gloomy view, tries "to lead them to adopt *his views of truth and right*" on moral matters. "Then he daily has all the opportunities indicated [through local examination]. Does anyone need more than to hear these facts to know what the not unfrequent results must be?" she ominously concludes (136). By the time she is through with this subject, she is calling the female patients "victims" and lamenting their "entire helplessness" (137). She refers the reader to an appended letter from a woman doctor, Mrs. R. B. Gleason of the Elmira Water Cure in New York, who solemnly testifies that manual replacement for *prolapsus uteri* was "in most cases totally needless, and in many decidedly injurious" (6*). After such evidence, Beecher can hardly avoid "the painful inquiry": "how can a woman *ever know* to whom she may safely entrust herself . . . in such painful and peculiar circumstances?" (138).

Gilman, a brilliant theorist and critic on women's role in American society, went through periods of nervous prostration strikingly similar to those of her aged relative's.[47] She sampled the fruits of medical wisdom a few decades later, undergoing Mitchell's rest cure. She expressed the result in a story entitled "The Yellow Wall Paper," published in 1890, and designed to convince Mitchell "of the error of his ways."[48]

The story concerns a married woman, the mother of a young child, suffering from "nervous" disorders, and clearly laboring under disguised but immense (and justifiable) hostility for both her spouse and her offspring. Her husband, John, who is a doctor, is ostensibly overseeing her cure, but is in reality intent with sadistic ignorance on destroying her body and soul. John, apparently modeled on Mitchell himself, confines his wife to a country house, which to her seems "haunted," remote from friends or neighbors. Presumably hoping to force her back to her feminine and maternal functions, he symbolically makes her sleep in an old nursery. With its barred windows, rings attached to the wall, bed nailed to the floor, and disturbing and torn yellow wallpaper, this nursery all too significantly and frighteningly resembles a cell for the insane. Treating her like a pet, the doctor alternates condescending tenderness ("Then he took me in his arms and called me a blessed little goose" [323]) with threats of punishment ("John says if I don't pick up faster he shall send me to Weir Mitchell in the fall"[326]). Since John "never was nervous in his life" (323), and is a doctor "of high standing" (320) to boot, he can "laugh" at her fears because he "knows there is no *reason* to suffer, and that satisfies him" (323). Complacently smug in his masculine insensitivity and his professional superiority, he is totally obtuse about the nature of her suffering and its possible cure. An early-day "mad housewife," she has been so browbeaten by his calm assumption of superiority that she can only timidly air the frightening truth:

> John is a physician, and *perhaps*—(I would not say it to a living soul, of course, but this is dead paper and a great relief to my mind)—*perhaps* that is one reason I do not get well faster. (320)

He has left her with only one recourse, and she takes it. Slowly but steadily, she goes mad, thus dramatically pointing up the results of his "cure." At the story's close, she is creeping on hands and knees with insane persistence around the walls of her chamber. In a symbolic moment, her husband, suspicious about her behavior, breaks down the door she has finally locked against him. His act is the essence of his "cure" and her "problem"; like Cath-

arine Beecher, Gilman sees the doctor "treating" his patient as violating her. But this patient is finally beyond feeling. When John faints away in shock at her state, their roles have been reversed: *He* has become the woman, the nervous, susceptible, sickly patient, and she wonders with a kind of calm, self-centered vindictiveness fully equal to his former arrogance: "Now why should that man have fainted? But he did, and right across my path by the wall, so that I had to creep over him every time!" (337). She has won, because she can ignore him now as completely as he ignored her, but she has won at the cost of becoming what he subconsciously sought to make her—a creeping creature, an animal and an automaton.

Beecher's *Letters* and Gilman's story are both intended to convey a nightmare vision of sick women dependent on male doctors who use their professional superiority as a method to prolong their patients' sickness and, consequently, the supremacy of their own sex. Both writers also hint, however, at a possible escape for such feminine victims. Beecher, according to her account, was finally cured by a timely tip from a *woman* physician, Dr. Elizabeth Blackwell. Gilman's heroine knows what her cure should be—work and intellectual stimulation—although she is too cowed and powerless to insist on it. Both Gilman and Beecher simply in writing their works are implying that the untutored common sense of two women can outdo the professionally trained brains of those male doctors who labored in vain to cure them. Both are thus in essence urging that a woman should be independent, that *she be her own physician*, so that the real business of healing can get under way.[49]

After all, Beecher and Gilman realized, there might be two possible ways of looking at the much-advertised problem of the increasingly bad health of middle-class American women. Doctors like Clarke and Mitchell liked to think that the fault lay with the women themselves, who were neglecting their homes and pursuing such an unfeminine goal as higher education. Women like Beecher and Gilman, shrewdly reversing the charge, queried whether the blame might not belong to the men who were supposed to cure them and to the professional training which was supposed to enable them to do it. Harriot Hunt, one of the most impressive of the early women doctors in America, put the challenge succinctly: "Man, man alone has had the care of *us* [women], and I would ask how *our health stands now.* Does it do credit to *his* skill?"[50] Hunt is clearly aware that what had been a condemnation of women (the charge of ill health) could be used as a powerful weapon in their defense. The women doctors who began to appear on the American scene in the 1850s saw women's diseases as a *result* of submission, and promoted independence from masculine domination, whether professional or sexual, as their cure for feminine ailments.[51]

In dealing with these pioneer women doctors and their theories, one is at once aware that here, too, the issues are inevitably cultural rather than scientific. Their primary aim, often an unconscious one, was to free ailing women from male control. On the one hand, this desire could and did further scientific advancement, for their distrust of the male doctor made them eager to reject aspects of medical practice that were in fact unscientific, if not harmful. Their paranoid fear that the male doctor was degrading his female patient paradoxically led them to some sound conclusions about the worthlessness of many drugs and the necessity of sanitation and preventive medicine. On the other hand, the same fear also made them, on occasion, throw out the baby with the bath water. Their hostility to the male doctor too often became a hostility to any scientific practice which appeared to their oversensitive consciousness as an invasion of the patient's privacy. Gynecological surgery, for example, which, despite undoubted abuse, represented a significant step in medical treatment of women, was often rejected by these early pioneers. Yet one must keep in mind that what is unwitting stupidity from a scientific point of view can be (albeit equally unwitting) shrewdness from a social or political point of view. These women bypassed science in large part because they had a goal quite distinct from its advancement: namely, the advancement of their sex.

Nowhere is this aim clearer than in the work of Hunt, a well-known, if home-trained, Boston practitioner and the most outspoken of the first generation of women doctors. Her autobiography, *Glances and Glimpses* (1856), published when she was forty-one, is clearly oversimplified, one-sided, and sentimentalized, but one must keep in mind that she was writing not a scientific report, or even a history, but rather a special kind of mythologized propaganda, scenario for a sexual revolution.

The ritualized drama begins with Hunt's explanation of why she chose medicine for a career—her stunned realization of the profound ignorance of the male doctors treating feminine diseases (81).[52] Her ailing sister was put through a course of remedies somewhat similar to the one Beecher tried, and she, and Harriot, came away having "lost all confidence in medicine" (85). The male practitioner here emerges as one of the villains of Hunt's piece. According to her testimony, he usually made his living by creating false dependencies in his female patients, by keeping them ignorant and totally reliant on his shortsighted or even harmful remedies (32, 89). Indeed, Hunt insinuates, his professional training led him actually to want his patients to be sick so that he would have something to do with all the games he had learned.

Professional exploitation by the doctor of his female patient was a mask, in Hunt's opinion, for a deeper and more humiliating sexual exploitation. Like Catharine Beecher, Hunt was publicly and loudly aghast at local examinations. They were "*too often unnecessary*" (271) and their moral effects were terrible. Many medical men, in her view, were skeptics, who lived "sensually" (177), and contaminated their patients. At this point, Hunt's scenario grows both alarmist and lurid. A woman once forced to submit to local examination, Hunt reveals, was well on the road to ruin: She felt "disgraced, and a don't careativeness [*sic*] and sort of sullen desperation" settled on her (184). Yet this fantasized sexual violation was dreadful, according to Hunt, not so much because of the moral degradation involved as because of the patient's loss of control and her consequent dependence on the doctor's will. In describing a physician who took advantage of a patient and left her with an illegitimate child, she explains significantly: His "will overmastered the weaker will of his patient" (376).

The doctor's was not the only malevolent will pitted against his woman patient's will in Hunt's story. The villainous physicians who kept women sick were only collaborating with the villainous husbands who had caused their illnesses in the first place. In her favorite role as minister-doctor, she collected many of what she called the "heart-histories" of her women patients, and publicized them as evidence that women's "physical maladies" stemmed from "concealed sorrows" (139), often at the "sins" of their spouses (159).[53] Hunt never married, but she was always ready with sympathy for those who had. One married patient after another apparently confided to her: "I thank heaven, my dear doctor, that you are a woman; for now I can tell you the truth about my health. It is not my body that is sick but my heart" (120).

Hunt's vision, so filled with villains and victims, has a savior to offer as well. This heroine is of course Hunt herself, as a woman doctor and simply as a woman. As a doctor, she dramatically renounced "medical science" as "full of unnecessary details," but without "a soul . . . a huge, unwieldy body—distorted, deformed, inconsistent and complicated" (121). Medicine was generally "worse than useless" (371), she remarked; moreover, it did not meet her "perception of the dignity of the human body." She did not enter "the medical life through physics, but through metaphysics" (127). She was only too eager to announce her disavowal of "science," because she considered her disrespect precisely her strongest claim to respect. Flaunting her antiprofessionalism like a medal of honor, she loved to proclaim herself an eclectic, as indeed she was, the "disciple of no medical sect" (171), but the sworn servant of her sex.[54]

Hunt's treatment consisted of telling her patients to throw away their medicines, begin a diary, and think of their mothers (401). The last item of this prescription is not simply the pure sentimentalism that it might appear. Hunt was symbolically turning her patients' thoughts to an acceptable but potent emblem of *female strength*.[55] It was from this source that she expected her patients to find their cure—not in the arms of their husbands, or under the hands of the male doctor. The medicine that she gave her patients as a sure antidote to the wares peddled by her masculine colleagues was the example of her own ample and self-sufficient womanhood. Could they forget their mothers with Hunt before them?

Hunt was an ardent and proclaimed feminist and suffragist, but other women pioneers in medicine who did not share, or did not avow, such sympathies were almost without exception part of her crusade.[56] The most famous of these was Elizabeth Blackwell, usually considered the first woman doctor in America. In her girlhood an avowed admirer of the fiercely virginal goddess Diana, Blackwell always loved to project an almost monstrous force as woman's natural dowry.[57] Yet she was clearly

drawn to such fantasies precisely because of her deep-seated perception and fear of the dependent role women usually played. With paradoxical logic, she explained that precisely *because* she was very "susceptible" to men and perpetually in love, she had determined never to marry. Not initially attracted to medicine, she deliberately chose it as a potentially "strong barrier between me and all ordinary marriage. I must have something to engross my thoughts, some object in life which will fulfill this vacuum and prevent this sad wearing away of the heart."[58]

Professionally, despite her soft-spoken, conciliating manner, she fought the code of the male medical establishment which in her view victimized women as surely as did matrimony. During medical school, she was shocked at the "horrible exposure" of women to male physicians, finding it "indecent for any poor woman to be subjected to such a torture."[59] In her later years, when local treatment was less common, Blackwell crusaded against its medical descendant, ovariotomy, or as she called it with characteristic dramatic flair, "the castration of women." Estimating that 1 of every 250 women in Europe had been "castrated," she collected newspaper clippings which supported her belief that young doctors were performing this operation needlessly on unsuspecting women just to obtain professional practice.[60]

The validity of Blackwell's fears is hard to estimate. Many reputable people shared them. Yet Dr. Marie Zakrzewska lamented the fact that women had come to her Boston hospital insisting that their ovaries be removed as a birth control device.[61] Nonetheless, in Blackwell's eyes, male doctors were performing a kind of "vivisection"—a practice that she violently opposed in any form—on their female patients.[62] Ovariotomies for her simply dramatized the antiwoman bias of much of modern science. If man were going to dedicate himself to cold-blooded experimentation, would not woman be his ultimate subject? Consequently, despite her fine mind and excellent training, Blackwell, an incipient Christian Scientist, obstinately opposed not just the usual run of drugs and medication, but vaccination and "all medical methods which introduce any degree of morbid matter into the blood of the human system."[63] All such practices were "especially antagonistic to women."[64] Blackwell's medical shortsightedness seems ludicrous, perhaps culpable, but it furthered her underlying and nonmedical goals.

To distrust science was to distrust masculinity, and to create an apparent immediate and desperate need for women doctors. She saw these projected new physicians, moreover, as undercover agents in enemy territory. Her advice to them reads a bit like a lesson in subversion. Proud that she had determined early in her career to *"commit heresy with intelligence"* to escape the perils of professionalized medicine, she declared that women doctors should not countenance practices like ovariotomies, vaccination, and vivisection.[65] In a crucial essay entitled "The Influence of Women in the Profession of Medicine" (1889), she urged women medical students, unfortunately, like all of their sex, trained to "accept the government and instruction of men as final" (20), to exercise a "mild skepticism" (21).[66] Their task was quite simply to revamp the whole medical profession, for, as she explained, "methods and conclusions formed by one half the race only must necessarily require revision as the other half of humanity rises into conscious responsibility" (20). They had a sure guide in this apparently momentous undertaking: Nothing that revolted their "moral sense as earnest women" could be scientifically true, and no "logical sophistry" (30) could make it so. In a letter to a medical colleague, she echoes Emerson as she anticipates a day when women will plant themselves firmly "on the God-given force of their maternal nature" and oppose the male intellect in its too restless search for scientific truth.[67]

Blackwell was very clever. Male doctors had indirectly told their women patients that their procreative femininity was their dearest treasure. Coining that treasure into current cash, Blackwell pointed to her sacred maternal nature as justification for a revolt against the ways of the male doctor. For the woman physician of Blackwell's vision, womanhood was hardly a liability, and very much a weapon. She was no subordinate, but an aggressive censor of the masculine world.[68] Blackwell herself was only too ready. Calling herself a "Christian physiologist," she fought prostitution, masturbation, and obscene literature in addition to various medical abuses. It was in these crusades that her underlying antimale bias most dramatically expressed itself. With so many of her feminine peers, she liked to see male sexuality, like male science, as one more method used by men to debase women to their own level by seducing them, and to keep them dependent by forcing them into parasitism. Blackwell's target in the antiprostitution campaign organized by the Purity Alliance was not the prostitute, but her exploiter.[69] "Male lust must be restrained in order to check female obscenity"[70] was the telling slogan Blackwell issued in one of her many essays on the subject. It is not too much to say that the paid whore whom Blackwell wished to regenerate was simply another version of the female patient corrupted by immoral medical practices whom Beecher and Hunt had sought to redeem.

It is telling that Blackwell, like most of the first generation of women doctors, chose hygiene, or preventive medicine, as her chosen field, and she made great contributions there, despite her distrust of vaccination. There can be no doubt, furthermore, that she and her feminine colleagues contributed significantly to improve treatment of women's and children's diseases.[71] But they also answered a different and more subtle need strongly felt by some members of their sex. If the woman patient dependent on the male doctor had seemed to feminists like Beecher and Gilman emblematic of the most degrading elements in woman's relation to man in nineteenth-century America, the woman doctor, able to take care of herself and cure the world's ills, appeared to them not only as a beacon of hope but as an avenger of the wrongs of all those prostrate women, whether victimized in an office or in their own homes.

Elizabeth Stuart Phelps, an immensely popular post–Civil War author who knew personally every variety of nervous disorder in its most acute form, celebrated this revengeful angel in *Dr. Zay* (1882), a novel about a woman doctor.[72] Dr. Zay's first name rather appropriately is Atalanta. Totally self-confident, direct, brilliant, and rather unpoetic although womanly, she exudes the independence and the self-sufficiency that Elizabeth Blackwell and Harriot Hunt had so longed to see in their sex. Like them, she has devoted herself to relieving the sufferings of women and, a Christian physiologist of the first order, she even brings off shotgun weddings as part of her healing mission. The novel centers on her relationship with her only male patient—a young man named Waldo Yorke, poetic and unmotivated, although attractive and personally charming. He falls deeply in love with her, and Phelps devotes most of the plot to the resulting role reversal which apparently fascinates her. Convalescent and ironically suffering from "nervous strain" (69), Yorke needs Dr. Zay, but she, in splendid health, "leaned against her own physical strength, as another woman might lean upon a man's" (110).[73]

By a further twist of irony, a twist clearly delightful to Phelps herself, Dr. Zay, out of her superfluous strength and in her off-hours, can provide salvation for man in the shape of Yorke, but he has nothing to offer her except the so-called feminine gifts of devotion and sexual attractiveness. The circle of revenge is complete, for Phelps is implying through Atalanta that the truly diseased sex is not woman, woman with her radiant maternal strength, but man, man with his barren professional pretenses and sexual excess. And so the last act of mercy Phelps's rather sadistic angel performs is to consent to enter the marriage relation with a sex she has demonstrated so clearly to be the inferior of her own.

Phelps's superwoman Dr. Zay is clearly the ex-aggerated product of wish-fulfillment fantasies on the part of a lifelong invalid and feminist, but she forcefully symbolizes what some women wanted women doctors to prove to them. With this novel, the drama of women and medicine in nineteenth-century America has in a sense reached its extreme dénouement. Unlike the male and female physicians who preceded (and succeeded) her, Phelps makes no pretense of interest in medicine as science. Her only concern is with medicine as a weapon in a social and political struggle for power between the sexes. In *Dr. Zay*, Phelps has seized upon the cultural assumptions underlying contemporary male doctors' treatments of women's diseases in order triumphantly to reverse them. Dr. Zay's example is meant to testify that, far from being the constitutionally diseased and dependent creature that Dewees and Byford saw, woman could be self-reliant. In Phelps's vision, woman need not be a prisoner in her own sick body, awaiting the coming of her deliverer, man, but may be a healer herself, the support of her sex, and by caring for its members, the donor to them of a new kind of self-esteem.

NOTES

1   See Richard Huber, *The American Idea of Success* (New York, 1971), 124–86; Donald Meyer, *The Positive Thinkers: A Study of the American Quest for Health, Wealth, and Personal Power* (New York, 1965); David Rothman, *The Discovery of the Asylum: Social Order and Disorder in the New Republic* (Boston, 1971), xvi. For another treatment of insanity in the same period, see Norman Dain, *Concepts of Insanity in the United States 1789–1865* (New Brunswick, N.J., 1964).

2   G. J. Barker-Benfield has given consideration to these medical practices from a cultural point of view in an unpublished paper entitled "The spermatic economy: a nineteenth century view of sexuality," delivered at the Organization of American Historians meeting, April 15, 1971, at New Orleans. (Editor's note: in 1972, this was published under the name of Ben Barker-Benfield in *Feminist Studies 1*:45–74.) His primary focus is on masculine sexuality, however, while mine is on feminine sexuality. For a more general, and somewhat superficial, survey of American sex mores and roles in the nineteenth century, see Milton Rugoff, *Prudery and Passion* (New York, 1971).

3   Catharine E. Beecher, "The American people starved and poisoned," *Harper's New Monthly Magazine,* 1866,

32: 771; *Physiology and Calisthenics for Schools and Families* (New York, 1856), 164; *Letters to the People on Health and Happiness* (New York, 1855), 124. Her findings were still being referred to in 1870. See the popular manual, Edward B. Foote, *Plain Home Talk* (New York, 1880), 451.

4   For a popular satire on the subject, see Augustus Hopper, *A Fashionable Sufferer; or, Chapters from Life's Comedy* (Boston, 1883). There is an interesting chapter on the subject in Page Smith, *Daughters of the Promised Land: Women in American History* (Boston, 1970), 131–40. Wendell Philips's wife was a typical example of a long-suffering but equally longlived victim of nervous complaints. See Irving H. Bartlett, *Wendell Phillips: Brahmin Radical* (Boston, 1961), 79. One could multiply examples almost endlessly of women of this period who never expected to live through the next year and survived into their eighties and nineties. Still this evidence, like all the evidence in this area, is ambiguous. There are many diseases and ailments which, in the absence of sufficient medical know-how, can become chronic and make their victim's life a torment without ending it.

5   Meyer, *The Positive Thinkers,* 30.

6   See James Fenimore Cooper, *Gleanings in Europe*, ed. Robert E. Spiller (New York, 1930), 2: 92–97; Nathaniel Hawthorne, *Our Old Home*, in *The Complete Works of Nathaniel Hawthorne* (Boston, 1898), 7: 66–68, 390–91.

7   William A. Alcott, *The Young Woman's Books of Health* (Boston, 1950), 17; Edward H. Clarke, *Sex in Education; or, A Fair Chance for Girls* (Boston, 1878), 63. For the history of similar arguments, see Willystine Goodsell, *The Education of Women: Its Social Background and Problems* (New York, 1923). In 1868, Dr. F. Saunders wrote a book quite frankly pleading with middle-class American women to have more children. See *About Women, Love, and Marriage* (New York, 1868).

8   See George H. Napheys, *The Transmission of Life: Counsels on the Nature and Hygiene of the Masculine Function* (Philadelphia, 1889), 71 ff. This was a standard analysis and countless supporting sources could be cited. One of particular interest is Nicholas Francis Cook, *Satan in Society: By a Physician* (Cincinnati, 1872). See also George Beard, *American Nervousness* (New York, 1881).

9   See, for example, Alcott, *The Young Woman's Book of Health*; Frederick Hollick, *The Marriage Guide or Natural History of Generation* (New York, 1860); George H. Napheys, *The Physical Life of Woman: Advice to the Maiden, Wife and Mother* (Philadelphia, 1880).

10 Quoted in M. L. Holbrook, *Parturition without Pain: A Code of Directions for Escaping from the Primal Curse* (New York, 1875), 15.

11 William P. Dewees, *A Treatise on the Diseases of Females* (Philadelphia, 1843), 17, 14. For a discussion of attitudes toward menstruation in the period, see Elaine Showalter and English Showalter, "Victorian women and menstruation," *Victorian Studies*, 1970, *14*: 83–89.

12 William H. Byford, *A Treatise on the Chronic Inflammation and Displacements of the Unimpregnated Uterus* (Philadelphia, 1864), 22–41. For a similar discussion of symptoms, see S. Weir Mitchell, *Doctor and Patient* (Philadelphia, 1888), 25–27, and *Fat and Blood and How to Make Them* (Philadelphia, 1877), 35.

13 James Henry Bennet, *A Practical Treatise on Inflammation of the Uterus, Its Cervix and Appendages and on Its Connection with Other Uterine Diseases* (Philadelphia, 1864), 237.

14 Ibid., 224.

15 Ibid., 255; Byford, *A Treatise on the Chronic Inflammation*, 152.

16 Byford, *A Treatise on the Chronic Inflammation*, 103, 117, 158, 164.

17 Bennet, *A Practical Treatise on Inflammation of the Uterus*, 244.

18 G. L. Austin, *Perils of American Women; or, A Doctor's Talk with Maiden, Wife, and Mother* (Boston, 1883), 198, 158–60. See also Monfort B. Allen and Amelia C. McGregor, *The Glory of Woman; or, Love, Marriage, and Maternity* (Philadelphia, 1896), 241.

19 Mitchell, *Fat and Blood*, 7. This cure, since it did not focus directly on the uterus, could be used on men as well as women, but rarely was. Significantly, in twenty-four case histories described by Mitchell in an account of his method, only one involved was a male. Furthermore, this man was suffering from consumption rather than a nervous complaint. See *Fat and Blood*, 93.

20 See J. Marion Sims, *The Story of My Life* (New York, 1884).

21 Elizabeth Blackwell, *Pioneer Work in Opening the Medical Profession to Women* (New York, 1895), 257–59.

22 Quoted in Seale Harris, *Woman's Surgeon: The Life Story of J. Marion Sims* (New York, 1950), 181.

23 Charles D. Meigs, a conservative gynecologist of Philadelphia, wrote in 1848 that he "rejoiced" at the difficulty of making local examinations since it was "an evidence of a high and worthy grade of moral feeling" in American women (quoted in Harvey Graham, *Eternal Eve: The History of Gynecology and Obstetrics* [New York, 1951], 495).

24 Dewees, *A Treatise on the Diseases of Females*, 224–25, 242–43; Bennet, *A Practical Treatise on Inflammation of the Uterus*, 19. Another widely used foreign authority made the same point. J. W. von Scanzoni, *A Practical Treatise on the Diseases of the Sexual Organs of Women* trans. Augustus K. Gardner, (New York, 1861), 37–38. See also Byford, *A Treatise on the Chronic Inflammation*, 98.

25 Graham, *Eternal Eve*, 451. For an example, see Napheys, *The Transmission of Life*, 190–91.

26 Byford, *A Treatise on the Chronic Inflammation*, 22–41. Mitchell also testified to this pattern of moral degradation, *Fat and Blood*, 27, 28. One should add here that condemnation disguised as diagnosis and punishment offered as cure were hardly unique to medical treatment of women in this period. Napheys hints at "surgical operations" to curb masturbation in men and advocates blisterings and "infibulation" (*Transmission of Life*, 80–83). Rugoff discusses various painful contraptions used to prevent nocturnal emission (*Prudery and Passion*, 53). I am simply trying to show how two particular courses of punitive medicine reflected and supported culturally induced ideas about female sexual identity.

27 Edward H. Dixon, *Woman and Her Diseases from the Cradle to the Grave* (New York, 1857), 134, 140.

28 For a discussion of Stowe's marital problems and responsibilities, see the following biographies: Joanna

Johnston, *Runaway to Heaven: The Story of Harriet Beecher Stowe* (New York, 1963) and Forrest Wilson, *Crusader in Crinoline: The Life of Harriet Beecher Stowe* (Philadelphia, 1941). Also of value is Edmund Wilson, *Patriotic Gore: Studies in the Literature of the American Civil War* (New York, 1966), 3–58.

29 "Insanity: From Combe's Work on Mental Derangement," *Ladies' Magazine*, 1835, 8: 461–63.

30 W. A. Alcott, "Female attendance on the sick," *Ladies' Magazine*, 1834, 7: 302.

31 Byford, *A Treatise on the Chronic Inflammation*, 15.

32 S. Weir Mitchell, *Roland Blake* (Boston, 1886), 254.

33 Anna Robeson Burr, ed., *Weir Mitchell: His Life and Letters* (New York, 1929), 374. Mitchell makes the same point in *Doctor and Patient*, 13.

34 Burr, *Weir Mitchell*, 37. The best recent biography is Ernest Earnest, *S. Weir Mitchell: Novelist and Physician* (Philadelphia, 1950).

35 Mitchell, *Fat and Blood*, 48.

36 Mitchell, *Doctor and Patient*, 48.

37 Quoted in Burr, *Weir Mitchell*, 290.

38 There are striking similarities between Mitchell's conception of his role, and that of Freudian psychiatrists. See Earnest, *Weir Mitchell*, 250.

39 Mitchell, *Fat and Blood*, 39.

40 He tried hypnosis in his practice, though with little success. See Earnest, *Weir Mitchell*, 229. Robert Herrick was to dramatize this aspect of the physician's role in *The Healer* (New York, 1911) and in *Together* (New York, 1909).

41 For examples of these weight gains, see Mitchell, *Fat and Blood*, 80–94. One 5′ 8″ woman went from 118 lbs. to 169 lbs.

42 Quoted in Harris, *Woman's Surgeon*, 181.

43 Both the homeopathic school, with its distrust of drugs and violent remedies, and the hydropathic school, with its reliance on the efficacy of water, advocated relatively mild treatments for women's ailments. For examples, see John A. Tarbell, *Homeopathy Simplified; or, Domestic Practice Made Easy* (Boston, 1859), 214–28; R. T. Trall, *The Hydropathic Encyclopedia: A System of Hydropathy and Hygiene* (New York, 1852), 2: 285–96. It must also be added, however, that such doctors were outside the higher echelons of American medicine. Furthermore, it is striking how many women turned to such doctors as a result of bad experiences at the hands of more orthodox doctors. In other words, it seems likely that the lady at the water cure had also sampled other forms of treatment.

44 Angelina Grimké, for instance, a famous abolitionist and speaker for women's rights, suffered terribly from *prolapsus uteri*. See Gerda Lerner, *The Grimké Sisters from South Carolina* (Boston, 1967), 288–92.

45 See Austin, *Perils of American Women*, 94–95.

46 All page references will be to the edition already cited.

47 See her own account in her autobiography, *The Living of Charlotte Perkins Gilman* (New York, 1935), 90 ff. She may have felt her similarities to Beecher since she named her daughter after her.

48 All page references will be to Charlotte Perkins Gilman, "The Yellow Wall Paper," in *The Great Modern American Short Stories*, William Dean Howells, ed. (New York, 1920), 320–37; Gilman, *Living of Charlotte Perkins Gilman*, 121.

49 The demand for women doctors could be quite explicit; See Julia Ward Howe, ed., *Sex and Education: A Reply to Dr. E. H. Clarke's "Sex in Education"* (Boston, 1874), 158.

50 Harriot K. Hunt, *Glances and Glimpses; or, Fifty Years Social, Including Twenty Years Professional Life* (Boston, 1856), 414.

51 For the history of women doctors in America, see Kate Campbell Hurd-Mead, *Medical Women of America: A Short History of the Pioneer Medical Women of America and of a Few of Their Colleagues in England* (New York, 1933); Esther Pohl Lovejoy, *Women Doctors of the World* (New York, 1957).

52 All page references will be to Hunt, *Glances and Glimpses*. For similar motivation in another woman doctor see Helen MacKnight Doyle, *A Child Went Forth* (New York, 1934), 15–18.

53 There was some medical truth underlying this apparently sentimental declaration. Aside from subjecting women to the perils of childbirth, men not infrequently unwittingly gave them syphilis. See Elizabeth Blackwell, *Essays in Medical Sociology* (London, 1902), 1: 90–91.

54 Antiprofessionalism in women doctors had another complex side which mainly lies outside the scope of this article. Women had been active medical practitioners in America as midwives until the time of the Revolution. Then licenses, obtainable only in the newly opened medical schools, which did not take women, began to be required. So, in effect, professional requirements had spelled the demise of the woman physician in the late eighteenth century. Hence, the mistrust felt for such training by her nineteenth-century feminine successor was not surprising. Unquestionably, late-eighteenth-century and early nineteenth-century American doctors had welcomed and even pushed for this change (see Victor Robinson, *White-Caps: The Story of Nursing* [Philadelphia, 1946], 137), although a few regretted it (see A. Curtis, *Lectures on Midwifery and the Forms of Disease Peculiar to Women and Children* [Columbus, Ohio, 1841], 9). On the whole question of women

and the professions in this period, see Gerda Lerner, "The lady and the mill-girl: changes in the status of women in the age of Jackson," *Mid-Continent American Studies Journal,* 1969, *10:* 5–15.

55 American society throughout this period agreed on the importance and potency of motherhood. In part this was a simple rationale of the fact that, since the American father was at work, the American mother was raising the children. See Anne L. Kuhn, *The Mother's Role in Childhood Education* (New Haven, 1947); Bernard Wishy, *The Child and the Republic: The Dawn of Modern American Child Nurture* (Philadelphia, 1968), 24–29. Contemporary paeans to motherhood are legion, but see Jabez Burns, *Mothers of the Wise and Good* (Boston, 1850); Margaret C. Conklin, *Memoirs of the Mother and Wife of Washington* (Auburn, N.Y., 1851).

56 I have picked the two most famous of the early women doctors in America, but most of the others fall into similar patterns. All of them devoted themselves professionally almost exclusively to women, few of them married, and most met determined opposition from the majority of their male colleagues, in some cases amounting to what Elizabeth Blackwell called "medical starvation" (unpublished letter of Jan. 23, 1855, to Emily Blackwell in Blackwell Collection, Radcliffe Archives, Cambridge, Mass.). For works on and by the other three most famous women doctors of the period, Emily Blackwell, Mary Putnam Jacobi, and Marie Zakrzewska, see the Blackwell Collection; Ruth Putnam, ed., *Life and Letters of Mary Putnam Jacobi* (New York, 1925); *Mary Putnam Jacobi, M.D.: A Pathfinder in Medicine: With Selections from Her Writings* (New York, 1925); Rhoda Truax, *The Doctors Jacobi* (Boston, 1952); and the Jacobi Papers, also at Radcliffe.

Jacobi was one of the most brilliant doctors of her day, and her monograph, *The Question of Rest for Women during Menstruation* (New York, 1877), an answer to Clarke, won the Harvard Boylston Medical Prize. For Zakrzewska's autobiography, see Caroline H. Dall, ed., *A Practical Illustration of Woman's Right to Labor; or, A Letter from Marie E. Zakrzewska, M.D.* (Boston, 1860); Agnes C. Vietor, ed., *A Woman's Quest: The Life of Marie E. Zakrzewska, M.D.* (New York, 1924). Also of great interest, although falling outside of official professional ranks, were Lydia Folger Fowler and Mary Gove Nichols. See Frederick C. Waite, "Dr. Lydia Folger Fowler: the second woman to receive the degree of doctor in the United States," *Annals of Medical History,* 1932, *4:* 290–97; T. L. Nichols and Mary S. Gove Nichols, *Marriage: Its History, Character and Results* (New York, 1854); Mary S. Gove Nichols, *Mary Lyndon; or, Revelations of a Life: An Autobiography* (New York, 1855); Helen Beal Woodward, *The Bold Women* (New York, 1953), 149–80.

57 Ishbel Ross, *Child of Destiny: The Life Story of the First Woman Doctor* (New York, 1949), 43.

58 Blackwell, *Pioneer Work,* 28, 32. She consistently opposed the marriages of the male members of her large family; the women all stayed single. See Elinor Rice Hays, *Those Extraordinary Blackwells: The Story of a Journey to a Better World* (New York, 1967), 155. Zakrzewska felt the same way. See *A Woman's Quest,* 193.

59 Blackwell, *Pioneer Work,* 72.

60 "Increase of operations," undated paper in the Blackwell Collection. See also Elizabeth Blackwell, *Essays in Medical Sociology* (London, 1902), *2:* 120.

61 Letter of March 21, 1891, in the Blackwell Collection.

62 See Blackwell, *Essays, 2:* 119 ff. Antivivisection had many passionate feminine adherents, medical and lay. Elizabeth Stuart Phelps, a popular writer and feminist of Blackwell's era, devoted much of her later work to the cause. See especially *Though Life Do Us Part* (Boston, 1908), 54–55, where she explicitly links male cruelty in vivisection with male cruelty in marriage, and *Trixy* (Boston, 1904) in which a girl refuses to marry a vivisectionist.

63 See Blackwell, *Pioneer Work,* 178, 157, 240. See also Blackwell, *Essays, 2:* 69 ff.

64 Blackwell, *Essays, 2:* 26. Jacobi seems to be making a similar point about the male intellect in "The Mad Scientist," in *Stories and Sketches* (New York, 1907).

65 Blackwell, *Pioneer Work,* 173.

66 All page references for this essay are to Blackwell, *Essays,* vol. 2.

67 Undated letter to Dr. McNutt in the Blackwell Collection.

68 Blackwell nowhere makes this more clear than in *The Human Element in Sex: Being a Medical Enquiry into the Relation of Sexual Physiology to Christian Morality* (London, 1884).

69 A good introduction to the spirit and work of the Purity Alliance is Aaron M. Powell, ed., *The National Purity Congress: Its Papers, Addresses, Portraits* (New York, 1896).

70 *Wrong and Right Methods of Dealing with Social Evil as Shown by English Parliamentary Evidence* (New York, n.d.), 41. See also "The purchase of women: the great economic blunder" in Blackwell, *Essays, 1:* 133–74.

71 See Hurd-Mead, *Medical Women of America,* and Robinson, *White-Caps.*

72 For her own account see Elizabeth Stuart Phelps, *Chapters from a Life* (Boston, 1897), 228–42. Her most

important fictional accounts of illness are "Shut In" in *Fourteen in One* (Boston, 1891), 66–99, about an invalid's recovery, and *Walled In* (New York, 1907), about the relationship between a nurse and a male patient.

73 All page references are to Elizabeth Stuart Phelps, *Dr. Zay* (Boston, 1886). I owe much of my thinking on Phelps to Christine Stansell's "Elizabeth Stuart Phelps: a study in female rebellion," *Massachusetts Review,* 1972, *13:* 239–56. For other contemporary fictional works on women doctors, see William Dean Howells, *Dr. Breen's Practice* (Boston, 1881), and Sarah Orne Jewett, *A Country Doctor* (Boston, c. 1884).

17

The Perils of Feminist History

REGINA MARKELL MORANTZ

The Victorian period holds a particular fascination for the sympathetic historian of women's history. On the surface, at least, women were obviously "oppressed" by society's narrow definition of their role. Torn by the harsh realities of industrialization and the uncongenial atmosphere of Social Darwinism, nineteenth-century Americans sought refuge in a cult of domesticity which exalted Woman and Home. Woman's psychological and cultural burdens consequently became more onerous, even as her legal rights remained circumscribed. Her image was shot through with contradictions: Guardian of the race, yet wholly subject to male authority; preserver of civilization, religion, and culture, yet considered intellectually inferior; the primary socializer of her children, yet with no more real responsibility and dignity than a child herself. Woman was inevitably tormented by the ambiguities of her position.

In the wake of the renewed feminist consciousness of recent years, it is tempting to locate the source of twentieth-century problems in the apparent injustices of nineteenth-century society. Many current feminist histories of the period do just that. One way or another each plays upon a single theme: Woman as Victim. The problem such works present for the historian are obvious: They are not history, but polemics.

Fortunately, Ann Douglas Wood's treatment of the "fashionable diseases" manages to avoid the worst defects of recent feminist writing.[1] But it, too, suffers from a presentism which makes the

REGINA MARKELL MORANTZ is Associate Professor of History at the University of Kansas, Lawrence, Kansas.

Reprinted from *The Journal of Interdisciplinary History*, IV (1973), 649–660, by permission of *The Journal of Interdisciplinary History* and The M.I.T. Press, Cambridge, Massachusetts. Copyright © 1973 by the Massachusetts Institute of Technology and the editors of *The Journal of Interdisciplinary History*.

author often too willing to distort historical evidence and lay blame, while missing a larger opportunity to explore the immense complexities which lie at the root of Victorian attitudes toward women. The article is at its weakest in its discussion of two major points: nineteenth-century medical therapeutics in the treatment of women's diseases, and the attitudes and self-images of pioneering women doctors. Wood's handling of both these problems is predicated on what seems to be a false and dangerous set of assumptions. Let me begin, therefore, by taking issue with her underlying point of view.

In a recent article on psychohistory Robert Coles cogently observed: "Will the application of psychological 'insight' to history or the arts be done in such a way as to produce caricatures of human beings—and those only to be turned into proof of some larger generalization about the 'laws' that govern the human mind?"[2] Coles recognizes the need for more psychologically sophisticated historians who, skilled in several disciplines, can help us to view human experience more broadly. The problem arises, he would argue, when psychologizing becomes rigid and narrow, even polemical, and the moral judgments made are based on the biases of a narrow, psychoanalytic formulation. Wood's treatment of the male medical practitioner suffers from just this kind of psychological "insight," and the portrait that emerges might well be termed a "caricature."

Often cruel, perhaps even sadistic, the nineteenth-century physician viewed the terrible suffering of his female patients "rather complacently" (224). He was guilty of countless acts of torture, sometimes leaving his patients "raw and bleeding" after cauterization or leeching (224). Constantly engaged in complex "psychological warfare" with the women they treated, even the "best-intentioned" practitioners were "in part hostile" to them (226). What else but ill will can explain the stubborn insistence of the majority of medical men that women would be safe from conception squarely in the middle of their menstrual cycles, when their patients, from empirical evidence, knew better?[3]

Male animosity derived from fear. The *form* of treatment for women's diseases evolved, Wood stresses, because "on some unacknowledged level" the doctor "feared his female patient"; he worried "that his sex, the constant companion of hers, was in some way menaced" (227). Although by 1870 young physicians like S. Weir Mitchell had abandoned gross physical torture for the more ingenious method of psychological cruelty, the "rest cure" was merely a "sophisticated culmination" of earlier methods. Mitchell was still the spiritual brother of his predecessor, "the cauterizer, with his injections, leeches, and hot irons" who spitefully nurtured a "veiled but aggressively hostile male sexuality and superiority" (228).

Wood's handling of Mitchell is based on a similarly simplistic Freudianism which makes for interesting reading but faulty history. Certainly he was very much the Victorian patrician—vain, stubborn, self-satisfied, and patronizing toward women. His ideal woman was well sheltered from the degrading influences of the modern age. Yet, he cannot be dismissed so easily. He conscientiously sought and relished the company of educated, intelligent, strong-minded women. He was a close friend of Agnes Repplier, who characterized their relationship as "the perfect flowering of sentiment and understanding." Nor did his disapproval of higher education for women interfere with a lifelong intimacy with Agnes Irwin, the Dean of Radcliffe College. Highly critical of the weak-limbed, nervous, delicately neurasthenic ideal of Victorian Womanhood, Mitchell was an early advocate of more physical activity for women. He even argued that no distinction should be made in the physical training of boys and girls until adolescence.[4] Although he clearly preferred that the majority of women should confine their interests to the home, he respected the right of individual women to opt for higher education.[5]

I dwell on these aspects of Mitchell's personality because he is so utterly distorted in Wood's characterization. Admittedly, he was a domineering figure who believed that a self-willed and forceful

personality made a better, more objective man of science. Convinced that overindulgence by well-meaning relatives exacerbated rather than cured the nervous condition of his patients, his first step was to substitute for this misplaced concern "the firm kindness of a well-trained hired nurse." His refusal to pamper his patients, and his insistence that they obey him, were a deliberate part of his therapy. Mitchell had apparently learned from experience that a stern, impartial demeanor was highly successful with certain kinds of patients. He doubted whether women doctors were always capable of this "needed control" over other women in "such cases"; yet, he was quick to assert that many male doctors also failed to achieve the proper distance. Nowhere in his discussion of this problem can I find the claim that "women doctors would always be inferior to male physicians" (228). Except for these specific cases, which required absolute obedience, women, he conceded, were "in all other ways capable doctors." Nor does he ever boast of "reducing his patients to the docility of children" (228). Rather, in describing the full trust placed in him by one particular woman patient he recalled that "she obeyed, or tried to obey me, like a child." Finally I can find no statement of Mitchell's to the effect that he felt that a doctor could or should become "godlike," or that he himself "skated on the edge of a theory of primitive healing through mesmeric sexual powers" (228).[6]

Wood wants to give special status to the "sadism" of men and male doctors when it is not at all certain that they are inherently more "sadistic" than women. Is it a special kind of "sadism" that leads more men than women to become surgeons? Can we label open heart surgery, or even mastectomy, "sadistic" and leave it at that? Alternatively, what *appears* as sadism may very well be a quality inherent in the "doctor role," or at least in the way that the patient perceives the physician. It is characteristic of Wood's approach that she is willing to draw the broadest possible conclusions concerning Mitchell's personality, based almost exclusively on her reading of Charlotte Gilman's "The Yellow Wall Paper," although the obvious question of Gilman's own neurosis is passed over as if it did not exist!

Mitchell was a neurologist, not a "woman's doctor," as Wood labels him (225), and his rest cure was never confined to women.[7] His first experience with rest as a treatment for "acute exhaustion" came during the Civil War, when he dealt with soldiers suffering from battle fatigue. In accord with the most advanced neurological thinking of his day, Mitchell saw the symptoms of exhaustion as somatic in origin; thus, it was to the physical symptoms that his rest cure addressed itself. Too much strain and too little relaxation taxed the limited resources of energy that each individual had at his or her disposal. Absolute rest was a logical and pragmatic answer to the problem. Excessive feeding to replace the needed "red corpuscles" was proposed to counteract the loss of weight which usually accompanied nervous illness. Massage was performed by experienced women and was added as an afterthought to achieve the benefits of "exercise without exertion." Such therapy is still practiced today with long-term hospital patients. Of highly questionable value to the modern neurologist, Mitchell's cure was nevertheless often successful. For a time it was adapted and used by Freud.[8] Mitchell himself saw it as a welcome departure from the excessive and indiscriminate drugging of the age. In his case report of the first patient whom he treated in this manner, he described with utter contempt the way in which she had "passed through the hands of gynecologists, worn spinal supporters, and taken every tonic known to the books."[9]

Wood's handling of medical therapeutics does not take into account that treatment of disease in nineteenth-century America cannot be viewed properly apart from the broad context of scientific ignorance which was displayed at midcentury. Medicine was clearly in a period of transition and crisis. For decades pioneer researchers centered in Paris had been concentrating their energies on the systematic identification and description of specific diseases in terms of a localized, structural pathology. It was slow and painstaking work: Bedside symptoms uncovered through careful observation had then to be correlated with lesions discovered at autopsies. Although the future therapeutic implications of such research were momentous—doctors could not cure *any* disease until they could isolate and diagnose it—the immediate results were discouraging. One by one the traditional methods of treatment—bleeding and heavy ("heroic") dosing with such dangerous substances as mercury, lead, and calomel—were discredited. Medical science, in short, found itself in the painful position of having advanced far enough to discard ancient

methods of therapy without being able to offer anything new to take their place. The patient and his inept but well-meaning physician were left to fend for themselves. In despair, many physicians surrendered to therapeutic nihilism.[10] Controversy increased within the profession. Rival medical sects and illegitimate quacks, promising success where regular medicine had failed, proliferated in the United States and abroad.

The problem was exacerbated in America by the social and political climate. Well-trained physicians from high-quality medical schools were ignorant enough, but only a minority of American doctors were well trained in this period. Quality medical education had fallen victim to the leveling forces of Jacksonian democracy. Proprietary schools, operated for profit by enterprising physicians swept up in the materialism of the age, competed with each other for students. Strict requirements were relaxed as medical training was made as quick and as easy as possible. Clinical facilities were virtually nonexistent, and mediocre personnel did little to advance research. Hundreds of graduates were licensed yearly without ever having treated a patient or witnessed a childbirth.[11]

Poor training on the one hand, and therapeutic nihilism on the other, led inevitably to a widespread loss of prestige for doctors.[12] It is in this context that the criticism of the profession by health reformers like Catharine Beecher and Harriot Hunt must be viewed. Much of their faultfinding was based on a realistic perception of the inability of medical men to cure *most* disease—not just those of women, but of everyone. Why so many physicians persisted in the use of heroic medicine in spite of its obvious inefficacy is a complicated issue. The answer lies not in their antipathy to women, but, again, in ignorance and poor training. Doctors, also, were prisoners of their own theoretical constructs. Medical science had left them no alternative in the 1850s except to admit to their patients and themselves that they were helpless. Was it not more comforting to persist in the practices that one had taken for granted in the past? This natural conservatism resulted in much unnecessary suffering. Yet, to attribute such behavior to "veiled hostility" rather than to the imperfections of a premodern discipline which hardly merits the adjective "scientific" is surely misguided.

The assumption that male physicians, like everyone else, were very much the products of their cultural milieu is unquestionably sound. But what does this mean? At times Wood seems to define Victorian culture in terms of male hostility rather than the reverse. Her presupposition of male antagonism is painfully simplistic. True enough, Victorian society exhibited a deep-seated ambivalence toward women, symbolized by its obsession with two dominant polar images—the Angel and the Prostitute. There was much apprehension about the necessity of keeping woman confined to her "sphere." But before drawing over-hasty conclusions, we need to know much more about the relationship of industrialization to changes in the family structure, and how this larger development altered attitudes toward sex roles and practices. As she asserted more and more exclusive control over the rearing of her children, woman, in some sense, gained power within the family. Historians have already begun to investigate the ramifications of the "feminization" of literature and morality in the nineteenth century.[13] How did this growing influence affect the relationship between the sexes within and without the family? What was woman's own self-image; how and in what degree was it shaped by society's view of her? It is with questions like these that we can move beyond accusation to deeper understanding.

Another major point of Wood's with which I must take issue is her portrayal of the attitudes and beliefs of the first-generation women doctors. It is curious that she chose Harriot Hunt, whom she characterizes as "one of the more impressive of the early women doctors in America," to represent that group (230). Hunt was never a licensed physician. She and her sister studied medicine in Boston in the 1830s with an itinerant English couple who practiced their own peculiar form of healing. Their methods of treatment combined several of the sectarian practices then in vogue—water therapy, homeopathy, eclecticism, and personal hygiene— and were probably far less harmful than the heavy dosing of some licensed medical men. Consequently, Hunt had a flourishing practice among women and children in Boston. Nevertheless, she herself must have sensed a gap in her medical education, for, in the 1850s, she twice applied for admission to Harvard Medical School and was refused, once by the trustees and once by the students. The Female Medical College of Pennsylvania

awarded her an honorary degree in 1853. Like many women's rights advocates who believed that women, in order to be better wives and mothers, should learn more about physiology and hygiene, she became an energetic and indefatigable lecturer on such subjects in the decade before the Civil War. Hunt maintained warm contacts with many of the first women physicians—the sectarians as well as the orthodox. A significant and interesting figure, she is often cited by feminists as the first woman doctor.[14]

Compared to the other women doctors whom Wood cites in her footnotes, however, Hunt's medical credentials were at best questionable. She was not a scientist, and it is not surprising that she eschewed scientific medicine, even in its still primitive form. She preferred, instead, the role of supportive therapist, and her deep insights into the psychological aspects of women's ailments are noteworthy. Justifiably bitter about the exclusion of women from medical training, she also seemed equally vexed by the fact that as an "irregular" practitioner, she was shunned (probably unjustly) for her unorthodoxy as well as for her womanhood. To suggest that her medical attitudes were representative of such highly trained and skillful physicians as Emily Blackwell, Marie Zakrzewska, Mary Putnam Jacobi, Ann Preston, and others does an injustice to these capable women, all of whom won the respect, although not the approval, of their male colleagues. These women did not "throw the baby out with the bath water" (231); they embraced scientific knowledge as much for its own sake as for what it could do to improve the lot of their sex.

Even Elizabeth Blackwell was not entirely typical of her more scientific sisters. A towering figure whose contributions to the furtherance of medical education for women were prodigious, she was never a physician by temperament. Her decision to become a doctor had little to do with an interest in the medical discipline itself, and her primary aim was to use medicine as a moral platform to further the causes in which she believed. Her opposition to such practices as vivisection and vaccination can be labeled "unscientific" even for the mid-nineteenth-century, and her outspokenness concerning these issues was tolerated, but never condoned, by her female colleagues.

Although the attitudes of Hunt and Blackwell toward medical science were somewhat idiosyncratic, their arguments for the entrance of women into medicine can properly be treated as representative of the thought of early women doctors. Yet, even here, Wood misreads her evidence. The discussion of Hunt's theories often turns on quotations taken out of their proper context.[15] The resulting portrait detracts from Hunt's well-deserved position as an important and significant figure in the women's movement. She emerges as a shrill and bitter woman who was somewhat "paranoid" in her relationships with the male profession and who dwelt on "alarmist and lurid" descriptions of the humiliating sexual exploitation of unsuspecting female patients by "malevolent" medical men. Husbands, too, were "villainous," and marriage an abomination. Wood's description would have us believe that Hunt was a man-hater (231–32).

Such a portrayal of Hunt lacks the richness which more attention to the historical background can provide. Let us take, for example, Hunt's denunciation of local examinations as "too often unnecessary" (231). In making this statement she was giving voice to a complex, sensitive, and much debated issue with which physicians themselves grappled throughout the century. As Victorian prudery reached its peak at midcentury, the importance of coming to terms with female modesty became increasingly apparent. Middle- and upper-class women often declined to consult physicians for gynecologic problems except in extreme cases. Even when they overcame their misgivings and sought professional services, it was difficult for doctors to get a proper history—the embarrassment of discussing her bodily functions being too much for the woman of refinement to bear. Ambivalent themselves over the dictates of Victorian morality, medical men did not deal adequately with the problem. Most denounced what they termed "false modesty"; yet, a minority agreed that female morality was being compromised. A few of this group advocated some sort of professional training in medicine for women as a solution.[16] Women's rights advocates had the perfect answer: Admit women to medical schools and give the modest woman the opportunity to seek aid from her own sex in her time of need. The argument was based on a full acceptance of Victorian delicacy which had hitherto kept woman out of the professions and confined to her "own sphere," and was, consequently, not without special irony.

Hunt's hostility to marriage is overdrawn. She had a blissful home life, reverently depicted in her autobiography; she adored her father and respected her brother-in-law. She had no reason to be as antagonistic to men as Wood suggests. Assuredly, she was critical of Victorian marriage but not simply because women were dominated. What bothered her most was something which rankled many women doctors—that women were becoming increasingly frivolous, weak willed, and self-centered.[17] Women were as responsible for this trend as were men. Hunt had nothing but contempt for wives and mothers who wasted precious time in worthless pursuits. She expressed sympathy for the husbands who were often victimized by the emptiness and lack of real spiritual qualities in so many marriages. Her social criticism was acute and to the point. Women were being educated as

> appendages and dead weights to husbands ... without a knowledge of those domestic duties and responsibilities, which alone can fit them to live true to those relations, without those solid intellectual attainments and spiritual graces by which they are to educate their children and hallow the atmosphere of the home, and without those "attractions,"— enduring when youth and beauty are gone, which alone can win and keep for them the respect and love of any sensible, upright and noble man, worthy of the name of husband!

Such poor training for women was ultimately "traitorous to the virtue of both sexes"; neither suffered alone.[18]

What is perhaps most interesting about the thinking of Hunt and others is not their putative ill will toward men, or even their justifiable criticisms of the medical profession, but the degree to which their own attitudes toward women mirrored those of their male colleagues. These professional women were not modern-day feminists charging the barricades of male privilege, but were very much Victorian women, prisoners of their own time and culture.

Thus, they could advocate the training of female physicians on the grounds of propriety and morality. Even more fascinating was their contention that medicine was a natural extension of woman's sphere and peculiarly suited to the female character, which was self-sacrificing, empathetic, and altruistic. Glorying in motherhood, even those who never married viewed their own role as that of a "connecting link between the science of the medical profession and the everyday life of women."[19] Women doctors would become the professional allies of wives and mothers everywhere. In performing this task, their value to the community would be immense. Mothers desperately needed to be educated in sanitary matters, hygiene, and physiology. This was properly the work of female physicians. Elizabeth Blackwell understood that "comparatively few" women, even when given the opportunity, would choose to "devote themselves entirely to scientific pursuits." Nevertheless, the sex was so linked together that inevitably "every woman would be benefited by the scientific development of a class."[20] As a final contribution, women, because of their superior moral qualities, would "raise the moral tone

of the profession and teach reverence and purity to the grossness of the world."[21]

It is unfortunate that, in her eagerness to portray nineteenth-century American women as victims, Wood misses or consciously ignores these larger issues. Yet, the contention of these women that their medical training would bring benefits to civilization as a whole was at once an extremely forceful, yet ultimately self-defeating argument. Its power lay in its embracing the concept of the separation of the spheres. Nevertheless, not until their own Victorian attitudes gave way to the more egalitarian concepts of the twentieth century would the full acceptance of women as professionals be possible. For them, however, such arguments were never a mere question of tactics. Proper Victorians themselves, thoroughly immersed in the values that their society held dear, they could view these issues in no other way.

NOTES

1 Ann Douglas Wood, "'The fashionable diseases': women's complaints and their treatment in nineteenth-century America," in this volume, 222–38. See, for example, Barbara Ehrenreich and Deirdre English, *Witches, Midwives, and Nurses: A History of Women Healers* (New York, n.d.).

2 "Shrinking history, I," *New York Review of Books*, Feb. 22, 1973, 21.

3 Wood points out that doctors miscalculated the fertile period by reasoning by analogy with the animal world. To blame them for such unfortunate logic is unfair. I would question the implication that women themselves knew better. Is it not plausible that farm women, themselves surrounded by animals, were equally likely to make the same mistaken connection that physicians did?

4 For his close relationships with women see Ernest Earnest, *S. Weir Mitchell: Novelist and Physician* (Philadelphia, 1950), 128–29. "To run, to climb, to swim, to ride, to play violent games, ought to be as natural to the girl as to the boy." (S. Weir Mitchell, *Doctor and Patient* [Philadelphia, 1887], 141). See also "Outdoor and camp–life for women," ibid., 155–77.

5 Mitchell, *Doctor and Patient*, 149. Also interesting is his good-natured confrontation with a grandniece who was a student at Bryn Mawr, in *Weir Mitchell: His Life and Letters*, ed. Anna Robeson Burr (New York, 1929), 374.

6 *Fat and Blood* (Philadelphia, 1902), 42, 60–61, 76. Wood's fertile imagination leads her to elaborate her

theory with this questionable final statement, offered without evidence: "Mitchell, like his cauterizing predecessor, played the role of possessor, even impregnator, in the cure process. Dominated, overfed often to the point of obesity, caressed and (quite literally) vibrating, were not his patients returned to health—to womanhood?" (228).

7 Because of numerous psychological and physical stresses on the Victorian woman, of which we still know too little, women were plagued with nervous exhaustion, or "neurasthenia," more often than men. See Carroll Smith-Rosenberg, "The hysterical woman: sex roles and role conflict in 19th-century America," *Social Research*, 1972, *39*: 652–78.

8 Earnest, *Mitchell*, 227; Nathan Hale, Jr., *Freud in America* (New York, 1971), 47–68.

9 "The evolution of the rest treatment," *Journal of Nervous and Mental Disease*, 1904, *31*: 368–73.

10 Oliver Wendell Holmes, Dean of the Harvard Medical School, observed that if all of the various medicines used in the treatment of disease were immediately thrown into the sea it would be so much the better for mankind and so much the worse for the fishes. See Oliver Wendell Holmes, *Currents and Counter Currents in Medical Science* (Boston, 1861), 39.

11 Detailed and generally excellent is William G. Rothstein, *American Physicians in the Nineteenth Century* (Baltimore, 1972), 41–62. See also Richard Shryock, *Medicine and Society in America, 1660–1860* (Ithaca,

1962), 117–66; "Cults and quackery in American medical history," in Middle States Association of History and Social Studies Teachers, *Proceedings*, 1939, *37:* 19–30; "Sylvester Graham and the Popular Health Movement, 1830–1870," *Mississippi Valley Historical Review*, 1932, *18:* 172–83; William B. Walker, "The health reform movement in the United States, 1830–1870," Ph.D. diss., Johns Hopkins, 1955, 5; Joseph Kett, *The Formation of the American Medical Profession* (New Haven, 1968), passim.

12 Shryock, *Medicine and Society*, 137–166; "The American physician in 1846 and 1946: a study in professional contrasts," in *Medicine in America: Historical Essays* (Baltimore, 1966); "Public relations of the medical profession," *Annals of Medical History*, 1930, *2:* 319–30.

13 See Mary P. Ryan, "American society and the cult of domesticity," Ph.D. diss., University of California, Santa Barbara, 1971; Barbara Welter, "The feminization of American religion: 1800–1860," in *Insights and Parallels*, ed. William L. O'Neill, (Minneapolis, 1973), 305–32.

14 See her autobiography, *Glances and Glimpses* (Boston, 1856); her correspondence with the Grimké sisters in the University of Michigan Library, Ann Arbor, is also interesting. Kate Campbell Hurd-Mead, *Medical Women of America* (New York, 1933), 20–21; Mary Putnam Jacobi, "Women in medicine," in *Woman's Work in America*, ed. Annie Nathan Meyer, (New York, 1891), 147–48.

15 The remark "I thank Heaven, my dear doctor, that you are a woman; for now I can tell you the truth about my health. It is not my body that is sick but my heart," inadvertently attributed by Wood to Hunt ("'Fashionable diseases,'" 232) is in fact to be found in Marie Zakrzewska's autobiography, *A Woman's Quest* (New York, 1924), 97.

16 For an excellent discussion of this problem, see J. P. Donegan, "Midwifery in America, 1760–1860: a study in medicine and morality," Ph.D. diss., Syracuse University, 1972, 91–159; Shryock, *Medicine and Society*, 121; Thomas Ewell, *Letters to Ladies, Detailing Important Information concerning Themselves and Infants* (Philadelphia, 1817); Samuel Gregory, *Letters to Ladies in Favor of Female Physicians for Their Own Sex* (New York, 1850).

17 She criticized the Shakers for rejecting entirely the institution of marriage, although she recognized that such a policy arose from "that general *abuse* which has marked it [marriage] in the world." (Hunt, *Glances and Glimpses*, 233.) See her denunciation of the leisure-class woman's selfish exploitation of working women, ibid., 133–34.

18 Ibid., 50–52, 408–11. For similar observations from several first-generation women doctors see Zakrzewska, *A Woman's Quest*, 97; Elizabeth Blackwell, *Address on the Medical Education of Women* (New York, 1856), 7; Ann Preston, *Valedictory Address to the Graduating Class of the Female Medical College of Pennsylvania* (Philadelphia, 1870), 5–6.

19 Elizabeth and Emily Blackwell, *Medicine as a Profession for Women* (New York, 1860), 8–9, 15–19.

20 Blackwell, *Address*, 6–7; Preston, *Valedictory Address* (1870), 6–7; Preston, *Valedictory Address to the Graduating Class of the Female Medical College of Pennsylvania* (Philadelphia, 1864), 7.

21 Ann Preston, *Introductory Lecture to the Course of Instruction in the Female Medical College of Pennsylvania* (Philadelphia, 1855), 12; Preston, *Valedictory Address* (1864), 4.

18

"All Hail to Pure Cold Water!"

KATHRYN KISH SKLAR

A century and a half ago American women faced a very different life prospect than today. Without dependable birth control techniques they could expect to spend their prime years bearing children. Without modern medicine they frequently could anticipate painful and debilitating disorders arising from the rigors of repeated childbirth. Moreover, they lived in a world where the facts of life and the processes of procreation were shrouded in secrecy and not thought fit topics for female conversation.

Contemporary manuals of advice offered little help. They encouraged women to accept their God-given biological destiny and prepare for a life of self-sacrificing service to others. What information they did give was often faulty. Even into the twentieth century some of these manuals adhered, for example, to the widespread but mistaken view that conception was most likely to occur during menstruation and least probable during the time we now know as ovulation.

Under these conditions it is not surprising that women responded avidly to those who could give them real medical relief and a good dose of understanding. One major source of such sympathetic healing in the nineteenth century was an aberrant medical practice known as hydropathy, or the water cure. From 1843 to 1900, 213 water cure centers sprang up to treat Americans of both sexes with the beneficent effects of pure water, and the good news of the water cure spread rapidly, especially among women.[1]

Hydropathy was based on the belief that water

KATHRYN KISH SKLAR is Professor of History at the University of California, Los Angeles, California.

© 1974 American Heritage Publishing Co., Inc. Reprinted by permission from *American Heritage* (December 1974).

was the natural sustainer of life. It prescribed bathing, wet compresses, steam, massage, exercise, the drinking of cold water, and a spare diet. From the time of its founding in 1845 through the 1850s the *Water-Cure Journal and Herald of Reforms, devoted to Physiology, Hydropathy, and the Laws of Life*—its motto "Wash and Be Healed"—popularized the cure, listed new establishments, presented exemplary case histories, and promoted many corollary doctrines such as temperance, women's rights, dress reform, and medical reform. It strongly endorsed the need for women medical practitioners, believing that most male doctors were insensitive to the problems of women and poorly trained to treat these problems. The *Journal*'s campaign on behalf of women doctors in the 1850s kept close tabs on medical school admissions policies, and in bold type its readers were informed each time an institution opened its doors to women applicants.

The water cure, although it became especially meaningful to women, began as a phenomenon offered enthusiastically to all.

> All hail to pure cold water
> That bright rich gem from heaven;
> And praise to the creator,
> For such a blessing given!

So ran the first stanza of a musical testimonial composed by Mrs. A. J. Judson in the 1840s. Other water cure enthusiasts, more extravagant if less poetic in their praise, claimed to have witnessed miraculous recoveries among their patients. Catharine Beecher, a nationally known educator, daughter of the famous evangelical preacher and older sister of Harriet Beecher Stowe, observed "one friend, a confirmed invalid of fifteen or more years," who could not walk a half mile when he arrived at the cure, leave after four months "able to perform such exploits as climbing a mountain" and feeling "the health and elastic vigor of childhood." Another patient, "given over by all physicians as the victim of scrofulous consumption" and having "selected his place for burial," after seven months of the water cure "left, declaring himself a new man, and anticipating health and long life." Other "interesting cases" observed by Catharine Beecher included two little girls brought to the water cure "emaciated and helpless, one with a leg useless from infancy, the other with distorted spine." Restored to health, "they gambol together now," Beecher said, "with ruddy cheeks and vigorous health, so changed and improved that a certain cure is fully anticipated by the physician."

The most fashionable, most expensive, and best-known center of such restorative activity was located at Brattleboro, Vermont. There such notable Americans as Julia Ward Howe, Martin Van Buren's family, Francis Parkman, Henry Wadsworth Longfellow, Richard Henry Dana, Harriet Beecher Stowe, and Helen Hunt Jackson enjoyed the establishment's mountain environs, participated in a constant round of social activities, and generally gave themselves over to the serious business of improving their psychic and physical health.

In 1851 the railroad to Brattleboro was completed, and a golden decade began at the water cure center. Visitors were met at the depot by Tom Miner, who drove the village coach during that period—returning patrons were greeted personally—and trunks were piled high on the top of the coach for a precarious ride down Main Street to the Wesselhoeft sanitarium. The crack of the whip and the rumble of the coach daily announced new arrivals to those already sequestered in the center's commodious buildings—two large houses linked by a new dancing salon and parlor in the front and by bathhouses in the rear. The main buildings thus formed a square, enclosing a green courtyard with a fountain and surrounded on three sides by a broad piazza that served as a sheltered place of exercise for the patients in bad weather. One side of the buildings was reserved for women, the other for men. Behind this complex was another new building containing the kitchen, the dining hall, and the doctors' offices on the first floor, with a range of single and double rooms above. As a sign of the increasing prosperity of the center and its

growing resort atmosphere, an additional building containing a bowling alley, billiards room, and gymnasium was erected to serve the large numbers of new patients who arrived by rail.

The remarkable popularity of Brattleboro demonstrates how rapidly the water cure craze took hold of middle-class Americans. Opening in May 1845, with 15 patients, it expanded during its first season to accommodate 150. The next year it more than doubled its clientele and its staff. By the end of the 1850s the place attracted between 600 and 800 guests annually. The *Green Mountain Spring Monthly Journal*, edited by Brattleboro's chief doctor, Robert Wesselhoeft, claimed a circulation of thirty thousand copies in 1851; and Wesselhoeft's main assistant, Charles Grau, began another monthly in 1858, the *Brattleborough Hydropathic Messenger*. Dozens of other water cure establishments were equally successful as the craze extended from New England through the Middle Atlantic and Middle Western states.

Who were these water cure enthusiasts, and why were they so enthusiastic? Casual visitors to the cure sites made it clear in their letters home that the clientele was predominantly female. At Brattleboro roughly two-thirds of the patients seem to have been women. This proportion is astonishing in a period that discouraged women from traveling alone, and we might well assume that for every woman who came to the spa alone, there was one who persuaded her husband, father, or brother to accompany her there and make use of the resort facilities while she engaged in the full routine of the cure. The new bowling alley, billiards room, and gymnasium may indeed have been built to accommodate these male escorts. The costs were the same for all guests—ten dollars a week in summer and eleven dollars in winter—covering "medical advice, board, lodging, and attendance at baths." Wesselhoeft claimed that no patients were turned away for lack of funds, but his was obviously a profit-making enterprise designed primarily for middle- and upper-class patrons.

The cure put heavy emphasis on bodily sensation and physical exertion. As Dr. Wesselhoeft explained it, a typical day at the spa began at four in the morning, when the patient was awakened and wrapped in thick woolen blankets, leaving only the face or sometimes the whole head free. "All other contact of the body with air was carefully prevented." The patron was left to perspire "till his covering itself becomes wet." During this time the head "may be covered with cold compresses and the patient may drink as much fresh water as he likes." Windows and doors were opened wide during this process. When the attendant "observes that there has been perspiration enough, he dips the patient into a cold bath, which is ready in the neighborhood of the bed." This deliberate shock to the system was held to be highly restorative, and when it was over, patients said they felt a new "sense of comfort." A mysterious process of purging was believed to occur during the cold water plunge, the pores giving off "clammy" waste matter and absorbing the pure moisture of the spring water. "This is the moment when the wholesome change of matter takes place," Dr. Wesselhoeft wrote, "by which the whole system gradually becomes purified. In no case has this sudden change of temperature proved to be injurious."

When the bath was finished, the patient was sent out to walk and to drink the pure spring water from a variety of nearby natural sources. Meals were very simple and consisted of only a few varieties of food. At breakfast there was a choice between bread and milk and mush and milk; at dinner, soup, one kind of meat—usually beef or mutton—vegetables, and a plain pudding; supper was a repetition of breakfast with the addition of fruit. Tea and coffee were banned altogether. Like most water cure physicians Wesselhoeft preferred not to administer any drugs.

Besides rigorous bathing the cure had two other chief principles: a communal atmosphere and an emphasis on the curative powers of outdoor exercise. Situated among hills bordering the Connecticut River, Brattleboro's scenery "on every hand is of the most romantic and beautiful kind," Wesselhoeft wrote when he first discovered it. "Thus," he continued, "it offers inducements to the exercise which forms so important a part of the cure. Fresh springs issue from all the surrounding hills . . . beautiful natural walks lead to each spring. Hills and green woods invite the patient on every side." A half mile from the main buildings Wesselhoeft placed outdoor baths among the trees beneath a hill bordering the Whetstone Brook. A thatched summer shelter was built in another spot, provided

with seats, and given the enticing name "Eagle's Nest." Many paths wound along the hillsides, through the woods, and beside the waters of the Whetstone and along the West and Connecticut rivers. Possibly with an eye to his entrepreneurial responsibilities, Wesselhoeft instituted a rule that each patient should contribute a dollar toward keeping the paths in repair. "A regular account was kept of receipts and expenditures, and each contributor, becoming a stockholder, had the right of suggesting improvements," one of Dr. Wesselhoeft's patients explained. Additional bathhouses were fitted into the landscape during the 1850s and 1860s, indicating both the success of the doctor's plan and the cooperative spirit of his patrons.

Perhaps because they had adopted an adversary relationship to the wilderness for two centuries, Americans were less accustomed than Europeans to practicing "the art of life lived in the open air," but Wesselhoeft and other water cure practitioners were determined to show them that the outdoors could be the site of genteel leisure as well as hard work. These outdoor activities were particularly adapted to women. "Breakfast and luncheon on the veranda, needlework and reading aloud by groups in sequestered nooks, walking at all times and in all directions, archery and picnics in favoring weather were features of his curriculum," wrote one observer. "By means of open wagons, stage-coaches and horseback, where nature was most alluring," wrote another, "picnickers would gather."

This environment was structured to provide women with more physical freedom than they experienced in the polite Victorian society then taking shape in American towns and cities. Whereas tightly laced corsets, elaborate attire, and the myth of female fragility constrained the average woman during this period, water cure centers encouraged women to experience the psychic and physical relaxation that comes from healthy bodily exercise. Another structural advantage of the cure site for women was its rule against the admission of children. Admitted as patients but not as dependents of patients, children were kept at a distance. Boarding schools grew up in the area to accommodate them, but while at the cure itself mothers had to resign themselves to a sweet interlude of childlessness. Communing instead with adults, they could choose from a wide variety of social events ranging from amateur theatricals and musicals to "hydropathic balls." For unmarried women water cure establishments were congenial to courtship activities, and romance flourished among its young patrons.

Yet the water cures had more to offer women than a romantically restful resort atmosphere at the sanitariums. As the pages of the *Water-Cure Journal* proclaimed, gynecological medicine was a major concern of hydropathy. Discussions of childbirth, menstruation, and diseases and disorders of the generative process filled the *Journal,* and related topics such as frequency of sexual intercourse, masturbation, abortion, and barrenness also received discreet attention. In all these matters hydropathy lived up to its claim to be the friend of nineteenth-century women. Its sympathy for the special medical problems of women stood in stark contrast to the hostility and indifference characteristic of traditional contemporary medicine.

The basic attitude of hydropathists toward the health of women was most clearly revealed in its treatment of childbirth. In one of its early issues the *Water-Cure Journal* presented its views on the topic, saying: "It is very certain that woman's suffering in labor can be in a great degree prevented, and that she need not endure that weakness after child-birth which is so common." Far from accepting severe pain during childbirth as natural or following the biblical imperative as a sign of Eve's guilt in originating sin, water curists felt that "it was unnatural for woman to be so injured, so torn to pieces, so wrecked by natural pains." Hydropathy tried to reduce labor pains by encouraging women to relax with massage and warm baths during labor, and it sought to minimize the effects of childbearing on the female constitution by promoting extensive exercise during pregnancy and a prompt return to routine activities after delivery.

One of the reasons nineteenth-century women thought themselves frail and weak was that they *became* frail and weak during the protracted convalescence that orthodox medicine prescribed after childbirth. Most women remained in bed for several weeks and grew progressively enfeebled. Mrs. M. M. Gross, a doctor and a practicing hydropathist, believed that childbirth was a season of "purification" for a woman, and "it is absurd for her to envelope herself in blankets, and live for weeks in an unventilated room, where no air or water is permitted to clean her person, or purify her lungs." Women who had benefited from water cure principles during childbirth frequently compared its effectiveness to orthodox methods in the pages of the *Journal.* One Mrs. O. C. W. wrote that she was "kept confined to my bed nearly two months" with the birth of her first child, and "it was not until about the middle of the following summer that I attained my former health and strength." Wanting to avoid this "regular" treatment and "regular" results with her next child, she converted to "hydropathic, that is, natural principles."

Except for the heavy reliance on cold water those principles, as Mrs. O. C. W. describes them, bear a remarkable similarity to modern maternity care:

> At my confinement, I was attended by intelligent females of the Water Cure order. Of doctors we had no need. At the commencement of labor, I took a sitz bath, and an enema of cold water; these soothed me into a quiet sleep, and seemed to prepare me for my coming trials. After the birth of the child, I was allowed to remain about an hour; I was then bathed in cool water, and linen towels wet in cold water were applied to the abdomen. The next morning I was again bathed, and I arose from my bed, walked to a chair, and sat up while I ate my breakfast, which consisted of Graham bread, a glass of cold water, and a few stewed peaches. In the afternoon I again arose, and partook of similar refreshments.

On the third day after her delivery she walked outside, and within a week she was once more enjoying her "usual health," she wrote—a typical water cure recovery. So strikingly did her maternal care contrast with the usual experience of women in childbirth that this woman's daring became the talk of her upstate New York town. Originally she herself "could not . . . really believe that I should be quite so speedily raised up," and her neighbors had warned her of the "rashness, presumption and folly" of her water cure plans. Nevertheless her rapid recovery and sound health showed that her trust in the water cure had been well placed.

The success of hydropathy in gynecological treatment arose from its willingness to abandon orthodox theory and practice, its willingness to transcend contemporary stereotypes and conventions pertaining to women, and its belief that the best medical practices for women were those that the patients liked and that made them feel good. This new health care was based on what had been found to work rather than what physicians believed ought to work. In keeping with this pragmatism, hydropathy encouraged women to take an active role at all levels of their own health care—by becoming physicians themselves (the *Water-Cure Journal* anticipated that women would soon dominate medicine, it being a field properly theirs through its close association with qualities of nurture); by reforming their dress and abandoning the fashionable garb that deformed their ribs, impaired their internal organs, created chronic shortness of breath, and generally inhibited their free movement; and by taking personal charge of their own health after mastering the basic invigorating principles of bathing, exercise, and a spare diet. A revolutionary premise stood behind these hydropathic beliefs: that a woman's body belonged to herself—not to her doctor, not to her children, and not to her husband.

In fact, the control by women of their own bodies was a basic tenet of the water cure; its corollary was the regulation of male sexual impulses. While orthodox physicians "saw woman as the product and prisoner of her reproductive system," water curists tried to help women exercise control over this system. The *Journal* not only hammered away at their campaign for more women doctors but also exposed and ridiculed the growing tendency of the medical profession to treat women as ignorant children who must be guided by their betters—especially by their physicians. When a leading gynecologist attacked female midwives as "cold, hard, calculating," hence unwomanly, and hence dangerous, the *Journal* denounced such self-serving misogyny, pointing out that a struggle was being waged for the control of the medical treatment of women. The *Journal* vowed to resist orthodoxy's effort to "wrest from our hands the very-well-paying and correspondingly important practice of midwifery."

T. L. Nichols, a doctor, a frequent contributor to the *Journal*, and a supporter of women's rights, declared: "Women must become their own physicians, and the physicians of each other. They have

leaned too long upon a broken reed." He further insisted that every woman must have "control of her own [life]" before she could be cured of illness. The control of a woman's sexual life by her husband was especially pernicious, Nichols implied, since it subjected her to the potentially deadly abuse of her generative system. "By the sensual and selfish indulgences of those who claim the legal right to murder them in this manner, and whom no law of homicide can reach, and upon whose acts no coroner holds an inquest," Nichols wrote, "thousands of women are consigned to premature graves."

Although Nichols's language may seem exaggerated, it should be remembered that the sexual experience of nineteenth-century women occurred in a culture that attributed an almost insatiable sexual drive to males, but practically none to females. Acting on such cultural definitions, many men assumed that women had no sexual needs of their own and that their role in sexual intercourse was merely that of an agency through which male satisfaction could be achieved. In these circumstances it is not surprising that many women were dissatisfied with their sexual lives in the nineteenth century and that they began to speak by midcentury of controlling "conjugal excesses." In this effort to assert some female control over sexuality the water cure provided emotional support and medical documentation. Most important, it advocated sexual abstinence as an essential ingredient in the cure of a wide variety of female illnesses ranging from nervous prostration to inverted wombs. On the question of sexual expression itself the *Journal* decried "conjugal excesses" as "a shame to our race" as well as a danger to female health and maintained that "the true and only safe rule in the exercise of the propensities and instincts God has given us for the wisest of purposes, is *to be temperate in all things*."

To understand fully the eagerness with which middle-class nineteenth-century women flocked to water cure centers, it is first necessary to understand how widespread ill health—usually associated with the reproductive system—was among them. In fact, so general were physical disorders among women of childbearing age that invalidism often became both chronic and ritualized. Invalidism did offer certain compensations. The decline, convalescence, and recovery ceremonies of the female sickroom allowed women to communicate with one another about their physiological fears and to express their normally repressed emotions. Whether they were nurses, companions, or patients, women in the sickroom were freed from the usual taboos against intimacy between females.

Invalidism was also a means through which women could express their resentment at being excluded from the culture's dominant values of competition, achievement, strength, and self-assertion. If their sex disqualified them from full social usefulness, then it could also disable them for the performance of their unrewarding routine duties.

Harriet Beecher Stowe, after ten years of childbirth and marriage, retreated for nearly a year to Brattleboro's water cure, from which she declared her unhappiness to her husband, Calvin. Assessing her marriage, she recalled the "sickness, pain, perplexity, constant discouragement, wearing, wasting days and nights" of the early years when Calvin was often absent and of little help when he was present. "Ah, how little comfort had I in being a mother—how all that I proposed was met and crossed and in every way hedged up! In short," Harriet concluded, "God would teach me that I should make no family be my chief good and portion, and bitter as the lesson has been, I thank Him for it from my very soul."

Calvin managed the household as best he could in Harriet's absence. Remaining at Brattleboro months longer than she had originally anticipated, Harriet slowly but deliberately advanced through the steps leading to an invalid's cure. Defending her need for a prolonged stay, Harriet gave herself sufficient time to think through her attitude toward American society's treatment of women and her own response to that treatment. *Uncle Tom's Cabin,* written a few years later, was built on the premise that there was something basically incompatible between the insitutions of American society and the well-being of its oppressed minorities—especially of its women, both white and black.

The extent of female invalidism was recorded by Mrs. Stowe's sister, Catharine Beecher, in an 1855 publication, *Letters to the People on Health and Happiness.* In a personal poll that sampled a total of seventy-nine communities and over a thousand women, she found that the sick outnumbered the well by a ratio of three to one. In a typical community profile of Batavia, Illinois, she recorded:

> Mrs. H. an invalid. Mrs. G. scrofula. Mrs. W. liver complaint. Mrs. K. pelvic disorders. Mrs. S. pelvic diseases. Mrs. B. pelvic diseases very badly. Mrs. B. not healthy. Mrs. T. very feeble. Mrs. G. cancer. Mrs. N. liver complaint. Do not know one healthy woman in the place.

Surveying the health of her personal acquaintances, she concluded, "I am not able to recall, in my immense circle of friends and acquaintances all over the Union so many as *ten* married ladies born in this century and country, who are perfectly sound, healthy, and vigorous." Although Catharine Beecher's casually gathered statistics provide impressionistic rather than conclusive measurements of the health of her generation, they do show that great numbers of women perceived their health as precarious, and they demonstrate the ubiquity of the image that linked women with infirmity in the middle decades of the nineteenth century.

Catharine Beecher's remedies for this situation fell into three categories. First, she campaigned for dress reform and an end to the suffering women experienced through fashions that distorted their physiology and hampered their freedom of movement. Second, she urged women to exercise regularly and rigorously to restore the natural resilience of their bodies. Third, she recommended the water cure and its attendant comforts.

Not all water cure propagandists were as "respectable" as the Beecher sisters, however. Given hydropathy's emphasis on the physical emancipation of women, it is not surprising that women's rights advocates of all kinds should have been drawn to the movement. The career of Mary Gove Nichols—a leading water cure lecturer from 1845 to 1853—serves as an example.

Born to a freethinking father and a Universalist mother, Mary Neal married Hiram Gove in 1831 and bore their first child a year later. Four subsequent pregnancies were abortive or produced a stillborn child. While Gove grew increasingly tyrannical, petty, and economically dependent on her needlework during the 1830s, Mary began to administer cold water treatments to neighboring women; and by the end of the decade she began lecturing to women on anatomy, physiology, and hygiene. In 1838 the newly formed Ladies Physiological Society in Boston invited her to give a course of lectures, and this launched Mrs. Gove on a health reform career dedicated to relieving women from the suffering they experienced due to their ignorance of biology and especially of sex. In 1842 she published her *Lectures to Ladies on Anatomy and Physiology* and left her husband.

After lecturing to female patients at Brattleboro in 1845, she established her own water cure center in New York the next year and increasingly emphasized the necessity of mutual love for the procreation of healthy children. In 1848 she married Dr. T. L. Nichols, and together they opened a new water cure establishment in New York City, established a short-lived coeducational water cure medical school—the American Hydropathic Institute—in New York, and increasingly adopted radical answers to the questions posed by the status of women. She and Nichols planned a "School of Life," to be located at Modern Times, site of a Long Island utopian community. At the school complete freedom was to be practiced in every human relationship, including that of sex. Every woman was to have the right to choose the father of her child. In their joint work on marriage in 1854 and in *Nichols' Journal of Health, Water-Cure and Human Progress* they attacked marriage as the origin of most human misery and evil. This advocacy of "free love" was totally out of Victorian bounds, and from then on the Nicholses were ostracized by respectable water curists.

Mary Gove Nichols was one of several women who lectured to women audiences about their physiology at midcentury. Such lecture courses were a standard event at water cure centers, especially those designed primarily or exclusively for women. The Glen Haven Water-Cure of upstate New York employed Harriet Austin as resident physician for women, and her advertisements in the *Journal* stressed the fact that women at Glen Haven "walk erect as God made women to walk." Summing up the Glen Haven attitude toward women, Dr. Austin said: "We eat, we drink, we sleep, we work, we dress, we laugh, we pray *with freedom.*" She encouraged women to come to Glen Haven to learn "our ideas, our notions, our plans, our purposes" and to carry back "our forms of life into the centers where they dwell. . . . We propagate our principles

. . . we make thorough converts of those we have not seen."

Whether or not it was converting women sight unseen, hydropathy was encouraging new forms of freedom for women. Some of these were revealed in an article by Thomas Nichols in his *Journal* in 1851. There Nichols concluded by condemning (and at the same time probably informing most of his readers about) the shocking practices begun by "a mercenary and libidinous wretch" whose medical practice consisted in "manipulations and anointings, managed in such a way as to stimulate the passions and produce a temporary excitement of the organs which his deluded victims mistake for a beneficial result." This masturbatory cure was "extremely lucrative," Nichols said, deluding "thousands of women" in New York City alone, and "has been taken up in other places." He assumed that "every pure-minded woman" condemned these "shameful practices."

Perceptive readers of the *Journal* might have noticed, however, a great similarity between Nichols's methods and those he condemned. Sexual release through genital stimulation was a rudimentary water cure experience for women. In this same article Nichols described the most common water cure treatment for the most common female disability, *prolapsus uteri,* or fallen womb, thus: "The water-cure treatment for *prolapsus uteri* is the general treatment of invigoration; and the local treatment best fitted to give tone to the whole region of the pelvis." Prominent among the available options, he said, were wet bandages, "carefully and tightly applied," the "sitz-bath," and "frequent vaginal injections." As a general principle, he concluded, "whatever exhausts vitality in a woman causes *prolapsus uteri.* Whatever restores the tone of the nervous system cures it." Thus although Nichols drew the line at overt masturbation, he did encourage patients to experience release of tension through stimulation of the "pelvic" area.

While an air of Victorian repression hovered over the lives of most American women, those frequenting the water cure found a sympathetic sanctuary where they could be more expressive and feel more relaxed than they did at home. There was something profoundly comforting about these cure centers for women. There bodily sensuality could be more freely indulged, and female communality replaced the characteristic isolation of American domestic life. One patient's sketch captured this sense of release in the 1850s:

> The next morning, after visiting the lady physician in her neat little office, we made our first visit to the bathing rooms, and found the baths really agreeable. Figures gliding in and out draped in sheets. . . . One lady sat with sketch book in her hand and sketched her companions, amidst a burst of fun and laughter, herself the most comical of the group, her head turbaned with a crash towel and her robe hanging as gracefully about her little figure as the robes of Roman Senators in the days of the Empire.

An important part of the release women experienced was simply that of being able to talk about their bodies and their symptoms. "The experience of each individual gradually becomes known to most of [his or her] fellow patients," Catharine Beecher wrote in praise of the cure in the *New York Observer* in 1851. This communal aspect of the treatment could provide women with the psychologically reassuring knowledge that their problems were shared by others, and practitioners of hydropathy were fully aware of the therapeutic benefits of this kind of communication. "The hydropathic treatment differs from all others," the *Journal* maintained in 1850, "inasmuch as it is administered to hundreds of persons congregated in one place, who are in the constant habit of meeting and discussing its merits, so that there is nothing important that is not known to the whole body; whilst under the allopathian and homeopathian treatment, patients are treated at their own homes, so that none but their own families know the results of either mode of treatment."

Women who were ill may have chosen the water cure because it provided a supportive female environment and frequently employed women doctors, but in so doing they were probably also choosing the best medical treatment available to them at the time. In comparison with orthodox medicine the water cure at least provided the fundamentals of exercise, cleanliness, good diet, and a reassuring environment, rather than leeches, injections, and strong drugs in the isolation of one's usual domestic setting. One outstanding specialist in uterine

diseases still, in 1858, taught medical students to insert leeches into the womb even though he admitted that this could "induce a paroxysm of almost intolerable suffering." Thomas Nichols voiced an attitude typical of water cure advocates when he denounced the "tinkerings and torturings" of orthodox gynecological medicine, saying that "their scarifications, leechings, cauterizings" outrage human sensibilities and "produce the most deplorable results."

Nineteenth-century women could not, of course, rely on abstinence as their sole means of avoiding pregnancy. Abortive pills were widely advertised in spite of the new set of state regulations designed to prevent women from seeking this option. Typical of such advertisements was one that appeared in the *Milwaukee Sentinel* in 1857:

> Dr. Chessman's Pills. The combination of Ingredients in these pills are the result of a long and extensive practice. They are mild in their operation, and certain in correcting all irregularities. Painful Menstruations, removing all obstructions, whether from cold or otherwise, headache, pain in the side, palpitation of the heart, disturbed sleep, which arise from the interruption of nature. To MARRIED LADIES they are invaluable, as they will bring on the monthly period with regularity. NOTICE: they should not be used during pregnancy, as a miscarriage would certainly result therefrom.

Clearly women in the mid-nineteenth century were seeking contraceptive and abortive remedies. Here, too, hydropathy may have served as an important source of information and sympathetic treatment. One example of such support was that provided by Russell Trall, an early popularizer and leader of hydropathy, who in his *Hydropathic Encyclopedia* of 1853 mentions "the safe period" and other contraceptive devices. Trall believed, Norman Himes noted in his *Medical History of Contraception*, that "a woman had an absolute right to determine when she should, and when she should not conceive." And on a less formal level it seems probable that women doctors at water cure establishments in their lectures and conversations with their women patients shared what knowledge they had of the use of contraceptive techniques.

Orthodox medicine, by contrast, took a very negative view of efforts by women to control the birth of children. "The dread of suffering, fears respecting their own health and strength, the trouble and expense of large families, and professedly, also, the responsibility incurred in the education of children, these and other reasons equally futile and trifling ... induce them to destroy the product of that conjugal union for which marriage was instituted," Dr. Hugh Hodge asserted in lectures delivered at the University of Pennsylvania Medical School in 1839.

Given this hostility of orthodox medicine to the "trifling" problems of women, hydropathy must have seemed a tremendous blessing. Offering at least a temporary respite from their annual childbearing, offering sympathy for their pain, a chance to discuss their fears, and a recognition of their sensuality, it is no wonder that water cure establishments won the patronage and enthusiastic support of so many American women.

NOTES

1 References for this article may be found in Kathryn Kish Sklar, *Catharine Beecher: A Study in American Domesticity* (New Haven: Yale University Press, 1973).

19

The Woman behind the Trademark

SARAH STAGE

Generations of Americans grew up with Lydia Pinkham. Her face, kindly yet abstracted, her gray hair drawn back into a braided bun, the solid respectability of black silk and white ruching became as familiar as the daily newspaper or the neighborhood druggist's display where she advertised her Vegetable Compound for over eighty years. No advertising agent intent on creating the perfect grandmother could have done a better job. He didn't have to. Lydia Pinkham was authentic. And yet of the woman behind the trademark we know little. A few letters, a scrapbook, and a dog-eared set of cashbooks provide the only clues that help to separate the actual Lydia Pinkham from the advertisement of herself. Over the years the story of her life, like her famous photograph, has been continually retouched until the legend of Lydia Pinkham comes to us suspiciously cast in the language of a company advertisement. To discover the actual woman, we must place her against the social and intellectual landscape of nineteenth-century America and reconstruct her life by sketching in the background until the outlines of the woman emerge in relief.

Genealogical records provide the first clues. Born on February 9, 1819, in Lynn, Massachusetts, Lydia was the tenth of a dozen children in the family of William and Rebecca Estes. This prolific Quaker clan and their assorted kin counted themselves among the founding families of Lynn. When genealogy became fashionable, Lydia Pinkham's chil-

dren traced their ancestry back to the thirteenth-century Italian house of Este. In the political intrigues of Dante's day, the Estes had been forced into exile in England where they remained for four centuries, until 1676, when Quaker Matthew Estes migrated to America. The penchant for political and religious dissidence which marked the Esteses' long history continued unabated in Lydia's family.[1]

Billy Estes, Lydia's father, began his career as a shoemaker, or cordwainer, in the late eighteenth century when Lynn was already earning its reputation as "the city of shoes." During the War of 1812, Estes constructed a saltworks on the flatlands near his home, an investment which paid off handsomely and enabled him to escape the ranks of Lynn's independent shoemakers at a time when competition and repeated business depressions threatened to pauperize the cordwainers.[2] By the time Lydia was born, Billy Estes owned a substantial farm on the corner of Estes and Broad streets, ideally located in the path of the city's development. He became a gentleman farmer who made his fortune in real estate.

If, as some of the local reformers complained, Lynn Quakers too frequently lost their moral militancy when they achieved financial success, the pattern did not hold for Billy Estes and his wife. When the Lynn Friends refused to endorse the abolition of slavery in the 1830s, the Esteses joined the radical "Come Outer" faction, which left the meetinghouse in protest. Although Lydia was only in her teens when she put aside her Quaker dress, she always remained something of a Quaker in temperament, as evidenced by her distrust of ecclesiastical and secular authority.

Lydia's mother, Rebecca Estes, like so many other radical Quakers, turned to the writings of Swedish theologian Emanuel Swedenborg, and in her en-

SARAH STAGE is Associate Professor of History at the University of California, Riverside, California.

"The Woman Behind the Trademark" is reprinted from *Female Complaints: Lydia Pinkham and the Business of Women's Medicine,* by Sarah Stage, by permission of W. W. Norton & Company, Inc. Copyright © 1979 by W. W. Norton & Company, Inc.

thusiasm introduced Lydia and the family to his ideas. Swedenborg, an eighteenth-century scientist turned theologian, was viewed by many as a fanatical mystic. His claim to have been in communication with the angels led to his ridicule and persecution. In reality his theology was part of a broader reaction against the rationalism of his century. He sought not to reconcile religion to science, but science to religion—to get beyond the description of phenomena to first principles. American transcendentalists admired him because, as Ralph Waldo Emerson wrote, Swedenborg "saw and showed the connections between nature and the affections of the soul."³

Swedenborg's beliefs nicely suited the psychological needs of the nineteenth century. He insisted that he had visited a spiritual world—between heaven and hell—where men went after death. The dead, he promised, were not in the grave, nor did they await judgment before an angry God. Instead they were "resuscitated" after death and sent to "dwell in gardens where flower beds and grass plots are seen beautifully arranged, with rows of trees round about, and arbors and walks."⁴ Friends and acquaintances, wives and husbands, brothers and sisters met and conversed in the spirit kingdom. Children passed immediately into heaven where they became angels attended by a loving angel woman. His description of the spirit kingdom served to allay fears of damnation and helped to create an afterlife with an appealing human dimension. To the many nineteenth-century men and women who lost their children and loved ones to disease and hardship, his message came as a soothing balm.

It was a short step from Swedenborgianism to spiritualism. Although Swedenborg himself had inveighed against meddling with the spirits of the dead, many of his readers, Lydia Pinkham among them, could see nothing wrong with establishing contact with a spirit world so benign. In the 1850s, when the Fox sisters of Rochester created a sensation with their spirit rappings, many prominent Americans embraced spiritualism or flirted with seances and spirit boards.

Swedenborg's theology met the social as well as the psychological needs of nineteenth-century Americans. He replaced the harsh features of Calvinism with the portrait of a God at one with man and the promise that all men could win a place in heaven through love of God and fidelity to duty.

His was a commonsense salvation which contained in it the seeds of social reform. European Swedenborgians were among the first to champion the antislavery cause. By the 1840s, Swedenborg's American followers embraced not only antislavery but a host of seemingly disparate movements which they saw as flowing from the same "fruitful unity."⁵ Temperance, vegetarianism, homeopathy, and Fourierism, as well as spiritualism, won their support.

Although Lydia Pinkham never joined the Swedenborgian New Church and never formally claimed adherence to its doctrines, Swedenborgianism seems to have supplied the philosophical framework which held together her own commitment to movements which included antislavery, temperance, and spiritualism. Without an understanding of Swedenborg, it would be difficult to perceive a fruitful unity large enough to encompass her varied interests.

Lydia Pinkham grew up in the forcing house of New England reform. As Emerson wrote to Carlyle, "We are all a little wild here, with numberless projects of social reform. Not a reading man but has a draft of a new community in his waistcoat pocket."⁶ So, although the perimeters of her life were marked by Boston on the south and Bedford on the west, Lydia came to know a surprising number of the leading figures of her day. In the decades before the Civil War, Lynn provided a center seat for the drama of agitation and reform.

The social atmosphere of Lynn intensified the reform spirit. Unlike its wealthier neighbors Boston and Salem, Lynn prided itself on its working-class character. An editorial in the local paper boasted, "This is not a place for idlers and social parasites." The townspeople frowned upon aristocracy. Lynn boosters liked to claim that the town was "a well regulated republic in miniature," but in fact the disdain for everything that smacked of conservatism or elitism made it an exceptionally volatile community which one prominent abolitionist characterized as a "place of fearless discussion."⁷

The Estes household in Lynn served as one of the gathering places for antislavery leaders. William Lloyd Garrison, editor of the *Liberator* and one of the most hated men in America, counted Rebecca Estes among his friends and visited her when he spoke in Lynn. Lydia Marie Child, popular author of *The American Frugal Housewife,* and her husband, David, editor of the antislavery *Massachusetts Whig Journal,* found themselves ostracized from Boston society because of their radical views and were glad to find welcome in the Estes house on Broad Street. The fighting ministers Wendell Phillips and Parker Pillsbury, the Quaker poet John Greenleaf Whittier (a distant relative by marriage to Rebecca Estes), and Nathaniel Rogers, editor of the *Herald of Freedom,* all frequented the Estes drawing room.

Down the street lived the Singing Hutchinsons, a colorful family who became the balladeers of temperance, woman's rights, and abolition. Abby Kelley, later one of the most effective speakers on the antislavery platform, taught at the local Friends' school. And on Union Street lived Lynn's most famous resident, the fugitive slave Frederick Douglass.

Small wonder Lydia gave her allegiance early to the antislavery movement. At the age of sixteen she joined the Lynn Female Anti-Slavery Society. Lucretia Mott, the society's national founder, held a commitment to antislavery matched only by her belief in woman's rights. Abby Kelley, Lydia, her mother, and her elder sister were among the charter members of the Lynn group.

The Estes family and their friends to the contrary, antislavery was not a popular cause in the 1830s and 1840s. Abolitionist speakers often found themselves locked out of halls and churches and not infrequently met by angry mobs. On at least one occasion, an abolitionist orator had to seek protection behind the skirts of a cordon of Lynn girls. No doubt Lydia and her sister were among the group.[8]

The Estes family thrived on controversy. In 1842 Lydia's elder sister, Gulielma Maria (named for the wife of William Penn), was asked to leave the Methodist church because of her friendship with Frederick Douglass. The incident, recounted in the *Liberator* and the *Herald of Freedom,* began when Gulielma went walking with Douglass and took his arm. The Reverend Jacob Sanborn found her action scandalous. Summoning her to his study, he catechized her on her behavior. An indignant Gulielma scored him in kind for his bigotry. When the Reverend asked if she "was much acquainted with colored people," she responded, "not as much as I hope to be," and asked him point-blank if he thought it a crime to associate with Negroes. The flustered

minister blurted out, "I think them a different race—their features are different," and ventured that although he did not condone segregation, he thought when Negroes attended his church they should sit by themselves in the gallery. Sanborn brought the interview to a climax by putting to Gulielma the question, "Would you *marry* a colored man?" Color, she responded, would make no difference. She would look only on character. With that Sanborn dismissed her. Later he ordered her to come before the congregation and "confess that she had been imprudent in being in the company of colored men in the *manner* which she acknowledges, and promise that she will do so no more . . . or her connection with the Church must be dissolved." Gulielma scorned the invitation. At its next meeting, the Essex County Anti-Slavery Society resolved that the Methodist Episcopal church was not a church of Christ, but "a synagogue of Satan."[9]

Frederick Douglass remained a fast friend of the Esteses. Among Lydia Pinkham's few surviving possessions is a "Friendship Album" containing an entry written by Douglass in 1848 which begins, "My dear Friend, How unspeakably pleasant it is to meet old and dear friends after a long separation."[10] One story, probably apocryphal, recounted how Lydia once stood in the way of a conductor who threatened to evict Douglass to the Jim Crow car. Douglass resolutely refused to sit in the car reserved for blacks and Irish on the Boston and Lynn railroad. When an angry group of passengers tried to remove him, he clung so tightly to his seat that it was ripped from the floor.[11]

The segregation of public facilities extended to the churches, meetinghouses, and public halls. In 1842 the Lynn Lyceum barred the black speaker Charles Lenox Remond. Lydia and Gulielma Estes joined dissidents who boycotted the Lyceum and formed a new subscription lecture series under the auspices of a society called the Freeman's Institute. The group chose as its motto "No concealment— No compromise."[12]

The following year the membership of the institute, under the presidency of Douglass, elected Lydia Estes secretary. In her journal, she copied in her copperplate hand the constitution of the club which provided, "No person shall be excluded from full participation in any of the operations of the Society on account of sex, complexion, or religious or political opinions."[13] The emphasis on sexual as well as racial equality distinguished the Freeman's Institute and highlighted a significant aspect of the antislavery movement.

The "woman question" touched off controversy in the antislavery movement in the late 1830s. Garrison and Nathaniel Rogers insisted that the women who formed the backbone of the local societies should be allowed to hold national office. The notion that women should participate equally in the leadership of the American Anti-Slavery Society disturbed not a few of the organization's male members. The controversy reached a climax at the annual meeting in 1840 when Abby Kelley, with Garrison's support, was elected to the business committee and Lucretia Mott and Lydia Maria Child won places on the executive committee. The more conservative delegates walked out, claiming that Garrison's insistence on women's equality clouded the antislavery issue by raising an "extraneous novelty." The Bible, decorum, and social usage dictated that women remain silent in meetings. Led by Arthur and Lewis Tappan, the faction soon formed the American and Foreign Anti-Slavery Society, which excluded women from its councils.[14]

The woman's issue gained its greatest notoriety the following summer at the World Anti-Slavery Convention in London. America's representatives included seven women, among them Lucretia Mott. The British rejected the women's credentials and denied them seats on the convention floor. As one British clergyman explained, the admission of women would subject the convention to ridicule. When Garrison arrived a few days later and heard of the episode, he refused his seat and joined the women in the gallery. As far as he was concerned, a meeting which began by barring the representatives of half the human race made a mockery of its claim to be a world's convention. His defection cast a pall on the proceedings by robbing the convention of its most celebrated American delegate.[15]

Lydia Pinkham consistently backed the radical faction which put woman's rights on a par with abolition. As the antislavery ranks split and regrouped throughout the 1840s, she took as her guide Nathaniel Rogers, the intransigent editor of the *Herald of Freedom*. The handsome Rogers and his family summered in Lynn where they enjoyed the Esteses' hospitality. Lydia admired Rogers so much that she later named a son after him.

In the internecine rivalries of antislavery, Rogers proved a demanding idol. Each split in the movement found him farther from the center. Early on he drew the rancor of many New England ministers when he attacked them for their moral cowardice on the slavery issue. A master of polemical prose, Rogers once described the clergy as having "an ear as deaf as an adder's to the wail of the American bondsman."[16]

In the end, Rogers's refusal to deviate from his principles led to his split with Garrison. When Garrison adopted as his war cry the slogan "No Union with slaveholders," and called for the dissolution of the Union by political means, Rogers held fast to his belief in nonresistance and moral suasion. Rogers had always insisted that slavery was a "moral disease" that must be cured by moral and spiritual agitation. Political action, he argued, could not make the white and black man brothers. His uncompromising consistency so alienated his old allies that in 1845 they forced his removal from the *Herald of Freedom*. Sick in both body and spirit, Rogers went to Lynn where he spent the last year of his life. In the fall of 1846, he died at the age of fifty-two.[17]

In the meantime Lydia Estes had grown from a young girl to a young woman. She was strikingly tall for her day, standing five feet ten, with a spare build, solemn dark eyes, and auburn hair she wore drawn back in ringlets. Too tall and thin to be thought pretty, she may have suffered embarrassment over her gangling height, but she never slouched and is said to have carried herself with a calm composure. After graduating from the select Lynn Academy, she became a schoolteacher; her twenty-fourth year found her still in the classroom. During the spring of 1843, the Freeman's Institute absorbed much of her time, perhaps because there she had met Isaac Pinkham, a newcomer to Lynn.

Pinkham was a widower of twenty-nine with a five-year-old daughter. Shorter and stouter than Lydia, he had fair skin, light brown hair, and quizzical blue-gray eyes. He dressed formally, always in black, from his Prince Albert coat to his boots and tie. Affable, kindly, but with no great mental power or personal dynamism, he seemed an odd match for Lydia when compared to the fiery Rogers she so much admired. After a short courtship, Lydia and Isaac married in September of 1843.

Isaac Pinkham lived on great expectations. The speculative fever of the 1840s made him discontented with a trade. Instead he moved from one enterprise to another in the hope of striking it rich. Isaac started out in Lynn as a shoe manufacturer, but increasingly he dreamed of making money as Lydia's father had—in real estate. Billy Estes set the couple up in a house on Estes Street which, like all of his holdings, lay smack in the middle of what promised to become the trading center of Lynn.

Shortly before Christmas in 1844, Lydia gave birth to her first son, Charles Hacker Pinkham. The increased responsibility, instead of steadying Isaac, made him more determined than ever to get rich quick through speculation. Before the next year was out, he gave up the shoe business and launched another enterprise. The Estes family must have watched with concern as the young couple struggled under the burden of Isaac's dreams.

It was during the following summer that Nathaniel Rogers made his last visit to Lynn. Lydia, pregnant with her second child, renewed their friendship and when the baby was born in July she named him Daniel Rogers Pinkham. The child lived only a year longer than his namesake. In 1847 the baby died of cholera infantum, a form of gastroenteritis which raged during the hot summer months and brought grief to scores of Lynn mothers. Lydia passed Rogers's name on to her next son, born a year later. The birth of a new baby seemed to punctuate each year. A picture taken during the period shows a pale and vaguely melancholy Lydia holding a baby on her lap.[18]

While Lydia took care of the growing family, Isaac Pinkham's fortunes continued to zigzag. He changed occupations as often as some people changed clothes. Produce dealer, kerosene manufacturer, trader, laborer, farmer, builder were among those he listed in the Lynn *Directory*. His real dream was to become a landed squire. When Billy Estes died in 1848, Isaac's ambitions knew no bounds. Although the estate was ample, it had to provide for a widow and ten surviving children. Isaac could hardly hope to fulfill his dreams on the couple's share. But even before the estate was settled, he began borrowing, buying, selling—moving his family eight times in a dozen years. He always seemed about to grasp success. Yet he so frequently overextended himself that the family found itself constantly out at the pocket.

During those bleak years, Lydia Pinkham, mourning the deaths of her friend Rogers, her

father, and her infant son, not surprisingly turned to spiritualism for solace. The *Banner of Light*, Boston's spiritualist journal, supplemented the *Liberator* and the *Herald of Freedom* as regular reading in the Pinkham household. Lydia was not alone in her enthusiasm. Spiritualism swept the country in the 1850s. William Lloyd Garrison embraced it, as did Lydia's Lynn neighbors, the Singing Hutchinsons. And another Lynn resident, a Mrs. Mary Glover Patterson, better known in later life as Mary Baker Eddy, made a name for herself in local spiritualist circles. For a decade Mary Baker Eddy moved in and out of Lynn, once living on Broad Street in a house that had been part of Billy Estes's farmstead when Lydia was born. Their mutual interest in spiritualism may well have brought the two women together, but neither left a record of such a meeting.

In 1857 with the family fortunes at a low ebb, Isaac decided to quit the produce business and try his hand at farming. Lydia, pregnant again, removed the family which by now included three sons—William Pinkham had been born in 1852—to Bedford, Massachusetts, where a daughter arrived whom she named Aroline Chase Pinkham after her favorite cousin.

While in Bedford, Isaac Pinkham, perhaps smarting from a setback at the hands of an unscrupulous associate, set down in Lydia's journal a list of rules "To Secure Success in Business," which he ostensibly dedicated to his three sons but which read as if he were talking to himself. He wrote:

1. Make all your purchases as far as possible of those who stand the highest in uprightness and integrity. Men of character.
2. Enter into no business arrangements with anyone unless you are well satisfied that such person is governed by a strict sense of honor and justice.
3. Engage in nothing of business at arms length, and be sure you are well acquainted with whatever business you may engage in.
4. Be satisfied with doing well and continue well doing. A sure sixpence is better than a doubtful shilling, which motto, be governed by.[19]

How well Pinkham himself held to these rules after leaving Bedford is debatable. But without a doubt,

Lydia and her sons later violated every one of Isaac's prescriptions when they launched their patent medicine business.

In fact, if legend is correct, Isaac Pinkham's prodigality helped lay the foundation for the family's patent medicine success. Always freehanded as long as his credit was good, Isaac endorsed a note for a Lynn machinist named George Clarkson Todd. When Todd defaulted, Pinkham paid twenty-five dollars on the note. In partial payment Todd gave Pinkham the formula for a medicine. The recipe purported to cure female complaints—the catchall nineteenth-century term for disorders ranging from painful menstruation to prolapsed uterus.

Such cures were common. Lydia Pinkham lived at a time when housewives brewed home medicines as a matter of course. The therapeutic confusion of nineteenth-century medicine spawned a host of curative systems from homeopathy to the mind cure. With the doctor suspect, self-dosing became a logical and inexpensive substitute. Home doctoring claimed its own venerable tradition, but it received an added impetus from the reform spirit of the nineteenth century. A typical enthusiast like Lydia Pinkham embraced a wide series of reforms ranging from temperance to the Graham diet.

Lydia Pinkham kept a notebook labeled "Medical Directions for Ailments" in which she jotted down folk remedies. Some were commonplace. For dyspepsia she recommended pleurisy root steeped in boiling water. Others were outlandish. One entry read: "A hog's milt procured fresh from the slaughter house split in halves, one half to be bound on the sole of each foot and allowed to remain there until perfectly dry, will produce relief and in many cases effect a cure of the complaint called asthma."[20] Her well-thumbed copy of John King's *American Dispensatory*, the most complete listing of pharmaceutical botanicals in its day, testified to her personal experiments with home remedies, quite apart from her supposed debt to George Todd. Whatever the source of the recipe for her female weakness cure, the medicine proved her most popular remedy. She brewed it on the stove and soon kept enough bottles on hand to give to neighbor women.

After three years in Bedford, Isaac Pinkham tired of farming and returned the family to the house on Estes Street. On the eve of Civil War, Isaac took up kerosene manufacturing. When the death of Lydia's mother brought the final division of Estes property in 1862, Isaac sold out his downtown holdings and moved his family to Wyoma, on the outskirts of Lynn, into a house with a roof so steep and sharp the neighbors called it the "Lightning Splitter." Pinkham hoped to buy the surrounding farmland and sell for a profit in what he anticipated would be a postwar real estate boom.

The coming of the Civil War did not affect the Pinkhams greatly. None of the boys was old enough to be conscripted, although Charles chose to enlist when he turned seventeen. His life had been particularly hard and perhaps he saw the war as a chance to escape the drudgery of the Pinkham household. As the eldest son, he had taken on a disproportionate share of the family's burdens. Before the war, he left high school to help support his younger brothers and sister. The only job he could find was in Cambridge, and he sometimes walked the eighteen miles to save carfare.[21]

The two younger boys, Dan and Will, fared better. They helped out by peddling popcorn and fruit, but they stayed in school. Both placed high in their classes in spite of the fact that they were so poor they had to borrow their schoolbooks. Dan won the silver medal in 1866 for "scholarship and deportment" and chose for his valedictory address a plea for Negro suffrage. Will followed four years later with a gold medal and a speech on the inevitability of progress. Lydia Pinkham had an especially close relationship with these two bright middle children. A well-educated woman for her generation, she delighted in their academic success and encouraged them by coaching them in Latin and declamation. Her journal for these years is laced with translations from Vergil, popular poems, and exercises invented to stimulate the boys' interest.[22]

After high school, Dan, the most resourceful and outgoing of the boys, determined to go West. Traveling through Missouri, Kansas, and into Indian Territory, he worked for a time as a cattle drover and later as a schoolteacher in Texas. During his adventure he contracted "fever and ague" which permanently damaged his health. Dan returned to Lynn in 1870, thin and hollow eyed, but ebullient as ever. In 1872 he opened a grocery store in Wyoma which he soon turned into a forum for the political ambitions he had harbored since his days as class orator. At the age of twenty-two, he had already earned a reputation among local politicians as a young man to watch.[23]

Will, the handsome charmer of the family, possessed an intellectual bent. His friend and classmate Will Gove talked him into trying for Harvard and tutored him for the entrance examination. In the fall of 1872 the two friends took a walking tour of New Hampshire. Will Pinkham stayed on to teach at the Clinton Grove Quaker School. He hoped to enter Harvard the next year, but before he had completed his preparation the Panic of 1873 put an end to his plans.

On the eve of the Panic, the Pinkham family appeared to be prospering at long last. With real estate values soaring to dizzying heights after the war, Isaac Pinkham's property in Wyoma had more than doubled in value. He retired from the kerosene business and declared himself a builder in the next Lynn *Directory*, a claim he made good with the completion of Pinkham Hall, a business block with an auditorium on the second floor. In 1872 Isaac cashed in some of his profits and moved the family from the Lightning Splitter into one of the best houses in the Glenmere section of Lynn, complete with a fountain in the front yard and a grand piano in the parlor. For the first time since her marriage, Lydia Pinkham could afford a few luxuries.[24]

Behind the prosperous facade, Pinkham finances remained as shaky as ever. The amiable Isaac endorsed promissory notes for more and more of his acquaintances. Money was easy, and he plunged into land speculation—buying, borrowing, and juggling his holdings by transferring chunks of his property into Lydia's name. Isaac did not worry about his indebtedness. Lynn had grown since Lydia's birth in 1819 from a village of 4,500 to a city of almost 20,000. Growth meant prosperity, or so Isaac Pinkham reckoned as he acquired more and more land.

What Pinkham had not counted on was a new national economy which inextricably tied Broad Street in Lynn to Wall Street in New York. On September 18, 1873, the banking house of Jay Cooke failed and within three months the financial panic touched off the most devastating industrial depression the country had seen. Credit froze, factories shut down, businesses folded, and wage workers faced a winter of starvation. Isaac Pinkham and thousands like him saw their speculative bubbles burst in their faces. Isaac's lands and buildings were mortgaged to the hilt. When the Lynn banks began to foreclose, they threatened to arrest those unable to pay their arrears. No longer a young man, Pinkham broke under the strain. When the bank officer arrived to arrest Isaac, he found him sick in bed. The family prevailed on the bank's attorney, who turned out to be a distant relative, to drop the suit; Isaac was spared the indignity of arrest and jail. But he never regained his vigor. He lived on until 1889, a diminished figure. His grandson recalled him as a feeble old man, rocking in his chair by the fire.[25]

The year 1875 found the family struggling together, with Isaac increasingly incapacitated. Dan's grocery store had gone under in the Panic. His liberality with credit led to bankruptcy. Will had given up his hopes of Harvard and taken rough work as a wool puller. Together he and Charlie, who worked after his stint in the army as a conductor on the Lynn horsecars, pitched in to support the family. Aroline, who had graduated from high school with the predictable gold medal, helped pay her share by teaching school. The Pinkhams had given up their grand house in Glenmere and moved to a smaller home on Western Avenue.[26]

Facing hard times, if not actual destitution, the Pinkham family cast about for a money-making scheme and finally hit upon the idea of selling Lydia Pinkham's female remedy.

Always the hustler of the family, Dan was the first to see the possibilities of marketing his mother's female weakness cure. As the story later appeared in the local paper, the family was sitting around the kitchen one day in 1875 when a party of ladies from Salem drove up to the house and asked for a half a dozen bottles of Mrs. Pinkham's medicine. Generally Lydia Pinkham gave the medicine away, but sometimes she sold small lots, and, times being hard, she accepted five dollars from the Salem women. After they had left Dan blurted out, "Mother, if those ladies will come all the way from Salem to get that medicine, why can it not be sold to other people—why can't we go into the business of making and selling it, same as any other medicine?"[27]

Dan had a point. The newspapers were full of ads for remedies like "Wright's Indian Vegetable Pills," "Oman's Boneset Pills," "Vegetine," and "Hale's Honey of Horehound and Tar." Lydia Pinkham at first demurred, but the boys' enthusiasm won her over. And so in the spring of 1875, the family, ignoring Isaac's motto of a sure sixpence over a doubtful shilling, launched their patent medicine business.

From its beginning the business operated as a family venture. Everyone contributed to the enterprise. Dan and Will provided the brains and sinew. Lydia made the medicine. Charles and Aroline turned over their wages to help pay for alcohol and herbs. And together Will and Lydia worked up advertising copy and put out a pamphlet called "Guide for Women." Even Isaac contributed. Sitting in his rocker, he folded and bundled the pamphlets for Dan to distribute.

Casting about for a name for the medicine, the family came up with "Lydia E. Pinkham's Vegetable Compound." Vegetable remedies, or botanicals as they were called, had gained wide popularity in the nineteenth century in reaction to doctors' indiscriminate dosing with mineral medicines like calomel. The straightforward name, "Vegetable Compound," proved a fortunate if commonplace choice. When the government forced Pinkham competitors to change the names of their products to meet truth-in-advertising standards laid down in the twentieth century, the Pinkhams in this respect were above reproach.

Lydia, with Will's help, brewed the first batches of the medicine on a stove in the cellar. The original formula called for unicorn root, life root, black cohosh, pleurisy root, and fengugreek seed macerated and suspended in approximately 19 percent alcohol, for preservative purposes. Lydia Pinkham bought the herbs from local suppliers, measured her ingredients with kitchen measures, and after she had steeped and macerated the herbs, mixed them all together and dumped them into cloth bags through which the mixture percolated in much the same way that jelly was made. She then added additional alcohol to preserve the medicine, filtered it through cloth, and bottled it.[28]

The Pinkhams, like so many Lynn working-class families bent on self-improvement, were strict temperance advocates. Lydia and the children belonged to the local temperance society. When the boys were young they wore white ribbons on their coat lapels to indicate they had taken the pledge. Part of Dan's difficulty in the grocery business had stemmed from his insistence that the store sell only "dry goods," not rum or spirits. Yet the family saw nothing wrong with selling a medicine which contained enough alcohol to make it forty proof, stronger than table wine or sherry. Alcohol, as far as they were concerned, was a legitimate medicinal substance. When Lydia Pinkham came down with pneumonia in April of 1878, Will recorded in the "Medical Directions for Ailments" that she dosed with an herb decoction and "also took before each meal a teaspoonful of whiskey in two tablespoonfuls of milk."[29] Although Lydia Pinkham viewed the alcohol in her medicine as therapeutically valuable and necessary for preserving the compound, she also made pills and lozenges for cases where alcohol might aggravate menstrual disorders. But taken as directed, three spoonfuls a day, the vegetable compound posed no threat to temperance, or so the Pinkhams argued when critics chided them.

With a Yankee passion for exact accounting, Lydia Pinkham kept cashbooks in which she recorded the first meager sales of the vegetable compound alongside the family's debts. In these ledgers something of the woman behind the trademark emerges. Family accounts she kept with unsentimental exactitude. Each child she charged for rent, clothing, and personal expenses, which could be written off by hard work. ("Daniel Pinkham, $311.32 balanced off by services.") Generosity occasionally prevailed. Next to one entry she noted, "A poor fatherless girl I promised to send six boxes for $3"—a discount from the normal price. In the back pages she collected remedies: "For consumption Pyrola and White-pine bark, equal parts of each, steep, strain. . . ."[30]

When the Lydia E. Pinkham Medicine Company officially organized in 1876, the Pinkhams, worried that Isaac's creditors might try to claim the profits of the business, named Will Pinkham sole proprietor because he was the only member of the family (besides nineteen-year-old Aroline) with no outstanding debts. Together Dan and Will carried on the burden of drumming up trade. Lydia remained in the background, making the medicine, answering letters, and writing advertising copy. The four-page "Guide for Women" began the first modest advertising campaign. Dan, who worked as a mail carrier, distributed the pamphlet on his rounds. Will joined him and together they covered the towns surrounding Lynn. Finally they tackled

Boston. Riding into town on the ten-cent working-men's train, they carried a few thousand circulars a day in knapsacks slung over their shoulders and worked door to door. Slowly their efforts began to pay off. Druggists who had at first been reluctant to stock the unknown medicine began to place orders. The Boston wholesale house of Weeks and Potter ordered a gross. But for a long time the Pinkhams counted themselves lucky if they could sell a bottle a day.

During the spring of 1876, Dan plunged full time into the medicine business. Packing a goatskin trunk full of circulars, he set off for Brooklyn to create a wider market for the compound. In his mid-twenties by now and sporting a full beard, Dan was full of grit and not afraid of hard work. He took a two-dollar room on Willoughby Street and set out singlehandedly to advertise the compound in Brooklyn, New York, and New Jersey. Borrowing pen and ink from the post office to save money, he wrote to his family almost daily and sometimes twice a day. His letters home, addressed "Fellow Doctors," captured the spirit of the early enterprise.[31]

"There is work enough around New York and vicinity to keep ten like me working from now to eternity," Dan wrote after he had taken a day to look around. "Send me another 100,000 pamphlets as I intend to do a 'Devil of a Business' here if possible."

Brooklyn proved more difficult than Dan anticipated. "There are more high toned people here in Brooklyn than I like to distribute among and the churches take up a little too much room," he complained. Because of the explicit wording of the pamphlet, which contained a reference to "Prolapsed Uterus" on its cover, Dan encountered difficulty getting women to read his pamphlet. Casting about for a more genteel ploy, he landed on a scheme to advertise and cut printing costs at the same time. "I believe a good way to advertise and a cheap way would be to get out small cards with this inscription on ... and have them dropped around on parks and other places of resort, say, late Saturday night so people will pick them up on Sunday." He suggested that the family buy small calling cards and write on the back, "Try Lydia E. Pinkham's Vegetable Compound. I know it will cure you, it's the best thing for Uterine complaints there

is. From Your Cousin, Mary, P.S. You can get it at P. Jackson's on Fulton Street." Anticipating his family's disapproval he hastily added, "They're all such darned frauds as that."

The more Dan contemplated his brainchild, the more enthusiastic he grew. The plan would foil the sharp-eyed rag pickers who too often got the pamphlets before women had a chance to read them. For a moment he fantasized littering the Chelsea beach with cards, then he realized the tide would wash them away. But he thought of other possibilities. "Before Decoration Day," he urged, "just try it and drop a few cards all through the Cemeteries around there and I'll bet it will sell a few bottles."

When after ten days Dan had put out more than twenty thousand pamphlets only to discover that Jackson's pharmacy had sold but a dozen bottles of the compound, he searched for another way to get sales started. The boy he hired to help distribute pamphlets gave him one idea. "His mother is a dressmaker and knows a good many sick women and has commenced to blow for the medicine," he wrote the family. "If you can send me that keg full of medicine I think it would be well for me to put it out in trial bottles here in Brooklyn and let her give it to parties she knows; if you can we can't lose much and I think it would be a grand good thing as it would get these Millinery Store keepers and Dress-Makers to guzzling it." Dan grew so impatient waiting for Will to send the medicine that he threatened to "buy some herbs and alcohol and make some medicine" himself. Will dutifully forwarded a keg of the compound and Dan tried his experiment, which did not work as expected. "I haven't met with very good success on the trial bottles that I've given away," he confessed. "One of them made one woman a great deal sicker." Lydia, indignant, must have spoken her mind on the virtues of the compound. A mollified Dan observed later, "I'm glad to hear the medicine is curing them up so well."

When it rained so hard that Dan was forced to "loaf for a spell," he paced his room trying to come up with ideas to increase sales. After one rainy weekend he wrote Will excitedly, "I think there is one thing that we are missing it on and that is not having something on [the pamphlet] in regard to Kidney Complaints as about half of the people out here are either troubled with Kidney Complaints or else they think they are." Dan suggested that Will change the copy on the front page of the "Guide" to include the new claim so that he could give the pamphlets to men as well as women. As he shrewdly noted, "[M]en have more money to spare these times than women." Will followed his lead and soon copy headed "Weak and Diseased Kidneys" appeared alongside claims that the vegetable compound cured uterine complaints.

When druggists showed some reluctance to display Pinkham posters and women refused to read the pamphlets because the explicit language embarrassed them, Dan countered the criticism by placing an ad "in a little religious paper that nobody but women read." The ad, he told Will, would give "a kind of religious tone to our Compound and get the good will of a few Methodists." More important, "if any publisher or editor refused to put our advertisement into their paper, [we can] show them this Pious Sheet."

Despite his machinations, business lagged during the summer. Dan became exasperated with the family, who kept him supplied with pamphlets but were maddeningly slow in sending money for his expenses. "For God's sake! Whose management is it that keeps me from having what I actually need?" he exploded after opening Will's latest letter and finding no money. "Now in consequence of your cussed judgment I shall have to loaf tomorrow and live upon a cracker diet." To prove he wasn't extravagant, Dan recited his expenses which totaled $1.55 a day, including the wage he paid his helper. "There is no use in writing," he lamented, "I actually can't spare 3¢ to buy a stamp with and cramp my guts. I have got to get a job at something else in order to keep my belly full. . . . I should think you either were all crazy or else thought I was getting my meals at free lunch establishments." (This last jibe could be appreciated only by an earnest temperance family like the Pinkhams, for of course a free lunch establishment was a saloon.) Angrily he concluded, "If it is necessary to wear a shirt two or three weeks at a time in consequence of the business not being good enough to have a clean one, I am willing to put up with that, but if it isn't good enough to supply me with food, then I want to get out of it."

By the next day Dan had cooled off. He wrote that his landlady, confident of the Pinkhams' success, had loaned him a dollar to carry him through. But, he warned, "I can't go it on my cheek much longer so hurry up with some money." "It beats all that everybody should say we are going to make a fortune," he marveled. "They seem to believe it, too."

In the meantime he sewed his shoes together every night and tried to keep his one suit clean. "This business is tough on clothing," he complained. "I'm beginning to look so confounded seedy that I feel as though I ought to go into the country pasting up posters." No sooner had he voiced the idea than he warmed to it. Everything in the city had been "advertised to death," he maintained. Why not get a horse and wagon and travel through the countryside peddling the compound? "It seems to me," he predicted with some accuracy, "that cities and towns of less than 50,000 inhabitants are going to pay us the best." Dan never got his horse and wagon, although the time did come when Lydia Pinkham's face decorated barns and fences across the country.

Early in June, Dan came home for a stretch "to help recuperate on finances," and the Pinkhams put their heads together to figure out some way to make the business pay. Printer's ink was the life-blood of patent medicine. Dan, with his eye for advertising, saw that clearly. But his ideas, like his plan to run a Pinkham poster the full length of the Brooklyn Bridge, cost more than the struggling company could muster. While Dan spent his time dreaming up ideas and haggling with printers to bring down the price of pamphlets, Will made a shrewder gamble. One day after he had collected eighty-four dollars for the last gross ordered by Weeks and Potter, he dropped by the office of the *Boston Herald* and inquired the cost of running the whole four-page circular on the front page. The *Herald* manager quoted a price of sixty dollars and Will quickly struck a deal. When he returned home and told the family, they were incredulous. "That was like a thunderclap out of a clear sky," Lydia Pinkham recollected, "and we all sat down and had a good cry."[32] Will's expenditure struck the family as foolhardy. Sales of the compound barely paid for the ingredients and the cost of printing up pamphlets. Will had thrown away sixty dollars on a single advertisement which would run for only one day.

In the long run Will's arithmetic proved sounder

than the family's. The *Herald* reached a circulation of fifty thousand. To print and distribute that many pamphlets cost the Pinkhams almost a hundred dollars, not counting the labor the boys provided free. Newspaper advertising was not only cheaper but, as they soon discovered, it enhanced their credit. Within two days, the *Herald* ad brought orders from three different wholesalers. The family skeptics were won over and soon hired an agent, T. C. Evans, who began a modest newspaper campaign.[33]

Dan returned to Brooklyn in the fall. Rested and full of new ideas, he determined to stick it out "till we either get rich or bust."[34] He worked himself relentlessly putting out pamphlets. "Send me 300,000 more," he ordered Will. No one he hired could keep up his demanding pace. "I've got sick of boys," he confided. "Other boys fight them too much." Next he hired a man for ten dollars a week, only to let him go because, as he put it to Will, "the cussed fool was too proud to work." Exasperated with hired help, Dan urged Will to send Charlie. "Tell Charlie to let the HRR job go to the Devil and be out here by Saturday morning," he urged. In November his older brother joined him and together they tramped the length of Manhattan shoving out circulars.

Dan liked having company and never tired of trying to induce the family to move to Brooklyn. He tantalized them with tales of exciting things to do (like hearing Henry Ward Beecher preach at Plymouth Church or attending the political rallies at Cooper Union). But the real advantage, as he saw it, lay in the opportunity to talk with druggists and patent medicine men. "I actually think if the whole family should move here the learning and sharpening of us all up during two years time would be worth thousands of dollars to use in this business which I think depends almost wholly on discernment, keenness, and knowledge," he insisted. "Hang it! We've got to reduce this advertising down to a science instead of so much brute force." Try as he might, Dan could never persuade the family to leave Lynn.

He returned home for Christmas and shortly after brought a guest from New York, the remarkable Charles N. Crittenton. Crittenton, a patent medicine dealer, later became something of a merchant evangelist who devoted the waning years of his life to rescuing "fallen women." In the 1890s,

with the help of Frances Willard of the Women's Christian Temperance Union, he established National Florence Crittenton Missions in the United States and abroad.[35]

Crittenton seemed an odd friend for the free-thinking Dan, who once remarked that he would not mind church if "there's something else preached besides Come to Jesus gabble." Probably the druggist was more secular in the days when he met and took a fancy to Dan. He had come up the hard way himself, and he did not mind giving the younger man a hand, especially when he was peddling a product as promising as the vegetable compound. Crittenton's business gave the family its first break. Dan could tell other wholesalers, "Crittenton has got it, so you better hurry up."[36] Even better, Crittenton paid cash instead of taking the medicine on consignment. His money helped the Pinkhams over several bad stretches.

After Will's success with the *Boston Herald* ad, the Pinkhams turned more and more to newspaper advertising. They mortgaged their home on Western Avenue to pay for space in the papers. With newspaper ads replacing door-to-door advertising, Dan was free to stay home in 1878 and pursue his political ambitions. A major shoe strike had broken out during the summer. When the Republican mayor protected property by sending in police to break up strikers, the workingmen of Lynn responded by squaring off against the Republicans in the next election. A Workingmen's party ticket which included Dan Pinkham as representative to the state legislature triumphed in the fall of 1878. Dan quickly made a name for himself, and an odd one at that. His colleagues tagged him "The Fish-Ball Representative" after a speech he made in defense of the Lynn strikers. A Republican had argued that if the shoemakers could not live on their wages, they should cut their expenses. Dan countered hotly that they earned only twelve cents a pair for shoes they made. If his fellow representatives believed so firmly in cutting expenses, he suggested, they could cut their own salaries and live like the Lynn shoemakers, on fish balls instead of beefsteak.[37]

By the end of his first term Dan had built up an enthusiastic following. An ardent admirer of Ben Butler and the Greenback-Workingmen's coalition, he stumped the state preaching currency inflation as a cure for the plight of the workingman.

No wonder his party was dumbfounded to see him deliberately throw away his chance for a second term. When the Republican opposition put forth an unpopular measure called the Civil Damage Bill, which would have prohibited the sale of alcoholic beverages in the county, Dan deserted the Workingmen's party to remain loyal to his temperance convictions. He voted in favor of the Republican measure. After the bill passed by a narrow margin, the *Lynn Examiner* vented its anger on Dan. "How does Dan Pinkham expect his mother to keep her roots and herbs without alcohol?" the paper queried. "That was a mean piece, Dan, voting prohibition; you were not elected for that, and next year you will be elected to advertise cures for female complaints at home."[38]

The antiprohibition forces made good the threat. In the next election, rum dominated politics. Dan faced a young unknown named Henry Cabot Lodge, who made it perfectly clear that, although he was a Republican, he would not oppose the repeal of his party's prohibition bill. In a bitter personal campaign the Pinkhams combined politics and advertising in broadsides headed "Republicans! Democrats! Workingmen!" which urged voters to support the Greenback-Workingmen's ticket, and promised in the same breath that sufferers from kidney complaints and dyspepsia could find relief by taking Lydia E. Pinkham's Vegetable Compound. Their efforts proved futile. Lodge began his long political career, with the backing of North Shore brewers and saloon keepers, by defeating Dan Pinkham in a close race.[39]

Shortly after the election Dan returned to Brooklyn. Out of politics and able to devote his full mental energies to advertising, he hit upon the idea of his life. For three years Dan had searched for a gimmick that would put the compound out in front of its competitors. During his first stay in Brooklyn he had noticed that "folks seem to be all tore up on home made goods," an observation which led him to suggest that they advertise the compound as "The Great New England Remedy" and embellish the label with a picture of "a humble cottage." The family did not have money enough to alter the wrappers, so Dan's idea died stillborn. But he continued to ruminate and in 1879 came up with the idea of putting a picture of "a healthy woman" on playing cards with the caption, "She is now as healthy a woman as can anywhere be found/

Having taken four bottles of Mrs. Pinkham's Compound."[40] When he came home for Christmas and saw his mother, he realized he had found his "healthy woman." At sixty Mrs. Pinkham was a dignified, handsome woman who possessed a benign motherly countenance. No better advertisement could be imagined. So, after a family council, Lydia Pinkham posed for the photograph which made advertising history.

The picture conveyed the whole Pinkham message. At a glance it inspired confidence. The attractive woman, sagacious and composed in her best black silk and white lace fichu, appealed to her audience as an idealized grandmother, sympathetic and compassionate. Other advertisers had used pictures. The Smith brothers' bearded faces appeared on the glass jars which contained their famous cough drops, and in the newspapers Buffalo Bill Cody advertised his Wild West show. But no one had thought of using a woman and no one had used a portrait to such good effect. Lydia Pinkham not only identified her product, she came to embody it.

The picture ads did a good deal to authenticate the medicine in the eyes of the trade and the general public. Will Pinkham handled most of the business arrangements, and as a result skeptical druggists and editors, doubting there was a real Lydia Pinkham, had taken to calling him "Lyddy." Once the picture ads appeared and Lydia's face graced the trademark, the Pinkhams had the last laugh. According to the company's agent, H. P. Hubbard, the picture "boomed the sales immensely." About six months after the ad began to run, the family refused an offer of $100,000 for the business and the new trademark.[41]

Lydia Pinkham soon became a national figure. Editors used the electrotype of her picture whenever they needed a photograph of a famous woman, be it Queen Victoria or actress Lily Langtry. Her ever-present face, staring from newspapers and drugstore displays, led Dartmouth men in the 1880s to parody in song:

> There's a face that haunts me ever,
> There are eyes mine always meet;
> As I read the morning paper,
> As I walk the crowded street.
>
> Ah! She knows not how I suffer!
> Her's is now a world-wide fame,

But 'til death that face shall greet me.
Lydia Pinkham is her name.[42]

Soon other college glee clubs picked up the song, embellishing it with infinite ribald verses. Sung to the tune of "Our Redeemer" and ending with the refrain—"Oh, We'll sing of Lydia Pinkham / And her love for the human race / How she sells her Vegetable Compound / And the papers they publish her face"—the Lydia Pinkham song became part of the American folk tradition.

Amused, and with a sharp eye to the advantages of free advertising, Lydia Pinkham clipped the songs, jokes, and anecdotes which played on her name and carefully pasted them in her scrapbook. A favorite went: " 'Oh, I've smashed my bottle of Lydia Pinkham's!' 'Aha! A compound fracture!' "[43]

By 1881 sales of the compound amounted to almost $200,000 a year. Dan Pinkham, who had once written from New York that when he returned to Lynn he wanted to dress "as if I'd just bankrupted a Rainbow," lived to see the business established on a solid footing and his mother something of a national celebrity. But by the time he could afford a new suit, he was dying of tuberculosis. "Daniel sick in New York," Lydia Pinkham wrote in November 1879. "Recommended to take three of my Liver Pills, then steep one-half ounce of Pleurisy root and Bugle weed and one-half ounce of Marsh-mallows, taken one-half cup at a time three or four times per day." Dan returned home for Christmas "threatened with Pneumonia." His mother prescribed another dose of Pleurisy root and Bugle weed and resorted to the Indian treatment of "sweating" him with hot bricks wrapped in soaked flannel. "In two days he was decidedly better," she concluded. "Advised . . . to take when on feet again one or two bottles of Pierson's B[lood] Invigorator."[44]

When Dan's cough lingered on only to flare up a year later, Lydia Pinkham's letters took on a note of desperation. "If you have pain in your lungs I want you to come home immediately," she wrote. "Don't go to staying out there and running any risk. Dr. Mason can bring your blood in right condition in a month so that you won't have a cough or pain for years."[45]

In her anxiety Lydia Pinkham revealed her genuine faith in her own remedies, in patent medicines in general, and in Dr. Monica Mason, a local homeopath. But in the end she watched as her most trusted remedies proved futile. In the winter of 1880, Dan headed south, hoping to regain his strength. He returned home in the spring too weak to walk. Exhausted, he lay in bed reading from the spiritualist *Banner of Light* and trying his best to cheer the stricken family. Early in October, a month before his thirty-third birthday, Dan Pinkham died.[46]

The family scarcely had time to mourn his passing. A second shock followed almost immediately. Will Pinkham contracted consumption early in 1881, just months after his marriage to Emma Barry. The disease proved as quick in Will's case as it had been lingering in Dan's. By October, Will was too ill to attend his brother's funeral. His frantic wife moved him to California in December, but it was too late. Will died in Los Angeles less than two months after Dan, at the age of twenty-eight.[47]

Bright, energetic, and fired by the dream of success, the two brothers burned themselves out building up the business. The years of hard labor, long hours, and poor meals consumed their physical strength. Their work paid off handsomely. They lived to see the compound selling not just a bottle a day, but over two hundred thousand bottles annually. But six years of hard work won them only six months of security. They died, in the words of one obituary, martyrs to the cause of the great business they helped to start.[48]

The double blow shattered Lydia Pinkham and sent her retreating further into spiritualism. Both Dan and Will had been spiritualists and their belief, coupled with her own, must have given her some solace. The local medium, a Mrs. Sanborn, became a frequent caller at the Pinkham home. Charles and Aroline, although they did not share their mother's faith in the spirit world, dutifully participated in the seances that were held each Saturday in the Pinkham parlor. Successful at long last, they could afford to humor their mother.

Two days before Christmas in 1882, Lydia Pinkham suffered a paralytic stroke. During her last months she felt very close to Dan and Will. Mrs. Sanborn came almost daily for private sessions. On May 17, 1883, Lydia Pinkham died at the age of sixty-four. Her funeral was held in the spiritualist manner as she had requested. Instead of lamenting her passing, the friends who gathered in the Lynn cemetery celebrated her reunion with her sons. At the close of the service her old friend John

Hutchinson, last survivor of the Singing Hutchinson family, sang the sad but hopeful refrain "Almost Home."[49]

Lydia Pinkham combined a shrewd business sense with a penchant for reform—a penchant which led her from antislavery through a labyrinth of movements from temperance to the Greenback party. Without hesitation she would have placed her vegetable compound squarely in the reform tradition. Like many in her age she believed that women suffered needlessly at the hands of doctors. She offered her vegetable compound, convinced it was more effective and less dangerous than the treatments of the medical profession. Her advice to women who wrote to her was direct and commonsensical, drawing on the practical knowledge of diet, health, and exercise she had gained in years of domestic practice. Conviction coupled with the hustle and pitch of advertising when she proclaimed herself in banner headlines "Saviour of her Sex."

The glimpse we are able to get of the woman behind the trademark reveals an intelligent, sincere woman who possessed absolute confidence in the medicine she sold. It is unfortunate that in the years following her death, Lydia Pinkham became more and more a victim of her own advertising. The story of her life, like her famous portrait, has been touched and retouched until the actual woman has become obscured. Today she is remembered not as a reformer, but as a trademark—her legacy the benign countenance that sold millions of bottles of vegetable compound.

NOTES

1 Charles E. Estes, *Estes Genealogies 1097–1893* (Salem, Mass.: Eben Putnam, 1894), 1–28.

2 Paul Gustaf Faler, "Workingmen, mechanics and social change: Lynn, Massachusetts 1800–1860," Ph.D. diss., University of Wisconsin, 1971, 51; Alan Dawley, *Class and Community: The Industrial Revolution in Lynn* (Cambridge: Harvard University Press, 1976), 51–56.

3 Ralph Waldo Emerson, quoted in Joseph Kett, *The Formation of the American Medical Profession: The Role of Institutions 1780–1860* (New Haven: Yale University Press, 1968), 149–50.

4 Emanuel Swedenborg, *Heaven and Its Wonders and Hell* (New York: Swedenborg Foundation, 1974), 341.

5 Marguerite Beck Block, *The New Church in the New World: A Study of Swedenborgianism in America* (New York: Octagon Books, 1968, orig. pub. Holt, Rinehart and Winston, 1932), 130.

6 Ralph Waldo Emerson to Thomas Carlyle, October 30, 1840, in *The Correspondence of Emerson and Carlyle*, ed. John Slater (New York: Columbia University Press, 1964), 283.

7 Faler, "Workingmen, mechanics and social change," 76 and 215; Nathaniel P. Rogers, letter from Lynn in *Herald of Freedom*, May 27, 1842.

8 Alonzo Lewis and James R. Newhall, *History of Lynn, Essex County Massachusetts, Including Lynnfield, Saugus, Swampscot, and Nahant* (Boston: John L. Shorey, 1865), 401–2.

9 "Clerical impudence—the climax," from the *Liberator*, quoted in the *Herald of Freedom*, September 2, 1842; "Resolution of the Essex County Anti-Slavery Society," quoted in the *Herald of Freedom*, October 14, 1842.

10 "Album of Lydia E. Pinkham," vol. 538, papers of the Lydia E. Pinkham Medicine Company, Arthur and Elizabeth Schlesinger Library on the History of Women in America, Radcliffe College, Cambridge, Mass. [hereafter cited as LEP SL].

11 Frederick Douglass, *Life and Times of Frederick Douglass* (Boston: De Wolfe, Fiske and Company, 1895), 277–79.

12 Letter from William Bassett, quoted in the *Herald of Freedom*, March 11, 1842.

13 "Journal of Lydia E. Pinkham," Box 180 (Folder 3365), LEP SL.

14 *Herald of Freedom*, May 23, 1840.

15 Ibid., June 13, 1840, and September 18, 1840.

16 Nathaniel P. Rogers, *Collection from the Miscellaneous Writings of Nathaniel P. Rogers* (Manchester, N.H.: William H. Fisk, 1849), xxi; *Herald of Freedom*, March 21, 1840, and April 4, 1840.

17 John Pierpont, "Introduction," in *Collection from the Miscellaneous Writings of Nathaniel P. Rogers*, xiii–xxiii.

18 "Picture of Lydia E. Pinkham at the age of 25," Box 119 (Folder 2379), LEP SL.

19 "Journal of Lydia E. Pinkham."

20 "Medical directions for ailments," vol. 537, LEP SL.

21 Arthur W. Pinkham, *Reminiscences* (Lynn, Mass.: published by the author, 1954), 34–35, listed as vol. 531, LEP SL.

22 "Journal of Lydia E. Pinkham."

23 "Obituary, Daniel Rogers Pinkham," *Lynn Transcript*, October 15, 1881, in "Lydia Pinkham's scrapbook," vol. 556, LEP SL.

24 "Photographs," Series IV, Oversize 5, LEP SL.
25 Arthur W. Pinkham, *Reminiscences*, 28, Vol. 531, LEP SL.
26 Robert Collyer Washburn, *The Life and Times of Lydia E. Pinkham* (New York: G. P. Putnam's Sons, 1931), 91.
27 Daniel Rogers Pinkham, quoted in *Lynn Daily Item*, January 23, 1893.
28 "History and development of the company's methods of manufacture," (Typescript, n.d.), Box 132 (Folder 2635), LEP SL.
29 "Medical directions for ailments."
30 "Cashbook," vol. 74, and "Cashbook," vol. 69, LEP SL.
31 Daniel Pinkham's letters often lack a full date. For convenience I refer the reader not to individual letters, but to the entire collection and will therefore refrain from noting the letters separately. *See* "Letters: thirty-eight original letters from Daniel Rogers Pinkham to William H. Pinkham, 1876–1879," Box 167 (Folder 3117), LEP SL.
32 Lydia Pinkham, quoted in Harlan Page Hubbard, "The true story of Lydia Pinkham," *Fame* 1 (November 1892), in Box 164 (Folder 3035), LEP SL.
33 Ibid.
34 The quotations that follow are from Daniel Pinkham's letters, see Box 167 (Folder 3117), LEP SL.

35 Charles N. Crittenton, *The Brother of Girls, The Life Story of Charles N. Crittenton as Told by Himself* (Chicago: World's Events Company, 1910), 195–205.
36 Daniel Pinkham's letters.
37 Newsclipping in "Lydia Pinkham's scrapbook."
38 Ibid.
39 Handbill in "Lydia Pinkham's scrapbook."
40 Daniel Pinkham's letters.
41 Hubbard, "True story."
42 Newsclipping in "Lydia Pinkham's scrapbook."
43 Ibid.
44 "Medical directions for ailments."
45 Lydia E. Pinkham to Daniel R. Pinkham, n.d., illustration in Eleanor Early, "The true life of Lydia E. Pinkham," clipping in Box 164 (Folder 3028), LEP SL.
46 "Obituary, Daniel Rogers Pinkham."
47 William H. Gove, "In memoriam," obituary of William H. Pinkham, clipping in "Lydia Pinkham's Scrapbook."
48 Washburn, *Life and Times*, 166.
49 John Wallace Hutchinson, *Story of the Hutchinsons: Tribe of Jesse* (Boston: Lee and Shepard, 1896), 2: 110.

20

The Rise and Fall of Battey's Operation:
A Fashion in Surgery

LAWRENCE D. LONGO

During the latter nineteenth century many women underwent bilateral oöphorectomy for amenorrhea, dysmenorrhea, menometrorrhagia, and a variety of other conditions variously termed pelvic neurosis, oöphoromania, and ovarian epilepsy. Generally these women were relatively young—the average age estimated to be thirty years—and their ovaries were free from overt pathology. The avowed purpose of this procedure was to produce a surgical menopause in an attempt to alleviate the patient's debilitating symptoms. This operation originated with Robert Battey, a surgeon in Rome, Georgia, and became popular not only in America, but in England and on the Continent. Among its proponents were J. Marion Sims and Lawson Tait.[1] On the one hand the operation was hailed as one of the unequaled "triumph[s] of surgery."[2] And Battey was described as leaping "over the legitimate bounds of surgery and traveling in paths hitherto untrod."[3] Physicians who failed to perform the procedure when such conditions were indicated were cited as "wanting in humanity"[4] and accused of criminal neglect of their patients.[5] On the other hand, this procedure was dubbed "castration,"[6] "spaying,"[7] "desexing," and "unsexing," and decried as a pernicious and dreadful operation.[8] Moreover, surgeons who carried out such procedures were labeled "gynecological perverts."[9]

Because since the turn of the century bilateral ovariotomy, or "Battey's operation," has attracted little attention, this essay considers problems relating to the origin and development of Battey's pro-

cedure: exactly what constituted Battey's operation and the indications for which it was employed; the origin of the term "Battey's operation"; the surgical results and postoperative sequelae; the extent to which it was practiced in America and Europe; the factors which accounted for its popularity; the reasons that it fell into disfavor and ultimate rejection; and the extent to which Battey's operation contributed to advances in pelvic surgery and an understanding of ovarian function and endocrinology.

Although Ephraim McDowell performed his first ovariotomy in 1809,[10] this operation only rarely was performed during the remaining first half of the nineteenth century. However, with the advent of anesthesia, by the mid-1860s many surgeons were performing ovariotomy, or oöphorectomy as it later was called.

Battey himself was an accomplished surgeon. Although this essay makes no attempt to review his life per se, some aspects of his career are relevant to his surgical contributions. Battey spent two sessions at Thomas Jefferson Medical College, part of the time studying under Charles D. Meigs[11] and graduating in 1857. The same year he also received a diploma from the Obstetrical Institute of Philadelphia.[12] In 1859 he toured Ireland, Great Britain, and the Continent, where he met, among other great surgeons, Spencer Wells, who was just commencing his brilliant career in ovariotomy. Battey is recorded to have determined to try the next case for which ovariotomy was indicated.[13] With the outbreak of the Civil War in the spring of 1861, Battey entered the Confederate Army and during the four years of the war served in several capacities, both in the field and as chief surgeon of several army hospitals, thus establishing his surgical reputation.[14] Following the Confederate sur-

LAWRENCE D. LONGO is Head of the Division of Perinatal Biology and Professor of Obstetrics and Gynecology and Physiology at Loma Linda University School of Medicine, Loma Linda, California.

Reprinted with permission from *Bulletin of the History of Medicine* 53 (1979): 244–267.

render in April 1865, Battey returned to Rome to resume his practice. In May 1869, he performed his first ovariotomy, successfully removing a thirty-pound dermoid cyst from a physician's wife. By August 1872, when he performed his first "normal" ovariotomy, Battey was considered one of the foremost surgeons in Georgia, if not in the South.[15] He established a gynecological infirmary in Rome where he kept his patients, later enlarging this to the Martha Battey Hospital, named in recognition of his wife, who assisted him with the operations and nursed the patients postoperatively. For two years starting in 1873, he held the chair of professor of obstetrics at the Atlanta Medical College, but apparently this aspect of medicine held little attraction for him. During the same period he also served first as corresponding editor and then as editor-in-chief of the *Atlanta Medical and Surgical Journal*. He was a founding member of the American Gynecological Society, a group of the most prestigious gynecologic surgeons in the country, and in 1888 served as its president.

Battey's idea of normal ovariotomy developed following the death of a patient. In 1865 two young women consulted him for amenorrhea with severe symptoms associated with the molimen (i.e., laborious performance of a normal function). The first woman soon died, and he operated on the second. Because these women's illnesses profoundly influenced his thinking, I shall detail their records.

The first patient, a 21-year-old woman, Mary ————, consulted Battey for primary amenorrhea associated with "violent perturbations of her nervous and vascular system."[16] For five years she had experienced regular bouts of extreme mental and physical suffering at the time of the menstrual molimen. In addition, she was said to have symptoms of "endocarditis" with cardiac hypertrophy. Physical examination revealed no evidence of a uterus. Otherwise, she was described as being "in the bloom of early womanhood—gifted with charms beyond the lot of the majority of her sex." Battey reasoned that "if she could be relieved of her ovaries . . . the menstrual molimen would cease; the violent strain upon the heart would be at an end; there might be hope for her." He searched in vain for a precedent—an authority who advocated ovariotomy. For unexplained reasons this patient grew worse and she died. That Battey was affected deeply by the death of this model southern belle is

evidenced by his repeated reference to her for over three decades. He resolved that "another such case should not perish in my keeping without my reaching out a friendly hand in the hope of rescue."

About the same time a 23-year-old woman, Julia Omberg, with somewhat similar complaints, came under his care. She, too, suffered from severe molimenal symptoms and had experienced only two "normal" menstrual periods since her menarche. Menstruation was accompanied by epileptiform convulsions which left her in a semicomatose state.[17] She also developed pulmonary congestion with occasional hemorrhage, and acute articular rheumatism. Repeatedly she experienced debilitating bouts of gastric and rectal bleeding with debilitation at five-to-eight-week intervals, and developed a pelvic abscess which ruptured into the rectum. The patient later reported that "her sufferings were most intense . . . [she] felt there was no future for her in this life, and that death would be a relief."[18]

Battey diagnosed chronic corporeal endometritis and treated the patient with intrauterine silver nitrate and other measures. As with many of the patients upon whom he and other surgeons were to operate, she "had become habituated to the use of morphia—taken to mitigate her long years of suffering—and her usual dose [was] a full grain of the sulfate." In the spring of 1872 the patient, who by now was thirty years old, improved following one of these particularly severe crises and Battey broached the idea of "a normal ovariotomy for her radical cure." He observed that this concept was "the creature of my own thought," and following long and deliberate contemplation[19] Battey wrote to several noted gynecologists seeking advice on the propriety of such a procedure. For instance, his inquiry addressed to members of the Gynaecological Society of Boston was discussed at its meeting of 4 June 1872.[20]

After some delays because of the patient's condition, Battey finally operated on 17 August 1872. He removed both ovaries, which appeared grossly normal. Although the patient apparently developed peritonitis, she recovered. Battey later recounted not only that postoperatively he personally had housed the patient, "spending ten days at her bedside, without leaving the house for a moment, even for a change of linen," but also that during this time "in the office of one of my brother practitioners were held nightly meetings of the profession of my town . . . awaiting her demise with anxious longings in order to institute proceedings in our court and put me before the bar as a criminal."[21]

Within a month Battey's report of "normal ovariotomy" with a description of the patient's course during her first thirty-one postoperative days appeared in the *Atlanta Medical and Surgical Journal*, and the same account was published the following January in the *Richmond and Louisville Medical Journal*.[22] Subsequently he described the patient's continued improvement for seven months.[23] Following ovariotomy the patient's "menstrual" molimen disappeared, as did her nervous phenomena, convulsions, pelvic inflammations, abscesses, and hematocele. In a brief, independent report W. F. Westmoreland, a friend (and co-editor of the *Atlanta Medical and Surgical Journal*) observed[24] that Miss J[ulia] presented "all the evidences of the most perfect health," despite her claim that her previous sufferings had been even greater than those recorded by Battey.

Subsequently Robert Battey reported cases of this operation in more than twenty publications over a period of almost two decades from 1872 to 1890. Although he continued to stress that he was removing only normal ovaries to produce an artificial menopause, he later[25] noted that the term "normal ovariotomy" was an "unfortunate and obsolete" choice and he stressed that the ovaries so removed were distinctly abnormal. His operative technique itself underwent several changes. During the first few years he performed ovariotomy in some instances using a vaginal approach. These early operations included numerous instances of unilateral oöphorectomy, and he recommended the use of the écraseur. Later, as the results became manifest, he stressed the importance of an abdominal approach for bilateral oöphorectomy in which the ovarian pedicles were ligated with silk sutures. At no time did he advocate removal of the fallopian tubes, as did Lawson Tait (see below), nor did he practice clitoridectomy or other "desexing" procedures. While he desired to produce an artificial menopause, originally he was somewhat ambivalent on whether a bilateral oöphorectomy was necessary for this effect. In his early cases in which he believed only one ovary was "viciously or abnormally performing its functions,"[26] Battey removed only that single organ. However, he later confessed

that these very patients were the least benefited by the procedure. Undoubtedly, a single ovary was removed in some of those cases because of the inadequate operative exposure through the vagina.

Undoubtedly, a major problem with Battey's operation was that its indications never were defined explicitly. Although Battey repeatedly presented indications that he considered valid they remained rather ill defined. In addition, while he stated that his procedure was a *dernier ressort* for desperate cases, many of the procedure's advocates, if not Battey himself, tended to regard it as a panacea. Initially (in 1872) he removed normal human ovaries "with a view to establish at once the 'change of life' for the effectual remedy of certain otherwise incurable maladies."[27] He wrote, "I have hoped, through the intervention of the great nervous revolution which ordinarily accompanies the climacteric, to uproot and remove serious sexual disorders and reestablish the general health."[28] Battey distinguished between his "normal ovariotomy" and the ovariotomy performed by the successors to McDowell. He stated, "it was I who had really and truly done an ovariotomy, rather than Dr. Ephraim McDowell, . . . I felt that my operation was *regular* ovariotomy, and McDowell's [for ovarian tumors] *irregular*." Although defending the expression "normal ovariotomy," he confessed that this term met with no favor from his professional brethren, noting that because it served to obscure rather than elucidate his meaning, he would abandon it even though he was unable to find a suitable substitute.

Originally Battey presented the prime indication for surgery as "any grave disease which is either dangerous to life or destructive to health and happiness, which is incurable by other and less radical means."[29] At the American Gynecological Society meeting in 1877, Battey presented four indications for surgery: (1) when life is endangered in the absence of the uterus; (2) with obliteration of the uterine cavity or vaginal canal that cannot be surgically restored; (3) in cases of insanity or epilepsy caused by uterine or ovarian disease; and (4) in cases of protracted physical and mental suffering associated with monthly nervous and vascular perturbations.[30] However, he confessed that in some cases he experienced great difficulty in reaching a decision on whether to operate. Later Battey further refined the indications for surgery as oöphoromania, oöphoroepilepsy, and oöphoralgia.[31] In ascribing the cause of mania and epilepsy to the ovaries rather than to the uterus as was the more accepted practice of the time, he perhaps set the stage for the wholesale abuse the procedure was to suffer. Indeed, what woman with pelvic pain, hysteria, or a convulsive disorder might not be a candidate for ovariotomy? Although he stated that he would never operate on a patient for nymphomania,[32] he did in fact operate for this condition.[33] When physicians would inquire, "[Do you] operate for dysmenorrhea, for amenorrhea, menorrhagia, for bleeding myoma, for epilepsy, for nymphomania, or for oöphoromania," he would answer, "Both yes and no. Yes under certain circumstances, and no under other conditions."[34] He attempted to resolve this seeming paradox by basing his decision to operate upon three questions: (1) Is this a grave case?; (2) Is it incurable by other means?; and (3) Is it reasonable to expect a cure by this method?[35] Battey concluded that if one could reply in the affirmative to these questions the case was a "proper one."[36] However, he maintained that he operated on only a small percentage of the cases offered. His thesis at this time appeared to be that if the patient's health was "broken down by the vitiated function of her ovaries" and she was "utterly miserable and without remedy," he would remove the offending organs unhesitatingly. Battey boasted, "I decide, in such cases that the sacrifice of the ovaries shall be made, and I believe I do God a service when I sacrifice them."[37]

Despite this list of broad indications, Battey occasionally admitted that the operation was being performed too frequently and that the indications had become too general. He also confessed that in several cases he had recommended the procedure prematurely, for the patients had improved despite their refusal of surgery.[38] Finally, in an almost prophetic note, he inquired "whether in cases of hysterectomy extirpation of the ovaries should not be a part of the operative procedure."[39]

At the 1886 International Medical Congress, Battey gave the only gross description of the ovarian pathology in his cases.[40] He noted that the organs often contained numerous small cysts, the lining of some of which appeared inflamed. He described other ovaries with a thickened, blanched, corrugated, sclerotic surface and fibrous stroma. Many appeared shrunken and "senile." (He included no microscopic findings.) The following year

he noted[41] that the two characteristic pathologic findings were cystic degeneration of organs that were but little enlarged although attended by great pain, and "a sort of sclerosis" with thickening of the surface and degeneration of the stroma.[42] On the other hand, he declared that the presence of ovarian pathology was not necessary for the operation. "I will interfere without hesitation. I ask nobody whether her ovaries are diseased or not. Of course, when I take them out, if I find those ovaries diseased, I felicitate myself that I have come within everybody's rule when that is the case, but I should not hesitate a moment, if I was satisfied that the patient was incurable, that her case was an extreme one."[43]

The eponymic appellation of bilateral ovariotomy first appeared in the title of Battey's presentation before the American Gynecological Society when he considered the question, "Is there a proper field for Battey's Operation?"[44] A few months later Sims, who had assisted Battey with several of his cases,[45] also used the term "Battey's operation,"[46] after noting that Battey had asked him to name the procedure. Sims stated that Battey was the first to recognize the systemic effects of an "unrelieved menstrual molimen," the first to suggest a method of cure, and the first to carry out his own suggestion. He continued: "I have always thought that 'Battey's operation' would be the most appropriate name for it, and cherish the hope that the profession in Europe will unite with us in America in giving it the name of the man who originated the operation, and who has, by the most indomitable courage, succeeded in proving its usefulness."[47] Undoubtedly, as an early champion of bilateral ovariotomy, Sims, one of the world's leading gynecologic surgeons, helped make the procedure respectable.

An additional consideration is the end result of Battey's operation. Battey summarized the outcome of his cases in numerous reports.[48] Although he explicitly described only about seventy cases, he is believed to have performed the procedure on several hundred women.[49] Of his first seven cases of bilateral ovariotomy, three women were cured completely, two were improved only slightly, and two women died postoperatively, apparently from peritonitis. The mortality rate in this first group was 22 percent, a not unreasonable rate when compared with about 30 percent for ovariotomy in general.[50] Despite the fact that these were not general. ovarian tumors, the operative procedure was fraught with difficulty. Battey recalled one case thus: "the ovary [was] found to be imbedded in pelvic lymph. The identification of the ovary [Battey himself being in doubt] was confirmed by the practical touch of Dr. Sims, and proved beyond controversy by portions of the stroma brought out upon my fingernail. . . . It was found impracticable to isolate the gland entirely and I contented myself with such disintegration as I could effect with my fingernail."[51] By 1880 Battey reported that in the eight years since he had invented the procedure, over one hundred cases had been performed among three surgeons, and probably more than two hundred cases were recorded.[52]

In a report to the 1881 International Medical Congress in London,[53] Battey tabulated 193 cases of bilateral oöphorectomy by 47 different operators. Although the overall mortality was 18 percent, he recorded that Lawson Tait and Thomas Savage had each performed the procedure 26 times without a single death. (In this same report he recorded perhaps the strangest postoperative sequela of his procedure, a patient who subsequently bore a living child. Presumably one ovary was removed only incompletely.)[54] A few years later he reported 36 consecutive personal cases[55] (in most of which he had employed Listerian antisepsis) without a death. For the first time Battey also presented results for the various indications of ovariotomy. His most favorable results were in the nine cases of oöphoroepilepsy, all of whom Battey claimed were promptly and completely cured of their epileptiform manifestations and neurotic symptoms. He noted that of twenty patients with oöphoralgia, thirteen were cured, but four women failed to be relieved of their pelvic pain and persisted in "their opium habit." The poorest results were noted in seven women with oöphoromania. Most of these latter patients had been ill for from three to fourteen years, and three had been institutionalized in an "asylum." Only one patient was "cured," four were improved somewhat, and two showed no improvement. In later reports he included up to 72 patients, noting that many of the failures were associated with opium and morphine addiction. He also recorded that cessation of menses occurred in all but 7 percent of these patients. By 1888, the year of his last substantive paper,[56]

one of Battey's admirers stated that among Battey's last 100 cases of bilateral ovariotomy the mortality rate was 3 percent.[57]

In addition to Battey's personal experience, it is appropriate to consider the extent to which Battey's operation was practiced elsewhere in America and Europe. During the last three decades of the nineteenth century, the removal of normal ovaries for various maladies, real or imagined, gained widespread popularity. One writer estimated that by 1906 about 150,000 women had undergone the procedure,[58] but the basis for that estimate was not given. Even allowing that only one out of every one hundred cases was reported, that estimate would appear inflated about tenfold. Undoubtedly, to a large extent the appeal of ovariotomy followed the surgeons' attempts to develop procedures that would cure supposed derangement of the body's "special nerve force." Such alterations were believed commonly to result in hysteria in women and spermatorrhea in men.[59] Some of the procedures employed included clitoridectomy, operations for vaginismus and cocyodynea, and forcible dilatation of the sphincters of the vagina and rectum.

Battey's interest in normal ovariotomy developed during the renaissance of ovarian surgery. The publication in the same year of Battey's first report of Peaslee's opus on ovarian tumors[60] (1872) and the following year of the monograph by W. L. Atlee[61] undoubtedly helped establish the acceptability of ovariotomy in America.[62]

Apparently James Blundell of London first suggested extirpation of healthy ovaries. In a paper read to the (Royal) Medical and Chirurgical Society,[63] he concluded, from experiments on rabbits, "That the womb, spleen, and ovaries may be taken away . . . without the necessity of destroying life." He continued[64] that the operation . . . would probably be found an effectual remedy in the worst cases of dysmenorrhea and in periodic bleeding from an inverted womb which could not be removed. Apparently, however, he did not regard this suggestion as very practical for he noted that the procedure "can scarcely in any instance be necessary."[65] Actually, previous writers had suggested male castration for the cure of satyriasis[66] and it was carried out as a cure of insanity,[67] but apparently it had not been performed to any great extent.

The first public discussion of Battey's operation

occurred at the 4 June 1872 meeting of the Gynaecological Society of Boston[68] following Battey's inquiry regarding his idea. Several of the members looked with favor on Battey's proposal and declared that a surgeon was unjustified in withholding relief for want of a precedent.[69] In fact, one member suggested that because the ovaries played the most important role in the female, the society's motto should be changed to "Propter Ovarium" from "Propter Uterum."

Battey's initial case report received a mixed reception. Within two months of its publication, the editor[70] of the *Richmond and Louisville Medical Journal* insisted that since bilateral ovariotomy was well known to have no effect on the menstrual cycle, Battey was incorrect in believing that it could, and "regretted" that he had failed to publish the views of many authorities to this effect. Only four months after Battey's first case, J. T. Gilmore, professor of surgery at the Medical College of Alabama, successfully performed normal ovariotomy.[71] The *American Practitioner* of December 1875[72] carried a rather remarkable ten-page interview with Battey by Drs. D. W. Yandell and Ely McClellan of Louisville, who had observed Battey perform several operations. In closing their report, these writers noted the procedure's simplicity and the facility with which Battey worked. They also observed: "Any tyro may perform the initiatory steps, but it requires a profound gynecologist to complete the operation,"[73] adding that the operation demanded a thorough knowledge of anatomy and an "educated" finger.[74] Although unwilling either to advocate or to decry the procedure, they quoted T. Gailliard Thomas that it could be greatly abused. Within a few years, reports of successful cases appeared from at least three surgeons in New York City—T. T. Sabine,[75] Edmund R. Peaslee,[76] and T. G. Thomas[77]—and from Trenholme of Montreal.[78] Several of these cases were patients with bleeding uterine leiomyoma, a condition which became, until the more general use of hysterectomy, one of the common and widely accepted indications for bilateral oöphorectomy.[79]

In 1877 James Marion Sims published his account of Battey's operation[80] in which he reviewed Battey's cases and presented seven of his own. Of his own series, one patient died, two became worse, and one of the other four improved. (Sims was forced to abandon the procedure in mid-operation

for one patient). Despite these somewhat disastrous results, Sims championed the procedure, declaring that if he had removed both ovaries (other than in the one who died) and used the abdominal approach (rather than a transvaginal route in four women) in all these patients, the results would have been different. He concluded by recommending bilateral ovariotomy for a wide variety of indications similar to those of Battey.

Subsequently the operation was performed widely by urban as well as rural physicians,[81] not only for ovarian neuralgia and severe dysmenorrhea, but epilepsy, nymphomania, and insanity.[82] Both the Chicago Gynecological[83] and New York Obstetrical[84] Societies recorded cases and discussed their indications and merits. Social class distinctions may have had some bearing on the performance of the procedure. Apparently most of the patients were from the middle (and upper) class or institutionalized (see below). Some reports included glowing testimonials from patients to bolster recommendation of the procedure. For instance, one patient observed:

> No pen can write the sufferings I endured in the five years previous to my operation. At times I became almost desperate enough to take my life and end my sufferings. . . . My life now seems a new one, and I am getting along splendidly. . . . I am now a well, happy, and cheerful girl, and do not feel like the same person at all.[85]

In contrast, several reports sounded a more cautionary note. For instance, Engelmann, who had three patients die following the procedure,[86] noted the mortality rate of 30 to 33 percent of all cases reported and the fact that only another third seemed to be improved appreciably. Engelmann also took issue with Battey's argument that this procedure should be associated with little more risk than the spaying of domestic animals[87] (Hegar later espoused a similar view [see below]), stating that such a comparison was totally unjustified[88] because the operative conditions were less favorable than in cases of ovarian tumors and the small ovaries lay deep in the pelvis, perhaps buried in bowel or omentum, with a pedicle that was difficult to ligate. Amazingly, Engelmann concluded his reports by advocating the procedure, echoing Battey in concluding, "However great the dangers, I can but again repeat 'they are not out of proportion to the severity of the malady, and the magnitude of the results.'"[89]

As late as 1893, H. Marion-Sims reported that he had performed bilateral oöphorectomy for epilepsy,[90] and in 1887 Howard A. Kelly reported that he had performed Battey's operation "many times with most happy results."[91] Other less renowned operators testified to similar success.[92] It probably never will be known how many patients underwent Battey's operation, as many reports mentioned large numbers of cases almost as an aside,[93] and undoubtedly many cases went unreported.

"Battey's operation" actually was performed first by Alfred Hegar of Germany three weeks prior to Battey's on 27 July 1872, in a patient with menstrual neuralgia. However, the patient died and Hegar waited until after five years and numerous other cases before reporting his results.[94] Hegar explicitly stated that by castration he hoped to suppress ovarian function and its influence on the body.[95] In an 1878 monograph Hegar recorded his series of cases and exhaustively reviewed the literature.[96] Although Hegar unquestionably led the Continental surgeons in ovariotomy and other pelvic surgery, his colleagues were not far behind.[97] However, surgeons in France were slow to espouse "Batteyism."

In Great Britain, Alexander Russell Simpson, presumably influenced by Sims's report the year earlier, reported to the Edinburgh Medico-Chirurgical Society a case performed in 1878.[98] Unquestionably, other than Battey himself, the leading advocate of bilateral oöphorectomy was Robert Lawson Tait, surgeon to the Birmingham and Midland Hospital for Women. Tait first performed double ovariotomy to arrest the growth of a bleeding leiomyoma five days after Hegar and sixteen days before Battey performed theirs.[99] Again, however, only in response to Simpson's report did Tait recount this experience in a brief note. An ovariotomist of first rank, Tait's experience with Battey's operation has several points of interest. Initially, he reported that his first three cases died,[100] but later he reversed himself, stating that the first patient recovered and regained her health.[101] In his magnum opus, *Diseases of the Ovaries*,[102] he claimed priority for the procedure for himself;[103] then later he credits Battey as the originator of this procedure.[104] Strangely, he failed to

mention his original operation in his Hastings Prize essay on ovarian disease (1873), which was a precursor to his 1883 work.[105] Tait reported numerous cases of the procedure and when Battey visited Manchester "demonstrated nine or ten [cases] of his own [Battey's] operation."[106] One of England's staunchest champions of ovariotomy, Tait was engaged in numerous controversies, both in the medical journals and public press, regarding the merits of ovariotomy.[107] In addition to numerous contributions to ovarian surgery, Tait developed the technique and espoused the removal of diseased uterine appendages, which, with the removal of the ovaries, became known as Tait's operation.

In light of this wave of enthusiasm it is appropriate to examine the factors that led to the "downfall" of Battey's operation. Despite Battey's enthusiasm for and advocacy of bilateral ovariotomy, he not infrequently sounded a cautionary note. On at least one occasion he admitted that the operation was being performed too frequently and that the indications had become too general.[108] At the International Medical Congress of 1886, he protested the operation's abuse and recorded that up to that date he had met with only fifteen cases in which he believed the procedure was justified.[109] Undoubtedly, to a great extent it was the flagrant abuse of the procedure and its performance for questionable indications that soon led to its loss of favor in the eyes of leading surgeons and the public. During the latter part of the 1870s and the 1880s an increasing number of reports advocated Battey's operation for "ovaralgia,"[110] "hystero-epilepsy,"[111] nymphomania,[112] and moral insanity.[113] This is perhaps understandable when one realizes that many authorities both in America and abroad[114] regarded insanity as a result of pathology of the ovaries, or kidneys, or even of intestinal putrifaction.[115] In fact, William Goodell, professor of gynecology at the University of Pennsylvania, advocated Battey's operation for all cases of insanity,[116] and this indication quickly was espoused by others[117] including Battey himself.[118] Goodell wrote:

> If the operation be not followed by a cure, the surgeon can console himself with the thought that he has brought about a sterility in a woman who might otherwise have given birth to an insane progeny. In fact, I am not sure but that, in this progressive age, it may

not in the future be deemed political economy to stamp out insanity by removing the ovaries of insane women.[119]

Goodell justified this approach by his belief that such a woman "is liable to transmit the taint of insanity to her children, and to her children's children for many generations."[120] As late as 1891 one writer[121] noted, "hundreds of unfortunate women are today languishing in insane asylums, who might be cured by [Battey's] operation." Enthusiasm for this approach reached such proportions that removal of both normal ovaries and ovarian tumors became regarded as a cure for insanity.[122] However, most advocates of such an approach presented little evidence for their thesis. Generally, the period of postoperative follow-up was only a few weeks[123] and the number of cases few.[124]

As might be expected, a reaction to indiscriminate castration caused Battey's operation to fall into disrepute. As early as 1874 the medical board of the Women's Hospital (New York) opposed Sims's performance of controversial procedures such as Battey's operation. In fact, this constituted part of the controversy that led to Sims's resignation from the Women's Hospital staff.[125] In 1879 Thomas Addis Emmet, in his textbook of gynecology,[126] criticized the procedure, noting that the mortality rate was high and the success rate had not exceeded 25 percent.[127] A few years later he expanded this view, stating that more harm than good had been done by Battey's operation and that the procedure was frightfully abused.[128] Emmet tempered these remarks by recommending that rather than totally abandoning the procedure, only a few experienced surgeons should perform it.[129] Regarding the operation, Thaddeus A. Reamy noted "a tendency, in certain quarters, to recklessness," cautioning that it would "do no harm to apply the breaks [sic] until the gentlemen have time to remember that the ovaries . . . should not needlessly be sacrificed."[130] He later observed that many a "sinless ovary" was being sacrificed because of the very brilliance and facility of the operation, and its comparative safety. Considering the "painful want of familiarity with its minor pathologic changes," he thought it "painfully suggestive of too much freedom with the ovary" to remove it when the disease could be cured by some less radical procedure. Although Reamy conceded that the operation might add years to female life, he warned that some day a statistician would compute the years of human life lost to the race by destruction of ovaries whose "structure yet bears many possibilities for population."[131]

Other writers took up the debate. Reports of the failure of Battey's operation appeared more frequently,[132] but so did successes.[133] Dr. Wharton Sinkler[134] reviewed the published reports and concluded that the opinions of different observers varied to such an extent that one might believe that totally different beings and conditions were being considered.

Probably the most important factor in the demise of Battey's operation was its almost wholesale use for the cure of convulsive disorders and insanity. From Catonsville, Maryland, George H. Rohé reported[135] that he had examined under anesthesia thirty-five females from a hospital population of about two hundred patients. He stated that he had found evidence of pelvic disease in twenty-six (74%) and removed the adnexa in eighteen of these women. His indications for surgery included melancholia, "simple" mania, puerperal mania, hysterical mania, hysteroepilepsy with mania, and epilepsy. Shortly thereafter he attempted to justify this approach, noting that a "prominent attorney" had given the opinion that an insane person "having lucid intervals could give a valid consent to any operation during said interval, being at that time considered by the law as sane."[136]

Perhaps this approach to insanity reached its apogee when at the Norristown, Pennsylvania, State Hospital for the Insane, a separate annex ward was established for women undergoing bilateral oöphorectomy. Dr. Joseph Price of that institution, with consent of the hospital trustees, already had performed at least four such procedures, and had fifty more patients "marked for operation" when the Committee on Lunacy of the Pennsylvania State Board of Public Charities investigated the institution. Their report[137] seems to have considered seriously for the first time the medicolegal aspect of oöphorectomy in institutionalized patients. The committee declared:

> The zeal of the gynecologist is being carried to an unusual extent when it proposes to use a State Hospital for the Insane as an experimental station, where lunatic women are to

be subjected to doubtful operations for supposed cures. If it is to be permitted in some forty or fifty cases, as proposed, it might be well to practice the experiment upon the entire female lunatic population, so that the gynecologist may have the large opportunity he doubtless craves to see just what would happen. At the expense of some lives, the continued and aggravated insanity of most of his subjects, with a few supposed cures and improvements, he could read his conclusions learnedly to his gynecological brethren, with the resultant added forward movement up his ladder of fame.[138]

The committee concluded that the operation was "illegal, . . . experimental [in] character, . . . brutal and inhumane, and not excusable on any reasonable ground." Although proponents of Batteyism protested this report,[139] the pendulum was swinging away from "normal" ovariotomy.

An additional factor in the demise of Battey's operation was increasing opposition by some leading gynecologists. Sir (Thomas) Spencer Wells, one of England's greatest ovariotomists, who had performed Battey's operation himself[140] in 1865, in the preface to his *Diseases of the Ovaries*[141] had forwarned of the potential for abuse:

A discovery which has triumphed over opposition of all kinds, honest and scientific, prejudiced and ignorant, may still be ruined by the support of rash, inconsistent, thoughtless partisans, whose failures do not reflect so much discredit on themselves as on the operation they have badly performed in unsuitable cases. Indications are not wanting that ovariotomy has entered on this phase of progress, and there is reason to fear that judicious men may be influenced by the outcry of the foolish, and that a triumph of British surgery, which has been won by such great labor and care, may be arrested before it is complete—may even be converted into temporary defeat—by the indiscriminate support of zealous but injudicious advocates.

Later, Wells explicitly stated that the procedure should not be performed for nymphomania, insanity, or any other form of mental disease, noting that

in many instances of supposed mental instability due to ovarian disease the patients undergo spontaneous cure, and . . . it cannot be determined to what extent the relief reported results from the removal of the ovaries and how much is psychical phenomenon. . . . gynecologists will never empty the lunatic asylums.[142]

Other gynecologists argued[143] that even if the ovaries were diseased many small ovarian cysts could be treated by simple puncture rather than oöphorectomy. John Whitridge Williams[144] of the newly founded Johns Hopkins Hospital recounted his pathologic findings over three or four years during which he examined the more than three hundred ovaries of nearly all the operative specimens. Williams recalled that in most cases the pathologic findings failed to justify the procedure. Other pathologic studies supported this conclusion.[145] Subsequently, only occasional case reports advocated the removal of relatively normal ovaries,[146] while most reports emphasized the futility of the procedure.[147] Howard A. Kelly in 1896, the year of Battey's death, expanded his essay on ovarian conservatism of a few years earlier,[148] and by the end of the century many textbooks, including Kelly's *Operative Gynecology*,[149] did not even mention Battey's operation. During the first decade of the twentieth century leading gynecologists preached conservatism in surgery. In recalling the previous years J. Thomas Kelly[150] observed:

one might see in almost any hospital numbers of normal organs sacrificed . . . so rabid were gynecologists to do surgery that there was nearly a wholesale wiping out of gynecological therapeutics.

Emil Novak, in a thoughtful essay, "The Hormone Theory,"[151] attempted to put ovariotomy in perspective and weigh the relative merits of the new conservatism. He wrote:

The time has passed when healthy ovaries were ruthlessly sacrificed to cure dysmenorrhea, obscure pelvic pains, etc. It is true, of course, that the saner and more conservative methods of the modern gynecologist were literally forced upon him by a realization of the futility of the irrational and mutilating measures of former days, as well as by the awakening of the surgical world to the fact that it is only rarely in accordance with the principles of true surgery to remove tissue which is not the seat of disease, especially when such tissue can be shown to possess a definite and useful function. A restraining influence of not little importance has therefore been imposed upon us by the knowledge that the ovary, in addition to its well known function of ovulation, plays another more subtle role in the processes of the woman's body. At the same time, it is only fair to present the other side of the picture also. . . . [it has been] shown that however important the hormones of the female generative organs may be, they are not by any means indispensable to life, or even usually to comparative comfort, and hence, from this standpoint there would seem to be no physiological basis for such ultraconservative operative measures as some would advise. . . . it would seen that radical conservatism, as it has been called, is scarcely less commendable than that unreasoning radicalism, pure and simple, which will not brook the restraint that knowledge and reason would impose.

A final consideration is the historical significance of Battey's operation and the extent of its contribution to the development of surgery and to the emerging science of endocrinology. Coincident with and following the publication of papers by Battey on ovarian surgery and by Robert Lawson Tait on tubal and ovarian operations, surgeons became more courageous in attempting pelvic surgery for various indications. Numerous writers maintained that Battey's operation contributed not only to an understanding of diseases of the female genital tract and the advancement of pelvic surgery, but to a popularization of laparotomy and abdominal surgery in general. Battey's name has been linked with that of Hegar and Tait as one who developed the whole field of pelvic operations for conditions other than gross ovarian or uterine pathology.[152] Following Battey's death (8 November 1895), an era of surgical conservatism ensued, with preservation of normal ovaries. "We now are in an era of renewed advocacy of the removal of normal ovaries, especially near or after the menopause, as a prophylaxis for ovarian cancer, . . . it has been recognized

that the ovaries elaborate little estrogen after the menopause." It is of interest that in an almost prophetic note Battey asked "whether [in cases of hysterectomy] the extirpation of the ovaries ought not to form a normal part of the operative procedure."

The related problem concerns an understanding of the ovaries' role in menstruation. Strangely, perhaps this was not firmly established until the late nineteenth century. Although the ovaries were conceded to influence the body through the medium of the sympathetic nerves, knowledge was so sparse that in 1885 as eminent a gynecologist as Emmet, in objecting to Battey's operation, suggested that dysmenorrhea had no relation to the ovaries.[153] At the same time another leading surgeon stated that if gynecologists wished "to have a clear idea of the true physiological position of the uterus, we must emancipate it from the thraldom of the ovary, in whose firm grasp for the last fifty years it has been secretly held."[154] While many individuals subscribed to the ovarian theory of menstruation,[155] others, including Lawson Tait,[156] held that this physiologic function lay under control of the fallopian tubes, the ganglion of nerves alongside the uterus,[157] or even the uterus per se.[158] As late as 1891 T. A. Reamy, president of the American Gynecological Society, observed with naïve surprise that in his experiences with 144 cases of bilateral removal of the ovaries[159] menstruation ceased within six months in every instance.

Thus, perhaps one of the most important contributions of Battey's operation was indirect, in that it helped establish the realization that development of the genital organs and of secondary sexual characteristics and menstruation depends on functioning ovarian tissue. In his reports Battey repeatedly stressed that the rationale and purpose of his operation were to "arrest ovulation and produce the change of life." He confessed that he could not explain why the menses stopped, but by reasonably careful analysis of his cases he demonstrated that indeed menstruation did cease following bilateral ovariotomy, and reemphasized that his procedure had as its goal production of the menopause. Additionally, both Battey[160] and Hegar[161] demonstrated the dependence of large vascular uterine leiomyomata on ovarian function by their decrease in size and sloughing following ovariotomy. One of Battey's admirers remarked: "It was Battey who invaded the hidden recesses of the female organism and snatched from its appointed place those delicate little glandular bodies whose mysterious and wonderful functions are of such high interest to the human race."[162] Fielding Garrison[163] credited Battey with "the first experiment in physiological surgery upon human beings," and noted its significance in connection with the development of ideas on internal secretions.

In conclusion, Battey's operation serves as an example of changing fashions in the practice of clinical medicine. The procedure represents a paradox of sorts because its major contributions occurred incidentally to its purported objective. For instance, it unquestionably served as an important factor in the development of abdominal surgery in general, and pelvic surgery in particular. In addition, "Battey's experiment" played an important role in the evolution of the concept of the relation of ovarian function to menstruation. However, these achievements were somewhat serendipitous or accidental by-products of the procedure. On the other hand, the enthusiastic manner in which Battey's operation was received by leading gynecologic surgeons and a large fraction of the profession illustrates the Achilles' heel of medicine: its too frequent and ready espousal of untested procedures or unproved theories. Yet, to relegate Battey's operation to the dustbin of passé procedures would be a mistake, for it unquestionably constitutes an important segment of the evolution of surgery and understanding of ovarian physiology. However, the extent to which it actually contributed to the physical, mental, and emotional well-being of the women on whom it was performed is difficult to evaluate. In fact, this remains as a problem for future solution.

NOTES

This is an expanded version of a paper presented at the 51st annual meeting of the American Association for the History of Medicine, Kansas City, May 12, 1978.

1 J. Marion Sims, "Remarks on Battey's operation," *British Medical Journal*, 1877, *2*: 793–94, 840–42, 881–2, and 916–18; Lawson Tait, "Removal of normal ovaries," ibid., 1879, *1*: 813–14.

2 E. W. Cushing, "Report of a case of melancholia; masturbation; cured by removal of both ovaries," *Journal of the American Medical Association*, 1887, *8*: 441–442.

3 E. P. Becton, "Batty [sic] and Batty's [sic] operation," *Texas Courier-Record of Medicine* (Dallas), 1888, *6*: 34–35.

4 Cushing, op. cit. (n. 2 above).

5 H. H. Carstens, "Three cases of Battey's operation," *American Journal of Obstetrics and Diseases of Women and Children*, 1883, *16*: 266–71.

6 A. Hegar, *Die Castration der Frauen vom physiologischen und chirurgischen Standpunkte aus* (Leipzig: Breitkopf und Hartel, 1878).

7 E. H. Trenholme, "Two cases of ovariotomy or spaying," *Obstetrical Journal of Great Britain and Ireland*, 1876, *43*: 425–35; J. H. Aveling, "The spaying of women. A note historical and philological," *Obstetrical Journal of Great Britain* (London), 1879, *11*: 617–21.

8 C. Tyrone, "Certain aspects of gynecologic practice in the late nineteenth century," *American Journal of Surgery*, 1952, *84*: 95–106.

9 N. Barnesby, *Medical Chaos and Crime* (New York: Mitchell Kennerley, 1910), 231–52.

10 E. McDowell, "Three cases of extirpation of diseased ovaria," *Eclectic Repertory and Analytic Review*, 1817, *7*: 242–44.

11 R. Battey, "Address by Dr. Robert Battey, Rome Georgia," *Transactions of the South Carolina Medical Association*, 1889, 61–68.

12 J. A. Eve, "A sketch of the life and labors of Dr. Robert Battey of Rome, Georgia," *Virginia Medical Monthly*, 1878, *5*: 1–8.

13 Ibid.

14 Ibid.

15 Ibid.

16 R. Battey, "Normal ovariotomy-case, *Atlanta Medical and Surgical Journal*, 1872/3, *10*: 321–29, and *Richmond and Louisville Medical Journal*, 1872, *14*: 711–29.

17 R. Battey, "Extirpation of the functionally active ovaries for the remedy of otherwise incurable diseases," *Transactions of the American Gynecological Society*, 1876, *1*: 101–20.

18 W. F. Westmoreland, "Report on Battey's operation," *Atlanta Medical and Surgical Journal*, 1872/3, *9*: 231.

19 R. Battey, "Battey's operation," in *A System of Gynecology, by American Authors*, ed. M. D. Mann (Philadelphia: Lea Brothers and Company, 1888), *2*: 837–49.

20 R. Battey, "The propriety of the performance of normal ovariotomy in a case of absence of the uterus with excessive nervous irritation," *Journal of the Gy-*

naecological Society of Boston, 1872, 7: 331–35 and 339–40.

21 R. Battey, "A history of Battey's operation," *Atlanta Medical and Surgical Journal*, 1886/7, n.s. 3: 657–75, and T. A. Reamy, "In memoriam, Robert Battey, M.D., LL.D., Rome, Georgia," *Transactions of the American Gynecological Society*, 1896, 21: 467–72.

22 R. Battey, op. cit. (n. 16 above).

23 R. Battey, "Normal ovariotomy," *Atlanta Medical and Surgical Journal* 1873/4, 11: 1–22 and 65–84, and *Transactions of the Medical Association of Georgia*, 1873, 24: 36–69.

24 W. F. Westmoreland, op. cit. (n. 18 above).

25 R. Battey, "Castration in mental and nervous diseases. A symposium," *American Journal of the Medical Sciences*, 1886, 92: 483–90.

26 R. Battey, op. cit. (n. 17 above), 112.

27 R. Battey, op. cit. (n. 16 above), 321, and "Normal ovariotomy," *Transactions of the Medical Association of Georgia*, 1873, 24: 36–69.

28 R. Battey, op. cit. (n. 17 above), 102.

29 Ibid., 113.

30 R. Battey, "Is there a proper field for Battey's operation?" *Transactions of the American Gynecological Society*, 1877, 2: 279–305.

31 R. Battey, op. cit. (n. 25 above), 484.

32 R. Battey, op. cit. (n. 17 above).

33 R. Battey, "Battey's operation—its matured results," *Transactions of the American Gynecological Society*, 1887, 12: 253–74.

34 R. Battey, "Battey's operation: its object, results, etc.," *Transactions of the Medical Society of the State of Virgina*, 1887, 10: 188–93.

35 R. Battey, "Occlusion of the entire utero-vaginal canal, following labor, with distressing sequelae of unrelieved menstrual molimen—Battey's operation—cure," *Transactions of the Medical Society of the State of Virginia*, 1879, 2: 432–38.

36 R. Battey, op. cit. (n. 34 above), 190.

37 R. Battey, "Discussion: pelvic inflammations; or cellulitis versus peritonitis, T. A. Emmet," *Transactions of the American Gynecological Society*, 1886, 11: 111–14.

38 R. Battey, op. cit. (n. 37 above), 112.

39 R. Battey, "What is the proper field for Battey's operation?" *Transactions of the American Gynecological Society*, 1880, 5: 38–43.

40 R. Battey, op. cit. (n. 25 above).

41 R. Battey, op. cit. (n. 34 above), 188.

42 R. Battey, op. cit, (n. 34 above), 191.

43 R. Battey, op. cit. (n. 21 above), 665.

44 R. Battey, op. cit. (n. 30 above), 279.

45 R. Battey, op. cit. (n. 17 above).

46 J. M. Sims, op. cit. (n. 1 above).

47 Ibid., 918.

48 R. Battey, op. cit. (n. 11 above, n. 17 above, n. 19 above, n. 21 above, n. 25 above, n. 33 above, n. 34 above, n. 39 above); "Summary of the results of fifteen cases of Battey's operation," *British Medical Journal*, 1880, i: 510–12; "Oöphorectomy—Battey's operation—spaying-castration of women," in *Transactions of the International Medical Congress, Seventh Session* (London: J. W. Kolckmann, 1881), 4: 279–88 and 291–97; "Antisepsis in ovariotomy and Battey's operation—eighteen consecutive cases—all successful," *Virginia Medical Monthly*, 1883/4, 10: 291–304; "Antisepsis in ovariotomy and Battey's operation—thirty consecutive cases—all successful," *Transactions of the Medical Association of Georgia*, 1884, 35: 151–65; "Conditions of success in ovariotomy," *Atlanta Medical and Surgical Journal*, 1885, n.s. 2: 1–7.

49 E. P. Becton, op. cit. (n. 3 above).

50 E. R. Peaslee, *Ovarian Tumors: Their Pathology, Diagnosis and Treatment, Especially by Ovariotomy* (New York: D. Appleton and Company, 1872).

51 R. Battey, op. cit. (n. 17 above), 104–5.

52 R. Battey, op. cit. (n. 39 above), 38.

53 R. Battey, "Oöphorectomy—Battey's operation—spaying-castration of women," in *Transactions of the International Medical Congress, Seventh Session* (London: J. W. Kolckmann, 1881), 4: 279–88 and 291–97.

54 Ibid., 284.

55 R. Battey, op. cit. (n. 25 above), 483, and "Antisepsis in ovariotomy and Battey's operation," *Kansas City Medical Index*, 1887, 8: 1–12.

56 R. Battey, op. cit. (n. 11 above, n. 19 above).

57 E. P. Becton, op. cit. (n. 3 above), 35.

58 E. Van de Warker, "The fetich [sic] of the ovary," *American Journal of Obstetrics and Diseases of Women and Children*, 1906, 54: 366–73.

59 J. T. Gilmore, "Normal ovariotomy," *Atlanta Medical and Surgical Journal*, 1873/4, 11: 175–76.

60 E. R. Peaslee, op. cit. (n. 50 above).

61 W. L. Atlee, *General and Differential Diagnosis of Ovarian Tumors, with Special Reference to the Operation of Ovariotomy; and Occasional Pathological and Therapeutical Considerations* (Philadelphia: J. B. Lippincott, 1873).

62 As an aside, Peaslee pointed out the barbarous Latin and Greek conjugate in the word "ovariotomy" (cutting an ovary), which had been introduced by James Young Simpson. Peaslee compounded from Greek roots the more proper term "oöphorectomy" (to cut out the ovary). Some surgeons then adopted the term "oöphorectomy" when referring to Battey's operation, and retained the term ovariotomy for removal of ovarian tumors (A. J. C. Skene, *Treatise on the Diseases of Women for the Use of Students and Practitioners* [New York: D. Appleton, 1888]).

63 J. Blundell, *Researches Physiological and Pathological: Instituted Principally with a View to the Improvement of Medical and Surgical Practice* (London: E. Cox and Son, 1825).

64 Ibid., 26.

65 Ibid., 26.

66 H. Bigelow, "Castration as a means of cure for satyriasis," *Boston Medical and Surgical Journal*, 1859/60, *61:* 165–66.

67 J. H. Marshall, "Insanity cured by castration," *Medical and Surgical Reporter*, 1865, *13:* 363–64.

68 R. Battey, op. cit. (n. 20 above), 331.

69 Ibid., 334.

70 Editorial, *Richmond and Louisville Medical Journal*, 1872, *14:* 828–29.

71 J. T. Gilmore, op. cit. (n. 59 above), 175, and "Normal ovariotomy," *Atlanta Medical and Surgical Journal*, 1874/5, *12:* 321–30.

72 D. W. Yandell and E. McClellan, "Battey's operation," *American Practitioner* (Louisville), 1875, *12:* 200–214.

73 D. W. Yandell and E. McClellan, "Battey's operation," *Atlanta Medical and Surgical Journal*, 1875/6, *13:* 481–92.

74 Ibid., 491.

75 T. T. Sabine, "Case of normal ovariotomy recovery," *New York Medical Journal*, 1875, *21:* 37–41.

76 E. R. Peaslee, "A case of solid uterus bipartitus: both ovaries removed for the relief of epileptic seizures, ascribed to ovarian irritation," *Transactions of the American Gynecological Society*, 1876, *1:* 340–53.

77 T. G. Thomas, "Obstetrics and gynecology," *American Journal of the Medical Sciences*, 1876, *72:* 133–70.

78 E. H. Trenholme, op. cit. (n. 7 above), p. 425.

79 S. C. Gordon, "Hysteria and its relation to diseases of the uterine appendages," *Journal of the American Medical Association*, 1886, *6:* 561–67.

80 J. M. Sims, op. cit. (n. 1 above), 793.

81 E. P. Becton, op. cit. (n. 3 above); J. H. Carstens, op. cit. (n. 5 above); C. Cushing, "What are the conditions that justify oophorectomy?" *Western Lancet, Journal of Medicine and Surgery* (San Francisco), 1883, *12:* 97–105; R. A. Kitto, "Ovariotomy as a prophylaxis and cure for insanity," *Journal of the American Medical Association*, 1891, *16:* 516–17; E. C. Mann, "Removal of both ovaries of hystero-epilepsy, without controlling the convulsions; rapid improvement under central galvanization followed by general faradization, nerve tonics, full feeding, and rest," *New York Medical Journal*, 1881, *33:* 16–20.

82 W. Goodell, "Clinical notes on the extirpation of the ovaries for insanity," *Medical Society of the State of Pennsylvania Transactions*, 1881, *13:* 638–43.

83 A. R. Jackson, "Battey's operation. Discussion before the Chicago Gynaecological Society, September 17th, 1880," *Chicago Medical and Surgical Examiner*, 1880, *41:* 456–61.

84 B. McE. Emmet, "Battey's operation," *New York Medical Journal*, 1882, *36:* 283–84.

85 J. T. Johnson, "Battey's operation," *Virginia Medical Monthly*, 1895/6, *22:* 1012–33.

86 G. J. Engelmann, "Battey's operation; three fatal cases, with some remarks upon the indications for the operation," *American Journal of Obstetrics and Diseases of Women and Children*, 1878, *11:* 459–81, "The difficulties and dangers of Battey's operation," *Transactions of the American Medical Association*, 1878, *29:* 463–73.

87 R. Battey, op. cit. (n. 23 above), 51.

88 G. J. Engelmann, op. cit. (n. 86 above), 471.

89 Ibid., 473.

90 H. Marion-Sims, "Hystero-epilepsy. Report of seven cases cured by surgical treatment," *Transactions of the American Gynecological Society*, 1893, *18:* 282–98.

91 H. A. Kelly, "Discussion: 'Battey's operation—its matured results' by Robert Battey," *Transactions of the American Gynecological Society*, 1887, *12:* 272.

92 Y. H. Bond, "Must the ovaries go?" *Weekly Medical Review,* (St. Louis), 1887, *16:* 62–69; P. F. Mundé, "My experience with oöphorectomy for the cure of hystero-epilepsy," *American Journal of Obstetrics and Diseases of Women and Children*, 1892, *25:* 454–60; J. T. Johnson, op. cit. (n. 85 above).

93 S. C. Gordon, op. cit. (n. 79 above); G. H. Rohé, "The relation of pelvic disease and psychical disturbances in women," *American Journal of Obstetrics and Diseases of Women and Children*, 1892, *26:* 694–726; J. T. Johnson, op. cit. (n. 85 above).

94 A. Hegar, "Ueber die Extirpation normaler und nicht zu umfänglichen Tumoren degenerierter Eierstöke. I. Die Bedeutung des Eierstocks für den Organismus," *Zentrablatt fur Gynäkologie*, 1877, *1:* 297–307.

95 A. Hegar, "Castration in mental and nervous diseases. A symposium," *American Journal of the Medical Sciences*, 1886, *92:* 471–83.

96 A. Hegar, op. cit. (n. 6 above).

97 A. Martin, "Ueber partielle Ovarien- und Tubenexstirpation," *Sammlung Klinischer Vortage* (Leipzig), 1889, *343 (Gynäk 3):* 2481–2498.

98 A. R. Simpson, "History of a case of double oöphorectomy, or Battey's operation: with remarks," *British Medical Journal*, 1879, *1:* 763–66.

99 L. Tait, "Removal of normal ovaries," 813–14.

100 Ibid.

101 L. Tait, "Discussion: 'Oöphorectomy' by Thomas Savage," in *Transactions of the International Medical Congress, Seventh Session* (London: J. W. Kolckmann, 1881), *4:* 293.

102 L. Tait, *The Pathology and Treatment of Diseases of the*

Ovaries (Being the Hastings Essay for 1873), 4th ed. (Birmingham: Cornish Brothers, 1883).

103 Ibid., 107.

104 Ibid., 326.

105 L. Tait, "The Hastings Prize Essay, 1873: the pathology and treatment of ovarian diseases," *British Medical Journal*, 1874, *1:* 701–3, 733–36, 765–68, 798–800, 825–27; and *2:* 8–10, 27–29.

106 H. A. Kelly, "A diary of Robert Battey, M.D.," *Therapeutic Gazette*, 1921, *45:* 612–20.

107 L. Tait, "Casey v. Imlach," *Lancet*, 1886, *2:* 375–76; "'Spaying,' or removal of the uterine appendages?" *Lancet*, 1886, *2:* 557; "Presidential address. On some pending questions in gynaecology," *British Medical Journal*, 1887, *1:* 145–48.

108 R. Battey, op. cit. (n. 53 above).

109 R. Battey, op. cit. (n. 25 above).

110 F. West, "History of a case of spaying for ovaralgia, accompanied by epileptiform convulsions," *Maryland Medical Journal*, 1879/80, *6:* 315–17.

111 E. C. Mann, op. cit. (n. 81 above); J. G. Brooks, "Castration for hystero-epilepsy (Battey's operation)," *Medical and Surgical Reporter*, 1885, *52:* 230–32.

112 J. G. Brooks, op. cit. (n. 111 above).

113 W. B. Goldsmith, "A case of moral insanity," *American Journal of Insanity*, 1883, *40:* 162–77.

114 R. Barnes, "On the correlations of the sexual functions and mental disorders of women," *British Gynaecological Journal*, (London), 1890/1, *6:* 390–406; C. E. L. Mayer, *Die Beziehungen der krankhaften Zustände und Vorgänge in den Sexualorganen des Weibes zu Geistesstörungen* (Berlin: A. Hirschwald, 1869).

115 G. H. Rohé, op. cit. (no. 93 above).

116 W. Goodell, "A case of spaying for fibroid tumour of the womb," *American Journal of the Medical Sciences*, 1878, *76:* 36–50; *Lessons in Gynecology* (Philadelphia: D. G. Brinton, 1879), 267–88; op. cit. (n. 82 above).

117 M. A. Pallen, "Some suggestions with regard to the insanities of females," *American Journal of Obstetrics and Diseases of Women and Children*, 1877, *10:* 206–17; R. A. Kotto, op. cit. (n. 81 above).

118 E. D. Bondurant, "Two cases of oöphorectomy for insanity," *Journal of Insanity*, 1886, *42:* 342–45.

119 W. Goodell, "Discussion: 'Oöphorectomy' by Thomas Savage," in *Transactions of the International Medical Congress, Seventh Session* (London: J. W. Kolckmann, 1881), *4:* 295.

120 W. Goodell, op. cit. (n. 82 above), 639.

121 R. A. Kitto, op. cit. (n. 81 above).

122 W. P. Manton, "A contribution to the history of ovariotomy on the insane," *Transactions of the American Association of Obstetrics and Gynecology*, 1889, *2:* 262–65; G. H. Rohé, op. cit. (n. 93 above); G. H. Rohé, "Further observations on the relation of pelvic disease and psychical disturbances in women," *American Journal of Obstetrics and Diseases of Women and Children*, 1893, *28:* 423–25.

123 R. A. Kitto, op. cit. (n. 81 above); J. M. Baker, "Oöphorectomy, or Battey's operation," *North Carolina Medical Journal*, 1883, *12:* 61–65.

124 W. Goodell, op. cit. (n. 82 above).

125 S. Harris, *Woman's Surgeon: The Life Story of J. Marion Sims* (New York: Macmillan, 1950), 297.

126 T. A. Emmet, *The Principles and Practice of Gynaecology* (Philadelphia: H. C. Lea, 1879).

127 Ibid., 775.

128 T. A. Emmet, "Discussion: 'Four cases of oöphorectomy, with remarks' by J. T. Johnson," *Transactions of the American Gynecological Society*, 1885, *10:* 135.

129 Ibid.

130 T. A. Reamy, "Discussion: 'Four cases of oöphorectomy, with remarks' by J. T. Johnson," *Transactions of the American Gynecological Society*, 1885, *10:* 140–41.

131 T. A. Reamy, "The President's annual address," *Transactions of the American Gynecological Society*, 1886, *11:* 41–59.

132 Luilam, "Failure of the Battey-Tait operation to cure epilepsy," *Clinque*, 1891, *12:* 471–73; A. Church, "Removal of the ovaries and tubes in the insane and neurotic," *American Journal of Obstetrics and Diseases of Women and Children*, 1893, *28:* 491–98 and 569–73.

133 G. H. Rohé, op. cit. (n. 93 above, n. 122 above); J. Meyer, "A case of insanity, caused by diseased ovaries, cured by their removal—a phenomenal triumph for operative treatment," *Transactions of the American Association of Obstetrics and Gynecology*, 1894, *7:* 503–4.

134 W. Sinkler, "The remote results of removal of the tubes and ovaries," *University Medical Magazine* (Philadelphia), 1891/2, *4:* 173–86.

135 G. H. Rohé, op. cit. (n. 93 above).

136 G. H. Rohé, "Letter to the editor," *Journal of the American Medical Association*, 1893, *20:* 182–83.

137 Editorial, "Removal of the ovaries as a therapeutic measure in public institutions for the insane," *Journal of the American Medical Association*, 1893, *20:* 135–37.

138 Ibid.

139 G. H. Rohé, op. cit. (n. 136 above); H. B. Young, "Letter to the editor," *Journal of the American Medical Association*, 1893, *20:* 258.

140 T. S. Wells, "Case of removal of both ovaries for dysmenorrhea (Battey's operation)," *Transactions of the American Gynecological Association*, 1879, *4:* 198–220.

141 T. S. Wells, *Diseases of the Ovaries*, 2 vols. (London: J. Churchill, 1865/72).

142 T. S. Wells, "Castration in mental and nervous diseases. A symposium," *American Journal of the Medical Sciences*, 1886, *92:* 455–71.

143 W. M. Polk, "Operations upon the uterine appendages with a view to preserving the functions of ovulation and menstruation," *Transactions of the American Gynecological Society*, 1893, *18:* 175–99.

144 J. W. Williams, "Discussion: 'Operations upon the uterine appendages with a view to preserving the functions of ovulation and menstruation' by W. M. Polk," *Transactions of the American Gynecological Society*, 1893, *18:* 192.

145 H. C. Coe, "Diseases of the ovaries," in *A System of Gynecology, by American Authors*, ed. M. D. Mann (Philadelphia: Lea Brothers and Company, 1881), *2:* 850–91.

146 J. Meyer, op. cit. (n. 133 above).

147 A. Church, op. cit. (n. 132 above); R. T. Edes, "Ovariotomy for nervous disease," *Boston Medical and Surgical Journal*, 1894, *130:* 105–7; W. S. Playfair, "Remarks on the systematic treatment of aggravated hysteria and certain allied forms of neurasthenic disease," *British Medical Journal*, 1882, *2:* 309–12; N. Barnesby, op. cit. (n. 9 above).

148 H. A. Kelly, "Conservatism in ovariotomy," *Journal of the American Medical Association*, 1896, *26:* 249–51, and "The ethical side of the operation of oöphorectomy," *American Journal of Obstetrics and Diseases of Women and Children*, 1893, *27:* 206–8.

149 H. A. Kelly, *Operative Gynecology*, 2 vols. (New York: D. Appleton and Company, 1898).

150 J. T. Kelly, Jr., "How far is the so-called conservative pelvic surgery conservative," *American Journal of Obstetrics and Diseases of Women and Children*, 1909, *60:* 94–100 and 145.

151 E. Novak, "The hormone theory and the female generative organs," *Surgery, Gynecology and Obstetrics*, 1909, *9:* 344–50.

152 M. D. Mann, "The early days of ovariotomy," *Buffalo Medical Journal*, 1904, *n.s. 13:* 510; Anonymous,

"Robert Battey, M.D.," *Southern Surgical and Gynecological Association Transactions*, 1902, *15:* 415–17; J. L. Baer, "A century of obstetrics and gynecology," *Illinois Medical Journal*, 1940, *77:* 468–70; R. S. Sutton, "A brief review of the growth of McDowell's operation done at Danville, Kentucky, in 1809; its present status," *Journal of the American Medical Association*, 1885, *4:* 563.

153 T. A. Emmet, op. cit. (n. 128 above).

154 A. W. Johnstone, "The infantile uterus," *Transactions of the American Gynecological Society*, 1887, *12:* 275–85.

155 R. Battey, op. cit. (n. 27 above), 40.

156 L. Tait, *Diseases of Women and Abdominal Surgery*, vol. 1 (Leicester: Richardson and Company, 1889).

157 A. W. Johnstone, op. cit. (n. 154 above).

158 J. T. Gilmore, op. cit. (n. 71 above), 323; C. Rauschenberg, "Ovulation and menstruation and Dr. R. Battey's operation of normal ovariotomy," *Atlanta Medical and Surgical Journal*, 1875/6, *13:* 713–27; A. R. Jackson, "The ovulation theory of menstruation: will it stand?" *American Journal of Obstetrics and Diseases of Women and Children*, 1876, *9:* 529–60.

159 T. A. Reamy, "Some clinical testimony as to the ultimate results from the removal of the uterine appendages," *Transactions of the American Gynecological Society*, 1891, *16:* 230–47.

160 R. Battey, "Discussion: 'An experience with sloughing intrauterine fibroids' by Ely Van De Warker," *Transactions of the American Gynecological Society*, 1889, *14:* 165–67.

161 A. Hegar, op. cit. (n. 6 above).

162 E. P. Becton, op. cit. (n. 3 above), 34.

163 F. H. Garrison, *An Introduction to the History of Medicine with Medical Chronology, Suggestions for Study and Bibliographic Data*, 4th ed. (Philadelphia: W. B. Saunders Company, 1929), 695.

PART II

PICTORIAL ESSAY

Rima D. Apple

RIMA D. APPLE is Project Coordinator at the Center for Photographic Images of Medicine and Health Care at the State University of New York at Stony Brook, New York.

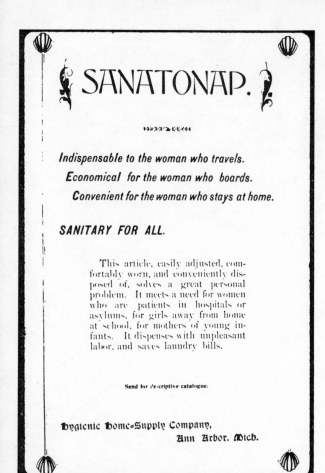

SANATONAP.

Indispensable to the woman who travels.

Economical for the woman who boards.

Convenient for the woman who stays at home.

SANITARY FOR ALL.

This article, easily adjusted, comfortably worn, and conveniently disposed of, solves a great personal problem. It meets a need for women who are patients in hospitals or asylums, for girls away from home at school, for mothers of young infants. It dispenses with unpleasant labor, and saves laundry bills.

Send for descriptive catalogue.

Hygienic Home-Supply Company,
Ann Arbor, Mich.

Advertisement for Sanatonap (*New Crusade*, 1899, 9:9)

Cultural stereotypes of femininity, and particularly menstruation, influenced the content and rhetoric of advertisements for "female personal products." Thus, nineteenth-century promotions were more circumspect than twentieth-century advertisements.

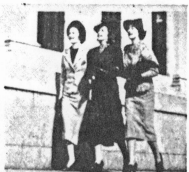

Make the best of
Nature's bad bargain

It's no news to you that ordinary sanitary pads bulge and give off embarrassing odors. For complete comfort on every "difficult day" try Cashay ... the new *internal* sanitary tampon. Made of highly absorbent surgical cotton and gauze. *Sterilized after wrapping.* Recommend Cashay to your patients, too. 35c for 12. For free booklet, write Cashay Corp., Dept. M., 19 West 24th Street, New York, N. Y.

Cashay

Accepted for Advertising by the Journal of the American Medical Association

Guaranteed by Good Housekeeping

Advertisement for Cashay (*American Journal of Nursing*, 1937, 37:48)

Advertisements by abortionists (*New York Herald Tribune*, April 9, 1864, 6)

The fact or possibility of pregnancy dominated a significant portion of most women's lives until the advent of reasonably safe, relatively dependable, widely available contraceptives in the twentieth century. In the nineteenth century, many women sought out abortifacients and abortionists to end life-threatening and unwanted pregnancies. Margaret Sanger used the media, most especially her own Birth Control Review, *to promote the need for and desirability of contraception.*

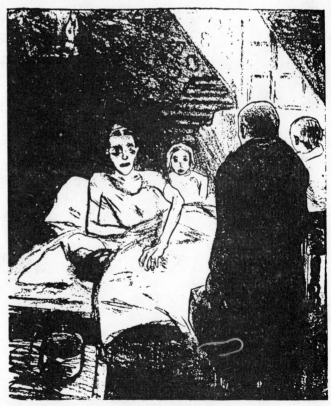

"Remember, Mrs. Judd, another child will kill you—"
"But, doctor, tell me— —"
"I cannot." (*Birth Control Review*, 1919, *3, no. 8*:9)

287

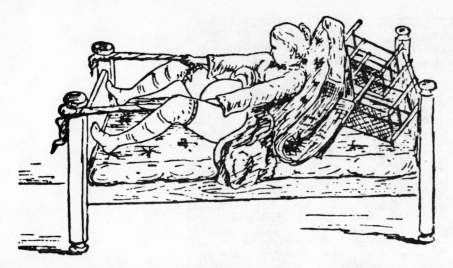

Woman birthing without the assistance of attendants, Virginia, late nineteenth century (G. J. Engelmann, *Labor among Primitives* [St. Louis: J. J. Chambers, 1883])

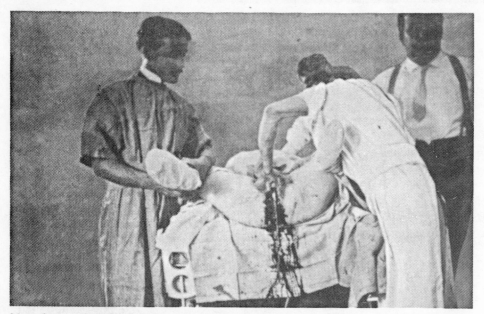

Manual expression of the placenta (Ebert H. Grandin and George W. Jarman, *Pregnancy, Labor and the Puerperal State* [Philadelphia: F. A. Davis, 1895])

Midwives attended most births in the United States before the twentieth century. Occasionally, women found themselves alone for the event and devised ingenious techniques for support during labor. Physicians, who increasingly participated in deliveries, gained their obstetrical knowledge from didactic lectures and textbooks, often illustrated with photographs and drawings.

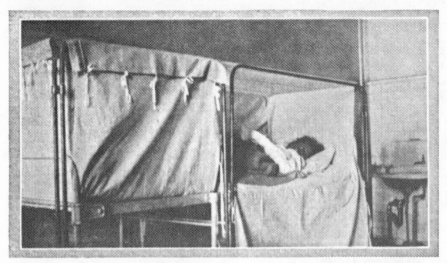

Since patients frequently experienced uncontrollable thrashing under the influence of scopolamine-morphine, physicians placed women in canvas cribs (Bertha Van Hoosen, *Scopolamine-Morphine Anaesthesia* [Chicago: House of Manz, 1915])

Lay women and some physicians in the early twentieth century promoted "twilight sleep," the controversial use of scopolamine and morphine designed to alleviate women's pain in childbirth.

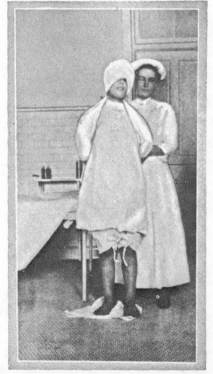

To insure that the patient did not interfere with the sterile field during delivery, physicians dressed a birthing woman in a continuous sleeve (Bertha Van Hoosen, *Scopolamine-Morphine Anaesthesia* [Chicago: House of Manz, 1915])

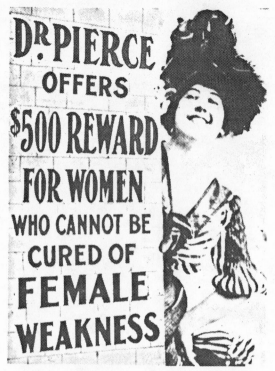

Advertisement for Dr. Pierce's patent medicine (History of Medicine Department, University of Wisconsin—Madison)

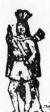

R. GREEN, M.D.
INDIAN PHYSICIAN,
No. 38 BROMFIELD STREET,
BOSTON,

Has, with his INDIAN REMEDIES, treated with complete success more than 50,000 cases of CHRONIC DISEASES His practice is attended with complete triumph in cases of CANCER, SCROFULA, and all CHRONIC DISEASES.

    The discovery of a plaster that will draw out CANCERS, with all their roots, without injury to the surrounding parts, and a remedy like the INDIAN PANACEA, which will cleanse the blood of all humors, are triumphs in medical science never before achieved.

    His medicines are all VEGETABLE, and act in harmony with the laws of life; and so perfectly do they cleanse the blood of all disease, that out of several thousand cases of CANCER and SCROFULA which he has cured, not a case can be found where the disease has ever troubled them afterwards.

    Consultations, personally or by letter, upon all diseases, free of charge. Circulars with full reference, sent by mail free.

Advertisement for Dr. Green and his "Indian remedies" (History of Medicine Department, University of Wisconsin—Madison)

Why did women buy patent medicines guaranteeing cures for vaguely defined diseases like "female weakness" and specific conditions like cancer? Perhaps they could not afford medical care. Maybe their modesty prevented them from consulting male physicians. Conceivably fear of surgery or other radical procedures made commercial promises preferable to medical treatment.

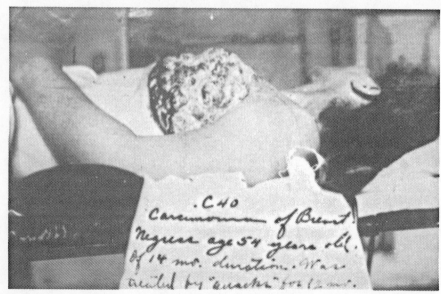

Case of breast cancer, "of 14 mo. duration. Was treated by 'quacks' for 12 mo.," St. Louis City Hospital, 1906 (Courtesy of St. Louis Society for Medical and Scientific Education)

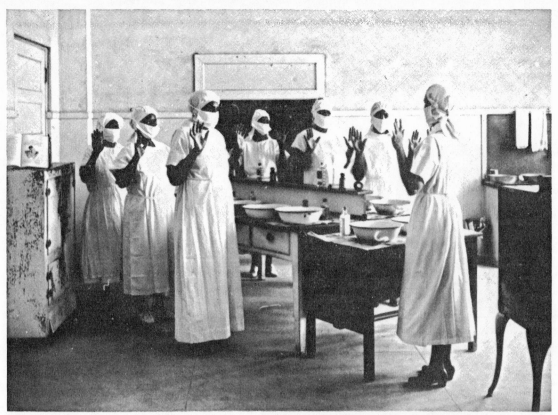

Midwife training class, Florida, 1935 (Courtesy of Rockefeller Archive Center, Rockefeller Foundation [211J])

Though physicians attended most obstetric cases by the early decades of this century, in many sections of the country women continued to rely on other birth attendants. Various organizations developed programs to train midwives and nurse-midwives, especially for rural areas.

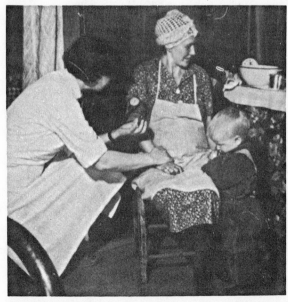

Prenatal examination in the home, Kentucky, c. 1930 (Courtesy of Frontier Nursing Service)

The Dress Reform.

AN APPEAL TO THE PEOPLE IN ITS
BEHALF.

BY MRS. E. G. WHITE.

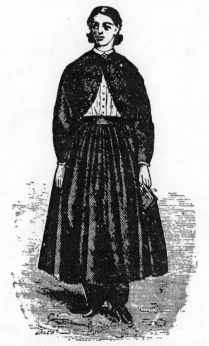

Illustration, accompanying an article by Ellen G.
White, advising women to adopt her dress standards (*Health Reformer*, 1869, *3, no. 2:*21)

*Responding to what they perceived as unhealthful life-
styles and possibly deleterious effects of contemporary
medical practice, health reformers promoted various
alternatives for American women.*

MARY B. G. EDDY,

PROFESSOR OF

OBSTETRICS,

METAPHYSICS AND CHRISTIAN SCIENCE,

*Receives calls TUESDAYS and FRIDAYS,
from 3 to 5 P.M.*

571   COLUMBUS   AVE.,

(MASS. METAPHYSICAL COLLEGE,)

BOSTON.

Professional listing for Mary Baker Eddy (*Christian Science Journal*, 1885, *3,
no. 1:*19)

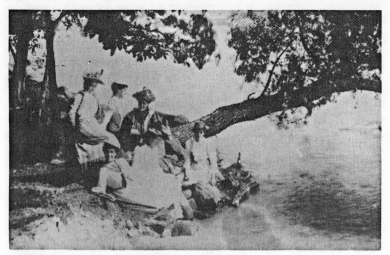

Guests at Lakeside House, originally a "water cure," on Lake Monona near Madison, Wisconsin, c. 1890 (Courtesy of State Historical Society of Wisconsin [WHi(x3)39594])

Many health reformers acclaimed the invigorating and healthful effects of fresh air and exercise. Hydropaths and others recommended visits to sanataria such as Lakeside House.

At the University of Michigan, Dr. Eliza Mosher, Dean of Women Students (1896–1902), required a rigorous physical education program, implemented in Barbour Gymnasium, the first gymnasium designed specifically for women.

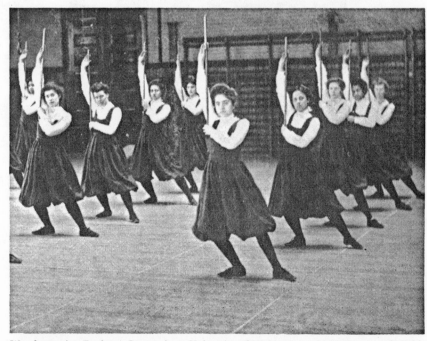

Wand exercise, Barbour Gymnasium, University of Michigan, c. 1910 (Courtesy of Michigan Historical Collections, Bentley Historical Library, University of Michigan)

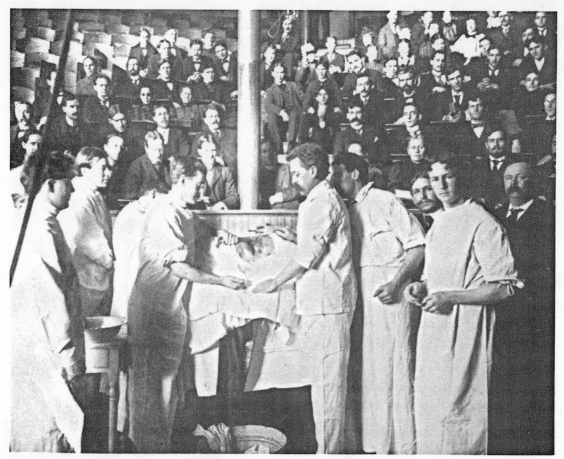

Surgical clinic, Hahnemann Medical College, Chicago, 1899 (*Prominent Physicians, Surgeons, Medical Institutions of Cook County* [Chicago: Redheffer Art, 1899])

Some sectarian schools prided themselves on admitting women "on equal terms with men." The women attending this surgical clinic at a homeopathic college were not segregated.

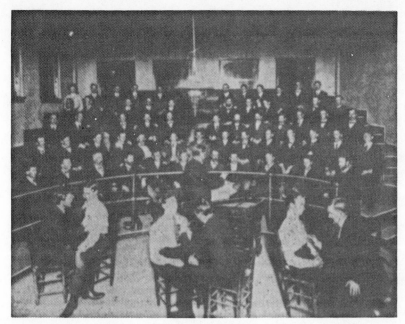

Auscultation class, Chattanooga Medical College, 1903–04 (Courtesy of National Library of Medicine)

Women who entered predominately male medical schools could find themselves isolated emotionally and even physically from their fellow students. Note the lone woman standing in the upper row, left, observing this class.

At female medical colleges, students often developed a sense of camaraderie and competence difficult to achieve in coeducational institutions.

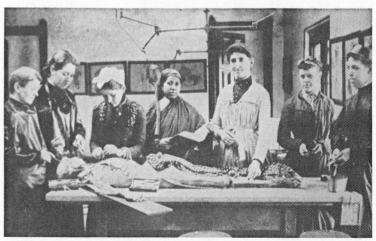

Anatomy class, Woman's Medical College of Pennsylvania, c. 1890 (Courtesy of Smithsonian Institution, Medical Sciences Division)

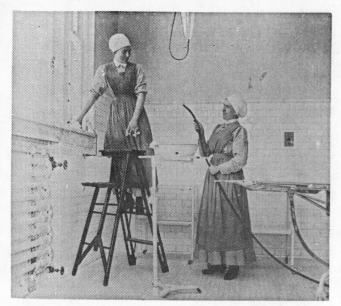

Through the early decades of this century, students of hospital nurse training schools typically provided the bulk of patient care and maintenance work in hospitals

Student nurses cleaning the operating room, Milwaukee Hospital, Wisconsin, 1912–13 (Courtesy of Good Samaritan Medical Center, Milwaukee, Wisconsin)

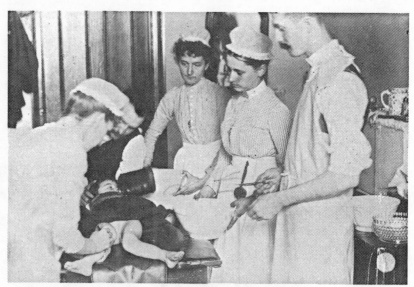

"Osteotomy for Genu-Valgum by head nurse," Bellevue Hospital, New York, 1890–91 (Courtesy of Edward G. Miner Library, University of Rochester Medical Center)

Graduate nurses in hospitals found that their role was not yet clearly defined at the turn of the century. Most directed nurse training programs, but some apparently undertook tasks usually considered outside the province of nursing.

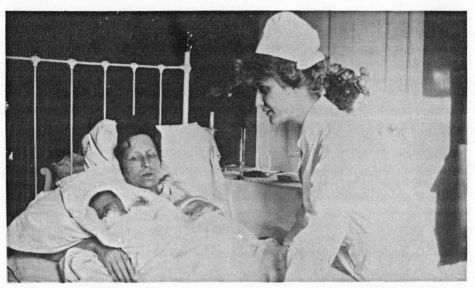

Private duty nursing, maternity care, Milwaukee, Wisconsin, c. 1916 (Courtesy of Signe Cooper, R.N.)

In the late nineteenth and early twentieth centuries, most trained nurses left the hospital after graduation. They entered private duty nursing and later public health nursing.

PART III

WOMEN IN THE HEALTH PROFESSIONS

MIDWIVES

Midwifery is the most traditional of women's healing occupations. For millennia women have attended other women as they labored to bring new life into the world. During the colonial period in America midwives, helped by other women neighbors and relatives, attended all birthing women except those few whose emergency problems led them to call in physicians. Beginning in the 1760s, however, some male physicians entered the practice of normal obstetrics and began replacing female midwives in the birthing rooms of those urban women who could afford to pay the doctors' higher fees. Jane B. Donegan writes of the early midwives and analyzes some of the social and medical forces that encouraged the growth of physician attendance.

Despite the attraction of male accoucheurs for some women, large numbers of American women, probably increasing with the rising immigration after 1840, continued to call midwives when their labors began. By 1910 midwives, many of whom were trained in Europe before they came to the United States, still delivered approximately half of America's babies. But the midwives could not withstand the increasing medical competition that arose at the turn of the century. As Frances Kobrin explains, the result of this second "midwife controversy" was the virtual elimination of the practice of midwifery except in small pockets of rural America. Nancy Schrom Dye analyzes the emergence in the twentieth century of the nurse-midwife, who combined familiar characteristics of the older midwife with a more professional demeanor, but who also encountered significant social and medical resistance even within the renowned Frontier Nursing Service of Kentucky.

Midwives were vulnerable in America throughout the nineteenth and early twentieth centuries because they were not organized, either locally or nationally, and they frequently spoke in their own native languages, which made communication among them unlikely. The majority probably were literate, but the lack of common training and standards, coupled with the existence of informal "granny" midwives alongside more professionally oriented women, produced an environment that made organization impossible. The fact that midwives were women also worked against them, especially since in America the feminist movement tried to get women admitted to medicine but did not identify with or support midwifery as a woman's health occupation.

The quality of midwife practice remains largely unanalyzed by historians. While we know that many midwives remained relatively noninterventionist birth attendants, providing psychological support more than physical aids, we do not know very much about the lengths to which midwives acted to help women suffering difficult labors. Podalic version (turning the fetus) and manual stretching of the cervix were probably common midwife techniques; but to what extent did midwives also administer ergot, potentially a very dangerous drug, or try too early to pull the baby out, causing unnecessary harm to the perineum? Midwifery practices must have varied enormously over time and from individual to individual, and historians need to examine the positive and negative in order to restore the midwife to her rightful place in the historical record.

21

"Safe Delivered," but by Whom?
Midwives and Men-Midwives in Early America

JANE B. DONEGAN

In the United States today the term *midwife* suggests disparate images. It is not surprising that confusion exists, given the fact that for many years standard medical histories either neglected to mention her at all, or dismissed her as a relic discarded not a moment too soon in the name of medical progress. Consequently, some people continue to think of the midwife as an ignorant, slovenly crone whose ministrations women were forced to accept in the remote past as an essential feature of the trauma of birthing. Others, familiar with the current work of midwives in Great Britain, Europe, and Third World countries may regard them as exclusive inhabitants of foreign shores. Few Americans realize that programs to train professional nurse-midwives have been available in this country for nearly half a century.

Nevertheless, in recent years several elements have combined to generate interest in what was once known as the "mysterious office of women." The coming of age of the "new social history," with its emphasis on illuminating the lives of ordinary people, has encouraged scholars to look beyond history's "great figures" to the anonymous and inarticulate, and to reassess interpretations within a general framework of shared experiences. Within this context the midwife has been rediscovered, and her work examined more carefully from the perspective of the parturient, rather than exclusively from that of the male physician with whom she eventually competed. Resurgent feminism, evident since the 1960s, has played a significant part in this rediscovery as women have sought to reclaim their lost heritage. Increasing numbers of Americans, moreover, have begun to question many

JANE B. DONEGAN is Professor of History at Onondaga Community College, Syracuse, New York.

aspects of institutionalized childbirth and to insist on their right to exercise choice in the selection of birthing attendants. In so doing some have turned to professional certified nurse-midwives, who usually practice in a hospital setting, and in lesser numbers to lay midwives without formal training, who attend the client in her home. Additional support for this renaissance of American midwives has resulted from the persistent economic and social problems posed by inadequate health care delivery systems and escalating medical costs.[1]

Historically midwifery was the exclusive province of women. The very term "midwife," literally "a woman who is with the mother at birth," suggests the existence of this female monopoly. For centuries European tradition dictated that men absent themselves from scenes of childbirth, and this tradition was extended into colonial America. The general rule was that no males, whether husbands, surgeons, or physicians, were welcome in the lying-in chamber. In her travail the parturient sought help and comfort from the presence of other women, preferably those who had themselves experienced childbirth. In most of the world today midwives still dominate childbirth, although their roles are undergoing change.[2] In Great Britain and on the Continent, for example, they attend at home or in hospital almost 80 percent of all births. This contrasts sharply with data for the United States. Although as late as 1910 American midwives reported approximately 50 percent of all births, a recent survey conducted by the American College of Nurse-Midwives disclosed that the estimated twenty-five hundred trained nurse-midwives in the nation attended only about 2 percent of American births.[3] The percentage for the more controversial, usually unlicensed lay midwives is undoubtedly much smaller, although the underground nature of their work precludes acquisition of reliable data.

How can this very marked difference in American birthing practices be explained? Of what did the role of the midwife consist in early America? Why was it that in the nineteenth century—an age characterized in many ways by increasing prudishness—more and more upper- and middle-class women abandoned their traditional midwives in favor of the services of attendants known for a time by that incongruous term, "men-midwives"? What were the ramifications of this trend in a society that claimed to revere modesty and to respect the concept of the "delicacy of the sexes"? These are questions considered in the following examination of the evolution of obstetrics from a woman-controlled "art" to a man-controlled, and officially acknowledged "legitimate," branch of medical science.

A brief historical survey of the English midwife is useful, for she represents the model introduced into England's North American colonies. In the seventeenth and eighteenth centuries childbirth had not yet been labeled inherently dangerous, and even pathological, as it would be in the nineteenth. Instead, it was recognized as a normal biological function for which women normally required little active assistance. Bearing children could be terrifying, perilous, and even life threatening. Yet midwives and patients could deduce from the experiences of other women that complications and death did not represent the norm. Accordingly, the midwife's role was confined primarily to offering the laboring woman comfort and reassurance, encouraging and supporting the mother's own expulsive efforts without interfering in the parturient process. The experienced, able midwife learned the value of patience, for in ordinary cases time was on her side. Once the child had been born, she tied off the umbilical cord, supervised the expulsion of the placenta, and put the mother and infant "to bed" for the lying-in period. Her tasks were done more often than not in the presence of the patient's female relatives and friends. They offered the parturient important emotional support and gave the midwife practical assistance, as needed.

Those who wrote about the "mysterious office" stressed the value of emulating nature by permitting the birth to unfold with little or no inter-

ference. Percival Willughby, a physician whose daughter was a midwife, advised attendants to "observe the waies and proceedings of nature for the production of her fruit on trees, or the ripening of walnutts and almonds, from their first knotting to the opening of the huskes and falling of the nutt." Nature separated the fruit without "enforcement," and so it was to be with the midwives. All nature's signs seemed designed to "teach midwives patience, and persuade them to let nature alone to perform her own work, and not to disquiet women by their strugglings." Attempts to hurry the process, warned Willughby, "rather hinder the birthe than any waie promote it, and oft ruinate the mother and usually the child."[4]

The ideal midwife, usually a mother in her own right, was expected to be at once mature, compassionate, pious, and, in general conduct, above reproach. John Maubray, an eighteenth-century surgeon, summarized this ideal in *The Female Physician:*

> SHE ought not to be too *Fat* or *Gross,* but especially not to have thick or fleshy *Hands* and *Arms,* or large-*Bon'd Wrists;* which (of Necessity) must occasion racking *Pains* to the tender labouring Woman. . . . SHE ought to be *Grave* and *Considerate,* endued with *Resolution* and *Presence of Mind,* in order to foresee and prevent ACCIDENTS. . . . SHE ought to be *Patient* and *Pleasant; Soft, Meek,* and *Mild* in her *Temper,* in order to encourage and comfort the *labouring* Woman. She should pass by and forgive her small *Failings,* and peevish *Faults,* instructing her gently when she does or says amiss: But if she will not follow *Advice* . . . the MIDWIFE ought to reprimand and put her smartly in mind of her *Duty;* yet always in such a manner, however, as to encourage her with *Hopes* of a happy and speedy DELIVERY.[5]

In brief, the midwife was to be a paragon of virtue, a primary source of strength and reassurance to the woman in travail.

In London, three groups of medical practitioners, i.e., physicians, surgeons, and apothecaries, were licensed by their own corporations and subject to self-regulation.[6] Midwives constituted a separate group. They did not fall under the jurisdiction of the medical corporations, nor did they have a guild or corporation of their own. Throughout the country, however, they were licensed by Anglican bishops. Churchwardens, ministers, and licensed midwives attested to a candidate's loyalty, piety, and place of residence, as well as to her "known & experienced ability in her pfession of Midwifery," relying in part on "sufficient testimony of many persons she hath delivered." One license extant includes statements taken from several women whom the candidate had delivered safely, and notes that she was "most apt and able through five years of practice."[7] Evidence suggests that many women practiced unlicensed for years, and that a great many more were never licensed. Those who did take the license were required to swear an oath, the contents of which changed little in more than a century. The fifteen items it separately detailed illustrate the stress placed upon the midwife's character and moral conduct. Details spoke to matters such as assigning rightful paternity to the child, not abandoning poor laboring women for the rich, baptising newborns near death, and seeing that stillborn infants were buried properly, rather than being "cast in the jaques [privy] or any other inconvenient place." Midwives were enjoined from exercising "witchcraft, charm, or sorcery" and from administering "any herb, medicine, or potion . . . to any woman being with child" in an effort to shorten labor in exchange for a higher fee. If, having exhausted her own skill, the midwife suspected the life of either mother or child to be in jeopardy, it was her duty to "send for other midwives and expert women in that faculty," relying on their advice and counsel.[8]

It is difficult to assess with accuracy the strengths and limitations of the midwives' skills, but surely these must have varied greatly. Formal training was not available to women, and what they learned about childbirth came primarily from observation and practice. Those fortunate enough to work closely with experienced, knowledgeable midwives could learn their craft well. A few midwives wrote midwifery manuals, and from these we can glimpse their methods.[9] It is not easy, however, to separate the ideal techniques described in these texts from those the women actually employed. Other contemporary sources dealing with the midwives' competence fall into several categories: the complimentary and critical references to midwives found in cases reported by male surgeons and physicians; midwives' oaths, and official licensing require-

ments, drafted and enforced by an establishment, whether church or state, that was male defined and controlled; accusations founded in male suspicions that the "mysterious office" encouraged sorcery, witchcraft, abortion, and infanticide; and occasional mention of midwives in letters and autobiographies. Added to these late in the eighteenth century and on into the nineteenth were, on the one hand, exaggerated claims asserting the midwives' competence in all cases, made in defense of woman's domain against the encroachments threatened by the man-midwife, and, on the other hand, equally unreliable accusations alleging the incompetence of women midwives made by those promoting the cause of the accoucheur. All of these sources have limitations, yet even the midwives' staunchest defenders agreed that many in practice knew little or nothing of their field.[16] Still, when one encounters a reference to the "ignorant" midwife in medical literature, it is well to keep in mind realistic comparisons with the abilities of other medical practitioners of the period. To comment that the midwife knew little about anatomy or physiology in an age when these areas of knowledge were only then emerging into the world of modern medicine is less a condemnation of the midwife than it would be once surgeons and anatomists had made their tremendous strides in the eighteenth century.

So long as childbirth continued to be defined as a normal physiological process, and its nuances remained generally unrecognized, society did not expect its midwives to be highly specialized. The entire process of reproduction, from gestation through parturition, was still imperfectly understood as late as the middle of the eighteenth century. Considered nature's assistant, rather than a primary agent, the acceptable midwife was the respectable older woman who carried herself correctly, encouraged and supported the mother, watched and waited, and interfered as little as possible in the actual mechanics of the birth. The overwhelming majority of cases were uneventful, just as they are today. If, therefore, she did not resort to meddling tactics through some misguided effort to shorten the duration of labor, or to ease the mother's travail, the midwife was on safe enough ground, provided the fetus presented normally and complications such as hemorrhaging or tedious labor did not develop. Indeed, a midwife might well practice her art for many years without ever encountering a single case of malpresentation, tedious labor, or other abnormality. Usually the midwife practiced her profession as an adjunct to other economic activities; in no sense was she a career-oriented medical expert. Regardless of licensing requirements or training—indeed even in the absence of both—her reputation among the local women would be the chief element in determining the size and duration of her practice. This is not to deny that many women who practiced the craft possessed only minimal skills, but merely to insist that those fortunate enough to learn from a competent, experienced midwife were capable of managing the normal birth, despite the absence of formal training.

Had all births been normal, the disparities among midwives would have been less crucial. Regrettably, there was no guarantee that complications would not arise, even though in comparison to normal births their occurrence was relatively rare. In ordinary, historically known as "natural," births, the fetus begins its passage through the birth canal head first. This cephalic presentation is the most common. In some cases, however, another part of the fetus may present, such as a foot, an arm, a shoulder, or the buttocks. Among these preternatural presentations the podalic, or feet first, was the least likely to provoke serious consequences provided the attendant knew how to seize the infant's feet and complete the delivery. Risks were substantially greater when another portion of the fetus presented. The knowledgeable midwife would then attempt version. This procedure consisted of turning the fetus, manipulating it, either externally or internally, into a podalic presentation, and then proceeding to deliver the child by its feet.

Jane Hawkins, the English midwife who attended Mary Dyer in seventeenth-century Massachusetts, probably performed this procedure, for Governor John Winthrop recorded of one birth she attended that the child "came hiplings till she turned it."[11] Nicholas Culpeper, author of a practical, self-help manual for midwives first published in 1651, insisted that women should learn this skill. Asserting that the attendant should always "labour to put the child in a right Posture," he directed the midwife to "reduce . . . [the fetus] into the cavity of the Womb when it comes not forth right, and place it right." Augmenting these directions he suggested, "When the Feet cannot be thrust upwards, let the Midwife supple the Parts with Oil, . . . take hold of the Part . . . help it and give Sneezings."[12]

Apart from administering "sneezings" to encourage the mother to bear down, this advice at first glance appears straightforward enough. It is important to remember, however, that because midwives had no access to formal anatomical study they were largely uninformed as to the location and functions of the internal organs. Thus, laboring to put the child in a "right posture" could take many forms among the uninitiated. In 1731 the British surgeon Edmund Chapman described one case to which he had been called. A fetal arm had presented, and the midwife, unable to cope, finally sent for Chapman. When he arrived the arm alone "had been 18 hours in the world, and [was] much swelled by the long Time and the Ignorance of the Midwife, who pulled violently at the Arm [with] every Pain; not knowing that it was altogether impossible to extract a full grown Infant by that Method."[13] According to Chapman, who authored a manual specifically for the edification of experienced midwifery attendants of both sexes, there were other birthing attendants who employed equally futile tactics. Insisted Chapman, there was no "Excuse for the Folly of dipping the Infant's Hand, . . . hanging out of the Womb, in *Cold Water*, rubbing it with Ice, or touching it with a wet Cloth, which some ignorant Midwives practice in hopes that the Child, upon perceiving the Cold, will presently draw it in again."[14]

Although, as the surgeon Benjamin Pugh wryly observed, "some Authors" had written about "Turning Children with as much Ease as though they were upon a Table," podalic version was always a difficult operation. It required the attendant to insert her hand into the uterus and turn the fetus during uterine contractions. So great was the tremendous pressure exerted on the operator's arm and hand that Pugh warned the reader, "sometimes you will hardly be able to move a single Finger."[15]

Midwives were expected to recognize signs indicative of abnormality. Confronted with complications requiring skills greater than hers, the wise, careful midwife would send for "seasonable help." Such help might come in the form of a more experienced woman, but gradually some midwives began to follow the French example by summoning the surgeon, or "man-midwife." Arriving at these decisions could not have been easy for the midwife. Calling the surgeon meant not only admitting her own limitations—an admission that might lead to loss of face and reputation among the other midwives—but, inasmuch as only men were surgeons, it also meant breaking the taboo against male presence at childbirth. At least one male author assured women that if they followed his midwifery instructions carefully they would never need to "call for the help of a Man midwife," an action he considered "a Disparagement" to both midwives and their profession.[16] Far more typical, however, were exhortations aimed at encouraging midwives to recognize their limitations and sharpen their abilities to discriminate between "a right Labour" and one demanding a call for help. Guidelines varied with surgeons, but essentially they agreed that malpresentations, hemorrhaging, and tedious labors required their assistance, even if the midwife were skillful.[17] An obvious underlying theme was the sexism typical of the age which assumed that although a few women might occasionally succeed at difficult tasks, women as a class lacked the requisite strength, judgment, and ability to remain calm in crisis. Illustrative of this reasoning was John Maubray's comment: "MEN . . . being better versed in *Anatomy*, better acquainted with *Physical helps*, and commonly endued with greater *Presence of Mind*, have been always found readier or discreeter, to devise something more new, and to give quicker *Relief* in Cases of *difficult* or *preternatural* BIRTHS, than common MIDWIVES generally understand."[18]

It was true that surgeons were better versed in anatomy because men had access to formal study and women did not. Yet because men had no opportunities to attend normal cases, they knew little about the normal birth process itself. Moreover, as midwife Jane Sharp acerbically observed, it was not "hard words that perform the work, as if none understood the Art that cannot understand Greek."[19] Even the best surgeons could perform only a limited number of operations. In faulty presentations they attempted version, but they did not always succeed in turning the child, nor could they prevent the development of other complications. When labor was tedious and the woman's contractions ineffectual, when the pelvis was malformed and perhaps too narrow to accommodate the fetal head, when flooding threatened, or the

child was hydrocephalic they then resorted to their bags of iron implements.

The surgeon's bag typically contained "a sharp pointed extractor called the crochets, . . . [along] with a pair of long small scissars [*sic*] with stops in the middle of their blades, for drawing the dead child from the womb [and] a double blunt hook for assisting in the delivering of the child, whether it be alive or dead in the womb."[20] These instruments were designed to enable the operator to save the life of the mother by sacrificing that of the child. When protracted labor or some other cause resulted in the death of the fetus in utero—indeed even in cases where the fetus was not yet dead— the attending surgeon would perform an embryotomy (usually a craniotomy) to relieve the mother's suffering. Using these devices singly or in combination, he would decapitate the fetus in utero, perforate the skull, and empty it of its contents. Alternately, he might first amputate the protruding portion of the fetus that impeded progress through the birth canal before proceeding with the necessary reduction of the fetal skull.[21] Horrifying as these painful and perilous operations were, they remained for many years the only practical alternative to certain death for both mother and child.

The caesarian section, i.e., removing the fetus from the uterus through an incision made in the lower abdomen of the mother, was not yet a satisfactory substitute for the embryotomy. Caesarian sections were almost never attempted while the mother was still alive. In an age lacking anesthesia and knowledge of antiseptic and aseptic techniques, the accompanying shock to the patient and the high risk of infection were so horrendous as to cause all but the most foolhardy to avoid this operation.

In view of the unsatisfactory procedures available to surgeons it is little wonder that men-midwives carried with them the aura of death. As one of them explained, "the frequency with which surgeons performed embryotomies hath very much caused the Report, that where a *Man* comes, one or both must necessarily die; and is the reason why so many forbear sending for the surgeon until the child is dead, or the Mother dying."[22] This negative view first began to give way when innovative surgeons developed the obstetric forceps. By reaching into the birth canal with these instruments, grasping the fetal head and pulling gently, surgeons were able to draw the fetus along. This was especially useful when the mother's strength was exhausted from protracted labor, or when her contractions proved too weak to accomplish an unassisted birth.

The forceps first had been utilized by various members of the Chamberlen family in England. They kept the invention secret, employing it as a nostrum and advertising that they could deliver women in tedious and difficult cases without resorting to embryotomies. Hugh Chamberlen, Jr., having no male heir, let the general design of the family secret be known before his death in 1728, but by then other surgeons had begun to develop similar instruments of their own. Once the forceps came into general use they revolutionized obstetrical practice, paving the way for men to move into general midwifery.[23] Physical possession of these instruments was merely the first step. Practitioners required detailed instruction in their use, as well as considerable understanding of anatomy and physiology. The forceps were developed and improved upon by surgeons for their exclusive use in performing surgical midwifery operations. They did not contemplate placing them in the hands of women, who were expected to continue to call upon surgeons for help as needed. Women midwives were not taught to use forceps, for surgeons argued that women lacked the necessary strength, courage, and requisite anatomical knowledge. The continuing development of improved procedures and equipment, therefore, widened the existing disparity between midwives and surgeons. The more sophisticated the technique, the greater the need for formal instruction of a type not available to women. So long as surgeons limited themselves to attending abnormal cases the midwives could continue to control the normal cases that constituted the majority of the practice. In the second half of the eighteenth century, however, men began to attend these normal cases, thereby posing a potentially serious threat to the women's domain.

Many surgeons participated in these changes, but no figure looms so large as that of William Smellie. His work revolutionized Anglo-American obstetrics, and the consequent effects upon the midwives were of enormous import. After twenty years of experience attending tedious and preternatural cases, this logical and mathematically oriented surgeon determined to investigate scientifically the mechanical process that constituted normal childbirth. Delivering poor women in London gratis, Smellie was able to take careful, precise measurements of the normal female pelvis and to investigate its shape and dimensions. He also studied the external shape of the fetal head. This information enabled him to arrive at an accurate explanation of the manner in which the head passes through the pelvic basin in normal childbirth. Further studies revealed the existence of various types of malformed pelves. Since the distorted pelvic basin was a cause of many cases of preternatural births, this information was requisite for an operator faced with complicated cases.[24]

The results of Smellie's work were of incalculable importance to the development of scientific midwifery. With this new knowledge, as Smellie explained, not only was he able to deliver "with greater ease and safety than before," but he also found in teaching students that he could "convey a more distinct idea of the art in this mechanical light than in any other," and particularly "give more sure and solid directions for applying the forceps." He used this information to improve upon the design and dimensions of the forceps, and discovered, further, that "mechanics applied to midwifery" could be useful when performing podalic version.[25] Equally important is the fact that Smellie taught midwifery to men (and a few women) in London, and by the middle of the century had trained well over nine hundred men-midwives.[26] Many of these men gained clinical experience in normal cases by delivering poor women without fee. In 1774 one of Smellie's students, the gifted anatomist William Hunter, produced the results of twenty years' research with the publication of *The Anatomy of the Human Gravid Uterus*. The importance of this work to the new obstetrics may be appreciated when one realizes that until Hunter began his investigations, few anatomists had ever had opportunities to dissect the bodies of pregnant women.

Another major element in the rapidly developing science of obstetrics was the establishment of lying-in hospitals in London to receive parturient women. These institutions provided care for poor women while at the same time affording men-midwives greater opportunities to attend normal childbirths. Significantly, it was now becoming fashionable for upper-class women to employ an accoucheur, or man-midwife, even in a normal case on the presumption that he was more skillful than the women. William Hunter, for example, who had attended Queen Charlotte in her first confinement, enjoyed a thriving clinical midwifery practice among the aristocracy.[27] Thus it was that significant advances in British medicine led to the development of the new obstetrics, with its promise of greater safety and ease of delivery.

In America colonial midwifery followed lines of development similar to those in the mother country. During the seventeenth and eighteenth centuries women controlled the field, and social norms dictated that male physicians or surgeons[28] be called in only as a last resort to manage abnormal cases. In the still comparatively unstructured world of English America, attempts to license or regulate medical practice of any type were rare. When such attempts were made, however, the midwives were included. Because the Anglican Church had not extended its episcopal supervision of midwives to the colonies, this responsibility fell to local civil authorities. As early as 1649 a Massachusetts law ordered that "persons . . . employed . . . about the bodyes of men, women or children . . . as Chirurgeons, Midwives, [or] Physicians" refrain from acting "contrary to the known approved rules of art, in each mistery or occupation," and that in "difficult and desperate cases" they seek the "advice and consent" of wiser, more skillful persons. A few years later the Duke's Laws in New York included similar provisions.[29] Early in the next century New York's Common Council enacted a law designed specifically to regulate midwives. Based largely on the episcopal model cited above, this law made no mention of skill, suggesting that in America, as in England, an important part of the midwife's role was to regulate social behavior. The version enacted several years later contained the requirement that midwives swear not to "open any mystery appertaining to . . . [their] office, in the presence of any Man." The exception was the case that threatened life. It is curious that even after men-midwives had begun to practice in New York, the prohibition against them remained in the oath.[30] It seems clear that any attempt to supplant the midwives, or even to supplement their practice with men, would need to offer clients inducements potent enough to overcome these tenacious cultural attitudes. Nor would the mere passage of time make

this less problematical, for the highly prized attributes of modesty and delicacy appear to have become increasingly desirable by the opening of the nineteenth century.

Few records have come to light to supply us with detailed insight into the activities and skills of individual colonial midwives, but it does appear that many of the women were highly regarded. Bridget Lee Fuller (d. 1664) practiced for more than forty years after arriving in Plymouth Colony on the *Mayflower*. The third wife of Deacon Samuel Fuller, who had studied medicine at the University of Leyden, she may have acquired some of her medical knowledge from him. When she was widowed in 1663 the magistrates of Rehobeth tried to lure her to their town, but without success. Another woman, identified only as Mrs. Wiat of Dorchester (d. 1705), attended over one thousand births, according to her epitaph. Ruth Barnaby (1664–1765) practiced the art for more than forty years. Remarkably alert, at the age of one hundred she had herself inoculated against smallpox. Elizabeth Phillips (1685–1761) was born in London. In 1718 she received a midwifery license from the lord bishop of that city. The following year she came to Boston with her husband, John, and began to practice midwifery. Her practice, which lasted more than forty years, was extensive, for her epitaph indicates that she had "by the blessing of God brought into this world above 3,000 children." Ann Eliot, married to the missionary and physician John Eliot, was another prominent midwife who may have acquired medical skills from her husband, but little is known of her practice. Survivors of another midwife, Mrs. Thomas Whitmore, of Marlboro, Vermont, claimed that she had never lost a patient in the course of attending more than two thousand births![31]

One of the most important sources for colonial and early national midwifery extant is the diary of Martha Moore Ballard for the years 1785–1812. Although Ballard does not elaborate the specifics of her cases, her diary reinforces earlier impressions that childbirth was as much a social as a medical occasion. It was unusual indeed for a woman to deliver without the presence of a female network of supportive relatives and/or friends. Once a woman found herself "in travail," she would have "her women called," and they would gather at her home to offer comfort and help.[32] In 1789, for example, when Mrs. Sherburn went into labor on

Sunday, she had midwife Ballard summoned. Upon her arrival Ballard found five women already present. Despite this assemblage, however, it was not until after 3:30 A.M. on Tuesday, when Mrs. Sherburn was finally "safe delivered" of a daughter, that the busy midwife seized the opportunity to take her "first nap of sleep" in more than two days.[33] On another occasion, when the wife of Thomas Hinkley was "in travail," the midwife traveled through "boisterous wind and rain" to be with her. Mrs. Hinkley had her women called at seven o'clock the following evening and was "safe delivered" of a daughter at 11:00 P.M. Notwithstanding the presence of the other women, Ballard "tarried" all night with her patient.[34] Sunday evening, April 13, 1800, Ballard was called to "see the wife of Abraham Davenport, who was in labour." On her arrival she found "old Mrs. Davenport, Mrs. Lee and wido Patin." In time "the patient's illness came on," and she was under Ballard's "immediate care" at 11:50 P.M. With the birthing thus supervised by the midwife, Mrs. Davenport's third son and eleventh child was delivered at one o'clock in the morning. The patient and child having been "put to bed" in customary fashion, the women "took b'fast and afterwards attended prayers." Only then did the midwife, assured of her patient's "cleverly" condition, take her leave.[35]

Martha Moore Ballard began to practice midwifery in 1777 and kept a tally of her cases until 1812. Shortly before her death at the age of seventy-six she recorded having attended her 996th birth. The vast majority of these were normal; repeatedly her diary indicates that the patient was "safe delivered" of a son or daughter, even when the infant weighed between ten and fourteen pounds.[36] Occasionally she supervised preternatural or complicated cases. She discovered one patient "in a deplorable situation," but managed nevertheless to "put her safe to bed[,] . . . the living mother of a fine daughter." Similarly, the case of Captain Springer's wife was "supernatural," but Ballard saw her through. Although Mrs. Randal had "suffered" before Ballard's arrival, the midwife preserved "the life of mother and child," as she did in 1797 in the "somewhat singular" case of Mrs. Abraham Davenport. Ballard also supervised the "preternatural" case of Mrs. Trask, whose labor lasted more than three days. Called to Mrs. Preskott on May 18, 1792, Ballard found her in

labor. The next morning Preskott's "illness came on" (a euphemism for advancing labor). Ballard, sensing trouble, "desired Doctor Hubard might be sent for." Her request was honored, but before the doctor could arrive she "performed the operation," saving both mother and infant son. For some time the midwife had expected both to die, and observed in retrospect that this case had encompassed "the most perelous sien" she had ever encountered in the course of her practice.[37]

In addition to supervising birth, Mrs. Ballard occasionally provided nursing care for mothers and infants, and when death took its toll she dressed the child in its grave clothes.[38] Nor were the midwife's problems confined to the infrequent difficult birth. At times she was called upon to undertake arduous journeys under extremely adverse conditions in order to reach a laboring woman. In April 1789, for example, Ebenezer Hewen called her during a severe rainstorm to attend his wife. Accompanied by Hewen, Ballard crossed the river by boat while "a great sea [was] going." Safely over, the two proceeded along their way, encountering a stream with "floting logs," which they negotiated successfully. As they continued their journey "a lardg tree blew up by the roots" in front of Ballard, causing her horse to spring back, thus sparing her life. Assisted over the fallen tree she went on, only to discover that the bridge over the next stream had been washed out. Hewen led her horse across by its reins and remarkably the midwife arrived in time to assist his wife in the safe delivery of a daughter. For her efforts Ballard received a mere eight shillings, the value of which was diminished considerably by the fact that while at the Hewen's her "cloak was burnt" so badly that it was unwearable. Calls in winter could be even worse, and when several women went into labor within a day or two of one another Ballard worked to exhaustion with little or no sleep. Vermin in the patient's home sometimes added to the midwife's problems. After tarrying all night at the home of Mrs. Savage, Ballard lamented, "O the flees."[39]

Of far greater concern than fleas and fatigue, of course, were dangerous cases requiring an attendant's active intervention. As in England, colonial doctors at first limited their attendance to these abnormal cases. Occasionally, as in the tedious labor of Mrs. Robbins, a physician was called, only to learn that the patient refused to see him. Robbins sent him home, preferring to rely instead on the midwife. More typical was the complicated case to which Doctor Coney was called in November 1789. The patient, Mrs. Densmore, endured a tedious labor lasting two days. Coney assisted with the delivery, but lost his patient. Often, too, physicians were called upon to assist with the delivery of stillborn infants. On occasion they might give a case up to the midwife, or cooperate with her. For example, in July 1798 Ballard was called to attend Mrs. Ansel Neys. Upon her arrival she discovered the patient already in the hands of Doctor Page. He "gave the case up" to her, however, and once Ballard had "removed obstructions," the woman was safely delivered of a son. At still another labor Page was called before Ballard could arrive. Once there, however, she "extracted the child," Page electing then "to close the loin."[40]

Yet despite the esteem in which a capable midwife such as Ballard was held, the "new obstetrics" gradually unfolding in England late in the eighteenth century proved the key to reversing the traditional midwifery pattern in America. Objections citing the impropriety of employing men to conduct ordinary labors notwithstanding, the newer ways had begun to take root even before the American Revolution. As young American men found sufficient means to attend medical lectures abroad, either at the University of Edinburgh or on the Continent, to walk the wards of the London hospitals, and study as private pupils with the celebrated London practitioners, they were thrust headlong into the dynamic medical revolution. Their exposure to the stimulating climate of scientific inquiry then nurturing the new obstetrics made it natural for them to fix on this field once they returned to America.

Midwifery was, therefore, the branch of medicine most immediately affected by British trends. The graduates who returned to settle in the major northern cities—Philadelphia, New York, and Boston—found among their established colleagues many persons of ability and experience who shared their enthusiasm for upgrading American medicine. One result, as in England, was that American women midwives soon found themselves under attack.

The initial position of those seeking change seems to have been not that men were preferable to women as birthing attendants, but rather that trained attendants were preferable to the untrained. Unfortunately for the midwives and the women who relied on them, only a few physicians attempted to educate rather than to replace them. All such efforts were privately financed. At no time did the colonial, state, or national governments attempt to follow the Continental plan by establishing schools where midwives could receive formal instruction. While it is equally true that no governmental support was forthcoming for male medical education in the period, one important difference may be noted. Society expected that men would become self-supporting. The family that could manage to do so was willing to secure a son's future by investing in his training. Privately financed education, whether through apprentice programs or formal schooling, was a realistic possibility for upper- and middle-class young men. On the other hand, society defined women as dependent and weak. They were expected to move from dependence on fathers to dependence on husbands. They were viewed primarily as wives and mothers, and their work was thought to be home centered. In all periods of our history some women have worked outside the home. Still, even in the frontier environment of colonial America, before urbanization and industrialization imposed distinct divisions between work done within the home and that performed away from it, woman's employment was regarded as auxiliary to her role as wife and mother. Families of means might send daughters to school with the expectation that they would acquire the charms and graces designed to increase their value in the marriage mart. They were not disposed to invest in a daughter's specialized training, even had it been available, since her future security was predicated on satisfactory marriage, not on any career. The women who did seek employment, in midwifery as in other fields, normally did so out of financial necessity. Midwives already in practice had little money, and even less incentive, to invest in upgrading their skills, especially since they could scarcely have realized the depths of their own limitations any more than self-made, untrained physicians were able to realize theirs.

The implications of this are as obvious as the results are predictable. Although some midwives received excellent training through private sources, the majority continued to learn their craft empirically in the traditional manner of observing other midwives. Criticism directed at some of them probably hit close to the mark. In New York, Dr. Valentine Seaman supported the midwives' cause. Yet, after inquiring extensively into the means by which women moved into midwifery, he concluded that most were first "*catched,* as they express it, with a woman in labour." Having managed to receive the child without incident, they considered themselves competent, and thus, almost by accident, they were "immediately established in the profession."[41] As more and more male practitioners introduced instruments into the practice, women midwives lacking both the instruments themselves and the knowledge necessary to use them effectively were placed at a further disadvantage.

The establishment of proprietary medical schools gave man-midwifery another important boost. In Philadelphia, William Shippen, trained in Edinburgh and London, had taught midwifery privately to a few women and men students. In 1765, with the opening of the all-male medical school of the College of Philadelphia, Shippen abandoned his private course and accepted an appointment that permitted him to teach midwifery as an adjunct to anatomy and surgery at the college. New York's King's College Medical School, established two years later, maintained a separate chair in midwifery. Not all of the later medical colleges included midwifery in their curricula; enough of them did, however, to contribute to the idea that medical school graduates were experts in childbirth, whether or not they were in fact. And all of these medical graduates, of course, were men.[42]

Between 1760 and 1800 in the northern cities, lying-in customs evolved from the almost exclusive employment of women midwives for all but the most exceptional cases, to the growing tendency among families of standing to send for a man-midwife, in the normal as well as the abnormal case. Midwives, threatened with loss of livelihood, insisted that only they could preserve the modesty of delicate women, but male practitioners continued to add obstetrics to their repertoire, both for profit and in the name of what they insisted was progress.

An examination of the private course for midwives offered in New York by Valentine Seaman in the 1790s suggests that misogynistic assumptions also contributed to this trend. Seaman made it clear that his women students were never to attend any but normal cases. To enable them to make intelligent judgments so that they might send for timely help, he provided a useful guide to the classification of labors. All but the normal cases he considered "diseases"; as such, insisted Seaman, they were beyond the province of midwives. He instructed women in the techniques utilized by men-midwives in preternatural births. He even permitted them to practice version on the leather manikin. Yet it is clear that he never expected these women to put this part of their training to practical use. Cautioned this doctor in unmistakable language, this is "a part of the business, well for you to know, but not politic for you to practise."[43] To avoid confusion Seaman carefully delineated the duties of the ideal woman midwife: to bolster her patient's morale during labor, to examine her to determine the degree of dilatation achieved, to support the perineum at the moment of birth, to tie off the umbilical cord, and above all, to refrain from pulling on the umbilical cord in an effort to hasten expulsion of the placenta.[44]

As the fashion to employ general practitioners as birthing attendants became prevalent in northern cities, midwives lost their upper- and middle-class clientele. Contemporary opponents and supporters of the midwives were agreed on this point. In 1820, alarmed by the implications of a proposal to revive female midwifery in Boston, Dr. Walter Channing, Harvard's first obstetrics professor, explained how it was that in Boston, "this branch of medical practice has become confined entirely to male" attendants. "It was one of the first and happiest fruits of improved medical education in America," Channing boasted, "that ... [women] were excluded from practice; and it was only by the united and persevering exertions of some of the most distinguished individuals our profession has been able to boast, that this was effected."[45]

By the second decade of the nineteenth century, then, upper- and middle-class northern urban women, convinced that the superior training of doctors equipped with instruments meant safer and shorter labors, hardly ever employed a midwife. Despite this, however, the doctors' grasp on midwifery was still tenuous. General practitioners were very much aware of the rewards that could accrue to them as accomplished obstetricians. It was not that midwifery itself was especially lucrative, although physicians probably received higher fees for this service than had the midwives.[46] Greater financial rewards could be obtained from a varied practice ranging from vaccinations and treating minor ailments to surgical operations and the treatment of serious diseases. Midwifery's attraction for the doctor was that it fed this general practice; the man who acquitted himself well in the lying-in chamber earned the enduring gratitude of patient and husband alike. Obstetrics became a highly competitive field precisely because, as one medical committee report stated, it led "to the highest success in medicine, more certainly than any other department of practice."[47] Even physicians who opposed man-midwifery despaired of accomplishing reform, owing to the common boast of the doctor that "if he can attend one single case of midwifery in a family, he has ever after secured their patronage."[48]

Consequently, most physicians were eager to add normal cases, which constituted the majority of deliveries, to the abnormal ones for which they would almost always be called. To accomplish this they attempted to reinforce the growing acceptance of the idea that the pregnant woman's best prospect for eliminating the hazards of childbirth and postpartum complications lay in employing the accoucheur. It would have been strange, indeed, had these physicians not played their strongest suit. In emphasizing the element of safety, they stressed the potential for danger that accompanied every normal case. The pregnant woman, vulnerable in her understandable wish for a shorter, safer delivery, permitted the man-midwife to be called because she was convinced that he offered the best chance for both. In the process childbirth, traditionally a social event managed by women, eventually was transformed into an institutionalized medical event over which the male physician assumed control.[49]

Despite the repeated claims and promises of the profession, however, evidence suggests that this belief was not always warranted. In the better medical colleges midwifery and the diseases of children constituted one separate department. Yet, even in these schools it was not required that students complete this course for the medical degree. Although medical students studied female anatomy and physiology, they often had little or no clinical experience in obstetrics. Dr. Daniel Drake, surveying medical education in the 1830s, noted that the

young practitioner would embark on his career with less practical knowledge in obstetrics than in any other branch of medicine. He urged the student to be especially diligent in acquiring theoretical information in midwifery in order to avoid being "thrown into situations of responsibility most harrowing to his feelings, if not fatal to his patient."[50]

Most obstetrics cases were normal, however, and the actual services performed by a knowledgeable physician should not have differed appreciably from those that a competent midwife would provide. These were limited to interacting with the patient and her female attendants with a view toward making the patient as comfortable as circumstances permitted, lending encouragement without giving false hope of a rapid delivery, supporting the woman's perineum at the moment of birth to prevent rupture of the tissue, tying off the umbilical cord, and supervising the expulsion of the placenta. The fact that the physician was equipped with obstetrical instruments, however, held a potential for disaster. Doctors tended to resort to mechanical aids in cases where their use was completely unnecessary. Many men poorly trained in midwifery and lacking in experience did not hesitate to use the lever or forceps with appalling disregard for the consequences. Indiscriminate "meddlesome midwifery" persisted, despite the repeated warnings of authorities that such interference was potentially harmful to mothers and infants.[51]

Had the deficiencies in medical education been common knowledge, women might have shown greater reluctance to employ men as midwives. As it was, doctors faced a more formidable obstacle to continued dominance in obstetrics in the form of the cultural mores of the period. With the growing urbanization of American life that accompanied nascent industrialism, upper- and middle-class women were confined to a narrow sphere of home and family. There they were expected to cultivate the virtues of "true womanhood"[52] and warned of the dire consequences of immodesty. A society that grew increasingly prudish as the century progressed could not be expected to look with equanimity upon the presence of accoucheurs in the lying-in chamber, regardless of their training. The idealized concept of delicate American woman—modest, docile, submissive, and gentle—is by now a familiar one. Of chief interest here is the incongruity of the expectation that, despite the "innate" modesty and delicacy of her character, the enceinte woman would suspend her prejudices and inhibitions—at least temporarily—on the questionable promise that her male attendant could make her delivery safer and more rapid. The physicians' task in overcoming woman's timidity was made all the more complex by their own recognition of the need to bow to propriety and decorum. To minimize the "embarrassments of the practice," they devised methods that enabled them to deliver patients who were clothed and covered completely with blankets or sheets.[53] The editor of the *New York Medical Gazette* articulated the doctors' dilemma by insisting that exposure of the patient was "never necessary" and could not be condoned. Continued the editor, "Catheterism, vaginal exploration, manipulations ... whether manual or instrumental, delivery by the forceps and embryotomy itself, can all be performed by a competent man as well without the eye as with it."[54] One obvious solution to the dilemma was to provide society with medically trained women attendants. The same cultural attitudes that bound women to their "natural sphere," however, made it increasingly difficult to accept the notion that "true" women could be trained to perform the delicate tasks of obstetrics and still retain their modesty and virtue. Physicians, not unexpectedly, capitalized on this in their determined efforts to keep women out of medical practice.[55]

In this same interest of morality, critics of man-midwifery attempted to drive men from the field and restore midwifery to the women. These critics argued that men-midwives, regardless of whether they called themselves accoucheurs, obstetricians, or general practitioners, undermined the very foundations upon which "civilized" society rested. They charged that men practiced obstetrics to satisfy their prurient lusts, and warned that unwarranted "meddlesome midwifery" inflicted great physical harm. Some argued against the value of instruments altogether, and only a very few sought to give women the thorough training they would have needed in order to compete successfully. Most of the anti-man-midwifery reformers shared a sex-based view that denied women's ability to learn the procedures requisite to their becoming the technical equals of men.[56]

The relationship between the women's rights movement and the entrance of women into the medical profession has been noted by historians.[57]

Obstetrics and gynecology seemed especially suited to the feminist cause. Yet it would be wrong to conclude that the anti-man-midwifery movement stemmed from the same origins as did the women's rights crusade. Supporters of the former were not necessarily motivated by a desire to broaden the professional opportunities available to women, but rather by a wish to remove from society that paradox created by the conflicting demands of modesty and safety. These reformers sought to bar men from the lying-in chamber only incidentally to give employment to women. Their principal goal was to eradicate a practice which to them clearly violated the claims of decorum.

In the 1840s, egalitarian impulses, attacks on orthodox medicine, and emergent feminism all joined with the reactionary forces to produce a threat to man-midwifery more potent than any the doctors had encountered previously. By then the physicians' argument that competence in obstetrics required a thorough education in all branches of medicine contributed to the idea that women who wished to practice midwifery must first qualify as physicians. In this way, the reactionary goals of the anti-man-midwifery forces ultimately became intertwined with the radical objectives of feminists who sought to open the medical profession to women as a matter of right.

Neither the critics of man-midwifery nor their feminist allies succeeded in restoring obstetrics to women. Yet, their activities did focus attention on the incongruity of expecting women to accept the services of male attendants and at the same time observe the dictates of a rigid moral code. Moreover, it was they who provided a much-needed support network for the few pioneering women who managed to enter the medical profession in antebellum America.

Nor had the midwives faded away completely. Although almost entirely replaced by physicians in upper-class urban practice, midwives continued to serve rural, working-class, immigrant, and black women well into the twentieth century.[58] Viewed from the perspective of self-conscious medical professionals desirous of fostering specialized obstetric care and institutionalizing childbirth, these attendants posed a menace to public welfare. Seen from the perspective of parturients, however, these "forgotten women" were a welcome presence in the birthing chamber, by virtue of both their sex and their valuable empirical knowledge. Until the twentieth-century campaign to eradicate them eventually succeeded, these attendants continued to provide laboring women with the comfort, re-

assurance, and support that over time have formed an integral part of the midwife's "mysterious office."

NOTES

An elaboration of the themes and ideas discussed in this article is contained in my book *Women and Men Midwives: Medicine, Morality and Misogyny in Early America* (Westport, Ct.: Greenwood Press, 1978).

1 For a review of recent scholarship on childbirth see Nancy Schrom Dye, "The history of childbirth in America," *Signs: Journal of Women in Culture and Society* 6 (Autumn 1980): 97–108. Discussions of nurse-midwives and lay midwives are found in newspapers and lay periodicals as well as in professional journals. See, for example, "Midwife births gaining wider acceptance," *New York Times*, Jan. 24, 1981; "No place like home," *Syracuse Herald-American*, Sept. 27, 1981; Patrick Young, "The thoroughly modern midwife," *Saturday Review* 55 (Sept. 2, 1972): 42–43; N. Ander, "Return of the midwife," *Good Housekeeping* 183 (September 1976): 198–200; H. Kaminetzky, "New midwife—sophisticated and caring: training program at the College of Medicine and Dentistry of New Jersey," *Intellect* 104 (March 1976): 417–18. Discussions in the professional literature include *The Midwife in the United States: Report of a Macy Conference* (New York: Josiah Macy Jr. Foundation, 1968); Ruth W. Lubic, "Myths about nurse-midwifery," *American Journal of Nursing* 74 (Feb. 1974): 268–69; Janice T. Kuhlmann and Edward G. Kuhlmann, "Nurse-midwifery: a new concept for middle class Americans," in *16th International Congress of Midwives, New Horizons in Midwifery*, ed. Alice M. Forman et al. (Baltimore: Waverly Press, 1973), 107–10; Judith Bourne Rooks and Susan H. Fischman, "American nurse-midwifery practice in 1976–77: reflections of 50 years of growth and development," *American Journal of Public Health* 70 (Sept. 1980): 990–96.

2 On recent changes in the scope of the practice of European and British midwives, see Margaret K. Willett, "Midwifery in seven European countries—a surprising spectrum, Part I," *Journal of Nurse-Midwifery* 26 (July–Aug. 1981): 28–33. Attempts to upgrade the skills of traditional midwives in India are discussed in H. N. Mathur, DAMODAR, and P. N. Sharma, "The impact of training traditional birth attendants on the utilization of maternal health services," *Journal of Epidemiology and Community Health* 33 (June 1979): 142–44.

3 Judy Barrett Litoff, *American Midwives: 1860 to the*

Present (Westport, Ct.: Greenwood Press, 1978), 27; cited in Alfreda Dempkowski, "Future prospects of nurse-midwifery in the United States," *Journal of Nurse-Midwifery* 27 (Mar.–Apr. 1982): 9–10.

4 Percival Willughby, *Observations in Midwifery*, quoted in Irving S. Cutter and Henry R. Viets, *A Short History of Midwifery*, 1st ed. (Philadelphia and London: W. B. Saunders Co., 1964), 7.

5 John Maubray, *The Female Physician* (London: James Holland, 1724), quoted in ibid., 13.

6 Medical licensing in London and the provinces underwent substantial alterations between the sixteenth and nineteenth centuries. See Wallace Notestein, *The English People on the Eve of Colonization, 1603–1630* (New York: Harper & Brothers, 1954), chap. 9; Joseph Kett, "Provincial medical practice in England, 1730–1815," *Journal of the History of Medicine and Allied Sciences* 19 (Jan. 1964): 17–29; Bonnie Bullough and Vern Bullough, "A brief history of medical practice," in Elliot Friedson and Judith Lorber, *Medical Men and Their Work* (New York: Aldine-Atherton, 1972), 86–102.

7 J. H. Aveling, *English Midwives: Their History and Prospects* (London: Churchill, 1872), 93; Thomas R. Forbes, *The Midwife and the Witch* (New Haven and London: Yale University Press, 1966), plates 1–8, facing 144–45. See also the copy of midwife Ellen Perkins's license, in Jean Donnison, *Midwives and Medical Men: A History of Inter-Professional Rivalries and Women's Rights* (New York: Schocken Books, 1977), 229–31.

8 Aveling, *English Midwives*, 90–93; Forbes, *Midwife and Witch*, 146–47.

9 See, for example, Jane Sharp, *The Midwives Book; or, The Whole Art of Midwifery* (London, 1671); Sarah Stone, *A Complete Practice of Midwifery* (London, 1737); Margaret Stephen, *The Domestic Midwife* (London, 1795); and Elizabeth Nihell, *A Treatise on the Art of Midwifery* (London: Morley, 1760).

10 An evaluation and discussion of these sources is found in Donegan, *Women and Men Midwives*, 15–25.

11 John Winthrop, *History of New England*, vol. 1, quoted in Francis R. Packard, *History of Medicine in the United States*, (New York: Hafner, 1963), 1: 45.

12 Nicholas Culpeper, *A Directory for Midwives; or, A Guide for Women, in Their Conception, Bearing, and*

Suckling Their Children . . . (London: Norris, Bettesworth, Ballard, and Batley, 1724), 297. Sneezings were induced by blowing snuff into a woman's nostrils by means of a quill. See Harold Speert, *Obstetrics and Gynecology: A History* (Chicago: American College of Obstetricians and Gynecologists, 1980), 11.

13 Edmund Chapman, *Treatise on the Improvement of Midwifery . . . A Work Particularly Adapted to Improve Such, of Either Sex, Whose Profession Has Already Led Them to Make Some Progress in This Science*, 3d ed. (London: L. David and C. Reymers, 1759), 111.

14 Ibid., 113.

15 Benjamin Pugh, *A Treatise of Midwifery, Chiefly with Regard to the Operation, with Several Improvements in That ART* . . . (London: J. Buckland, 1754), 44.

16 Culpeper, *Directory*, A-3.

17 See, for example, Hugh Chamberlen, "Translator to the reader," in François Mauriceau, *The Diseases of Women with Child, and in Child-bed*, 2d ed., trans. Hugh Chamberlen (London: John Darby, 1683), no pagination; William Giffard, *Cases in Midwifery* (London: B. Motte, T. Wotton, & L. Gulliver, 1734), quoted in Cutter and Viets, *Midwifery*, 18–20; Chapman, *Treatise*, xi–xii, 139, 142.

18 John Maubray, *The Female Physician* . . . quoted in Cutter and Viets, *Midwifery*, 12.

19 Jane Sharp, *The Midwives Book* quoted in Hilda Smith, "Gynecology and ideology in seventeenth century England," in *Liberating Women's History: Theoretical and Critical Essays*, ed. Berenice A. Carroll (Urbana, Chicago, London: University of Illinois Press, 1976), 112.

20 John Memis, *The Midwife's Pocket Companion; or, A Practical Treatise of Midwifery on a New Plan . . . Adapted to the Use of the Female as Well as the Male Practitioner in That Art* (London: Edward and Charles Dilly, 1765), 91–92.

21 Ibid.; I. Snapper, "Midwifery, past and present," *Bulletin of the New York Academy of Medicine*, n.s. 39 (August 1963): 507.

22 Chamberlen, "Translator to the reader," no pagination.

23 For a discussion of various types of obstetrical forceps and their historical development, see Donegan, *Women and Men Midwives*, 47–59.

24 William Smellie, *A Treatise on the Theory and Practice of Midwifery*, 3d ed. (London: D. Wilson & T. Durham, 1756), 251–53, 78–82, 281–82; Robert W. Johnstone, *William Smellie: The Master of British Midwifery* (Edinburgh and London: E. & S. Livingstone, 1952), 42–45.

25 Smellie, *Theory and Practice*, 252–53.

26 Ibid., v.

27 John L. Thornton and Patricia C. Want, "William

Hunter's 'The Anatomy of the Human Gravid Uterus,' 1774–1974," *Journal of Obstetrics and Gynaecology of the British Commonwealth*, n.s. 81 (January 1974): 1–3.

28 In America the terms physician, surgeon, and doctor were often used interchangeably, owing in part to the absence of separate guilds. Benjamin Rush, reviewing earlier norms, observed that in the 1760s physicians "were seldom employed as man-midwives except in preternatural and tedious labours." Benjamin Rush, "An inquiry into the comparative state of medicine, in Philadelphia, between the years 1760 and 1765, and the year 1805," in Benjamin Rush, *Medical Inquiries and Observations*, 2d ed. (Philadelphia: J. Conrad, 1805), 4: 375.

29 *The Colonial Laws of Massachusetts*, 137–38, quoted in Henry B. Shafer, *The American Medical Profession, 1783–1850* (New York: Columbia University Press, 1936), 205; *The Colonial Laws of New York from the Year 1664 to the Revolution*, (Albany: Lyon, 1894), 1: 27.

30 *Minutes of the Common Council for the City of New York, 1675–1776*, (New York: Dodd, Mead & Co., 1905), 3: 121–23; *Laws, Orders and Ordinances of the City of New York* (New York: Bradford, 1731), 27–29; *Laws, Statutes, Ordinances and Constitutions . . . of the City of New York* . . . (New York: Holt, 1763), 34–36; Richard H. Shryock, *Medical Licensing in America, 1650– 1965* (Baltimore: Johns Hopkins Press, 1967), 16.

31 Francis R. Packard, *History of Medicine in the United States*, (New York: Hafner, 1963), 1: 44; Kate Campbell Hurd-Mead, *Medical Women of America* (New York: Froben Press, 1933), 17; Rhoda Truax, *The Doctors Warren of Boston: First Family of Surgery* (Boston: Houghton Mifflin, 1968), 5; Cutter and Viets, *Midwifery*, 143–44; Speert, *Obstetrics and Gynecology*, 9–10.

32 *The Diary of Mrs. Martha Moore Ballard (1785–1812)*, in Charles Eleventon Nash, *The History of Augusta: First Settlements and Early Days as a Town* (Augusta: Charles E. Nash & Son, 1904). Ballard frequently recorded the presence of women as "assistants" to the midwife. See, for example, 285, 294, 296, 305, 307–8, 310, 313. Their absence is noted in ibid., 298, 406, as is that of husbands, who generally did not enter the birthing chamber. See 298, 311, 319, 329, 331, 367.

33 Ibid., 274, 311, 284.

34 Ibid., 274.

35 Ibid., 391.

36 Ibid., 232, 350, 279, 283, 285, 286, 309, 321, 351, 376.

37 Ibid., 287, 341, 313, 363, 364, 314. The "operation" may have been version.

38 Ibid., 329, 350, 386, 388, 361.

39 Ibid., 279–80. On travel, see, for example, 278, 286, 311, 334, 369, and on lack of sleep, 352–53, 358, 371. On fleas, see 316, 352.

40 Ibid., 338, 286, 355, 373–74, 327. Possibly a reference to a torn perineum. On other colonial men-midwives, see Donegan, *Women and Men Midwives*, 110–23.

41 Valentine Seaman, *The Midwives Monitor, and Mothers Mirror* . . . (New York: Isaac Collins, 1800), viii.

42 Advertisement, *Pennsylvania Gazette*, January 31, 1765, quoted in Cutter and Viets, *Midwifery*, 149. At King's College the midwifery post was held first by John Van Brugh Tennent, followed by Samuel Bard. See Baron Stookey, *A History of Colonial Medical Education in the Province of New York, with Its Subsequent Development, 1767–1830* (Springfield, Ill.: Thomas, 1962), 50–51.

43 Seaman, *Midwives Monitor*, 101–2.

44 Ibid., 90–99.

45 [Walter Channing], *Remarks on the Employment of Females as Practitioners in Midwifery, By a Physician* (Boston: Cummings and Hilliard, 1820), 3.

46 Midwife Martha Moore Ballard, for example, usually charged nine shillings for her services. At times she received less, and occasionally more; she sometimes accepted amounts of tobacco, rum, coffee, and salt, a pair of shoes, a thimble, or in one instance twenty four shillings, a pattern for a calico gown, a yard of cloth, and some lining. See Ballard's diary in Nash, *History of Augusta*, 233, 238, 248, 258, 310, 321, 336. On occasion an experienced and respected midwife might command much higher fees. Janet Cumming, who practiced midwifery in Charleston during the 1770s, claimed an annual earned income in excess of £400 sterling. See Mary Beth Norton, *Liberty's Daughters: The Revolutionary Experience of American Women, 1750–1800* (Boston and Toronto: Little, Brown, 1980), 140. In 1766 the New Jersey Medical Society established a fee table for physicians setting a fee of £1.10.0 for natural deliveries, £3.0.0 for preternatural and laborious cases. In Philadelphia Thomas and Phineas Bond charged "£2 or £3" for a delivery in 1766, but their fee was not broken down into specific charges for normal and abnormal cases. Physicians in New York City set the following rates in the 1790s: "Ordinary cases in Midwifery £4.0.0; Extraordinary do. from £5 to £10." Maurice Bear Gordon, *Aesculapius Comes to the Colonies* (Ventnor, 1949), 350; Rates of Medical Charges, New York, 1798, MSS, New-York Historical Society. Whitfield J. Bell, Jr., *John Morgan, Continental Doctor* (Philadelphia: University of Pennsylvania Press, 1965), 153. In the nineteenth century, of the three northern cities considered— New York, Philadelphia, and Boston—physicians in

New York received the highest midwifery fees. The New York City Fee Bill of 1816 set fees of $25 to $30 for common cases, and $35 to $60 for tedious or difficult ones. In 1817 the Boston Medical Association established fees of $12 for day cases and $15 for night cases, without apparent regard for the nature of the case. In 1834 the fee table for the College of Physicians in Philadelphia listed $8 to $20 for midwifery. Detailed discussion of fees appears in Shafer, *American Medical Profession*, 154–60.

47 "Report of the College of Physicians, November 15, 1835," in W. R. Penman, "The public practice of midwifery in Philadelphia," *Transactions of the College of Physicians of Philadelphia* 37 (October 1869): 129. See also, [Channing], *Remarks*, 19–20.

48 W. Beach, *An Improved System of Midwifery Adapted to the Reformed Practice of Medicine . . . with Remarks on Physiological and Moral Elevation* (New York: Scribners, 1851), 13.

49 In the nineteenth century this was a gradual transformation, for women continued to occupy birthing rooms, offering encouragement and support to laboring women even in the doctor's presence. See Judith Walzer Leavitt and Whitney Walton, " 'Down to Death's Door': Women's Perception of Childbirth in America," in this volume. In her essay, "Science enters the birthing room: obstetrics in America since the eighteenth century" *Journal of American History* 70 (September, 1983): 281–304, Judith Walzer Leavitt analyzes the extent to which physicians were able to realize their promises to parturients. Other studies have examined the transformation of childbirth from essentially a social to an institutionalized medical event. See, for example, Datha Clapper Brack, "Displaced—the midwife by the male physician," in *Women Look at Biology Looking at Women: A Collection of Feminist Critiques*, ed. Ruth Hubbard, Mary Sure Henifin, and Barbara Fried (Boston: G. K. Hall & Co., 1979), 83–101; Catherine M. Scholten, " 'On the importance of the obstetrick art': changing customs of childbirth in America, 1760 to 1825," in this volume; Richard Wertz and Dorothy C. Wertz, *Lying-In: A History of Childbirth in America* (New York: Free Press, 1977), especially chap. 1; Donegan, *Women and Men Midwives*.

50 Daniel Drake, *Practical Essays on Medical Education, and the Medical Profession, in the United States* (Cincinnati: Roff & Young, 1832), 40–41.

51 See, for example, Samuel Bard, *A Compendium of the Theory and Practice of Midwifery . . .* , 5th ed. (New York: Collins, 1819), iv–vi, 240; William P. Dewees, *A Compendious System of Midwifery, Chiefly Designed to Facilitate the Inquiries of Those Who May Be Pursuing This Branch of Study*, 1st ed. (Philadelphia: Carey and Lea, 1824), 188; John G. Metcalf, "Statistics in mid-

wifery," *American Journal of the Medical Sciences,* n.s. 6 (October 1843): 327–30, 334.

52 See Barbara Welter's classic article, "The cult of true womanhood: 1820–1860," *American Quarterly* 18 (Summer 1966): 151–74.

53 For more on this theme, see Jane B. Donegan, "Man-midwifery and the delicacy of the sexes," in *"Remember the Ladies": New Perspectives on Women in American History,* ed. Carol V. R. George (Syracuse: Syracuse University Press, 1975), 90–109.

54 "Observations on Clinical Obstetrics," *New York Medical Gazette,* reprinted in *Medical News and Library* 8 (October 1850): 83–84. An interesting and revealing controversy developed within the medical profession around the issue of clinical teaching in midwifery. A discussion of the furor created by an experiment in "demonstrative midwifery" at Buffalo Medical College in 1850 and the libel trial that followed is found in Donegan, "Man-midwifery," 103–9. See also Virginia G. Drachman, "The Loomis trial: social mores and obstetrics in the mid-nineteenth century," in this volume.

55 See, for example, Mary Roth Walsh, *"Doctors Wanted: No Women Need Apply": Sexual Barriers in the Medical Profession, 1835–1975* (New Haven and London: Yale University Press, 1977), especially chap. 4.

56 These arguments are detailed in Donegan, *Women and Men Midwives,* chap. 6.

57 Recent examples include Regina Markell Morantz, "The 'connecting link': the case for the woman doctor in 19th-century America," in *Sickness and Health in America: Readings in the History of Medicine and Public Health,* ed. Judith Walzer Leavitt and Ronald L. Numbers (Madison: The University of Wisconsin Press, 1978), 117–28; John B. Blake, "Women and medicine in ante-bellum America," *Bulletin of the History of Medicine* 39 (March-April 1965): 99–123; Walsh, *"Doctors Wanted."*

58 An examination of the decline of American midwifery and the reasons behind it appears in Frances E. Kobrin, "The American midwife controversy: a crisis of professionalization," in this volume. The most complete study is Litoff, *American Midwives,* cited above. For a different resolution of the midwife controversy in Great Britain, see Donnison, *Midwives and Medical Men.*

22

The American Midwife Controversy: A Crisis of Professionalization

FRANCES E. KOBRIN

Although medicine itself has long been an established profession, many of the specialties within
medicine have a much shorter history. This diver-
sification is a result not simply of developments
within the field itself but has also depended upon
the attitude of potential patients—their feeling of
a need for such specialization and their ability to
take advantage of it. The role of this external factor, however, has varied considerably in the historical development of the several specialties. Surgery
became differentiated as soon as the techniques
developed enabling it to be practiced safely, whereas
other specialties, such as dermatology, plastic surgery, or orthodontics, had to wait until a public
attitude evolved which considered ills far less serious than malaria (itself once thought a natural state)
as unnatural conditions which require treatment.

Such a specialty was obstetrics, which dealt with
what many still consider to be the "natural process"
par excellence. In the obstetricians' struggle for
universal acceptance they faced both medical and
nonmedical competition and an almost insuperable economic problem; even the best obstetrical
work was almost more of a hindrance than a help.
The decade from about 1908 began the contest
between the increasingly self-conscious obstetrical
specialist and his adversaries, the midwife and her
advocates. That such a debate could be carried on
with great virulence is itself indicative of the importance of considerations other than the strictly
medical. The result, the complete defeat of the
United States' variety of midwife and the essential
triumph of a "single standard of obstetrics," was

not simply a function of the maturity of the obstetric profession.

In the United States in 1910, about 50 percent
of all births were reported by midwives,[1] and the
percentage for large cities was often higher. At the
same time, and continuing well beyond this peak
period, the maternal death rate in the United States
was the third highest of countries which kept such
records.[2] Midwives were employed primarily by
Negroes and by the foreign born and their children, and the midwives themselves usually shared
race, nationality, and language with their customers.[3] Because this was a period of unrestricted and
heavy immigration (one-third of the population was
foreign born or Negro),[4] the midwife population
was swollen considerably.

At this time also, various local medical units in
the nation began to assess the situation in their
areas, and this resulted in a flood of articles and
addresses on "the midwife problem in _____." The
big eastern cities, most affected by the heavy immigration, were the most diligent in this regard
and produced the bulk of the available data. In
1906, New York commissioned a study which revealed that the New York midwife was essentially
medieval, very different from European midwives,
for these did not emigrate as rapidly as those who
expected such service. According to this report,
fully 90 percent were "hopelessly dirty, ignorant,
and incompetent."[5] These revelations resulted in
the tightening up of existing legislation, and the
creation of new, for the licensing and supervision
of midwives, and eventually in the establishment
of the Bellevue School for Midwives, an institution
which lasted for thirty years. Other areas reported
similar conditions.

The major failing of the midwife, which this leg-

FRANCES E. KOBRIN is Associate Professor of Sociology at
Brown University, Providence, Rhode Island.

Reprinted with permission from *Bulletin of the History
of Medicine* 40 (1966): 350–363.

islation was to correct, was responsibility for maternal deaths from puerperal sepsis and for neonatal ophthalmia, both preventable with the knowledge available at the time. But it became clear during the controversy that occurred over how to deal with this problem that the midwife was by no means the sole offender in these matters. A survey of professors of obstetrics reached the conclusion that general practitioners were at least as negligent as midwives, as well as being equally responsible for preventable deformities.[6] The overall picture of the obstetrical possibilities open to a prospective patient was not very good. Hospitalization was impossible for all but the very rich or the charity cases in the wards, obstetricians were few, and general practitioners unreliable. Use of a midwife involved many hazards, despite the fact that she was usually a sympathetic woman who would wait and work with the natural labor process (often, of course, for too long) and would also in many cases be in regular attendance for more than a week afterward, not only caring for mother and infant, but also assuming such duties as were necessary to keep the household functioning normally.

The most obvious cause of this medically unsatisfactory situation was the general opinion that the midwife was an adequate birth attendant. Her success was due to the fact that the rigors of childbirth were still considered normal and risks in the process unavoidable. The general attitude was that nature really controlled the process so that there was little constructive assistance that could be given. This feeling was clearly dominant among the public, although there were signs of change; it was also an important attitude within the medical profession as a whole. One observer, in assessing the lack of interest in obstetrics generally, noted that the word "obstetrics" comes from a Latin word meaning "to stand before" and added, "or as a sneering colleague once said, 'to stand around.'"[7]

The best evidence that this was the judgment of the medical profession was the status of the teaching of obstetrics in United States medical schools. Dr. J. Whitridge Williams, professor of obstetrics at Johns Hopkins University, made a comprehensive report on obstetrics as it was studied in United States medical schools in 1912; he found that although medical schools had been improving rapidly, obstetrics was by far the weakest area.[8] He sent a questionnaire to professors of obstetrics of

61 schools rated by the American Medical Association as acceptable (they required entrants to have at least a high school degree) and to 59 nonacceptable schools, receiving 32 and 11 replies respectively. Among his results were the following: Of the 42 professors of obstetrics, only 5 limited their outside practice to obstetrics, 21 to obstetrics and gynecology, and 17 were in general practice. Only 10 had served in lying-in hospitals for more than six months. Only 9 had seen more than a thousand cases of labor as preparation for their post, 13 had seen fewer than five hundred, 5 fewer than one hundred, and 1 had never seen a woman deliver. Six schools had no connection whatsoever with a lying-in hospital for teaching purposes, and only nine had as many as five hundred cases a year for teaching material. The average medical student witnessed but one delivery, and the average for the best twenty medical schools was still only four. Half the schools required a period of service of less than a year in training assistants for their own staff, a level, according to Williams, at which a student is still unable to recognize, much less cope with, a serious emergency. Several of the professors admitted that they themselves were incapable of performing a caesarian section. Williams concluded that there was only one medical school in the country properly equipped for teaching obstetrics, and he regretted that it was not Johns Hopkins. The result of this neglect of obstetrics, he saw clearly, was that poor schools with poor facilities and poor professors were turning out incompetent products who lost more patients from improper practices than midwives did from infection.[9]

But the obstetricians themselves were fighting this conception of the insignificance of their field. They argued again and again that normal pregnancy and parturition are exceptions and that to consider them to be normal physiologic conditions was a fallacy.[10] It was this view which contributed to much of the unnecessary operative interference that occurred in this period. Amused critics pointed out that women often delivered themselves while their doctors were scrubbing up for a caesarian,[11] but other results, such as the use of high forceps previous to sufficient dilation, were less fortunate for the health of mother or child.

It was these two fundamentally different approaches to the process of childbirth, based on opposite views of its naturalness, which were responsible for many of the arguments which appeared during this period about the future of the midwife. At one extreme were those who advocated outright abolition of midwives, with legal prosecution of those who continued to practice. This was the official attitude of the state of Massachusetts and also that of most eminent obstetricians.[12] Less adamant was a second group, led by Dr. W. R. Nicholson of the Pennsylvania Bureau of Medical Education and Licensure, which favored eventual abolition, with the existing midwives closely regulated until substitutes could be furnished. A third group was pessimistic about ever abolishing the midwife and thus felt that regulation plus education would elevate the midwife to the relatively safe status she had achieved in England and on the Continent. This attitude was reported from Newark, New York State generally, and New York City and Buffalo particularly. Finally, there were those, especially in the South, who felt that if, somehow, midwives could be made to wash their hands and use silver nitrate for the babies' eyes, that would, because of a host of economic and cultural reasons, be the most that could be expected.[13]

Since all but those who held the first position believed that at present there really was no substitute for the midwife, and thus she had at least temporarily to be endured, their views can be conveniently called the public health approach. Their concern was for the immediate future. The first group based its arguments on the necessity of developing obstetrics for the long-term good of American mothers, and so can be identified with the professional approach. An early analyst of this division in medical opinion described it as a conflict between the practical and the ideal,[14] but the actual arguments involved a great deal more than that.

The public health exponents did, in fact, always claim to be realistic, and they accused the professionals of "criminal negligence."[15] The aspects of the situation which they were in a position to consider were certainly important. Since midwives were registering 50 percent of all births, it did not seem likely that the medical profession could expand sufficiently to take care of all. Some public health officials were not even sure that such expansion was desirable. Arguments against it included the record of the medical profession as a whole, the economic problem of supporting the higher prices

charged by doctors, and the attitude of the women themselves. There was also a subterranean problem of status: doctors were often considered less manageable than the more easily supervised midwife.[16]

With regard to the question whether the medical profession ever could absorb all the obstetric cases, Dr. Florence E. Kraker of the Children's Bureau in Washington felt that the midwife problem would actually grow as the preference for hospitals and laboratories among doctors increased, causing them to desert rural areas.[17] Even if sufficient expansion were possible, it would still be necessary, according to New York City public health official Dr. S. Josephine Baker, to keep midwives and make them safe, because immigrant women, and particularly their husbands, would allow no male attendants. They expected the simple nursing care and household help that a doctor would not provide, and for this they expected to pay the customary small fee. Providing only doctors for these groups would force them either to pay a higher fee or to use clinics with their implication of charity. Above all, they rejected hospital delivery, which would badly upset the home situation.[18]

What encouraged the proponents of the public health view most was the actual progress which had been made through legal recognition, education, and supervision of midwives. England was the chief source of inspiration, since Parliament had, as recently as 1902, established a Central Midwives Board "to secure the better training of midwives and to regulate their practice." Following this change, infant mortality, which had been 151 per 1,000 in 1901, dropped to 106 in 1910, with a commensurate decrease in maternal mortality.[19] A committee of the Russell Sage Foundation, after studying the results, was entirely in favor of the change. In particular, they found that rather than replacing obstetrical practice with trained midwives, it had "increased, improved, and upheld the work of the obstetrician."[20] Germany was also much admired by those of public health persuasion, since the midwife there was a scrupulously regulated institution, trained in government clinics and working in a set district in a defined relationship with a government doctor.[21] The level of obstetric training received by German midwives was recognized as superior to that of most United States doctors.[22]

Major progress had also been made in the United

States itself. Newark, after adopting a program of "conference, lectures and personal visits," reported a drop in the three years 1914–16 in maternal mortality from 5.3 to 2.2 per 1,000 for the city as a whole, and a level of 1.7 per 1,000 among mothers who "received prenatal supervision from the Child Hygiene Division and were delivered by midwives." This was aggressively compared with the rate of 6.5 for Boston, where midwives were banned. For 1916, again, Newark's infant mortality rate below one month was 8.5 for the special category, as opposed to a city rate of 36.4. The reporting of births was greatly improved, silver nitrate was in universal use, and Board of Health Officer Levy was highly pleased with his results.[23] In Philadelphia a similar program, which emphasized in addition control through registration, gave its director "hope to show statistics unequaled in the history of the world."[24] Midwives, more secure in their licensed status, were calling doctors earlier and oftener, neonatal ophthalmia had vanished, and all at relatively little cost.

Besides pragmatically recognizing the midwife's possibilities, many of her promoters felt a strong sympathy for her and her deficiencies. Ira S. Wile defended her on the grounds that it was "unfair to criticize the lack of an educational standard which has never been established." He felt that abolition was no more the answer than it had been for nurses of the "Sairy Gamp type," eighteenth-century doctors, or present-day obstetricians, all of whom, by absolute standards, were very bad indeed.[25] Midwives also gained sympathy from their adherents because of the rudeness with which the "arrogant," "unrealistic" obstetricians treated them. Those most in favor of the midwife seemed bent on elevating her to a professional status well above that of a nurse. Recognition was to build self-respect and pride; caste and dignity would bring a more intelligent type of woman into the profession.[26]

It was with these general attitudes that the public health exponents faced the task of elevating the American midwife. The consensus which developed was that midwives should have training for at least six months to a year, including instruction on pregnancy, asepsis, care of labor, and of mother and child confinement, and, above all, recognition of conditions that indicate when a doctor is needed. These requirements, coupled with legal proscriptions against vaginal examinations, drugs other than laxatives, douches, and the use of instruments, would, they felt, render the midwife a useful member of the community. The further elaboration of linking the midwife to a clinic and to a physician who would make examinations and be available for emergencies was advocated by some, but the problem of maintaining doctors in government employ presented such difficulties that many public health officials were forced to ignore the possibility that a doctor might not be available when needed.[27]

What is important in the plans discussed and occasionally established by public health officials is that in general these men were not simply embracing a distasteful necessity that would otherwise have been avoided. There were some, of course, who felt this way: the official who established the Philadelphia system was well aware of "the incongruity of allowing or actively sanctioning by license, the doing of distinctly medical work by non-medical persons. We cannot adduce a single argument in its favor except . . . *necessity*."[28] But the others were expressing an ideal of obstetric service whereby the ubiquitous process of childbirth could be carried on cheaply and easily, respecting modesty and the integrity of the household, and in a more natural and personal way than if rendered by doctors.

The solution offered by the obstetric profession, on the other hand, was not merely an ideal of obstetric care, but also a very realistic solution for the obstetricians' difficulties. Until this last great wave of immigration, graduating obstetricians had always found sufficient numbers of patients. J. L. Huntington, a Boston obstetrician who was partly responsible for Massachusetts's unique position and was the most vocally concerned of the professionals, observed that the midwife was not—yet—a native product of America. She comes with the immigrant, "but as soon as the immigrant is assimilated, . . . then the midwife is no longer a factor in his home."[29] It was this latest influx of immigrants from southern Europe which had given the midwife problem such dimensions, and, if left alone, her numbers would again dwindle with the slowing of immigration. But if she were given official recognition so that immigrants' sons and grandsons expected such service for their wives, the obstetric profession would, he felt, face grave difficulties. Huntington believed, therefore, that the greatest danger in recognizing the midwife lay in the effect of such recognition on the general public. If the midwife was sufficient, then calling a G. P. would be the height of caution, and there would be no need felt for obstetricians.[30] He and other obstetricians believed recognition of midwives would set the progress of obstetrics back tremendously. The 50 percent of all cases handled by midwives were useless for advancing obstetrical knowledge. Elevating the midwife and training her would decrease the number of cases in which the stethoscope, pelvimeter, and other newly developed or newly applied techniques could be used to increase obstetrical knowledge. The need for strengthening obstetrics courses in medical schools would diminish, and practicing doctors would think themselves so superior to the strengthened corps of midwives that they would feel no need for improvement.[31] Lowering the standard of adequacy would lower all standards.

Because they believed this situation existed, the obstetricians had very different perspectives from the public health exponents. Some physicians felt the arrangement in Germany was far from ideal, so that even if such a system could be transplanted to the United States the resulting standard of obstetrics would be inadequate. Although German midwives learned obstetrics of high quality in their six-month course, that time was considered insufficient to instill an "aseptic conscience." Further, even in Germany their relationship with the physician was not one of "perfect harmony." According to Huntington's analysis, since it was profitable for a midwife to deliver each case herself, she might postpone calling a physician in time of danger; the physician, as well, might also be insufficiently cautious if he were called in, since the responsibility for complications remained with the midwife. Huntington argued further that in the United States such a plan would be impossible because (stating clearly the issue which so troubled some public health officials) the American medical profession could never be forced by law to respond to the call of the midwife in trouble.[32]

From the professional standpoint, the solution in England was also a bad one. In fact, the more midwives there were, and the more successful they were, the worse the situation would be for the community at large, according to Huntington, because this would aggravate a "double standard of obstetrics." The thirty thousand English midwives had not only taken cases that would have been better cared for by doctors but had also taken enough practice away from physicians to obtain a livelihood.[33] Dr. Charles Ziegler, who was later to become cynical about the whole debate, also complained of the estimated five million dollars collected annually in the United States by midwives "which should be paid to physicians and nurses for doing the work properly."[34] The relationship between the ideal of a "single standard" and the issue of economic competition came up clearly again when obstetricians saw the midwife to be in league with "outside" influences—optometrists, osteopaths, neuropaths, Christian Scientists, and chiropractors—who were all invading the legitimate field of medicine.[35] Massachusetts had just licensed optometrists; "if the midwives are now to be recognized we may fairly ask, where is it going to end?"[36]

The professional ideal, of course, was that all women be delivered by an obstetrician, privately, or, if they could not afford such care, in a hospital–medical school complex. Thus, at a stroke, the midwife could be eliminated and the basis established for enormous advances in obstetrics, since students would then get ample training. In suggesting such a system for New York City, Dr. J. Van D. Young felt that even if it were inaugurated at state expense, "the ultimate good to the profession and to the people would be enormous" and rapidly repaid, and, also, that it would attract serious obstetrical students to New York.[37]

The professionals saw only one way by which their goals could be reached and those of the public health approach thwarted. There had to develop a demand from the public for a higher standard of obstetrics. "We can teach the expectant mother what she deserves, and when she demands it she will get it."[38] They urged accordingly that every mother has a right to such care as shall preserve her and hers in life and health, the care which, they said, the midwife cannot provide since the necessary skills are difficult to teach. Combating the "fallacy" of normal pregnancy and delivery was necessary not only to enhance the value of obstetric skills but also to make the American mother not merely respect, but fear, possible danger and so consider no precaution excessive.

Behind both these perspectives on the midwife problem was a complicating factor with which neither side dealt adequately. The economic realities of the situation and the costs of the various programs should have been given far more consideration. Since these economic aspects were working against the obstetricians in particular, they were the most guilty in this respect. In general, the public health approach overstated the economic obstacles to the realization of the obstetricians' ideal, whereas the obstetricians tended to ignore such obstacles, with one significant exception. The problem was that the training of an obstetrician was expensive, and his practice had to be sufficiently lucrative to draw able men into the field. In addition, the expansion of hospital and laboratory facilities to train new men was expensive. Public health officers, who always have many places to spend every appropriation, are not in a position to weigh these facts and their possible consequences; the chief attraction of the midwife for them was that she was cheap. Levy, who established the Newark system, considered as only rhetorical the question whether those who can afford only midwives "should be delivered in finely appointed hospitals at public expense."[39] Others presented the obstetric ideal as a sort of reductio ad absurdum. The obstetricians, on the other hand, ignored this difficulty altogether because of their hope of changing what was then a very annoying fact: the same family will pay easily for surgery but expect to pay meagerly for attendance during pregnancy and confinement.[40] All that would be needed was propaganda to solve what they felt was not really an economic problem.

Huntington felt he had another answer to the "economic necessity for the midwife." Boston Lying-In Hospital ran an outpatient department to provide obstetric training for medical students, and the patients, contributing an average of $1.28 each, in 1910 paid "all the expense" of the department, with a surplus of $807.82.[41] But his conclusion that the finest hospital care was itself inexpensive can be seriously questioned. The Boston medical school complex attracted prospective obstetricians from all over the country. Cases used for teaching amounted to nearly 20 percent of the total number of births in Boston in 1913.[42] Huntington thus claims an amazing percentage, and few other areas could hope to rival it, considering the scarcity of obstetricians at that time; yet it still left 80 percent of the births unaccounted for. It can perhaps be safely inferred that the costs of giving the rest similar treatment would rise rapidly, once deliveries had

to be accomplished without the help of unpaid medical students. Yet even if the costs were indeed relatively low for caring for everyone on such a basis, the necessary expenditures on facilities to make room for all would be beyond the economic horizon of public officials forced to account closely for their use of public funds.

Only two writers proposed a solution which would make ideal obstetric care possible for all, given all the existing conditions. A. K. Paine, Huntington's only apparent critic in his home state, said that our method of government was not suited to the rigid requirements which the properly regulated midwife demands, but that the "obstetric poor" could be handled on a community basis, if the community would assume the responsibility.[43] Because of the stress Paine gave community responsibility, his argument clearly implied public institutions staffed by government employees and run with tax funds on some level or another.

Charles Ziegler, who earlier had complained of the money wasted on midwives, was a Pittsburgh obstetrician who was concerned with the midwife problem. What happened to him when he attempted to approximate ideal obstetric care for all puts an interesting light on the importance of the "ideal" elements in the original professional argument. Ziegler's experiment also involved inexpensive delivery of the poor and, although he got his funds privately, he had even then the idea that what was essentially obstetric charity should not be borne solely by obstetricians, but should be subsidized by the community.[44] Although he had no access to public funds, he evidently could generate other sources of aid by his enthusiasm for his project. Ziegler wanted to establish a dispensary which could give the best care to those who usually did not get such care, i.e., those not in either of the extreme income categories. The aim was to demonstrate how much mortality statistics could be improved, in the hope, of course, that the result would provide encouragement for others to try to achieve the same result. Six years after opening the dispensary in 1912, $80,000 in contributions had been spent caring for 3,384 confinements on both an in- and out-patient basis. Fifty-six percent of the cases were foreign born and 16 percent were Negroes. There were two sets of results. First, maternal mortality was 17 per 10,000 as opposed to a national average of 88.5.[45] This was a remarkable result for the time and clientele. The other result was that the Allegheny County Medical Society found Ziegler guilty of breaches of professional ethics by "solicitation and attendance on cases in families able to pay for a physician [and] . . . solicitation and attendance on cases where a physician had previously been engaged."[46]

Ziegler himself was suspended from the society, and, in 1918, his hospital was commandeered for government service, finishing his experiment.[47] Ziegler concluded after all this that, given the existence of such patients, the cost of caring for them properly (about twenty times Huntington's figure of $1.28), and the strength of the enemies made in the process, the only solution would be municipal, state, and federal aid, not as charity, "but as a matter of wise public policy and of justice to those to whom we look for the perpetuation of our family and national life."[48] He saw the whole obstetric problem as an economic one in which many people could not pay for the services they deserved; an institutional redistribution of such services was therefore necessary.

He believed that his solution would bring opposition from the medical profession, "as they are opposed to any plan which includes municipal or state aid looking toward the solution of the problem on a public-health or public-welfare basis."[49] For although Ziegler's solution ostensibly fulfills the obstetric ideal by granting every American mother her "right," by his method the natural elevation in status of obstetricians which would otherwise have occurred might be jeopardized.

Today the prospective American mother theoretically has access to high-quality obstetric care. If she is from a relatively urban environment, this is available through clinics, or through a private obstetrician, for whom a group insurance plan might help pay. If she is from a rural area, a general practitioner graduated from a medical school, whose quality, both overall and in obstetrics, has greatly improved, is likely to be available. Obstetrics, both as a branch of medicine and in professional status, has advanced significantly. Can this result somehow be attributed to the developing superiority of obstetrics as performed by obstetricians, or could the forces arrayed against them have been exaggerated by the obstetricians, making the whole issue just a paper debate?

It appears that despite the potential obstetric superiority of obstetricians over midwives, the triumph of the former was probably due most to the fact that the circumstances debated in this period changed radically. It is certain that the relevant health conditions were not improving in those areas where the midwife was first being superseded. Although in Washington the percentage of births reported by midwives shrank from the 1903 high of 50 percent to 15 percent in 1912, infant mortality in the first day, the first week, and the first month of life had all increased in this period. Also, New York's dwindling corps of midwives achieved significant superiority over New York's doctors in the prevention of both stillbirths and puerperal sepsis.[50] Rather, the obstetricians triumphed because, before the public health programs became firmly established in the public mind, the obstetrician gained tremendous advantages from other sources. Immigration decreased significantly during the war and was afterward reduced legally to a small fraction of the numbers experienced just before the war. This put time entirely on the side of the physicians, a considerable advantage in itself, while concurrently the economic problem per se was greatly reduced. This did not occur simply because of the "prosperity" of the 1920s, which may have had no impact at all; rather, the secular trend toward limitation of family size accelerated to include nearly the entire population. In 1919 in New York City there were 1,700 midwives who were responsible for 40,000 births, or 30 percent of the total. In 1929, though there were still 1,200 midwives, they delivered but 12,000, 12 percent of the total.[51] Not only did the average deliveries per midwife shrink decidedly from 23 to 10 births a year, but also total births decreased by 25 percent. With the limitation of births, it is possible that pregnancy and anticipated delivery seemed sufficiently rare to be generally equated with major operations and worthy of greater expense.

The other secular shift in attitudes from which the obstetricians benefited was a new, general demand for improved obstetrics, the change for which they had been most devoutly hoping. The midwife controversy itself was in some ways a reflection of this change. It was not merely the benevolent concern of public health officials about their vital statistics which was instrumental in effecting all the legislation regulating the midwife. Also responsible was a growing public demand from women, who were becoming increasingly self-conscious about their own welfare, and who were still infected with the reforming zeal of the Progressive Era which was to lead to their enfranchisement. These were, after all, the women who shortly afterward were to deluge their congressmen and senators with pleas for the passage of the Sheppard-Towner Bill. This bill, which Ziegler worked for, provided federal money to the states for the "protection of maternity." With "womanhood" no longer rooted in the domestic, "natural" environment, or perhaps reflecting the struggle for release from such roots, the "natural" way of doing things was losing its appeal for the many emerging American women, and the obstetrician was increasingly there to reap the results of a growing anxiety about childbirth.

In summary, then, the professionalization process was very sensitive to external conditions and attitudes. If conditions had not changed so propitiously, if an economic problem and a conflict of attitudes had continued to exist, the obstetrician might well have found himself in the position of the present-day psychoanalyst with the public realizing that his skills solve but a small part of a complicated problem.

NOTES

1 Thomas Darlington, "The present status of the midwife," *American Journal of Obstetrics and Gynecology*, 1911, *63:* 870.
2 E. R. Hardin, "The midwife problem," *Southern Medical Journal*, 1925, *18:* 347.
3 See nearly any discussion of the subject at this period, e.g., Darlington, "Present status"; J. Clifton Edgar, "The remedy for the midwife problem," *American Journal of Obstetrics and Gynecology*, 1911, *63:* 882.
4 Darlington, "Present status."
5 Edgar, "Remedy."
6 J. Whitridge Williams, "Medical education and the midwife problem in the United States," *Journal of the American Medical Association*, 1912, *58:* 1–7.
7 C. E. Ziegler, "How can we best solve the midwifery problem," *American Journal of Public Health*, 1922, *12:* 409.
8 Abraham Flexner came to much the same conclusion in his discussion of the clinical years in American medical schools. *Medical Education in the United States and Canada: A Report to the Carnegie Foundation for the Advancement of Teaching*, Bulletin no. 4 (New York, 1910), 117.
9 Williams, "Medical education."
10 See for example, J. F. Moran, "The endowment of motherhood," *Journal of the American Medical Association*, 1915, *64:* 126; J. L. Huntington, "The midwife in Massachusetts: her anomalous position," *Boston Medical and Surgical Journal*, 1913, *168:* 419.
11 "Discussion—midwife problem," *New York State Journal of Medicine*, 1915, *15:* 300.
12 For an impressive list, see Huntington, "Midwife in Massachusetts," 420.
13 W. A. Plecker, "The midwife problem in Virginia," *Virginia Medical Semi-Monthly*, 1914–15, *19:* 457–58;

Jeidell and Fricke, "The midwives of Anne Arundel County, Maryland," *Johns Hopkins Hospital Bulletin*, 1912, *23:* 279–81.
14 A. K. Paine, "The midwife problem," *Boston Medical and Surgical Journal*, 1915, *173:* 760.
15 Clara D. Noyes, "The training of midwives in relation to the prevention of infant mortality," *American Journal of Obstetrics and Gynecology*, 1912, *66:* 1053.
16 See n. 11 above.
17 Hardin, "Midwife problem," 349.
18 Josephine Baker, "The function of the midwife," *Woman's Medical Journal*, 1913, *23:* 197.
19 Noyes, "Training of midwives," 1054.
20 Ibid., 1052.
21 A. B. Emmons and J. L. Huntington, "The midwife: her future in the United States," *American Journal of Obstetrics and Gynecology*, 1912, *65:* 395–96.
22 Harden, "Midwife problem," 347; Emmons and Huntington, "The midwife," 395.
23 Julius Levy, "The maternal and infant mortality in midwifery practice in Newark, N.J.," *American Journal of Obstetrics and Gynecology*, 1918, 77: 42.
24 W. R. Nicholson, "The midwife situation . . . ," *Transactions of the American Gynecological Society*, 1917, *42:* 632.
25 "Schools for midwives," *Medical Record*, 1912, *81:* 517.
26 Ibid., 518.
27 See, among others, Hardin, "Midwife problem," 349; Plecker, "Midwife problem," 457; J. A. Foote, "Legislative measures against maternal and infant mortality," *American Journal of Obstetrics and Gynecology*, 1919, *80:* 550; Edgar, "Remedy," 883.
28 Nicholson, "Midwife situation," 626.
29 Emmons and Huntington, "The midwife," 399.

30 Huntington, "The midwife in Massachusetts," 419.
31 Ibid.
32 Emmons and Huntington, "The midwife," 397–400.
33 Ibid., 394.
34 Charles E. Ziegler, "The elimination of the midwife," *Journal of the American Medical Association*, 1913, *60:* 34.
35 "Discussion—midwife problem," 299.
36 Huntington, "The midwife in Massachusetts," 419.
37 J. Van D. Young, "The midwife problem in the State of New York," *New York State Journal of Medicine*, 1915, *15:* 295.
38 George C. Marlette, "Discussion," in Hardin, "Midwife problem," 350.
39 Levy, "Maternal and infant mortality," 41.
40 Paine, "Midwife problem," 761.
41 Huntington, "The midwife in Massachusetts," 421.
42 Paine, "Midwife problem," 762.
43 Ibid., 763–64.
44 Ziegler, "The elimination of the midwife," 34.
45 Ziegler, "How can we best solve the midwifery problem," 407–8.
46 *The Weekly Bulletin: Official Journal of the Allegheny County Medical Society* 5, no. 7 (February 12, 1916), 5.
47 Ziegler, "How can we best solve the midwifery problem," 412–13.
48 Ibid., 407.
49 Ibid., 413.
50 Baker, "Function of the midwife," 196.
51 Hattie Hemschemeyer, "Midwifery in the United States," *American Journal of Nursing*, 1939, *39:* 1182.

Mary Breckinridge, the Frontier Nursing Service, and the Introduction of Nurse-Midwifery in the United States

NANCY SCHROM DYE

Since the early decades of the twentieth century, physicians have been the sole legitimate birth attendants in the United States. In contrast to Great Britain and many nations in Continental Europe, where trained midwives attend a significant percentage of births and where home delivery continues to be an accepted alternative to hospital confinement, the United States has little in the way of a tradition of professional midwifery, and most Americans regard the hospital as the only safe place to give birth. Early in the twentieth century, Mary Breckinridge attempted to transplant the European tradition of professional midwifery to the United States. To demonstrate the desirability of trained midwives, she established the Frontier Nursing Service (FNS) in 1925. Since that time, the FNS has provided maternal and infant care to many of the residents of Leslie County, Kentucky, an impoverished rural county in the heart of Appalachia. By establishing the FNS, Breckinridge introduced the profession of nurse-midwifery to the United States, pioneered in establishing an autonomous professional role for nurses, and helped demonstrate that the quality and consistency of care rather than surgical intervention or hospitalization were the critical factors in maintaining low maternal and infant mortality. Despite the success that the FNS has enjoyed and despite the fact that it has served as a model for health care organizations throughout the world, nurse-midwifery is still an anomaly in the American health care system. Nurse-midwives attend only 1 percent of American births.[1] The history of the establishment and early work of the Frontier Nursing Service illustrates some of

the difficulties nurse-midwifery has faced in the United States and sheds light on the question of why professional midwifery continues to be a relatively little known system of maternity care.[2]

During the 1920s, Mary Breckinridge often appealed to potential supporters of her nurse-midwifery organization in the Kentucky mountains by comparing childbirth to war. "The bearing and rearing of children," Breckinridge declared, "is as much a national service as fighting—and should receive equal recognition. . . . But up until now, although we have hospitalized and pensioned our soldiers . . . we have left our rural women and infants to die unattended or, far too often, to drag out a mutilated existence unrelieved. We have lost more women in childbirth than men on the battlefield, and exact the heaviest toll from our youngest and most defenseless citizens."[3]

In the years immediately following World War I, as the public became increasingly alarmed by the United States' high maternal and infant mortality rates, many found this analogy compelling. Until the mid-1930s, an American woman of childbearing age was more likely to die from complications related to parturition than from any other medical cause except tuberculosis. What was more, although the number of deaths from diseases such as typhoid, diphtheria, and tuberculosis had been steadily declining since the late nineteenth century, maternal and infant mortality remained persistently high. In 1923, when Mary Breckinridge began to make plans for the Frontier Nursing Service, the national maternal death rate stood at 6.7 per 1,000 live births, one of the poorest rates in the western world.[4] The United States' infant mortality record was also poor. Each year in the first decades of the twentieth century, more than 250,000

NANCY SCHROM DYE is Associate Professor of History at the University of Kentucky, Lexington, Kentucky.

Reprinted with permission from *Bulletin of the History of Medicine* 57 (1983): 485–507.

327

infants, nearly one of every ten born, died before they reached their first birthdays. By the twenties, infant mortality had begun to decline steadily, but the United States remained among the countries with the highest death rates.[5]

Mary Breckinridge founded the Frontier Nursing Service at a time when physicians, public health officials, and social reformers were engaged in a well-publicized debate over the causes and remedies for America's high maternal and infant death rates. The twenties also witnessed the first federal legislation, the Sheppard-Towner Maternity and Infancy Act, enacted specifically to provide public funds for maternal and child health programs. Although physicians and public health experts recognized that many factors, including poverty, lack of prenatal care, unsanitary living conditions, and contaminated milk and water, contributed to maternal and infant deaths, most focused their concern upon the competence of American birth attendants.[6] Who, they asked, was qualified to manage childbirth?

By the 1920s, three types of practitioners served as birth attendants. General practitioners cared for a significant majority of American women. Midwives still attended about 20 percent of American births, considerably lower than the 50 percent of births they had managed in 1910. Although their numbers had declined appreciably by the 1920s, they continued to be important birth attendants in cities with large foreign-born populations and in the rural south and west.[7] Obstetrical specialists attended a small but increasing number of urban women.

Obstetricians, striving to win full professional recognition for their new specialty and anxious to impress Americans with the necessity of skilled medical attendance for all births, argued that ideally every woman should be attended by a specialist. They were particularly vocal in identifying poor obstetrical technique and inadequate clinical training as the major reasons for the high American death rates. At least half of all maternal deaths, obstetricians pointed out, were preventable. Nearly 40 percent were due to puerperal sepsis, but the incidence of infection could be drastically reduced by observing aseptic technique. Other potentially fatal diseases and complications of pregnancy and labor—toxemia, pelvic disproportion, malpresen-

tations, and hemorrhage, for example—could often be prevented or remedied by conscientious prenatal care and skilled practitioners. According to obstetricians, however, the average American birth attendant's skills left much to be desired. Many general practitioners were apparently ignorant of the necessity of prenatal care, careless about asepsis, and ill prepared to handle any complication of pregnancy or labor.[8] Obstetricians argued that to remedy this situation the public must be educated to realize that obstetrics was a highly skilled branch of surgery, requiring "a surgical operating room, all the appliances of modern surgery, all the precautions of modern surgery."[9] Once that state of affairs was reached, they maintained, maternal and neonatal mortality would decline dramatically.

Physicians also blamed midwives for America's high death rates, although by the 1920s the midwifery controversy was considerably less heated than it had been in the previous decade. Obstetricians and general practitioners alike regarded midwives as ignorant, dirty anachronisms, incapable of appreciating the need for cleanliness or of understanding the basic anatomical and physiological principles of the birth process. Most advocated doing away with midwifery altogether, either by outlawing its practice or by licensing midwives and enacting requirements so demanding that few would be able to meet them.[10]

Many public health officials, particularly those in rural regions, disagreed. Pointing out that midwives still attended a significant percentage of American births, they argued that abolishing midwifery altogether was impractical, if not impossible.[11] Although urban midwifery patients might be accommodated by expanding public maternity clinics and hospitals, there were no alternatives to the midwife in rural areas, where doctors were scarce and hospitals virtually nonexistent. Kentucky, for instance, counted 2,500 practicing midwives in 1922. Although they attended only 18 percent of births in the state as a whole, they were the primary birth attendants in the thirty-six eastern mountain counties. Kentucky board of health figures for three rural Appalachian counties illustrate midwives' importance. In Leslie County, for instance, 43 midwives attended 265 births while the one physician in the county attended 40. In Knott County, 55 midwives attended 396 births; 5

doctors attended 37. In Owsley County, 53 midwives attended 163 births; 3 physicians attended 66.[12]

Public health officials also pointed out that despite midwives' lack of systematic training, many appeared competent. Early twentieth-century comparative investigations of physician- and midwife-managed births in Providence, R.I., Newark, N.J., and New York City found that midwives had fewer maternal deaths than general practitioners, reported births more promptly, and had fewer cases of infant ophthalmia, presumably because state health departments required them to use silver nitrate.[13] Educate and supervise rather than eliminate the midwife, the public health argument ran; upgrade her status and competence with required instruction and certification. In this way, intelligent young women, especially in rural communities where physician shortage made the need for skilled birth attendants most pressing, could be encouraged to take up midwifery as an occupation.[14]

Mary Breckinridge introduced a new alternative to this debate over who should manage childbirth. She argued that the major difference between countries such as the United States, with one of the highest maternal and infant death rates, and countries such as the Netherlands and Sweden, with the lowest, was the existence of skilled professional midwives.[15] If the United States would rely upon nurses with intensive postgraduate training in midwifery (i.e., nurse-midwives) to provide maternal and infant care, particularly in rural areas, the nation could significantly improve the health and survival rates of mothers and children. Nurse-midwives could effectively perform several essential functions. They could provide primary health and prenatal care in communities that lacked physicians and they could handle the great majority of normal, uncomplicated labors. At the same time, they could work as health educators, instructing families in the basic principles of sanitation, nutrition, and child care. It was to demonstrate the efficacy of nurse-midwifery as a system of maternity and infant care that Breckinridge established the Frontier Nursing Service in 1925.

Mary Breckinridge was herself a nurse and a trained midwife. Born in 1881 into one of the most politically and socially prominent of southern families,

she made the decision to become a nurse shortly after the untimely death of her first husband. She entered St. Luke's Hospital in New York for training in 1907, at the age of twenty-five. Upon her graduation in 1910 she did not pursue her new occupation, but returned to her parents' home in Fort Smith, Arkansas, to care for her invalid mother. There she met and married Richard Thompson, president of Crescent College in Eureka Springs, Arkansas. As Mrs. Thompson, Breckinridge postponed a nursing career indefinitely. In 1914, she bore a son, Clifton. Two years later, she bore a premature daughter who died shortly after birth.[16]

Although Breckinridge took great delight in her little boy, life in Eureka Springs proved unfulfilling and her marriage unhappy. To stave off discontent, she served as secretary for the local woman suffrage organization and as board member for several state public health committees. She also developed a course on child care for the students at Crescent College. In the midst of Breckinridge's involvement with these activities, her four-year-old son died. The tragedy changed the course of her life immediately and irrevocably. Determined to end her unhappy marriage and to break all ties with the past, she separated from Thompson and, after her divorce several years later, resumed her maiden name.[17]

When she left Eureka Springs in 1918, she had few concrete plans for the future. Her son's death, however, had rendered her fiercely determined to devote her life to child welfare. She worked briefly as a researcher for the federal Children's Bureau, took up nursing again during the influenza epidemic, and, shortly after the Armistice, left for France as a volunteer for the American Committee for Devastated France (C.A.R.D.), a private relief organization.

C.A.R.D. assigned Breckinridge to Vic-sur-Aisne, a town in a war-devastated area of northern France where she coordinated food and medical relief for some seventy villages. During her two years there, Breckinridge discovered and developed her considerable administrative abilities. Her primary achievement was organizing a visiting nurse service that offered both general and maternity nursing. This organization was the prototype of the FNS.[18]

In France, Breckinridge became well acquainted

with the European tradition of professional mid-wifery. Impressed by the work of both French mid-wives and British nurse-midwives, she wrote in her autobiography that "after I met British nurse-midwives, first in France and then on my visits to London, it grew upon me that nurse-midwifery was the logical response to the needs of the young child in rural America."[19] A major obstacle existed to introducing nurse-midwifery to the United States, however, for midwifery went unrecognized as a profession, and neither health care professionals nor the general public drew a distinction between professional and lay midwives.

When Breckinridge returned to the United States late in 1921, she began a systematic program of preparation for introducing nurse-midwifery to this country. Her schedule included graduate study in public health nursing at Columbia Teachers College, midwifery training at the British Hospital for Mothers and Babies and at the York Road General Lying-in Hospital in London, and an extended visit to Scotland to observe the operation of the Highland and Islands Medical and Nursing Service, a decentralized health care organization staffed by nurse-midwives that provided skilled care to an impoverished rural population.[20]

By 1923, Breckinridge had decided upon the eastern Kentucky mountains as the site for her nurse-midwifery demonstration. She chose this location for several reasons. Like many health professionals concerned with maternal and infant health, Breckinridge believed that rural women and children were at higher risk than urban ones. Although vital statistics consistently indicated that both infant and maternal death rates were lower in rural regions than in cities,[21] Breckinridge argued that the rural figures were unreliable. In keeping with the emphasis on the attendant as the critical variable in explaining maternal and neonatal mortality, she insisted that more rural mothers died because they often went without skilled care.[22]

Other factors influenced Breckinridge's choice. As a Breckinridge, she had political and social connections in Kentucky that would automatically ensure interest and support. Personal influence, she wrote in 1923, "counts for so much in the South. I would be too doubtful of success to push this project in Vermont or Michigan, but I *know* I can put it across in Kentucky—and probably anywhere in the South."[23] Then, too, Breckinridge emphasized the

geographical isolation, rugged terrain, and poverty of eastern Kentucky. If nurse-midwives could succeed in improving maternal and infant health under such adverse conditions, she argued, their success would be all the more impressive.

Breckinridge spent the summer of 1923 in eastern Kentucky, surveying the health needs of women and children. In Leslie County, where the FNS was eventually located, ten thousand people lived in scattered hollows, almost completely isolated from modern transportation and communication networks. "There was no motor road within sixty miles in any direction," Breckinridge recalled. "Horseback and mule team were the only mode of travel. Brought-on supplies came from distant railroad points and took from two to five days to haul in."[24] Hyden, the county seat, with 313 people, was the largest settlement. Without a railroad, Leslie County was not yet visibly penetrated by the coal industry that had already transformed the traditional culture and economic patterns of many Kentucky mountain counties. But by 1925, most of Leslie County's land was already owned by northern investors and industrialists, most notably Henry Ford, whose Fordson Coal and Timber Company made him the largest landowner in the county.[25]

The county ranked as one of the most impoverished in Appalachia as well as one of the poorest in the United States. Most families eked out a precarious living from the land, cultivating small crops of corn on tenant farms. In 1929, the average per capita income was $102 a year, compared with the southern Appalachian average of $433 and the national average of $776.[26]

Missionaries and settlement school teachers in the region described Appalachian families as patriarchal and invariably commented upon the hard life of mountain women. In this preindustrial mountain society, a woman's life was indeed hard. In addition to the daily domestic round of cooking (generally over an open fire), spinning, weaving, knitting, making quilts, hauling water, and chopping wood, women performed much agricultural labor, helping to plant corn on the steep hillside in the spring, hoeing throughout the summer, and helping to harvest the crop in the fall. Leslie County women married young and bore an average of nine children. Frequent childbearing, then, represented a central and virtually inevitable part of mountain womanhood.[27]

Because the great majority of women relied upon lay, or "granny," midwives as birth attendants, Breckinridge concentrated upon investigating these folk practitioners' practices. Not surprisingly, the fifty-three midwives whom Breckinridge interviewed in three mountain counties appear to have regarded her with considerable suspicion. None allowed her to be present while she attended a birth or confided any details about deaths or problems. Nevertheless, Breckinridge's report on mountain midwifery is valuable for providing information on the identity, economic status, and practices of early twentieth-century Appalachian midwives.[28]

Almost all of the mountain midwives with whom Breckinridge talked were elderly; their mean age was sixty. They delivered an average of nineteen babies a year in a small radius of territory around their homes. All but two had borne children themselves; most had eight or nine. Like the population they served, midwives generally made their living off the land. Those who were married had farmer husbands; eighteen widows cultivated land themselves. Their midwifery practices provided small supplementary incomes. Two of the four midwives who lived in the region's small towns kept boardinghouses; one served as county jailer.[29]

Unlike midwives in other parts of the American South, Appalachian midwives did not have a prescribed training system, although nine women in Breckinridge's sample were daughters of midwives and had worked as their mothers' assistants and almost all had observed other midwives at work before taking on cases of their own.[30] The one black midwife in Breckinridge's sample had been taught the rudiments of midwifery by her mistress when she had been a Virginia slave. A few had assisted physicians. Breckinridge made her survey just when the state had begun to regulate midwifery practice. The Kentucky legislature mandated midwifery registration in 1920, and in 1922, with Sheppard-Towner funds, the new Bureau of Maternal and Child Health instituted a series of one-day classes for mountain midwives. Ten of the women in Breckinridge's sample had attended these classes, where they had listened to lectures on how to equip and care for a regulation midwifery bag, maintain personal cleanliness, and administer silver nitrate. For the most part, though, these women were self-taught, and had taken up their occupation by accident. As they explained to Breckinridge, neighbors had turned to them for help in childbirth and they had discovered an aptitude for the work. Twelve of the midwives could read and write. Breckinridge stressed, however, that literacy was not necessarily a correlate of competence in a region in which the literacy rate, particularly among the older population, was low.[31]

One aspect of the granny midwives' care that most distressed Breckinridge was the lack of prenatal attention. Rarely did a mountain mother visit her midwife before delivery. A family did not summon the midwife until active labor began. Because travel was difficult, and often involved fording mountain streams and climbing steep slopes, a midwife could take hours to reach her patient. In spring, when floods made many creeks impassable, transportation was even more difficult.

Breckinridge found that eastern Kentucky midwives, like traditional folk practitioners elsewhere, relied upon empirical knowledge, local customs, and herbal remedies. Contrary to the notion of midwives as noninterventionist practitioners who "let nature take its course," however, Breckinridge found that most midwives actively managed their patients' labors.[32] Although few went so far as the one young midwife who employed pituitrin extract, all performed vaginal examinations to see if the baby was "coming straight" and if the "womb was open." Most examined women frequently, often trying to stretch the birth canal to speed labor. In the event of an abnormal presentation, midwives usually attempted to turn the baby, either by external or, more commonly, internal version. For complications of labor, they relied primarily upon a variety of herb, root, and spice teas. Usually midwives delivered women in a sitting position, either on the knees of their husbands or on a rude birthing chair. One sometimes delivered patients standing. Breckinridge believed that such birth postures caused perineal lacerations and prolapsed uterus.[33] Once a mother was "fixed up" and the baby dressed, the midwife collected her small fee, usually paid in kind, and took her leave. Unless a family called her back to deal with a postpartum complication, she did not return.

Midwives reported a variety of empirical and folk practices to deal with complications. Hemorrhage, the most dreaded, generated the greatest variety of responses. Some midwives relied upon a practice called "cording the leg" which involved binding the leg and hand on one side of a woman's body. Others employed ergot or paregoric or applied cold cloths to the woman's perineum. Teas of yellowroot, rattlewood, service bark, comfrey, pepper, assafetida, nutmeg, pine needles, and coal soot were also named as remedies to stop hemorrhage. An ax under the bed blade up, a practice found not only in Appalachia but throughout the rural United States, was believed to stop bleeding and alleviate labor pains. One midwife reported that she laid her hands upon a hemorrhaging patient and repeated Ezekiel 16:6: "And when I passed by thee, I saw thee polluted in thine own blood. I said unto thee when thou wast polluted in thy own blood, live."[34] For other complications of pregnancy and labor, such as the convulsions of eclampsia, the "granny" midwives had no remedies to suggest. Eastern Kentucky midwives only rarely sent for a physician. Because the region's few doctors lived in towns or coal camps, they were usually too far away to offer much help.[35]

Breckinridge was able to glean only an impressionistic sense of mortality and morbidity in this first survey. Kentucky had entered the birth registration area in 1915 and had been collecting its own vital statistics since 1912, but Breckinridge had no doubt that births and deaths in rural mountain counties were at best haphazardly recorded. She insisted that maternal mortality was exceedingly high, but had no statistics to document this assertion. The midwives she interviewed were reluctant to discuss deaths. As one stated, "Everybody lost women."[36]

As a professional nurse, Breckinridge felt little sense of sisterhood with these traditional female practitioners. The report that resulted from her survey was highly critical. She conceded that some midwives were clearly competent and knowledgeable, and acknowledged that they performed necessary services. They charged much less than the region's doctors ($2.00 to $5.00 for a delivery as compared to $30.00 to $35.00) and were willing to accept in-kind payments in lieu of cash, essential in a cash-poor region. Nevertheless, she judged most midwives and their houses dirty and assumed that because they lacked formal training their practices were harmful. "It is unthinkable," she concluded, "that childbirth should be without skilled care."[37]

In the fall of 1923, just before she sailed for England to take her own midwifery training, Breckinridge sent a copy of her report, accompanied by a detailed proposal for a maternal and child health project, to the American Child Health Association. Her proposal outlined a five-year demonstration project in eastern Kentucky to be called the Children's Public Health Service. The program would provide "each child from antenatal life through the school age free health facilities similar to the opportunities now provided for a free public school education" and would be staffed by public health nurses with specialized midwifery training. Breckinridge assured the Child Health Association that the region's few physicians had already expressed their support for such a program so that "such obstetrical cases as fall to the share of the Children's Nurses can be met legally and without friction." To fund the project, she estimated an annual budget of $16,300 to pay the salaries of six nurses and purchase supplies.[38]

Breckinridge stressed that the rural communities in need of such a program could never bear the greater part of its cost. But, she argued, "the bearing and rearing of children is not a local, or even a state, but a national function. Nobody," she concluded, "expects a poor city district to finance its health centers. Why should one expect it of a poor rural county which has already contributed to the wealth of the city?"[39] Although Breckinridge envisioned local taxes and charity eventually covering some of the expense, she stressed that the greater part of the cost should be assumed by public funds such as those provided through the Sheppard-Towner Maternity and Infancy Act.

The Child Health Association responded warmly to Breckinridge's proposal and indicated serious interest in sponsoring the Children's Health Service. Soon, however, the proposal ran into difficulties. The Commonwealth Fund, which underwrote Child Health Association projects, required the approval of the appropriate state health officials before financing a project. In this instance, Annie Veech, a physician who headed Kentucky's Bureau of Maternal and Child Health, was the individual consulted to evaluate Breckinridge's plan.

Veech was strongly and unalterably opposed to the Children's Health Service proposal, largely because it advocated the employment of nurse-midwives. Veech disagreed with Breckinridge's assessment of Kentucky's lay midwives and accused her of exploiting and misrepresenting mountain people. Many lay midwives, she maintained, were competent, as evidenced by the fact that the mountain counties had among the lowest maternal mortality and puerperal sepsis rates in the state. Rather than hire professional midwives, the state should recruit young mountain women for state-sponsored midwifery training programs. Such local midwives, Veech argued, would be far less expensive than trained nurses and would be content to reside permanently in the region. Implicit in Veech's argument, too, was the idea that lay midwives would be more amenable to state control and supervision than professional nurse-midwives would be.[40]

Professional rivalry and the customary opprobrium physicians displayed toward midwives also colored Veech's objections. "If high-type young women want to be of real value in isolated areas," she asked, "why do they not prepare themselves by taking a medical degree? They could then practice obstetrics instead of midwifery and meet the other medical needs of the people they wish to help. After all," Veech concluded, "a nurse-midwife is only a midwife. There appears to be a tendency among certain groups of nurses towards practicing medicine for which they are in no way prepared without graduating in medicine."[41]

Annie Veech's opposition proved to be an important and longstanding obstacle to Breckinridge's plans. Without Veech's support, Breckinridge had no choice but to withdraw her proposal from the Child Health Association. Nor could she look to the state for financial assistance. Thus, from the beginning, funding agencies, state officials, and health professionals viewed nurse-midwifery as an impractical, professionally questionable anomaly.

Breckinridge, a singularly strongminded individual, remained undaunted by Veech's hostility. When she returned to the United States in 1925, recently certified as a nurse-midwife by England's Central Midwives' Board, she was still determined to work in eastern Kentucky and chose Leslie County as the site for her project. Working with her wide network of personal friends and family connections, Breckinridge bypassed the state and established the Kentucky Committee for Mothers and Babies (renamed the Frontier Nursing Service in 1928) as a private philanthropic organization. She quickly won the support of some sixty of the state's

most influential citizens and social reformers, including Frank McVey, president of the University of Kentucky, and three of the most prominent individuals in mountain welfare work: William Hutchins, president of Berea College; Katharine Pettit, founder of the Pine Mountain Settlement School; and Linda Neville, well known for her efforts to eradicate trachoma, a disease then endemic to mountain communities.

The fledgling Committee for Mothers and Babies' first problem was funding. Breckinridge remained hopeful about receiving state or foundation support in the future, after her nurse-midwifery demonstration had proved itself, but she realized that in the short run she would have to depend upon individual donations and her own. She soon proved to be a talented fund raiser, persuading Appalachian coal operators and railroad officials to donate money and services and Lexington and Louisville physicians to promise free treatment. As it became apparent that large-scale support was not going to be forthcoming, Breckinridge established FNS women's committees in cities throughout the nation. The money they raised soon provided the basis of the FNS budget. Some of them, most notably those in Detroit and New York, served as a kind of women's auxiliary to industrialists with investments in the region. One of the largest contributors, for example, was Henry Ford's wife, Clara, who was active in the Detroit committee.

Breckinridge's success as a fund raiser was due partly to the fact that the establishment of the FNS coincided in time with rising interest in the people and culture of the southern highlands. As industrialists penetrated the region, attracted by its vast timber and mineral wealth, Americans created a romantic image of mountain people. Appalachia, according to this conception, was populated by rugged, self-reliant, but essentially childlike people, with quaint folkways, dialects, and rustic crafts.[42] Breckinridge capitalized upon this image to raise funds and attract attention to the FNS's work. In the strongly nativist decade of the 1920s, she also carefully presented a picture of mountain people as "the finest American stock" living on the "last frontier." As one FNS spokeswoman made this appeal, "They are the nursery of the race for children of the old American stock. Could money be better spent than in protecting the motherhood and infancy of such a race?"[43] In characterizing mountain culture in this nativist and stereotyped fashion, the FNS ignored the cataclysmic social changes that were reshaping mountain society in the early twentieth century, and remained aloof from the labor strife and economic exploitation of the region.

In the summer of 1925, two nurse-midwives, Edna Rochstroh and Freda Caffin, settled in Hyden. Both had worked as nurses with the Maternity Center Association of New York City, and taken their midwifery training in England. In Hyden, they confronted a second major problem: gaining community acceptance for a new and unfamiliar system of health care. Leslie County families were initially suspicious of the new nurse-midwives, and the region's "granny" midwives understandably felt threatened. As Betty Lester, an English nurse-midwife who joined the FNS staff in 1927, recalled, "At first they . . . questioned us. Did we know what we were talking about? And then, of course, the midwives who were here before us didn't like us very much because we were taking their work away from them."[44]

The first staff members worked gradually to win community acceptance. Their initial project was a house-to-house survey of maternal and infant mortality. The Kentucky Committee for Mothers and Babies was determined to compile accurate mortality statistics to serve as a baseline against which to evaluate future work.[45] At the same time, the nurse-midwives, under the auspices of the state department of health, initiated a general public health program, inoculating residents against typhoid, diphtheria, and smallpox, and treating the parasitical infections common in mountain communities.

From 1925 through 1927, the staff attended few deliveries. Although pregnant women began to register with the FNS for prenatal care, about one third of them called a local midwife during labor.[46] Betty Lester recalled, "They wanted their friends . . . the midwife they'd had for all their other babies. . . . So it was all right by us. And if a Midwife went to a call we never went. I mean, if we had done all the prenatals and . . . when the time came for the delivery, they called the local midwife, we didn't go; we just left it. But if a midwife got into trouble, if she needed us, or if the husband wanted us to go, then we would go and help out. . . . If they wanted them, it was all right . . . whoever they

wanted they had."[47] The FNS aimed to replace the granny midwives gradually. While significant numbers of them continued to practice in Leslie County, Breckinridge insisted that they be treated courteously and with respect. FNS facilities and services were always available to them.[48]

Women's reluctance to trust the FNS diminished rapidly. During 1928–29, only 15 of a total of 106 prenatal patients turned to lay midwives for delivery. By 1931, the FNS nurse-midwives averaged "a baby a day," and were attending the majority of reported births in Leslie County. The opposition of local midwives also seems to have declined, perhaps because few mountain midwives depended upon midwifery for their livelihoods, or because folk traditions associated with midwifery were not as strong in eastern Kentucky as they were in other parts of the South. By 1928, no new midwives were starting practice in the FNS area.[49]

The FNS expanded rapidly throughout the rest of the 1920s. By 1930, Breckinridge had a staff of more than thirty nurses. Because nurse-midwives were not trained in the United States, she recruited most of her staff from English lying-in hospitals, and required prospective staff members to be certified by the English Central Midwives' Board. The American nurses who worked for the FNS also took their training and certification in England.

By 1930, too, the FNS covered more than seven hundred square miles of territory in Leslie County and in neighboring Perry and Clay counties, had raised more than $40,000 toward a permanent endowment, and had arranged for Louis Dublin, a vice-president at the Metropolitan Life Insurance Company and a statistician well known for his knowledge of and concern for maternal and infant welfare, to tabulate the FNS medical statistics. Breckinridge, upon Dublin's advice, hoped to cover a thousand square miles by 1934. The expanse of territory, she maintained, "will give us the statistical data . . . necessary in order to demonstrate adequately that the work of nurse-midwives in remotely rural areas does lower the death rate of women and young children, and raise the general level of health of the population."[50]

The FNS's decentralized organization followed that of the Highlands and Islands Medical and Nursing Service that Breckinridge had studied in Scotland. FNS operations centered in Hyden, where a nursing center and, by 1928, a twelve-bed hospital were located. Most services were provided by teams of two nurse-midwives who lived and worked in outpost nursing centers. Five such centers opened between late 1925 and 1929. Each nurse covered approximately seventy-five square miles of territory in the district surrounding her center. To visit their patients, nurses rode horseback through the mountain creek beds and trails. Although maternal and infant care were the FNS's primary concerns, the district nurses also provided general health care, occasionally referring family members to periodic FNS specialty clinics in Hyden or to Lexington and Louisville physicians and hospitals.

Breckinridge was proud of the FNS's cost efficiency. For $1.00 a year, a family could register for general health care. The midwifery service cost $5.00. Both fees could be paid either in cash or, as was more common, in kind. As Breckinridge had predicted, these fees covered only a small portion—less than 10 percent—of the FNS's costs. However, despite the distances FNS nurses traveled to visit their patients, the costs of the FNS compared favorably to other health projects. The average per capita cost of an FNS visit in 1926–27 was $1.45, considerably lower than the costs of several other rural health projects. Breckinridge was convinced that decentralization and reliance upon nurse-midwives rather than physicians were important innovations in the economics of health care.[51]

Breckinridge was also proud of the maternity care her organization provided. The FNS nurse-midwives' management of pregnancy, labor, and the puerperium compared very favorably to and differed significantly from the care American women customarily received. The first FNS departure was in prenatal care. At a time when few physicians routinely monitored their patients' pregnancies and only an estimated 20 percent of American women received prenatal care of any kind,[52] the FNS urged women to register for care as soon as they believed themselves pregnant, and followed patients closely from the time their pregnancies were diagnosed. The nurse-midwives visited their patients biweekly until the seventh month, and weekly thereafter, concentrating upon remedying dietary deficiencies and parasitic infections. Once summoned during labor, the nurse-midwife stayed continuously with her patient. "We think the support and help given through the long hours

of the first stage [of labor] has a bearing on the outcome," Mary Breckinridge stated, explaining this hallmark of a nurse-midwife's care.[53] Although more than 90 percent of FNS-managed deliveries took place in patients' homes, Breckinridge's staff was rigorous in maintaining aseptic conditions. A nurse-midwife carried everything she needed to conduct an aseptic delivery in her horse's saddlebags.

FNS nurse-midwives' management of childbirth differed from contemporary practices in other ways as well. At a time when medical attendance at birth was becoming nearly universal, the FNS staff handled nearly 95 percent of its deliveries without medical assistance.[54] Initially, medical supervision consisted only of signed protocols drawn up by Lexington physicians. Regional doctors handled the small number of major complications. In the early 1930s, the FNS hired its first resident physician who served as medical director. Given the distances involved, the physician's presence could not be counted upon in the event of an emergency. In practice, then, FNS nurse-midwives were essentially autonomous practitioners, forced to handle most complications on their own.

At a time when surgical intervention increasingly characterized American obstetrics, and when approximately 25 percent of American hospital deliveries could be characterized as operative,[55] FNS nurse-midwives did little to interfere with the birth process. In its first three thousand deliveries, conducted over the years 1925 through 1937, intervention was minimal. Caesarian sections, which, of course, had to be performed by physicians, were very rare. Only six were performed during these years. Other operations were also uncommon. Forceps, which only physicians could employ, were used very infrequently. Only fourteen of the first three thousand deliveries involved forceps. Episiotomies, not general in obstetrical practice at the time, were extremely rare. In the first three thousand deliveries, only two were performed, although lacerations of the perineum were listed among the most frequent complications.[56] One nurse-midwife observed after a forceps delivery in 1938 that "this is my second forceps case in seven years. I know doctors and midwives will think this almost incredible. I do myself when I am in the cities and around hospitals. Of course in the mountains I only average around thirty deliveries in a year, but even so I think two forceps deliveries an unusual record for more than two hundred cases."[57]

How successful was the FNS in its original goal of reducing maternal and infant mortality? No reliable baseline figures exist for 1925. The mortality survey that the Kentucky Committee for Mothers and Babies conducted in that year has been lost.[58] It is clear, however, that the FNS maintained excellent maternal mortality and morbidity records. In its first two series of one thousand deliveries, spanning the years 1925 through 1934, the FNS did not have a maternal death; in its third series, covering the years 1935 through 1937, it had two. Its maternal mortality rate for these twelve years stood at .68 per thousand live births.[59] For white women in rural Kentucky, the closest comparable population for which figures are available, the maternal death rate during these years averaged from 4.4 to 5.3 per thousand live births. The maternal death rate for white women in the city of Lexington, where physicians attended almost all deliveries and where, by the 1930s, hospitalization was common, stood between 8 and 9. In the United States as a whole, the maternal death rate during these years ranged from 5.6 to 6.8 per thousand live births.[60]

The percentage of FNS patients who developed complications during pregnancy was also significantly lower than the general population. Toxic symptoms were the most common complication of pregnancy. In the first series of 1,000 deliveries, for instance, 172 women exhibited symptoms of toxemia, but only 2 developed eclampsia. This low incidence of eclampsia was one of the best indicators of the efficacy of FNS prenatal care.[61]

FNS patients also developed fewer complications during labor and the puerperium than the general childbearing population. The incidence of puerperal sepsis, the major cause of maternal death in the United States, was very low. In the first thousand FNS deliveries, for example, five women were judged to be suffering from a septic condition. By the third series, for reasons that are unclear, the incidence of sepsis had increased to twenty-five cases.[62] Finally, FNS end results were extremely favorable. In each of the first three series of one thousand deliveries, more than 95 percent of the patients were in satisfactory or better condition at the end of the puerperium.[63]

The FNS's strikingly low maternal death rate and its unusually good morbidity statistics must be set within the context of general health conditions in Leslie County. As John Kooser, the FNS's resident physician during the 1930s, summarized, "Our major problems are related directly or indirectly to poor diet, intestinal parasites, chronic infection, and to a high birth rate."[64] Many FNS mothers were high-risk maternity patients. The patient population included significantly greater numbers of very young and very old mothers than the national norm, and the number of women who were bearing their fourth or subsequent child was also greater than the national average. Then, too, the FNS came to believe that their patients' inadequate diets may have rendered them particularly susceptible to toxemia. Kooser reported that "there appears to be a direct relationship between the seasonal incidence of toxemia and the seasonal scarcity of food."[65]

During its first years, the FNS achieved an impressive neonatal mortality record also, although again, in the absence of reliable baseline figures, it is difficult to generalize. In the first 1,000 deliveries, 15 infants were stillborn and 25 babies died within a month of life; in the second thousand, 18 infants were stillborn and 26 died. In both these series, the incidence of stillbirths and neonatal deaths was one-third less than that of the surrounding population.[66] In the third series, covering the years 1935 through 1937, the neonatal death rate rose to 39.8 compared to the national figure of 33 per 1,000 live births. Two-thirds of these infants were premature.[67] This rise corresponds in time to the depths of the great depression. The FNS's greater difficulty in reducing neonatal mortality may well have been related to the closer and more direct connection between infant mortality and poverty.[68]

In its first years, then, when Mary Breckinridge was most determined to use the Frontier Nursing Service as an example of how efficacious nurse-midwives could be as providers of maternal and infant care, the FNS was clearly a successful organization. Its maternal mortality and morbidity rates, and the incidence of stillbirths and neonatal deaths, were considerably lower than those found in virtually any other patient population. Breckinridge attributed this success to the quality and consistency of care throughout pregnancy, labor, and the puerperium, and maintained that the FNS record

proved that nurse-midwives were highly competent professionals, able to handle the vast majority
of maternity cases without medical assistance.

The record of the FNS was well known and publicized. Several prominent American obstetricians,
including George Kosmak, editor of the *American
Journal of Obstetrics and Gynecology,* praised the FNS's
work. Statistician and maternal welfare expert Louis
Dublin was the most steadfast champion of the FNS
and of nurse-midwifery generally. After tabulating
the statistics of the first FNS series of deliveries, he
stated that "the first need today is to train a large
body of nurse-midwives." The Frontier Nursing
Service, he announced, demonstrated that "a decentralized service of nurses who are properly
qualified as midwives, under the general direction
of a competent obstetrically qualified doctor at a
central point . . . does effectually reduce our high
national maternal death rate to a negligible level."[69]

The FNS came in for a good deal of popular
journalistic coverage as well. Articles in the *Survey,*
the *Nation,* and *Harper's,* among many others, helped
give favorable publicity to its work. Ernest Poole's
Nurses on Horseback, serialized in *Good Housekeeping*
in the early 1930s, was widely read.[70]

Although the FNS was well known and regarded
as a highly successful health care organization,
nurse-midwifery was not adopted in the United
States to any significant extent. Why not? Part of
the answer to this question lies in the history of the
FNS itself. Developments and trends over which
the FNS had no control, however, were far more
important in explaining why nurse-midwifery has
not flourished. Specifically, funding problems, the
attitudes of leading nursing professionals toward
nurse-midwifery, physician opposition, and general trends in American obstetrics during the 1920s
and 1930s help explain why professional midwifery had such difficulty taking root.

Mary Breckinridge remained unable to find any
large-scale backing for the FNS's work. In 1927 she
appealed directly to the Commonwealth Fund. She
bolstered her proposal with testimonials from several leading public health experts and statisticians
who stressed their support for both the concept of
nurse-midwifery and the work of the FNS. Louis
Dublin, for instance, wrote that "I frankly do not
know of anything that has come to my attention in
the long list of health projects in the last year which
has stirred me so much and has made its appeal

with such intensity." The new type of midwifery
that Breckinridge was developing, Dublin stressed,
had "national implications with reference to the
health and welfare of mothers and children in our
frontiers."[71] The Commonwealth Fund, however,
rejected her proposal, arguing that her work was
too expensive, and ill suited for private financial
backing.[72] In 1929, Congress refused to extend the
Sheppard-Towner Act, thus ending all federal
spending for maternal and child welfare.

By the early 1930s, Breckinridge despaired of
receiving public funds and of convincing foundations to support nurse-midwifery. Accordingly, she
redoubled her efforts to find private philanthropic
backing for her work. Breckinridge's organization
remained dependent upon piecemeal private lar-
gesse. As Ellen Breckenridge has argued in her
work on the FNS as a rural health care demonstration, the FNS's permanent dependence upon private charity affected its image as a health care organization during a period in which large-scale
foundation and government funding was rapidly
becoming the customary means of financing major
health projects. Since the 1930s, the American
public has viewed the FNS primarily as a romantic
group of heroic "nurses on horseback," rather than
as a demonstration of a viable alternative in childbirth management.

The great depression also had a profound effect
upon the organization's history. The economic collapse hit the southern Appalachian region hard,
and exacerbated the FNS's already chronic financial difficulties. "Everything has been harder this
past year than before," Mary Breckinridge wrote
in the summer of 1930. "Thousands of mountain-
eers who sought better opportunities for their
families in the towns along the railroads have lost
their jobs and poured back into the mountains,
without cows, chickens, pigs, or gardens—seeking
subsistence in a county where the margin of living
is never far above the hunger level."[73] A severe
drought in 1930–31 added to the already desperate economic situation. By the winter of 1931, fa-
mine existed throughout Leslie County. The FNS
strained its existing budget to help families meet
their immediate needs. During the same years,
however, outside contributions began to diminish.
By 1932, despite salary cuts and staff layoffs, the
FNS was operating with a large deficit. Before the
Depression, Breckinridge had planned to expand

FNS services further into surrounding eastern Kentucky counties. In addition, in 1930, the FNS surveyed health conditions in the Ozark region of Arkansas and southern Missouri with the idea of establishing a second nurse-midwifery demonstration there. The Depression, however, ended these plans.[74]

Even had the FNS expanded, however, it is clear that neither Breckinridge nor her supporters advocated the FNS model for cities where physicians were plentiful or for middle-class women who could afford a doctor's care. In other words, she did not envision an organization that directly challenged the medical system. The Frontier Nursing Service, Breckinridge repeatedly stressed, was designed for impoverished "remotely rural areas" without physicians. Indeed, Breckinridge may well have realized that given many physicians' hostility toward nurse-midwifery and their fears of nurse-midwives as potential competitors, an impoverished rural area offered the only location in which she could carry out her project independently.[75] Breckinridge, then, may have had no choice but to advocate a two-tiered system of maternity care: private obstetrics for affluent women, nurse-midwifery for poor women. To the limited extent that nurse-midwifery has been adopted in the United States, it has been largely along such lines. The two other major nurse-midwifery organizations, the Maternity Center Association of New York and the Catholic Maternity Institute in Santa Fe, New Mexico, have existed primarily for women who could not afford a private physician or hospitalization.

Nurse-midwifery's difficulty in making headway was also due in part to the American nursing profession's ambivalence about this new specialty. Even nurse-midwifery supporters disagreed over how nurse-midwifery should be defined. Breckinridge and her predominantly British staff pushed for full recognition of nurse-midwifery as a profession. In 1928, the FNS staff founded the Kentucky State Association of Midwives (later renamed the American Association of Nurse-Midwives) to work for professional recognition and certification standards along the lines of those required by the English Central Midwives' Board. Breckinridge, however, stood largely alone in this early determination to professionalize midwifery, and in her insistence that nurse-midwives work as autonomous practitioners. Indeed, during these same years the Ma-

ternity Center Association took the opposite tack, stressing that nurse-midwives were "at best only careful conscientious routine assistants to the physician. None would attempt or pretend to be more. . . . Several have tucked away the title of midwife as, in some situations, it would be far more of a handicap than a help because of the prejudices it arouses."[76]

This ambivalence helps explain the slowness with which American nurse-midwifery training programs were established. In 1923, the Maternity Center Association contemplated starting a midwifery training program, but found that the obstetrical community and many leading public health nurses opposed the idea.[77] The Maternity Center Association reversed itself in 1932, when it established the first nurse-midwifery training program in the United States, although, in keeping with the association's ambivalence about professionalization, its graduates were not granted any sort of professional certification. During World War II, when the FNS lost the better part of its staff as its English nurse-midwives returned home, it, too, established a midwifery training program for registered nurses.

Finally, the FNS innovation of using nurse-midwives to offer complete care to women with normal pregnancies and labors differed too radically from the dominant trends being established in American obstetrics by the 1920s to make much headway. Certainly influential medical advocates of professional midwifery existed. Physician Dorothy Mendenhall, for instance, did much to publicize the desirability of professional midwives in her research and writing for the federal Children's Bureau.[78] Obstetricians such as Frederick Adair and Ralph Lobenstine, both of whom were concerned primarily with maternal welfare programs, were longtime proponents of nurse-midwifery. In its report on maternal mortality published in 1933, the New York Academy of Medicine recommended the training and employment of nurse-midwives.[79]

In practice, however, the possibilities for developing nurse-midwifery as a viable alternative in maternity care have been undermined by dominant medical conceptions of childbirth and its management. In the 1920s, medical attendance, preferably by an obstetrical specialist, was rapidly becoming the sine qua non of safe, competent care. A physician's attendance was mandatory at birth because birth had come to be defined as a medical crisis, always potentially pathological. As a result, many health care professionals came to believe that they "must eliminate midwifery entirely from our social scheme."[80] Medical practitioners who argued for nurse-midwifery were increasingly overshadowed by physicians such as Joseph DeLee who argued that ideally birth should be managed as a surgical procedure. "All my medical life," DeLee wrote in 1934, "I have striven to eradicate the low opinion of obstetrics. . . . It is therefore with great pain and some alarm that I notice a trend in Britain and in parts of our Eastern seaboard, a reactionary trend, toward the state of midwifery."[81] Thus, many obstetricians still refused to make much distinction between professional and lay midwifery and would always regard a midwife's care as inherently inferior to that provided by a physician.

The work of the Frontier Nursing Service became increasingly anomalous in another way as well. The FNS attended the great majority of its patients at home at a time when doctors began to insist that only in hospitals could birth be safe. Although only 36.9 percent of American births took place in hospitals in 1935, by 1950, fully 88 percent did.[82] The widespread construction of rural community hospitals in the late 1920s and 1930s also undercut this aspect of the FNS's care. Significantly, at the same time the Commonwealth Fund refused to consider a grant to the FNS, it underwrote a major rural hospital construction program.[83]

Thus, greater reliance upon operative intervention, hospitalization, and universal medical management became the hallmarks of American birth management during the 1920s and 1930s. In a system that emphasized the pathology of birth, nurse-midwifery had little role to play. Most health care professionals have seen the FNS model as a successful but marginal, even anachronistic system, useful for poor, geographically isolated Appalachian women, but with little relevance for the nation as a whole.

NOTES

This article is a revised and expanded version of a paper originally presented at the "Women and Medicine" conference held at Boston College, November 1980. I wish to thank Janet James, James Klotter, Anne Campbell, Eric Christianson, and Judith Walzer Leavitt for their helpful comments and suggestions at various stages of its evolution. I also wish to thank Ellen Douglas Breckenridge for sharing her work on the Frontier Nursing Service and Manfred Waserman for his help with manuscript collections at the National Library of Medicine.

1 American College of Nurse-Midwives, *Nurse-Midwifery in the United States, 1976–1977* (Washington, D.C.: American College of Nurse-Midwives, 1978), 1.

2 A second organization, the Maternity Center Association of New York City, has been closely identified with professional midwifery and active since the 1930s in training and employing nurse-midwives and exploring alternatives to physician-managed, hospitalized childbirth. Although the Maternity Center Association was established in 1918, it did not begin to make use of nurse-midwives as birth attendants until the 1930s. For a general overview of nurse-midwifery in the United States, see Judy Barrett Litoff, *American Midwives, 1860 to the Present* (Westport: Greenwood Press, 1978), chap. 7.

3 Mary Breckinridge, "Outline for a demonstration of a children's public health service," copy of proposal submitted to the American Child Health Association, 1923, 1. Frontier Nursing Service Papers, Special Collections, University of Kentucky Libraries, Lexington, Kentucky. (Hereafter cited as FNS Papers).

4 Carolyn Van Blarcom, "Provisions for maternity care in the United States," *American Journal of Obstetrics and Gynecology*, 1925, *9:* 697–703; Grace Meigs, *Maternal Mortality from All Conditions Connected with Childbirth in the United States and Certain Other Countries*, U.S. Department of Labor, Children's Bureau Pub. no. 19 (Washington, D.C.: G.P.O., 1917), 7–13, 51; Robert Morse Woodbury, *Maternal Mortality: The Risk of Death in Childbirth and from All Diseases Caused by Pregnancy and Confinement*, U.S. Department of Labor, Children's Bureau Pub. no. 148 (Washington, D.C.: G.P.O., 1926). For a brief historical overview, see Joyce Antler and Daniel M. Fox, "The movement toward a safe maternity: physician accountability in New York City, 1915–1940," *Bulletin of the History of Medicine*, 1976, *50:* 569–95, especially 569–77.

5 In 1915, the infant mortality rate stood at 99.9 per 1,000 live births. By 1934 the figure was reduced to 60.1 per 1,000 live births. These statistics cited from Robert Woodbury, "Infant mortality in the United States," *Annals of the American Academy of Political and*

Social Science, 1936, *188:* 94–106. Also see *Save the Youngest*, U.S. Department of Labor, Children's Bureau Pub. no. 61 (Washington, D.C.: G.P.O., 1920), 2–7. Infant mortality varied widely from community to community and was closely correlated with socioeconomic status. For specific community studies during this period, see, e.g., Elizabeth Hughes, *Infant Mortality: Results of a Field Study in Gary, Indiana, Based on Births of One Year*, U.S. Department of Labor, Children's Bureau Pub. no. 112 (Washington, D.C.: G.P.O., 1923), and Anna Rochester, *Infant Mortality: Results of a Field Study in Baltimore, Maryland, Based on Births in One Year*, U.S. Department of Labor, Children's Bureau Pub. no. 119 (Washington, D.C.: G.P.O., 1923).

6 Antler and Fox, "Movement toward a safe maternity," 569–77. See, e.g., "Minimum standards for the public protection of the health of children and mothers," *Standards of Child Welfare: A Report of the Children's Bureau Conferences, May and June, 1919*, U.S. Department of Labor, Children's Bureau Pub. no. 60 (Washington, D.C.: G.P.O., 1919); Julius Levy, "Maternal mortality in the first month of life in relation to attendant at birth," *American Journal of Public Health*, 1923, *13:* 88–95; Joseph B. DeLee, "Progress toward ideal obstetrics," *Transactions of the American Association for the Study and Prevention of Infant Mortality*, 1919, *6:* 114–23.

7 See Litoff, *American Midwives*, 114, for percentage of births attended by midwives. For good discussions of lay midwives' declining role as birth attendants, see Litoff, *American Midwives*, especially chap. 3, and Frances E. Kobrin, "The American midwife controversy: a crisis of professionalization," in this volume.

8 Antler and Fox, "Movement toward a safe maternity," 569–95; Kobrin, "The American midwife controversy," in this volume, 318–26; *Maternal Mortality;* New York Academy of Medicine Committee on Public Health Relations, *Maternal Mortality in New York City: A Study of All Puerperal Deaths, 1930–1932* (New York: Commonwealth Fund, 1933), 32–50, 183–212. For an early influential critique of American obstetrical education, see J. Whitridge Williams, "Medical education and the midwife problem in the United States," *Journal of the American Medical Association*, 1912, *58:* 1–7.

9 Comment by Dr. Mary Sherwood in response to Charles V. Chapin, "The control of midwifery," *Standards of Child Welfare*, 166.

10 See, for example, Chapin, "The control of midwifery," 157–63. For a detailed and illuminating discussion of physicians' attitudes toward midwifery, see Litoff, *American Midwives*, especially chaps.

5 and 6, and Kobrin, "The American midwife controversy."

11 Kobrin, "The American midwife controversy"; Annie Veech, "For blue grass and hill babies," *Survey*, 1924, *52:* 625–26.

12 Annie Veech, "A practical solution of Kentucky's midwife problem," typescript, William Hutchins Papers, Berea College, Berea, Kentucky (hereafter cited as William Hutchins Papers); Mary Breckinridge, *Midwifery in the Kentucky Mountains: An Investigation* (privately printed, 1923), Mary Breckinridge Papers, University of Kentucky Special Collections, Lexington, Kentucky. (Hereafter cited as Mary Breckinridge Papers).

13 Kobrin, "The American midwife controversy." The best known of these comparative studies is Julius Levy, "The maternal and infant mortality in midwifery practice in Newark, New Jersey," *American Journal of Obstetrics*, 1918, *77:* 41–53, and Julius Levy, "Maternal mortality and mortality in the first month of life in relation to attendant at birth," *American Journal of Public Health*, 1923, *13:* 88–95. For a critique of Levy's statistical methodology, see M. Pierce Rucker, "The relation of the midwife to obstetric mortality with especial reference to New Jersey," *American Journal of Public Health*, 1923, *13:* 816–22. See also Chapin, "The control of midwifery," and comments, 157–66, and S. Josephine Baker, "Schools for midwives," *American Journal of Obstetrics*, 1912, *65: 256–70.*

14 Veech, "A practical solution of Kentucky's midwifery problem," comments of S. Josephine Baker, *Standards of Child Welfare*, 165–66. See Kobrin, "The American midwife controversy," for a clear statement of the public health argument.

15 See, for example, Mary Breckinridge, "A Frontier Nursing Service," *American Journal of Obstetrics and Gynecology*, 1928, *15:* 667–72.

16 Mary Breckinridge's autobiography, *Wide Neighborhoods: A Story of the Frontier Nursing Service* (New York: Harper and Bros., 1952; reissued 1981, University Press of Kentucky, Lexington) remains the standard source for biographical information. She destroyed most of her personal papers, but a small collection of letters and memorabilia is preserved in the Mary Breckinridge Papers. The Frontier Nursing Service Papers and the Frontier Nursing Service Oral History Project interviews, both held by University of Kentucky Special Collections, also contain much biographical material. For published studies, see Drew Gilpin Faust, "Mary Breckinridge," *Notable American Women: The Modern Period* (Cambridge: Harvard University Press, 1980), 103–5, and Carol Crowe-Carraco, "Mary Breckinridge

and the Frontier Nursing Service," *Register of the Kentucky Historical Society*, 1978, *76:* 179–91.

17 Faust, "Mary Breckinridge."

18 Breckinridge, *Wide Neighborhoods*, 83–110; Faust, "Mary Breckinridge"; Anne Campbell, "Mary Breckinridge and the American Committee for Devastated France: Foundations of the Frontier Nursing Service," unpublished seminar paper, University of Kentucky, 1981. This period of Breckinridge's life is extensively documented in her correspondence, contained in the Mary Breckinridge Papers.

19 Breckinridge, *Wide Neighborhoods*, 111.

20 Faust, "Mary Breckinridge"; *Wide Neighborhoods*, 122–56.

21 See, e.g., Van Blarcom, "Provisions for maternity care," 689–99; Woodbury, "Infant mortality," 97; Frederick Adair, "Maternal, fetal, and neonatal morbidity and mortality," *American Journal of Obstetrics and Gynecology*, 1935, *29:* 384–94. In 1923, the urban maternal mortality rate was 7.7 per thousand live births; the rural rate was 5.9. Van Blarcom, "Provisions for maternity care," 699.

22 Mary Breckinridge, "Memorandum concerning a suggested demonstration for the reduction of the infant and maternal death rate in a rural area of the South," typescript, 1923, FNS Papers; Van Blarcom, "Provisions for maternity care," 698–99; Elizabeth G. Fox, "Rural problems," *Standard of Child Welfare*, 186–93.

23 Mary Breckinridge to Ellen Phillips Crandall, October 20, 1923, Mary Breckinridge Papers.

24 Breckinridge, *Wide Neighborhoods*, 169–74.

25 Harry Caudill, *Night Comes to the Cumberlands* (Boston: Little, Brown, 1962), 254–55.

26 Mary Willeford, "Income and health in a remotely rural area," Ph.D. diss., Columbia University, 1927, 37, 55.

27 For a typical description of Appalachian culture and gender roles, see John Campbell, *The Southern Highlander and His Homeland* (New York: Russell Sage Foundation, 1921), 126–42.

28 Breckinridge, *Midwifery in the Kentucky Mountains*.

29 Ibid., 5–7.

30 Ibid., 9. Also see K. Osgood, D. L. Hochstrasser, and K. W. Deuschle, "Lay midwifery in southern Appalachia: The case of a mountain county in eastern Kentucky," *Archives of Environmental Health*, 1966, *12:* 759–70. Black midwives in the Deep South often had to complete a prescribed apprenticeship and give evidence of a special calling in order to take on the role of midwife. See Beatrice Mongeau, Henry Smith, and Ann Maney, "The 'granny' midwife: changing roles and functions of a folk practitioner,"

American Journal of Sociology, 1961, *66:* 497–505; Molly Dougherty, "Southern lay midwives as ritual specialists," in *Women in Ritual and Symbolic Roles*, ed. Judith Hoch-Smith (New York: Plenum Press, 1978), 151–64; Linda Holmes, "Granny midwives in Alabama," paper delivered at the American College of Nurse-Midwives convention, Lexington, Kentucky, March 1982.

31 Breckinridge, *Midwifery in the Kentucky Mountains*, 7–8.

32 Ibid., 17–20. For discussion of midwives as noninterventionist practitioners, see Dorothy Wertz and Richard Wertz, *Lying-In: A History of Childbirth in America* (Glencoe, Ill.: Free Press, 1977), chap. 1.

33 Breckinridge, *Midwifery in the Kentucky Mountains*, 20.

34 Ibid., 22. The reading of Ezekiel 16:6 is also reported as a practice of black midwives in the Deep South. See Dougherty, "Southern lay midwives as ritual specialists," 161.

35 Breckinridge, *Midwifery in the Kentucky Mountains*, 20–25.

36 Ibid., 19–20.

37 Ibid., 27.

38 Breckinridge, "Outline for a demonstration of a children's public health service," 3, 7, FNS Papers; Mary Breckinridge to Ellen Phillips Crandall, October 20, 1923, November 14, 1923; Ellen Crandall to Mary Breckinridge, February 12, 1924, Mary Breckinridge Papers.

39 Breckinridge, "Outline for a demonstration," 2. This early emphasis on the necessity for public funding is very different from Breckinridge's later insistence that the FNS always remain privately funded. The FNS did not accept federal funds until 1965, the year of Breckinridge's death.

40 Annie Veech to Mary Breckinridge, October 31, 1923, FNS Papers; Annie Veech to William J. Hutchins, May 6, 1927, William Hutchins Papers; Annie Veech, "A practical solution of Kentucky's midwife problem."

41 Annie Veech to William Hutchins, May 6, 1927, William Hutchins Papers.

42 For a discussion of Appalachia's image, see Henry Shapiro, *Appalachia on Our Mind* (Chapel Hill: University of North Carolina Press, 1978).

43 Ella Woodyard, "Statement of costs of the Frontier Nursing Service during the fiscal year May 1, 1926–27," *Quarterly Bulletin of the Frontier Nursing Service*, 1928, *4:* 3–8. Also see Edna Rochstroh, "Enter—the nurse-midwife," *American Journal of Nursing*, 1927, *27:* 149–64.

44 Interview with Betty Lester, Frontier Nursing Service Oral History Project, FNS Papers.

45 Breckinridge, *Wide Neighborhoods*, 162–63; W. Bertram Ireland to Kentucky Committee for Mothers and Babies, September 1, 1925, FNS Papers.

46 *Quarterly Bulletin of the Frontier Nursing Service*, 1927, *3*: 3.

47 Betty Lester Interview, FNS Oral History Project, FNS Papers.

48 Mary Breckinridge to Louis Dublin, April 14, 1928, Louis Dublin Papers, National Library of Medicine, Department of the History of Medicine, Bethesda, MD. (Hereafter cited as Dublin Papers.)

49 *Quarterly Bulletin of the FNS*, 1929, *5*: 2; *Quarterly Bulletin of the FNS*, 1931, *7*: 3; Mary Breckinridge to Louis Dublin, April 14, 1928, Dublin Papers.

50 *Quarterly Bulletin of the FNS*, 1929, *5*: 1.

51 Woodyard, "Statement of costs of the FNS," 4. The best discussion of FNS costs within the context of rural health care generally is Ellen Douglas Breckenridge, "The Frontier Nursing Service: a demonstration project in rural health care," B.A. thesis, Harvard University, 1979, 40–43. This thesis is also on file in the Appalachian Collection, University of Kentucky Libraries, Lexington, Kentucky.

52 J. Stanley Lemons, *The Woman Citizen* (Urbana, Ill.: University of Illinois Press, 1973), 154.

53 Mary Breckinridge, "The nurse-midwife—a pioneer," *American Journal of Public Health*, 1927, *27*: 1149.

54 "Report on the third thousand confinements of the Frontier Nursing Service," compiled by Elizabeth Steele for the Metropolitan Life Insurance Company, 1937, 8, FNS Papers.

55 Ibid., 8–9; New York Academy of Medicine Committee on Public Health Relations, *Maternal Mortality in New York City*, 116–23.

56 "Report on the third thousand confinements," 8–9; "Analysis of the records of 1,004 women during pregnancy, labor, and postpartum," First Series, FNS Papers.

57 Nora Kelly, "Put out the fire and all the lamps," *Quarterly Bulletin of the FNS*, 1938, *14*: 12.

58 Although there are numerous references in early FNS publications and correspondence to this survey, its results were never reported upon in any detail, and all copies of the completed survey apparently have been lost. Although Breckinridge turned a copy of the compiled statistics over to the state health department, no state agency has a record of the transaction or a copy of the survey. There is no copy in the FNS records.

59 "Report on the third thousand confinements," 1, 8.

60 "Report on the third thousand confinements," 8–9, compares FNS mortality to that of rural white Kentucky women generally and to the United States as a whole. Lexington statistics compiled from State Board of Health of Kentucky, *Preliminary Vital Statistics Reports*, 1925 through 1938.

61 Louis Dublin to Mary Breckinridge, May 4, 1932, Dublin Papers; "Analysis of the records of 1004 women during pregnancy, labor, and postpartum"; "Report on the third thousand confinements," 3–9.

62 "Report on the third thousand confinements," 7, 9.

63 Ibid., 9.

64 John Kooser, "Rural obstetrics: a report of the work of the Frontier Nursing Service," *Southern Medical Journal* 35 (February 1942): 123–31, quotation from 130.

65 John Kooser, "Observations on the possible relationship of diet to the late toxemia of pregnancy," *American Journal of Obstetrics and Gynecology*, 1941, *41*: 288–94, quotation from 294.

66 "Report on the third thousand confinements," 2; Louis Dublin to Mary Breckinridge, May 4, 1932, Dublin Papers.

67 Ibid., 7–8.

68 The early twentieth-century infant mortality surveys made by the Children's Bureau are valuable for documenting the relationship between infant mortality and social class. See especially Anna Rochester, *Infant Mortality: Results of a Field Study in Baltimore, Maryland*, 105–6.

69 Louis Dublin to Mary Breckinridge, May 4, 1932, Dublin Papers; *Quarterly Bulletin of the FNS*, 1932, *7*: 3; George Kosmak, "The trained nurse and the midwife," *American Journal of Nursing*, 1934, *34*: 425.

70 See, for example, Mary Sumner Boyd, "Why mothers die," *Nation* 132 (March 18, 1931): 293–95; Dorothy Bromley, "What risk motherhood?" *Harper's* 149 (June 1929): 11–22; Mary Breckinridge, "An adventure in midwifery," *Survey* 57 (October 1926): 25–27; Ernest Poole, "Nurses on horseback," *Good Housekeeping* 94 (June 1932): 38–39, 203–10.

71 Louis Dublin to Barry Smith, February 10, 1928; Louis Dublin to Mrs. John Sloane, November 29, 1930, Dublin Papers.

72 Barry Smith to Louis Dublin, November 8, 1928; Barbara Quin to Louis Dublin, February 11, 1928, Dublin Papers. I am indebted to Ellen Douglas Breckenridge for her discussion of the FNS's difficulties with the Commonwealth Fund during 1927 and 1928 and for her perceptive discussion of the changing patterns of foundation funding and private philanthropy as they related to rural health care generally. Breckenridge, "The Frontier Nursing Service: a demonstration project in rural health care," 34–46.

73 "Fifth annual report of the Frontier Nursing Service," *Quarterly Bulletin of the FNS*, 1930, *6*: 1–2.

74 *Quarterly Bulletin of the FNS*, 1932, *8*: 2–3.

75 On physicians' attitudes toward nurse-midwifery, see Seth Goldsmith, John W. C. Johnson, Monroe Lerner, "Obstetricians' attitudes toward nurse-midwives," *American Journal of Obstetrics and Gynecology*, 1971, *111:* 111–18.

76 For information on the Kentucky State Association of Midwives, see "Kentucky State Association of Midwives, Inc.," *Quarterly Bulletin of the FNS*, 1939, *15:* 19–22; Hattie Hemschmeyer, "Midwifery in the United States," *American Journal of Nursing*, 1939, *39:* 1183; Interview with Hazel Corbin, FNS Oral History Project, FNS Papers.

77 *Maternity Center Association, 1918–1943* (New York: Maternity Center Association, 1943); Hemschmeyer, "Midwifery in the United States."

78 Dorothy Reed Mendenhall, *Midwifery in Denmark*, U.S. Department of Labor Children's Bureau (Washington, D.C.: G.P.O., 1929).

79 New York Academy of Medicine Committee on Public Health Relations, *Maternal Mortality*, 207–12, 221–22; Litoff, *American Midwives*, 125–26.

80 *Maternity Center Association, 1918–1943*, 25. The classic articulation of the idea that childbirth should always be regarded as a medical crisis is Joseph B. DeLee, "The prophylactic forceps operation," *American Journal of Obstetrics and Gynecology*, 1920, *1:* 34–44.

81 Joseph B. DeLee, "Obstetrics versus midwifery," *Journal of the American Medical Association*, 1934, *103:* 308.

82 For discussion and statistics concerning the increase in hospital birth, see Neil Devitt, "The transition from home to hospital birth in the United States, 1930–1960," *Birth and the Family Journal*, 1977, *4:* 47–58.

83 "Rural community hospitals established by Commonwealth Fund," *American Journal of Public Health*, 1926, *16:* 315; W. S. Rankin, "Rural medical and hospital services," *American Journal of Public Health* 17 (January 1927): 15–19; "Federal hospital construction act of 1940," *American Journal of Public Health*, 1940, *30:* 719.

HEALTH REFORMERS

Health reform flourished in the United States during the middle of the nineteenth century in part as a reaction against ineffective medical practice. Numerous Americans found existing heroic therapy—characterized typically by massive bleedings and dosings with emetics and cathartics—painful and dangerous, and they sought to avoid it by teaching the public physiology and hygiene to help them stay healthy. Regina Morantz explores the connection between the health reform movement and middle-class women, who, in emphasizing their nurturing abilities, became active reformers. Women expanded their domestic duties beyond their own homes when they traveled around the country giving lectures on hygiene and disease prevention, and in the process they helped transform society's view of the role and abilities of women in general.

John Blake's essay relates the story of Mary Gove Nichols, one of the most active and successful health reformers. Her activities proved that women could transcend their traditional boundaries and have a significant impact on the health of Americans. Ronald Numbers and Rennie Schoepflin explore the parallel careers of two important religious leaders, Ellen G. White and Mary Baker Eddy, who responded to health reform in distinctive ways.

Health reform was a subject that in some ways transcended socioeconomic divisions in society. While many of the health reformers were middle- or upper-class men and women, the movement consciously made connections with the masses of Americans for whom sickness was a particularly grim burden. Many of the sectarian reactions to regular heroic medicine not only fostered participation as practitioners but authorized a degree of do-it-yourself medicine, which encouraged people to take control of their own health. Such democratic appeals, especially during and after the Jacksonian period, in part accounted for the popularity and success of these reform groups.

In emphasizing equality, health reformers hit a particularly responsive chord among women. Whether consciously or not, women used their participation in the movement to move their sex a little closer to full citizenship. Even the women who remained within their traditional role found gratifying the positive efforts to gain control of their family's health through understanding physiology and practicing better domestic hygiene. In a society in which men still had to be prodded to "remember the ladies," in Abigail Adams's words, health reform promised full participation and acceptance of women.

24

Making Women Modern:
Middle-Class Women and Health Reform
in 19th-Century America

REGINA MARKELL MORANTZ

Social historians have yet to explore adequately either the connection between health reform and advances in nineteenth-century medicine or the role of women in the active promotion and adoption of rationalistic health practices. As life expectancy increased and infant mortality declined, sickness gradually ceased to be endemic. More important, fatalistic attitudes toward death and disease gave way to the conviction that good health was within the reach of each and every citizen. The nature and impact of these changes cannot be explained merely by recounting the heroic strides made by medical scientists during these years. While the work of Pasteur, Koch, and others was vitally important, advances in bacteriology and medical therapeutics do not tell the whole story. The nineteenth-century revolution in health was far more pervasive; its advocates were not only great men of science, but ordinary men and women who promulgated and implemented new attitudes toward public and personal cleanliness.

Beginning in the antebellum period, self-help in health matters, public hygiene, dietary reform, temperance, hydrotherapy, and physiological instruction merged as ingredients in a coherent and articulate campaign to save the nation by combating the ill health of its citizenry. Although such attention to personal health and hygiene was not wholly original, never before had the regard for good health given rise to such widespread public activity.[1]

In the modernizing world of the nineteenth-century, health reformers played a critical role in transforming traditional attitudes toward sickness and death. They promoted the active assumption by men and women of the responsibility for their own health, the health of their families, and the health of society at large. Itinerant speakers lecturing to enthusiastic audiences and dedicated to furthering common knowledge of health and hygiene traversed the cities and towns of the North and West. Hundreds of heuristic tracts instructed eager readers in the "laws of life." A handful of journals kept men and women informed of new developments. The popular *Water Cure Journal*, for example, boasted ten thousand subscribers in 1849, the second year of its publication.[2]

Although the movement held attractions for both men and women, and, as we shall see, the contributions of male spokesmen were vital, middle-class women, by virtue of their new roles in an increasingly complex society, became the health reformers' primary constituency. Because the changing structure of the nineteenth-century family increasingly required women to school their children in "modern" values, they welcomed with relief the practical solutions to bewildering problems offered in health reform journals and tracts.

The concern with hygiene was an integral part of the antebellum reformist world view. Indeed, the health crusade converged with several better-known radical concerns. Historians have been quick to point out this identity of ideas and personnel. No study of antebellum reform can ignore the fundamental role of hygienic and physiologic concepts. Abolitionist speakers, for example, lodged at health reform boarding houses, and a large number of women's rights advocates followed some

REGINA MARKELL MORANTZ is Associate Professor of History at the University of Kansas, Lawrence, Kansas.

Reprinted with permission from *Journal of Social History* 10 (1977): 490–507.

form of Sylvester Graham's vegetarian diet. Oberlin College, familiar as a breeding ground for abolitionism and women's rights, adopted strict vegetarianism in its dining room in 1835. Asa Mahan, the college's president, put a "reformation in food, drink, and dress" high on the list of important causes.[3]

Moreover, a cursory glance at the men and women who actively promoted the health revolution suggests that, like other reformers, they came from the northeastern, predominantly middle-class sectors of the American population. Sylvester Graham began his career in New Jersey as a Presbyterian minister and temperance lecturer. William A. Alcott, cousin of Bronson, was a thoughtful, Yale-trained physician. Joel Shew and Russell Trall graduated from regular medical schools in New York. James Caleb Jackson, a self-made man, was the son of a yeoman farmer in upstate New York. Mary Gove Nichols became a teacher in Maine. Rachel Brooks Gleason graduated from New York's Central Eclectic School of Medicine and ran a water cure establishment with her physician husband. Paulina Wright Davis and Elizabeth Oakes Smith both hailed from prominent New York landholding families. Harriot Hunt's father, a skilled navigator, invested his small capital in Boston's commercial shipping industry. Lydia Folger Fowler, wife of the phrenologist publisher Lorenzo, was the second woman to receive a medical degree in the United States. A descendant of the Puritan settlers of Nantucket Island and distant cousin of the astronomer Maria Mitchell, Lydia's father was a manufacturer, a shipowner, and a selectman of his native town. Recently, an intensive study of the rank and file of the Boston Ladies Physiological Society found that the large majority were predominantly the wives and mothers of Boston's middle class.[4]

Previous students of the health reform movement have offered us a number of useful insights. We know, for example, that health crusaders shared with other reformers of the period a fundamental Enlightenment rationalism. Implicit in their theory of sickness was a concept of self-help and a conviction that disease could be prevented by teaching people the "laws" of physiology and hygiene. Other scholars suggest that the rationalistic impulse in health reform rhetoric was overshadowed by heavy doses of Christian perfectionism. Preaching the interconnections of the moral and physical life, health reformers agreed that man could not achieve success in the one without total control over the other. Medical historians, in contrast, have emphasized a causal relationship between the rise of health reform and the decline of heroic medical therapeutics. Health crusaders stood united in their criticism of the bleeding, purging, and dosing of the professional practice of the day. Finally, a few scholars attribute the rise of the movement to the pervasive antielitism characteristic of the antebellum period, an atmosphere which fueled the public animus against established medical practice.[5]

While earlier work has been informative, two crucial questions remain virtually unexplored in the historiographical literature. The first concerns the relationship of health reform to modernization; the second relates to the connection between women's interest in health reform and changes in their status.[6] Although this essay will make some brief and admittedly speculative observations concerning the first of these problems, its primary focus will be to suggest a tentative framework for explaining women's role in the health reform movement. It is hoped that such a framework will aid others in further explorations of the subject.

Former accounts have only briefly acknowledged and never analyzed women's participation. We know a great deal about Sylvester Graham, William A. Alcott, and John Harvey Kellogg, but our information about the many women who preached, implemented, and occasionally elaborated on the ideas of these more prominent health reformers remains sketchy.[7] Yet a number of the most outspoken of the health crusaders were female, and women swelled the ranks of the new movement.

In 1837 the American Physiological Society was found in Boston to foster health by teaching physiology. Almost a third of its members were women, and at its second annual meeting the new organization acknowledged women's central role in promoting good health in the following resolution:

> *Resolved,* That woman in her character as wife and mother is only second to the Deity in the influence that she exerts on the physical, the intellectual, and the moral interests of the human race, and that her education should be adapted to qualify her in the highest de-

gree to cherish those interests in the wisest and best manner.[8]

Women took to the field as lecturers. Ladies Physiological Societies appeared throughout the Northeast. The names of Mary Gove Nichols, Harriot Hunt, and Lydia Folger Fowler are only the most familiar of the dozens of women who taught enthusiastic female audiences the "laws of life."

Profound changes in women's roles underlay their active interest in health reform. The social transformation touched off by industrialization and urbanization gradually forced them to redefine their responsibilities in an altered family setting. Since colonial times traditional verities had suggested that woman's place was in the home. But women had experienced family, home, and work as an integrated, stable whole. The heavy burden of household production and the immediate concern with economic subsistence left them little time and less inclination to question their duties. Moreover, social roles for women in the seventeenth and eighteenth centuries in reality remained quite fluid and imperfectly defined. It was left to the nineteenth century to institutionalize the concept of "woman's sphere."

As productive labor shifted from the home to the factory, men, acting on premodern conceptions of men's and women's responsibilities, increasingly sought outside employment. Masculine and feminine spheres became more rigidly separated. This development quickly colored nineteenth-century cultural expectations.

Economic changes suddenly made it possible for the first time for large numbers of women to become primarily wives and mothers. No longer did playing a vital role in the family economy compete for their time and attention. The ideal of the modern family—small in size, emotionally intense, and woman supervised—made its appearance as a distinctive emblem of middle-class culture.

Contemporaries noted these changes with satisfaction. In a letter to the *Water Cure Journal* in 1854, the reformer Frances Dana Gage observed:

Steam power suggested steam power, [*sic*] and one invention gave leisure for another; mind was released from physical labor, and gained time and leisure for higher and nobler development; woman was obliged to keep sight of the age. She was a help-meet, suggesting,

striving, planning, and executing; thinking for the young, and leading them to the depots of usefulness. . . . Woman . . . thirty years ago seldom went from the home, because she *could not be spared*, now that spinning-jennies and patent looms do the spinning and weaving, and sewing machines are doing the needle-work, steam-power does the knitting, and garments are made so cheap . . . it seems an idle waste of time to use 'Her needle'.[9]

Paralleling these economic developments was the desire to educate women to their duties as mothers which sparked the spread of female education in the first half of the nineteenth century. Enlightenment theorists had been the first to propose that, within the home, women should have primary responsibility for rearing the nation's young. Only an astute mother, they argued, could raise her sons to be proper citizens of the republic. Health reformers merely elaborated on this theme. "Now who," asked a typical contributor to the *Practical Educator and Journal of Health* in 1847, "is the best qualified to supervise a household? She who has been thoroughly trained . . . or she who knows practically nothing about it . . . Let woman be intellectually educated as highly as possible."[10]

Educational opportunity brought middle-class women into contact with Enlightenment ideas about progress and individual freedom. Such concepts colored their adjustments to underlying social changes and helped produce a talented minority with rising status expectations who came to feel frustration, distaste, anger, even desperation at the severe limitations imposed on them by the growing popularity of the "cult of the lady." Trained in a more ascetic Protestant tradition of usefulness, strength, duty, and good works, many middle-class women rejected the fashionable, indolent life of the leisured wife. Gradually two competing images of the ideal nineteenth-century woman emerged. On the one hand, woman was described as weak, sickly, dependent, and ornamental. On the other, she was exalted as highly spiritual and morally superior—confined to the home, yet invested with genuine power and responsibility within her sphere. Both health reformers and women's rights advocates would reject the first and seize on the second ideal—that of woman's moral power—using it effectively in this century to explore significant and divergent outlets for female energies. These women would practice domesticity, not as a cult, but as a science. Responding to changes in women's traditional role which left them devoid of adequate models and established forms of behavior, they sought to elevate and professionalize the domestic sphere as a means of seeking an effective and practical role for women in a new and unpredictable social setting.[11]

The middle-class woman's new domestic orientation required a single-minded concern with the problems of health and hygiene. Her own good health became a matter of conscious choice. She took an assiduous interest in questions concerning marriage, childbearing and child rearing, family health, sexuality and family limitation. Health reformers, both men and women, shared these interests and attempted to provide practical solutions to unsettling problems. Indeed, health reformers gave to the majority of their female constituents a justification for devoting their fulltime efforts to woman's traditional role of homemaking, recast, it is important to note, in a modern and scientific setting.

For the ordinary woman, the health revolution became a fundamental ingredient in women's modernization, allowing her to cope with the problems created by industrial and urban living and easing her transition into a more complex and modern world. Yet the movement also produced a smaller number of female activists who linked their concern with health problems to a more aggressive feminism. The health reform movement thus touched the average woman and the feminist in slightly different ways. Ironically, even as health reformers aided in readjusting female roles to coincide with traditional values concerning woman's place, they helped, sometimes unwittingly, to lay the groundwork for the eventual erosion of ancient pieties. To the female leaders of the campaign health reform offered a path out of the home and a more active role in social change.

Because woman's procreative role often made her health more precarious than man's, it seemed natural for the health reformers to begin their efforts with an aggressive concern for the state of female health. "If a plan for *destroying female health*, in all the ways in which it could be most effectively done,

were drawn up," announced Catharine Beecher, "it would be exactly the course which is now pursued by a large portion of this nation, especially in the more wealthy classes." Dr. James C. Jackson, founder of the Dansville water cure, agreed. "American girls," he lamented, "are all sickly." "You are sick," wrote Mrs. S. M. Estee to the feminine readers of the *Water Cure Journal*, "and have been for months, years, and some of you your whole lives."[12]

We cannot know for sure whether or not this generation of women was sicker than their grandmothers. What is certain, however, is that they *thought* they were. Indeed, they well may have been. Fashionable dress took its toll on female health; the corset and tight lacing did much to damage female anatomy. Increased urbanization brought crowded and unsanitary living conditions. More and more middle-class women denied themselves the fresh air and exercise experienced by the rural housewife out of necessity rather than by choice. And the psychological strains of dislocation may have prompted some women to opt for ill health, rather than stand and face changes which they could still barely comprehend.[13]

It soon became apparent that only healthy vigorous women could meet the challenges thrust upon them by a society in transition. Health reformers believed that woman was in the process of creating a new role for herself. "Woman . . . is a new element in society," wrote Dr. James Jackson to his associate Dr. Harriet A. Judd, "just emerging from her hybernation . . . and so much better fitted to take to herself *new* ideas, and develop them."[14] Good health was essential to woman's new self-expression and improved status. "Let mothers be educated in all that concerns life and health," insisted Mrs. Eliza de la Vergue, M.D. "Let them learn that *knowledge gives the highest order of power*."[15]

Good health became a prerequisite to woman's new place in the world. "Woman was neither made a toy nor a slave, but a help-meet to man," wrote "A Bloomer to Her Sisters," "and as such devolves upon her very many important duties and obligations which cannot be met so long as she is the puny, sickly, aching, weakly, dying creature that we find her to be; and woman must, to a very considerable extent, redeem herself—she must throw off the shackles that have hitherto bound both body and mind, and rise into the newness of life."[16]

Women could achieve none of these goals until they learned to dress properly. Health reformers made dress reform a symbol of women's new aspirations. Impractical clothes immobilized women and kept them from their responsibilities. Some regular physicians had linked fashionable dress to female ill health, but health reformers succeeded in making dress reform a moral imperative. Good health was doomed, they argued, as long as women clung to the dictates of French fashion. They called upon women to liberate their souls by freeing their bodies from the harmful effects of tight lacing and long, heavy, unhygienic skirts. "How . . . glorious," mused Rachel Brooks Gleason, M.D., "would it be to see every woman free from *every* fetter that fashion has imposed! Such a day of 'universal emancipation' of the sex would be worthy of a celebration through all coming time." "We can expect but small achievement from women," warned Mary Gove Nichols, "so long as it is the labor of their lives to carry about their clothes." "How in the name of common sense," asked Edith Denner, "is a woman with long full skirts, ever to become a practical Ornithologist, Geologist, or Botanist?"[17]

Health reform journals pressed the issue. Lengthy technical descriptions of the damage wrought on female anatomy by the corset appeared, complete with diagrams. Pictures entitled the "Allopathic Lady, or Pure Cod Liver Oil Female, Who Patronizes a Fashionable Doctor, And Considers It Decidedly Vulgar to Enjoy Good Health," were published side by side with those of women in reformed dress. A typical caption read "A Water-Cure Bloomer, Who Believes In The Equal Rights Of Men And Women To Help Themselves And Each Other, And Who Thinks It Respectable, If Not Genteel, To Be Well." Not content merely to admonish their readers, some journals printed sewing instructions. For a modest sum, the *Laws of Life* sold patterns to its subscribers.[18]

In a society where women were expected to play an increasingly complex role in the nurture of children and the organization of family life, health crusaders brought to the bewildered housewife, not just sympathy and compassion, but a structured regimen and way of life. William A. Alcott, as early as 1839, took for granted the mother's primary responsibility in child rearing and the father's extended absence from the home. "All, or nearly all,"

he wrote in his book *The Young Mother,* "must devolve on the mother. The father has not time to attend to his children."[19]

Burdened by this reorientation toward their family responsibilities, many ordinary women found in the health reform movement a means of coping with an imprecise, undependable, and often hostile environment. Lectures, journals, and domestic tracts provided friendly advice and companionship in an era characterized by weakening ties between relatives and neighbors. Women found a means to end their isolation and make contact with others of their sex. In study groups and through letters to the various journals, they shared their common experiences with other women. No longer must woman bear her burden alone. This collective sensitivity to the community among women was symbolized by the frequent references to "sisterhood" in health reform literature.[20]

"I wish, " wrote Mary Gove Nichols of her motives in becoming a health reformer, "to teach mothers how to cure their own diseases, and those of their children; and to increase health, purity, and happiness in the family and the home."[21] For some women, Mrs. Nichols and her fellow reformers achieved these goals.[22] Numerous articles on cookery, bathing, teething, care of infants, childhood, sexuality, cleanliness, and domestic economy carefully taught women how to manage their households properly. Itinerant physiological lecturers assaulted women's widespread ignorance of their bodies. Nichols relied heavily on discussion of anatomy and physiology in her lectures. She instructed her listeners in the formation of bone structure, the role of respiration and circulation, the anatomy and physiology of the stomach. The process of digestion was described in detail. The remainder of her course involved information on dietetics and the importance of physical education. The evils of "tight lacing," and dire warnings against the harmful effects of the "solitary vice" also proved popular topics for discussion.[23]

Advice on the supervision of pregnancy and childbirth was strikingly prophetic of today's feminist critique of professional obstetrical practice. Health reformers questioned regular physicians' very approach to the process of parturition, calling their treatment "unnatural and often outrageous." "Here," observed Thomas Low Nichols, where august nature should reign supreme, her laws are too often violated, and all her teachings set at naught. Instead of preparing a woman to go through the process of labor with all the energy of her vitality, she is weakened by medication and blood-letting. Instead of being put upon a proper regimen, and a diet suited to her condition, she is more than ever pampered and indulged. And when labor comes on, the chances are that it will be interfered with in the most mistaken, the most unjustifiable ... manner. The uterus will be stimulated into excessive and spasmodic action by the deadly ergot; the mother, at this most interesting and sacred hour of life, will be made dead drunk with ether or chloroform ... and if a weakened and deranged system does not act as promptly as the doctor wishes, he proceeds to deliver with instruments, with the risk, often the certainty of destroying the child, and very often inflicting upon the mother irreparable injury.

"Under the popular medical orders of the day," agreed Russell Trall, "pregnant females are regarded as invalids, and are bled, paregoric'd, magnesia'd, stimulated, mineralized and poisoned, just as though they were going through a regular course of fever."[24] In contrast, health reformers viewed conception, gestation, and parturition as natural functions. They rejected the notion that pain in childbirth was inevitable, labeling such a belief "an insult to Providence." They urged exercise, fresh air, proper diet, and cleanliness. Daily bathing was advised for infants, who were to be dressed in loose-fitting, comfortable garments to give plenty of opportunity for movement. No drugs were allowed for mother or child. Such attention to hygiene and diet probably improved the health of many, if we can believe the numerous testimonials from satisfied individuals to be found in the back pages of health reform journals.[25]

When the middle-class woman took possession of her life and the lives of those around her in the area of health, she also provided herself with a platform from which to effect other changes, both within the family constellation and in society at large. One doubts if this process was always conscious. Yet it seems equally clear that her psychological acceptance of various domestic responsibilities often led to subtle shifts in the power relationship between the sexes, giving rise to new attitudes toward what was, and what was not, acceptable in marriage. Nowhere was this process more apparent than in the health reformers' attitudes toward sexual intercourse.[26]

Health reformers were among the first nineteenth-century thinkers to prescribe restraint in sexual matters. Believing that good health required constant control, vigilant self-discipline, and vigorous dominion over man's animal nature, they warned that of all the sensual passions, "the sexual element" was the most difficult to subdue. "No other element in our own nature," wrote Henry G. Wright, "has so much to do in ... forming our character and shaping our destiny.... But what is done ... to bring the sexual element under the control of an enlightened reason and a tender conscience?"[27]

Reformers clearly intended sexual restraint to benefit women and urged them to assert their rights in the sexual sphere. Much of female ill health and infant mortality, they argued, could be attributed to husbands' sexual abuse of their wives. Believing that the male's passion for copulation far outdistanced his wife's, thinkers and educators urged men to follow the sexual rhythms of their more delicate spouses.[28]

Excessive childbearing endangered female health while it drained most women of the energy needed to perform the duties of scientific motherhood. Hence, health reformers linked their insistence on sexual restraint to family limitation. They were among the first to advocate birth control publicly. Children, they argued, must never be the result "of chance, of mere reckless, selfish passion." When, they asked "will men and women show a rational, conscientious, loving forethought, in giving existence to their children as they do in commerce, politics, and religion?" Every child should be a welcome child. "Welcome" became a code word for "planned." The "great object" of sexual intercourse, declared Henry G. Wright, was the *"perpetuation and perfection of the race."* Couples not ready to have children should remain sexually continent.[29]

In an era still largely ignorant of mechanical means of contraception, women benefited from such cautious attitudes in numerous ways. Historians have already documented women's profound fears of pregnancy in this period. Less frequent childbearing did improve female health. Furthermore, the desire to avoid conception probably colored women's enjoyment of coitus. Some undoubtedly followed the common belief that failure to achieve orgasm would prevent pregnancy. Moreover, lovemaking techniques were often brutal and aggressive.[30] Even nineteenth-century physicians, although aware of female orgasm, knew very little else about the intricate nature of female sexual response. One suspects that middle-class women instructed their husbands and sons in the laws of sexual continence with a degree of enthusiasm and a measure of self-defense.[31]

While exalting the rewards of parenthood and elevating the motherly role, health reformers enjoined couples to limit their offspring. The contradiction in such views remains more apparent than real. The ideal of educated motherhood eventually proved antithetical to large families. Women were simply incapable of achieving either the emotional intensity or the domestic expertise required of them when caring for a large brood. Margaret Sanger's injunction that parents should have "fewer and better babies" had its origins in the antebellum period, among these "enlightened" sections of the middle class.[32]

Rarely in any century have human beings been content to view health and disease as matters of mere chance. The health reformers' approach, however, was distinctly novel. To the Puritans and other colonials, sickness had been primarily a moral and spiritual dilemma which called for introspection and soul searching. But the nineteenth-century health reformers insisted that it resulted from a violation of God's and Nature's laws. Such laws were eminently sensible, and the individual could, indeed, he *must,* keep himself well. No longer were sickness and death to be tolerated with the stoicism and resignation that contrasted the limited moral choices of man with the all-powerful inscrutability of God. "Many people," observed Mary Gove Nichols, "seem to think that all diseases are immediate visitations from the Almighty, arising from no cause but his *immediate* dispensation. . . . Many seem to have no idea that there are established laws with respect to life and health, and that the transgres-

sion of these laws is followed by disease." Man, agreed Marie Louise Shew, was designed to live in good health to a ripe old age. Disease was man's doing, not God's. The prevention of disease and premature death was indeed within the control of mankind.[33]

The emergence of health reform as a coherent crusade cannot be understood apart from the gradual appearance of a novel set of assumptions about the world—an attitude which historians, for want of a more precise theoretical model, have attributed to the modernization process. Health reformers insisted upon the efficacy of individual action. They were certain that human beings could affect the future by manipulating the environment and controlling themselves. This was a conviction that they shared with all other reformers of the antebellum period. Yet this common outlook was itself a reflection of a more fundamental change in thought and feeling.

Even many critics of the concept of modernization agree that if used carefully it can serve as a helpful organizing principle for studying the social, political, and cultural fragmentation which accompanied industrialization.[34] The modernization model can be of aid in relating changes in individual and family dynamics to other aspects of social history.

Although we may differ as to the cause, most of us would agree that modern men and women behave differently from their ancestors: they exhibit high occupational and educational goals, they value mobility, personal freedom, and self-improvement, and their fundamental belief in progress leads to an implicit abandonment of passivity in the face of life's difficulties.[35] Health reformers filled their literature with such themes. Indeed, one could argue that health reform facilitated the adjustment of men and women in the nineteenth century to industrialization and urbanization.

Occasionally health tracts revealed the reformers' profound ambivalence toward social and economic change, and such equivocation was itself significant. By no means did all health crusaders welcome the new order with unbridled enthusiasm.[36] As other historians have shown, many individuals looked nostalgically backward to an idealized "republic of virtue" where the mutual interdependency of family members and society at large promoted "good health" in the form of physical and spiritual unity.[37] While they desired "progress," health reformers did not always realize that it would lead inevitably to changes in values. Arguing, on the one hand, that an excessive application to business led to insanity in men, while luxury and idleness produced nervousness in women, they simultaneously sought the creation of a personality type remarkably well suited to the competitive atmosphere of the industrial order.[38] Preaching moderation and self-control, reformers strove to provide men and women with a coherent mode of adjustment to the physical and psychological demands of an urbanizing environment. By helping, willy-nilly, to effect a transformation of personality which equipped individuals to deal with other aspects of modernization, health reform itself became a part of the modernization process.

By the end of the nineteenth century, reform ideas about personal cleanliness, public health, and family hygiene had become familiar axioms of middle-class American culture—a badge of distinction by which members set themselves off from "illegitimate" immigrant groups, many of whom retained distinctly premodern daily habits and attitudes toward disease. Indeed, those health reformers primarily concerned with public health had long been aware of the relationship between ignorance, immoral habits, poverty, and sickness. The allegedly "filthy" and "depraved" customs attributed to the immigrant poor proved particularly vexing. Health reformers of all persuasions believed that they worked to make good health a measure of middle-class respectability.[39]

To the middle-class women, troubled by the contradictory demands of urbanization and industrialization, health reform offered both physical and psychological relief. Holding out to confused wives and mothers the prospect of improving the quality of life, not merely by changing the environment, but by gaining control of themselves, health reformers promised women that they could raise their children healthy in mind and clean in body. Reformers offered wives the possibility of keeping their husbands moral by cooking the right foods. Preaching sexual continence and physiological knowledge, they helped to legitimate female rights in the bedroom at a time when sexual contact need not universally have been a positive experience. Indeed, health reform manuals supported women's right to limit the number of their children and

control their own bodies, though they accepted only sexual continence as a moral means of birth control. Nevertheless, the idea that fertility should, or even could, be consistently tampered with was distinctly modern, and neatly complemented other social and economic developments.[40]

For a minority of brave, ambitious, and talented women health reform also provided an outlet and an escape from an intolerably narrow and confining role. Health reformers shared with other nineteenth-century Americans the belief that women's role was invested with cosmic moral significance. But unlike many of their contemporaries, female health activists subscribed to the widest possible definition of woman's sphere. They understood that to purify society, women would indeed have to enter it. Admitting women into the masculine sphere, even in a limited way, would eventually have profound effects on future definitions of sex roles.

Most middle-class women, however, were not feminists. Health reform gave them a coherent program to ease their adjustment to a society in transition. Over and over again the reformers identified poor female health with underemployment and idleness. This familiar refrain suggests a lack of integration in the lives of middle-class women, a tenuousness and uncertainty about their role. Female health reformers especially addressed themselves to this problem. Elevating the art of domesticity to a science, they restored to their followers a sense of purpose and direction, while they preserved in a new form traditional assumptions about woman's role which were deeply imbedded in the culture. The health reform regimen established new standards by which ordinary women could measure their own respectability and worth.[41]

Reformers underscored woman's importance by emphasizing her central role in the task of human betterment. Improvement of female health, they argued, would lead to social regeneration. Woman was invested with awesome responsibilities. "There are no duties on earth so nearly angelic as those which devolve upon woman," declared Alcott. "If all wives loved and delighted in their homes as Solomon would have them, few husbands would go down to a premature grave through the avenues of intemperance and lust, and their kindred vices." The *Lily*, a feminist and temperance journal, emphasized woman's moral power. "Woman's influence is truly kingly in general society. It is powerful in a daughter and a sister; but it is the mother who weaves the garlands that flourish in eternity." The gravity of woman's influence went even beyond her own family, for health reformers shared a contemporary belief in the inheritance of acquired characteristics. "For the sake of the race," explained Mary Gove Nichols, "I ask that all be done for woman that can be done, for it is an awful truth that fools are the mothers of fools." James C. Jackson was even more blunt: "God punishes as well as rewards mankind *through woman*. . . . She is appointed to dispense divine retributions as well as divine blessings . . . through her does God visit the iniquities of the father on the children to the third and fourth generations."[42]

Though such attitudes gave women genuine responsibility and power, they also exacted a large measure of anxiety and even guilt. "Women are answerable, in a very large degree," admonished Paulina Wright Davis, "for the imbecilities of disease, mental and bodily, and for the premature deaths prevailing throughout society—for the weakness, wretchedness, and shortness of life—and no remedy will be radical till reformation of life and practice obtains among our sex."[43] Such a psychological burden might well have been unbearable had not health reformers given to women fellowship, moral support, and practical information.

The health reformers' emphasis on educated motherhood and scientific domesticity in a sense helped make middle-class women modern. But being modern did not necessarily mean being equal. If the concept of female moral superiority was a source of *power* for women in the nineteenth century, it cannot be confused with *liberation*.[44] Indeed, it may have merely guaranteed the perpetuation and elaboration of traditional assumptions about mothering and housekeeping in an altered social setting. Full equality for women continued to be undermined by a single-minded concern with woman's maternal role. Even the most feminist of health reformers failed to realize that women would never be equal as long as they remained confined to a sphere—no matter how expansively that sphere was defined.

NOTES

This article grew out of a paper presented at a symposium, "Medicine without Doctors: Home Health Care in American History," sponsored by the Department of the History of Medicine, University of Wisconsin, Madison, April 14, 1975. The author is grateful to Ellen Chesler, Rita Napier, Cliff Griffin, Eric Foner, John Clark, and Martin Pernick for reading and criticizing the manuscript.

1   The most recent treatments of the health reform movement include William B. Walker, "The health reform movement in the United States, 1830–1870," Ph.D. diss., Johns Hopkins, 1955. Richard Shryock, "Sylvester Graham and the Popular Health Movement, 1830–1870," in *Medicine in America, Historical Essays* (Baltimore, 1966), 111–25; John Blake, "Health reform," in *The Rise of Adventism: Religion and Society in Mid-Nineteenth Century America*, ed. E. S. Gaustad (New York, 1974), 30–49; H. E. Hoff and J. Fulton, "The centenary of the first American Physiological Society founded at Boston by William A. Alcott and Sylvester Graham," *Bulletin of the History of Medicine*, 5 (Oct. 1937): 687–734; Stephen Wilner Nissenbaum, "Careful love: Sylvester Graham and the emergence of Victorian sexual theory in America, 1830–1840," Ph.D. diss., University of Wisconsin, 1968; James C. Whorton, "Christian physiology: William Alcott's prescription for the millennium," *Bulletin of the History of Medicine*, 49 (Winter 1975): 466–81. Two lively popular works are James H. Young, *The Toadstool Millionaires: A Social History of Patent Medicines in America before Federal Regulation* (Princeton, 1961), and Gerald Carson, *Cornflake Crusade* (New York, 1967). The public health movement is dealt with in Charles Rosenberg and Carroll Smith-Rosenberg, "Pietism and the origins of the American public health movement: a note on John H. Griscom and Robert W. Hartley," *Journal of the History of Medicine*, 1968, *23:* 16–35; Richard H. Shryock, "The early American public health movement," in *Medicine in America*, 126–38. John Davies skillfully chronicles the phrenology movement in *Phrenology: Fad and Science* (New Haven, 1955).

2   *Water-Cure Journal*, 1849, 7: 18. (Hereafter cited as *WCJ*.) The Seventh-day Adventist publication, the *Health Reformer* claimed 11,000 subscribers in 1868. See Ronald L. Numbers, "Health reform on the Delaware," *New Jersey History* 92 (Sept. 1974): 7.

3   For the convergence of health reform with other reform movements, see Robert S. Fletcher, "Bread and doctrine at Oberlin," *Ohio State Archeological and Historical Quarterly* 49 (Jan. 1940): 58; Sidonia E.

Taupin, "'Christianity in the kitchen,' or a moral guide for gourmets," *American Quarterly*, 1963, *15:* 85–89; Thomas H. LeDuc, "Grahamites and Garrisonites," *New York History* 20 (April 1939): 189–91; Michael Katz, *The Irony of Early School Reform* (Boston, 1968). For a thoughtful and highly provocative recent treatment, see Ronald G. Walters, "The erotic South: civilization and sexuality in American abolitionism," *American Quarterly* 24 (May 1973): 177–201.

4 See Martha Verbrugge, "The Ladies Physiological Institute: health reform and women in ante-bellum Boston," Paper delivered at Third Annual Berkshire Conference on Women's History, Bryn Mawr, June 1976. The one exception to this middle-class analysis may have been the Thomsonians, a health reform sect which has been tentatively linked to working-class elements. I would contend that the Thomsonians do not fall out of the mainstream of the movement I am discussing, because health reform could very well have played a similar role in "modernizing" native American workers in the antebellum period as I will argue it played for the middle class. As Paul Faler and Alan Dawley have recently shown, the internalization of "modern" values often transcended class divisions. See "Working class culture and politics in the industrial revolution: sources of loyalism and rebellion," *Journal of Social History* 9 (June 1976): 466–79. I am indebted to Irene Javors of City College for discussing her preliminary findings on the Thomsonians with me.

5 For the influence of the Enlightenment, see Alice Felt Tyler, *Freedom's Ferment* (New York, 1944). For Christian perfectionism, see James C. Whorton, "'Christian physiology.'" For the decline of heroic therapeutics see Richard H. Shryock, *Medicine and Society in America, 1660–1860* (Ithaca, 1960). For antielitism, see Richard Shryock, "Cults and quackery in American medical history," *Middle States Association of History and Social Studies Teachers Transactions,* 1939, *37:* 19–30.

6 The most recent treatment of modernization in America does not refer to health reform at all. See Richard D. Brown, *Modernization: The Transformation of American Life, 1600–1865* (New York, 1976).

7 The one exception is John Blake's excellent article on Mary Gove Nichols, "Mary Gove Nichols: Prophetess of Health," in this volume.

8 Hoff and Fulton, "Centenary," 701.

9 On changes, particularly in New England, which touched the lives of many in the reform leadership, see the thoughtful introduction by Michael Katz to *The Irony of Early School Reform*. Also Stanley Engerman, ed., *The Reinterpretation of American Economic*

History (New York, 1971); Stephen Thernstrom, *Poverty and Progress* (Cambridge, 1964); Stephen Thernstrom and Richard Sennett, eds., *Nineteenth-Century Cities* (New Haven, 1969). Two recent articles on women and work before industrialization are Joan Scott and Louise Tilly, "Women's work and family in 19th century Europe," *Comparative Studies in History and Society* 17 (Jan. 1975): 36–64; Alice Kessler-Harris, "Stratifying by sex: understanding the history of working women," in *Labor Market Segmentation,* ed. Richard Edwards et. al (Lexington, Mass., 1975). For quote from Frances Dana Gage, see *WCJ,* 1854, *17:* 35.

10 Rev. H. Winslow, "Domestic education in females," *Practical Educator and Journal of Health,* 1847, *1:* 259–61.

11 The concept of the "republican mother," which was given life during the antebellum period, gained momentum through several permutations until progressive era reformers and social workers recast it in the 20th-century notion of "educated motherhood." See Linda Kerber, "Daughters of Columbia: educating women for the republic, 1787–1805," in *The Hofstadter Aegis* ed. Stanley Elkins and Eric McKitrick (New York, 1974), and "The republican mother," Paper read at the Southern Historical Association Meeting, November 1975; Jill Conway, "Perspectives on the history of women's education in the United States," *History of Education Quarterly* 14 (Spring 1974): 1–12. For the progressive period, see Sheila Rothman, "Social history and social policy: the case of women, children & the family," Paper read at the meeting of the Organization of American Historians, April 1976, St. Louis. For an excellent discussion of the social and economic roots of American feminism, particularly the influence of education, see Keith Melder, "The beginnings of the women's rights movement in the United States, 1800–1840," Ph.D. diss., Yale, 1964; Gerda Lerner, "The lady and the mill girl: changes in the status of women in the age of Jackson," *Mid-Continent American Studies Journal* 10 (Spring 1969): 5–15.

12 Catharine Beecher, *Letters to the People on Health and Happiness* (New York, 1856), 7. James C. Jackson, "Shall our girls live or die," *Laws of Life,* 1867, *10:* 2; Mrs. S. M. Estee "To Sick Women," *WCJ,* 1858, *26:*96. See also Augustus K. Gardner, "The physical decline of American women," *WCJ,* 1860, *29:* 21–22, 50–51.

13 Striking evidence for the conviction of many women writers that their grandmothers enjoyed better health can be found in Catharine Beecher, *Housekeeper and Healthkeeper* (New York, 1873), 424–28. Another possible explanation for the increase in complaints is that women were no longer willing to

tolerate their ill health. See also Carroll Smith-Rosenberg, "The hysterical woman: sex roles and role conflict in nineteenth-century America," *Social Research* 39 (Winter 1972): 652–78.

14   *WCJ*, 1854, *15:* 74, 94.

15   Italics mine. *WCJ*, 1855, *20:* 74.

16   *WCJ*, 1853, *15:* 131. See also Harriet Austin, "Woman's present and future," *WCJ*, 1853, *16:* 57.

17   "Woman's dress," *WCJ*, 1851, *11:* 30; "The new costume," *WCJ*, 1851, *12:* 30; "Science and long skirts," *WCJ*, 1855, *20:* 7.

18   *WCJ*, 1853, *16:* 120; 1851, *11:* 96, and passim. Most of the water cure establishments encouraged their female patients to wear reformed dress. Almost every issue of any health reform journal had something about dress: the *Water-Cure Journal* and the *Laws of Life* showed special interest in dress reform; the *Graham Journal* and the *American Vegetarian and Health Journal* less frequently. Dress reform was also a popular topic in women's rights journals like the *Una*, the *Lily*, and later the *Revolution*. Many of the articles in these journals pertaining to dress were written by health reformers. See especially *WCJ*, 1851, *12:* 33, 58; *WCJ*, 1862, *34:* 1–2; *WCJ*, 1853, *15:* 7, 10, 32, 34, 35, 131; *WCJ*, 1852, *13:* 111; *Laws of Life*, 1867, *10:* 93–94, 129–30, 145–46; *Revolution*, 1869, *3:* 149–50; *Graham Journal*, 1839, *3:* 301–2.

19   William A. Alcott, *The Young Mother* (Boston, 1839), 265–66.

20   *WCJ*, 1846, *1:* 29.

21   See "To her sick sisters," *WCJ*, 1858, *26:* 96. "A Bloomer to her sisters," *WCJ*, 1853, *15:* 131. There are many examples. For a possible meaning to this sense of community see Carroll Smith-Rosenberg "The female world of love and ritual: relations between women in 19th century America," in this volume. For Nichols quote, see *A Woman's Work in Water Cure and Sanitary Education* (London, 1874), 14. See also Mary Gove Nichols, "To the women who read the Water Cure Journal," *WCJ*, 1852, *14:* 68: "We do not consider ourselves doctors in the common understanding of the word—though we shall not neglect to do the highest good in this department, but we consider ourselves educators—set apart and qualified by Providence for the work. We will educate men and women for Physicians and Teachers of health, and young women to be wise wives and mothers. We will make the most beneficial impression on the world that is possible to us."

22   See Martha Verbrugge, "Ladies Physiological Institute." Hers is the first local study we have of the rank and file. One suspects others will yield similar conclusions.

23   Chapters on food, cooking, and domestic economy in William A. Alcott, *The Young Housekeeper* (Boston, 1849); *Graham Journal*, "Keep your children clean," 1837, *1:* 176; "Masturbation and its effect on health," 1838, *2:* 23. Mary Gove Nichols, *Lectures to Women on Anatomy and Physiology* (New York, 1846), passim. See also advertisement in the *Graham Journal*, 1838, *2:* 288. For articles on fresh air and bathing: *WCJ*, 1847, *4:* 161–68, 177; *WCJ*, 1847, *4:* 193; pregnancy, exercise and childbirth: *WCJ*, 1847, *3:* 145, 151, 183–84; "Our new cookbook," "How to can a fruit," *Laws of Life*, 1867, *10:* 12; "Cleanliness and healthfulness," *Laws of Life*, 1867, *10:* 16; "Teething and its management," "Children's dress," *WCJ*, 1851, *12:* 101, 104, Martha Verbrugge has emphasized this practical dimension of the health reform program. She contends that the Ladies' Physiological Institute helped ordinary middle-class women adjust to the opportunities and the limitations imposed on them by modern life. Verbrugge is impressed less with the radical elements of the Boston group and more with the organization's goal of easing women into traditional role patterns potentially disturbed by changing social conditions. Her study is significant because it suggests that health reform appealed to several different types of women. She argues, for example, that only a small minority of the members of the Boston society were outspoken feminists. See Verbrugge, "Ladies Physiological Institute."

24   Thomas Low Nichols, *The Curse Removed: The Efficacy of Water-Cure in the Treatment of Uterine Disease and the Removal of the Pains and Perils of Pregnancy and Childbirth*, (New York, 1850), 13; R. T. Trall, "Allopathic midwifery," *WCJ*, 1850, *9:* 121; Mary Gove Nichols, "Maternity and the water cure for infants," *WCJ*, 1851, *11:* 57–59. Eliza de la Vergue, M.D., "Infants, their improper nursing and medication," *WCJ*, 1855, *20*.

25   See an interesting autobiographical sketch by Mrs. Mary A. Torbit, "Reasons for becoming a lecturer," *WCJ*, 1851, *14:* 91. One of the health reformers' favorite arguments—that women had natural abilities to cure—led them to a desire to teach women medicine. Indeed, the entrance of women into the medical profession grew out of the cult of scientific domesticity popularized by the health reform movement. Reformers applauded the acceptance of women as medical students, chiding the regulars for their conservatism. In time these early female pioneers, who entered medicine convinced of their natural abilities, would be transformed into full-fledged professionals by their contact with an increasingly scientific and empirical discipline. They

became exposed to a more modern system of values, their outlook permanently altered in the process. See Regina Markell Morantz, "Daughters of Aesculapius: the entrance of women into the medical profession in 19th century America, ideology and social setting," Paper delivered at Women Historians of the Midwest Conference, Minneapolis, October 1975.

26 Indeed, the attitude of health reformers toward the relations between the sexes was innovative. They preached a version of companionate marriage. See Morantz, "Health reform and women: an ideology of self help," Paper presented at the symposium "Medicine without doctors, home health care in American history," Department of the History of Medicine, University of Wisconsin, Madison, April 14, 1975.

27 Henry G. Wright, *Marriage and Parentage* (Boston, 1855; Arno reprint, 1974), 5.

28 Ibid., 91, 257. See also Orson Fowler, *Love and Parentage* (New York, 1847), 272–74, passim. See Linda Gordon, "Voluntary motherhood: the beginnings of feminist birth control ideas in the United States," in this volume. Not all advisors proscribed sexual intercourse without procreation. However all agreed that coitus should be approached with caution. Mechanical means of contraception were an anathema because such methods degraded women by encouraging overindulgence.

29 Wright, *Marriage and Parentage.*

30 See Eliza B. Duffey, *The Relations of the Sexes* (New York, 1879), especially chap. 13, "The limitation of offspring."

31 Although Carl Degler has rightly pointed out that at least some women did have orgasms in the 19th century, a fact which it would be silly to dispute, I would suggest that female orgasm was inherently more problematical than that of the male, and that the 19th century was generally ignorant of the more subtle nature of female sexual response. Marriage counselors in the 1920s and 1930s documented this widespread ignorance and tried to correct it. Alfred Kinsey's statistics show a gradual increase in the number of married women achieving orgasm in the years after 1900. Carroll Smith-Rosenberg has examined possible differences in male and female approaches to sexuality in the 19th century in greater detail in a recent paper, "A gentle and a richer sex: female perspectives on nineteenth century sexuality," Third Berkshire Conference on Women's History, Bryn Mawr, June 1976. See also Regina Markell Morantz, "The scientist as sex crusader: Alfred Kinsey and American culture," *American Quarterly* (Fall 1977). See Duffey, *Relations of the sexes,* chap.

13. It should be pointed out that most health reformers were also eugenicists. See Henry G. Wright, *The Empire of the Mother over the Character and Destiny of the Race* (Boston, 1863).

32 Moreover, social reformers of all types recognized that large families hampered upward mobility. The reputation of the Irish for their alleged indulgence of the sensual passions was widespread. They had nothing but "large," "dirty" families to show for it: "Did wealth consist in children," asserted the *Common School Journal,* "it is well known, that the Irish would be a rich people; and if the old Roman law prevailed here, which granted special privilege to every man who had more than three, this people would be elevated into an aristocracy." Quoted in Katz, *The Irony of Early School Reform,* 123. Many of the early school reformers, including Horace Mann, had a lively interest in health reform. Largely because of this interest the Massachusetts legislature passed a law in 1850 requiring physiological instruction in the schools.

33 Nichols, *Lectures to Women,* 20. Marie Louise Shew, *Water Cure for Ladies,* Preface, iii. See Charles Rosenberg, *The Cholera Years* (Chicago, 1962).

34 See Christopher Lasch on the problems of the modernization model in the first of three articles on the historiography of the family in *New York Review of Books,* Nov. 13, 1975.

35 James T. Fawcett, "Modernization, individual modernity, and fertility," in *Studies in the Psychology of Population,* ed. J. T. Fawcett (New York, 1973); Alex Inkeles, "The modernization of man," in *Modernization: The Dynamics of Growth* (New York, 1966), 138–150, and "Making men modern: on the causes and consequences of individual change in six developing countries," *American Journal of Sociology,* 1969, *75:* 208–25; also Richard D. Brown, "Modernization and the modern personality in America, 1600–1865," *Journal of Interdisciplinary History,* 1972, *2:* 201–27.

36 See for example, David J. Rothman, *The Discovery of the Asylum* (Boston, 1971).

37 "Excessive application: a cause of insanity," *Monthly Miscellany and Journal of Health,* 1846, *1:* 212. See also Barbara Sicherman, "Paradox of prudence: mental health in the gilded age," *Journal of American History* 62 (Mar. 1976), 890–912.

38 For other discussions of this personality type, see Peter Cominos, "Late Victorian respectability and the social system," *International Review of Social History,* 1963, *8:* 18–48, 216–50; Herbert Gutman, "Work, culture, and society in industrializing America," *American Historical Review* 78 (June 1973): 531–587; Michael Katz, *The Irony of Early School Re-*

form; Alan Dawley and Paul Faler, "Working class culture and politics in the industrial revolution."

39 "Looking . . . at the social habits of the working people in some of our densely populated districts, it does indeed appear a hopeless effort to attack their vices, unless one could at the same time pull down their houses, and build them others adapted to a more perfect state of bodily and mental health," "Sanitary and social reform coeval," by Mrs. Ellis in *Practical Educator and Journal of Health,* 1847, *1:* 354–55. Charles Rosenberg has made this same point in connection with 19th-century prescriptions for male sexual purity. See "Sexuality, Class, and Role in Nineteenth-Century America," *American Quarterly* 25 (May 1973): 131–53; also William Coleman, "Health and hygiene in the Encylopedie: a medical doctrine for the bourgeoisie," *Journal of the History of Medicine* 29 (Oct. 1974), 339–412, applies a similar argument to the French bourgeoisie. See S. Weir Mitchell, "So great is my reverence for supreme wholesomeness, that I should almost be tempted to assert that perfect health is virtue." *Address on Opening of the Institute of Hygiene of the University of Pennsylvania,* Philadelphia, 1892, 4. A few health reformers merged the moral injunction to "guard the health of the race" with overt nativism. "Already," warned James C. Jackson,

> the decay of our women and the delicate constitutions of our young men are forcing the latter to seek revitalization by intermarriage with immigrant women from Europe. What with the decline of the Puritan and Cavalier stock on the one hand, and the great influx of foreign born on the other, it is not difficult to predict *our future.* In less than fifty years the New England type of manhood will have ceased to govern this Republic, and when once it ceases to govern it will cease to exist. . . . *Nothing but a bold and faithful advocacy of the laws of health can stop this ebbtide of human life.*

See *WCJ,* 1858, *26:* 4.

40 See James T. Fawcett, "Modernization, individual modernity, and fertility." Also see Robert V. Wells, "Family history and demographic transition," *Journal of Social History* 9 (Fall 1975), 1–20.

41 It should be pointed out that the domestic ideal had very different effects on working-class women. By encouraging them to aspire to an often impossible goal, the cult of domesticity helped keep married women out of the work force, or at least aspiring to be idle. This insured that working women would often be undependable allies in labor disputes. Believing that their primary commitment should be to the family, they accepted low-pay and low-status jobs, viewing their situation as only temporary. See Alice Kessler-Harris, "Stratifying by sex." The domestic ideology also increased women's perceptions of class differences among themselves. Middle-class women were often advised to be cautious about the health of hired servants. Advice literature warned of the dangers of immigrant girls' infecting the household. I am indebted to my colleague David Katzman for this information. For a stimulating discussion of the middle-class English woman's involvement in health reform, see Patricia Branca, *Silent Sisterhood: Middle Class Women in the Victorian Home* (Pittsburgh, 1976), especially pts. II and III. Branca argues that middle-class Victorian women were the first large group to establish a modern outlook toward life and death.

42 William Alcott, *The Young Wife* (Boston, 1837), 87–89; *Lily,* 1849, *1:* 52; Nichols, *Lectures to Women,* 212, and "Woman the physician," *WCJ,* 1851, *12:* 75; Jackson, "The women of the United States," *WCJ,* 1858, *26:* 3, and "Women's rights," *WCJ,* 1861, *31:* 61. For an excellent summary of hereditarian views in this period, see Charles Rosenberg, "The bitter fruit: heredity, disease, and social thought in nineteenth century America," *Perspectives in American History,* 1974, 7: 189–238.

43 *WCJ,* 1846, *1:* 29.

44 See Christopher Lasch, "The woman reformers' rebuke," in *The World of Nations* (New York, 1974).

25

Mary Gove Nichols, Prophetess of Health

JOHN B. BLAKE

"Happiness writes no story," wrote Robert Latou Dickinson.[1] In the unhappy childhood and marriage of Mary Gove Nichols may be found the origin of her own intensely personal autobiography, and of her revolt against the morals, customs, and laws of her day governing the status of women. "My mother told me often," she wrote, "that I was a fright; that my skin was yellow as a squash, my nose large enough for two, and that my eyes were not mates."[2] Constantly compared with her beautiful and popular older sister, rejected by her mother, Mary as a child withdrew into her own world of books and dreams. In chronic poor health and married at an early age to an opinionated, greedy dolt, Mary as a woman devoted her soul to promoting the health of women through education and liberation from the tyrannies of marriage.

Mary Sargeant Neal was born August 10, 1810, in Goffstown, New Hampshire, the second daughter and third child of William A. and Rebecca R. Neal, of Scottish and Welsh ancestry. About 1822, after the death of her favored older sister, the family moved to Craftsbury, Vermont, where they lived until after Mary's marriage.

Unlike her mother, who found virtue only in work, Mary's father was a strong partisan Democrat, who liked a good argument, and a "free thinker" who read such scandalous scribblers as Voltaire and Thomas Paine. He first sent Mary to school at the age of two with an "ancient Scottish maiden lady." At the age of five she went to the head of the class in spelling, and by the age of six she had read Plutarch. Mary continued in school about six or seven months of the year until the

family moved to Craftsbury, and thereafter sporadically. More decisive than this scant schooling was an ardent desire to learn and to do good, coupled with a religious, mystical bent. A shy and lonely child—"As odd as Mary Neal" was a neighborhood byword—able to express her capacity for love only to a succession of pets, she yet received kindly encouragement from adult book-loving friends. About the age of fifteen she underwent a sudden religious experience. A year later she borrowed a book on Quakers which told of prisons and persecutions. Little realizing that Quakers had changed since the reign of Charles II and wanting to love, worship, and believe, she combed back her now luxuriant brown curls, removed all ornament, and adopted plain dress. Only with time and experience did she learn that members of the sect to which her books had converted her were, like other human beings, subject to such failings as pride, vanity, and covetousness.

A voracious reader, Mary devoured as varied an assortment of volumes as she could find or borrow. Among these, at first by chance, were the *Anatomy* of John and Charles Bell and a number of other medical works; these she pursued in secret until she chanced to correct her medical student brother. Forced to give up studies so improper for one of her sex, she turned to Latin and French. By the time she was seventeen, Mary was writing stories and essays for newspapers and magazines. She began teaching, and the school board was pleased. Conscious at last of doing her part for the general weal, and enjoying it, her health and spirits soared.[3]

If Mary had not married, or if she had married happily, she might well have settled down as a successful teacher known only to her pupils and as a minor—a very minor—New England essayist and poet. But in 1830, on a visit to her uncle, he introduced her to Hiram Gove, of Weare, New Hamp-

JOHN B. BLAKE is Scholar in Residence, History of Medicine Division, National Library of Medicine, Bethesda, Maryland.

Reprinted with permission from *American Philosophical Society Proceedings* 106 (1962): 219–234.

shire, a Quaker with a mind to get married. Knowing as much about courtship and love as she had known about Quakers, Mary was persuaded to accept his persistent proposals. In a sense, Hiram was an apt teacher. Even before the wedding day Mary longed for the release of death, and only the certainty of eternal damnation as the consequence kept her from breaking her vow. The marriage took place on March 5, 1831. Their first child, Elma Penn, born March 1, 1832, lived to adulthood; four subsequent pregnancies were abortive or stillborn. A failure at his trade, Gove lived off his wife's desperate needlework and forbade her to spend a cent without his niggardly permission. When she became too fond of letters from a brother she adored, Gove burned them. Ignorant, tyrannical, jealous, and mean, Gove quickly taught Mary that marriage without love made each hour "an eternity of misery."[4]

Despite, or perhaps because of, her mental and physical suffering, which doctors could never assuage, Mary Gove returned to her medical reading until it possessed her with a "passion." A "Book of Health" which she read in 1832 and the works of John Mason Good convinced her of the virtues of cold water, and in 1832 she began using it therapeutically with occasional women patients. Though Elizabeth Blackwell had yet to breach the barrier against women in medicine, a number of friendly physicians aided Mary's pursuit of knowledge in books and even in pathological museums. "Kindness from the medical profession and the manifestation of a helpful disposition towards my undertakings," wrote Mrs. Gove, "were everywhere the rule."[5]

About 1837 the Goves moved from Weare to Lynn, Massachusetts, where Mary, prevailing over her husband's initial opposition, again took up teaching. Then she discovered the works of Sylvester Graham, who was at the height of his career in diet reform and whom Mary regarded as "one of the greatest benefactors the world ever had." Seeing herself surrounded by sin and ever anxious to do good, she was imbued with the true spirit of hygienic reform, an ardent ambition to teach others the way of moral and physical salvation through knowledge of physiology and the laws of health. At first she began lecturing on anatomy and physiology to a female lyceum in Lynn and to the pupils in her school. By March 1838, her young ladies were boarding "on the Graham system."[6]

In Boston, meanwhile, Dr. William Andruss Alcott, who had for years been promoting popular health knowledge, joined with a group of Grahamites in February 1837 to launch the American Physiological Society, for monthly meetings and popular lectures. Its unofficial organ was the new *Graham Journal.* By learning, experience, and temperament, Mrs. Gove was prepared as no one else to fill the quickly felt need for a woman to lecture to the ladies of the society on subjects too delicate for mixed audiences. Sponsored by a new Ladies Physiological Society, she presented her first course of lectures for ladies in Boston in the fall of 1838. A number of women would be presenting similar lectures in the 1840s, but Mrs. Gove was apparently the first to undertake this bold endeavor.[7]

The lectures were a success beyond all expectation. "Mrs. Gove is found to be very capable of giving instruction on the topics she has introduced," the *Graham Journal* commented staidly, "and as we are informed, is very acceptable in her manner as a lecturer." The professors of Harvard Medical School provided drawings and preparations and spoke "very encouragingly of the undertaking." Great must have been the interest when Mrs. Gove exhibited a skeleton "with the heart, arteries, &c. entire and injected." Her audience averaged four to five hundred at each lecture and the *Graham Journal* published synopses of them all, except, "of course," the tenth and eleventh, which were given to unmarried and married ladies separately. When Mrs. Gove repeated free her lecture on tight lacing, the crowd numbered no less than two thousand. As a testimonial of their respect, the ladies, at the close of the course, presented Mrs. Gove with a fine English silver watch, thinking gold too showy for a member of the Society of Friends. (Hiram considered it handsome enough, even so, to take it for his own.) Evidently she had found her calling. In December and January, Mrs. Gove repeated her course in Boston, Lynn, Haverhill, Providence, and New York, often to audiences with standing room only. The opportunity to stand at the door and pocket the fees seems to have reconciled Hiram to his wife's unseemly activities.[8]

Even aside from Mrs. Gove's abilities as a speaker, the causes of her success are not far to seek. For one thing, lectures were at that time a very popular form of entertainment,[9] and occasional lectures on health by men had helped to pave the way.[10] The 1830s and 1840s were a period of innumerable enthusiastic "causes," hopefully intended to reform everything from specific abuses like prison conditions or the treatment of the insane to the entire basis of society. In this respect, health reform conformed to the spirit of the age, partaking even in the same methods of enthusiastic public speakers, local and national societies, and a profusion of generally ephemeral journals. Moreover, at this very time European clinical-pathological research was showing the uselessness—the harm even—of much traditional therapy without offering as yet any effective replacement. The classic expression of this trend is the oft-quoted remark of Oliver Wendell Holmes in 1860 that "if the whole materia medica, *as now used*, could be sunk to the bottom of the sea, it would be all the better for mankind,—and all the worse for the fishes."[11] Therapeutic nihilism, however, seems to have been a luxury indulged in by relatively few physicians. For the tens or hundreds who turned to quacks or irregulars because the best physicians acknowledged the limitations of their art, there were thousands who turned away from the general run of poorly educated American practitioners because they continued relentlessly to prescribe mercurials, opiates, and bloodletting as taught by their teachers who were taught by Benjamin Rush. Most Americans, it is safe to say, knew little of French clinical research. But Jacksonian democracy made them suspicious of pretenders to exclusive learning or supporters of a monopolistic profession. Deathly sick of calomel, they turned in droves to the minute doses of homeopathy, the "vegetable" drugs of the Thomsonians and Eclectics, or the pure cold water of the hydropaths. Others turned to prevention—the more conservative, like Lemuel Shattuck, to state action, the more radical to individual, moralistic reform. Among the latter, Mary Gove, who had experienced too often during her sickly childhood the effects of blue pills and bloodletting,[12] was a leader. Many were prepared to attend her call.[13]

Praise for Mrs. Gove's efforts was not universal. She was promptly denounced by other Friends and eventually departed the society.[14] Newspaper editors whose moral sense, in the eyes of the *Lobelian, and Rhode Island Medical Review,* was "so blunted as to be incapable of seeing the difference between gratuitous obscenity and physiological truth," also denounced her lectures,[15] and in truth her remarks on the "solitary vice" and the evil effects of excessive indulgence in "amativeness" must have shocked many contemporary sensibilities. The strain of this opposition and of traveling and speaking told on her strength, and late in 1838, in the midst of a lecture, she was attacked by a severe pulmonary hemorrhage. Her thought was for her work.

> The darkness that then shrouded the land on the subjects of health and disease was palpable, [she later wrote] and I felt the importance of my mission to be in proportion to the evils I sought to remove. The thought of leaving my mission unfulfilled, of leaving woman to suffer and die under the black pall of ignorance that enveloped her then, was more than I could bear.

Convinced that she would "yet have a *name* and a *place* among the benefactors of our race," she was sustained by that sense of mission which welcomes the martyr's crown.[16]

Despite her sickness and collapse in the fall of 1838, Mrs. Gove was soon lecturing and writing again. She had published her lecture on the "solitary vice" in 1839,[17] and a number of articles—anonymously, because she was a woman—in the *Boston Medical and Surgical Journal.* Early in 1840 she moved to Worcester to edit the *Worcester Health Journal and Advocate of Physiological Reform,* a successor to the defunct *Graham Journal,* and prepare her lectures for the press. Publication of the latter was delayed while she looked for some way to keep her husband from garnering the profits and in November, needing the money, she gave up the *Journal* to concentrate on her more remunerative lecturing. With increasing boldness she spoke before a mixed audience in Philadelphia on the evils of tight lacing. "My tongue clave to the roof of my mouth," she wrote in her diary. "I trembled and grew sick at heart, but I rallied, and went through my lecture, my friends assured me, very well."[18] Mrs. Gove's *Lectures to Ladies on Anatomy and Physiology* was finally published by Saxton and Pierce in Boston early in 1842. In Dr. Alcott's phrase the book had "merit enough, at any rate, to excite opposition," and it received qualified support, except for its idolization of Graham, from even the *Boston Medical and Surgical Journal.*[19]

Blaming ignorance for most of women's ills, Mrs. Gove conceived her mission in life to be teaching women the rules of health in order to relieve them of a crushing burden of physical and mental suffering. To this end she advocated a Grahamite regimen and plain diet, including plenty of fresh air and exercise, cleanliness and daily cold bathing, whole wheat bread, and abstinence from flesh, tea, coffee, and alcohol. She inveighed repeatedly against the widespread use of opium and other powerful drugs, the ignorance that fostered quackery, and the evils of fashionable dress. Attributing her own ill health to tight lacing in her youth, she urged others to "loosen the death grasp of the corset, and send the now imprisoned and poisoned blood rejoicing through the veins of woman."[20]

Following Graham's *Lecture to Young Men on Chastity,* Mrs. Gove leveled some of her heaviest guns against the "solitary vice." Quoting liberally from the annual reports of the Worcester State Lunatic Hospital, she warned against masturbation as a major cause of insanity—a not uncommon theme in American psychiatry at that time—and of a host of other diseases. But fortunately such insanity, although incurable, could be prevented by timely moral instruction and a hygienic mode of life. Whatever others might think, Mrs. Gove was determined to speak plainly of the evils that threatened the children of heedless mothers. "I believe," wrote one of Mrs. Gove's auditors, "you are engaged in an important and holy work." Undoubtedly she felt so herself.[21]

Deploring the notion that Grahamism stood merely for a no-meat diet, Mary Gove took the broad view that physiological education and reform were destined to set women free. A call to loosen tight-laced stays was not aimed solely at the wasp-waist of fashion: "will our countrywomen," she asked, "ever be such servile slaves to customs they might reform? . . . Will not American females rise in the full vigor of intellectual majesty, and hunt from society constraint and compression, and the untold anguish they produce?"[22] She was becoming deeply interested in many women's rights, advocating in a Baltimore lecture in 1841 property

for married women, general education, and freedom of thought and action.[23] She knew from experience the gross inequity of the married woman's status before the law and in public opinion.

Added to her ill health was the increasing torment of life with Hiram. When she first asked for a separation soon after she began lecturing, Hiram threatened to destroy her reputation and take away her child, coldly and correctly pointing out that the law offered her no redress. Only after a long struggle to free herself from the accepted views of a woman's duty could Mary bring herself to leave her husband. Only when her father threatened in 1842 to sue Hiram for money lent him at various times was she free from his demands and fear for her child.[24] Even so, in the spring of 1845, after her father died, Hiram seized their child and held her for three months until some friends of the mother, finding no legal solution, spirited the daughter back. The climactic experience of her marriage, it was to cost her dearly in subsequent lawsuits as well as in peace of mind.[25]

Strongly as Mary felt in 1842 about physiological reform and the sin of a loveless marriage, the day was not far off when one Henry Gardiner Wright would open her mind and heart to new visions as no man had before. In 1838 James Pierrepont Greaves, an English educational reformer, had organized a school near London named in honor of Amos Bronson Alcott, whose educational experiments in Boston he greatly admired. Visiting England in 1842, Alcott met Henry Wright, the teacher at the school, and was soon "knit to him by more than human ties." He had "more genius for teaching," Alcott wrote, than anyone he knew. The group at Alcott House observed strict temperance in diet and regimen. Wright was co-editor of a journal called the *Healthian,* and the works of Sylvester Graham held an honored place on the library shelf.[26]

Alcott returned to Boston and Concord in October, bringing Wright and Charles Lane, also of Alcott House, with the intention of establishing an ideal community. A few months later Wright bowed out. His asceticism was not equal to Lane's, for whom brown bread and water were a sufficient diet, nor was his joy in manual toil equal to Alcott's.[27] Besides, he met Mary Gove at a lyceum picnic. Each discovering that the other ate only "beautiful food," they felt immediate spiritual kinship; that evening Mr. Wright came to call. Love, Mary later wrote, was "that day born in my heart, in a divine full-ness." Soon Wright was installed as a boarder in her parents' home in Lynn and Mary put curtains in the windows so neighborhood gossips could not see them holding hands. Her association with Wright drew Mary increasingly deep into reform-ist circles. From him she also learned that "the heavens were opened to mortals through love." Bronson Alcott and Lane went ahead during the summer of 1843 with their famous if short-lived community "Fruitlands," without Wright. In poor health, he recrossed the Atlantic in the fall, des-tined to die after a few short years. If Mrs. Gove ever knew he had a wife in England, she did not mention it in her autobiography.[28]

While teaching Mrs. Gove the meaning of love, Wright, an experienced contributor to reform journals, also assisted her in launching the *Health Journal, and Independent Magazine* as a successor to both the *Worcester Health Journal* and the *Healthian.* The first issue contained a variety of literary and "physiological" fare, including contributions from John Neal and Horace Greeley. Editorially, the new *Journal* stood foursquare for reform, promising "to discuss faithfully and fearlessly all questions and subjects that concern the great brotherhood of Man," including the

> regenerating power of Love, the Pharisaism of the age, the Tyranny of Public Opinion, the right of every Human Being to freedom of Thought and Action, the Divine nature of Marriage, . . . the Laws of Health, the Reor-ganization of Society or the Doctrine of As-sociation and the restoration of all things to the Divine order.[29]

Fortunately or unfortunately, the first issue of the *Independent Magazine* was also the last.

Wright also introduced Mrs. Gove to the work of the Silesian peasant Vincent Priessnitz and his theory of the water cure. Heretofore she had ad-vocated cold bathing as a hygienic measure and had used cold water in the treatment of fevers and some other diseases. Wright persuaded her that hydrotherapy was the proper treatment for all ail-ments.[30] After his departure, and more than a year lost in sickness and those harrowing months when Hiram abducted their child, she went in June 1845 to Dr. Robert Wesselhoeft's new water cure estab-lishment in Brattleboro, Vermont. Confident that

water cure promised a wider field of usefulness than lecturing, as well as a larger income, she spent three months observing his practice, and, as al-ways, lecturing to ladies. She then served as resi-dent physician for women at another new water cure house in Lebanon Springs, New York. But again her health failed, and in December she moved to New York. After a few weeks at Dr. Joel Shew's water cure house, she began seeing patients and giving lectures, illustrated now by a "splendid" manikin from Paris. In May 1846, she established her own water cure house, on Tenth Street in New York.[31]

The use of water in therapy has an ancient and honorable history extending back to antiquity, but its elevation to the level of a panacea was primarily the work of Priessnitz. Like a number of eminently respectable eighteenth-century systems, including that of Benjamin Rush, it was based on a monistic pathology and therapeutics. Indeed, the theories adopted by Mrs. Gove and her methods of treat-ment—which were largely derivative—are as logi-cal and as well supported by evidence as those so confidently espoused by Rush. Hydropathy, like homeopathy, lost caste because it came too late. By mid-nineteenth century a monistic pathology was no longer acceptable to well-educated medical minds.[32]

According to Mary Gove, health of body and mind resulted from balanced and legitimate action of the vital powers belonging to each faculty or passion; evil and disease resulted from action that was excessive, erratic, and unbalanced. Excessive action of a faculty wasted the vital energy, or ner-vous power. Indulgence in sources of false en-ergy—such as overeating, alcohol, opium, and other drugs—only induced further excessive action and waste of vital powers, leading to exhaustion of the nervous system and collapse of the vascular sys-tem. As the cause of disease was a deficiency of vital energy, restoration was the cure. But how? "We have reason to believe," she answered, "that there is an electricity or force in water which unites with the heat of the human system, when the water is properly applied, and that vital power, or life, is the result." Hydrotherapy, in Mrs. Gove's view, as-sisted the body to rid itself of a load of morbid matter (for example, the poisonous drugs of "al-lopathic" doctors) and simultaneously restored the vital energy. "Facts prove . . . ," she wrote, "that all curable diseases may be cured by water." "Truth is always simple. The cause of disease is one."[33]

The techniques of water cure were various. The patient might be wrapped in a wet sheet and then, perhaps, given a rubbing. There were foot baths, head baths, half baths, and plunge baths, and vaginal and rectal injections. The sitz bath—a powerful method subject to abuse—acted "almost miraculously" in "spinal affections, . . . female weaknesses, and piles." The douche, a stream of water as thick as the wrist projected from a height of ten to twenty feet, was considered a "powerful means of moving bad humors," but, cautioned Mrs. Gove, it must be used with care: "It may knock the patient down. . . ."[34]

Once established in New York, Mrs. Gove soon became a successful water cure physician. While continuing her lectures to classes of ladies, she also attended the sick in their homes or in her own establishment, including boarders from as far as Kentucky. During the first four years of her practice, so she claimed, only two patients died.[35]

Content at the age of eighteen to teach ordinary school, fired in 1837 with an ardent desire to teach health reform, Mrs. Gove now enlarged her mission to include the establishment of Woman as Physician. She had considered the calling unsuitable for her sex so long as it was thought necessary "to bleed and poison people into health." But the methods and philosophy of water cure—learned from Wright along with the divinity of love—entirely changed her views. Water cure, to Mrs. Gove, became "love and truth cure." Children who had been poisoned by medicines and given up to die were brought to her and saved. Mary, it will be remembered, had suffered the agonies of four successive stillbirths in a hateful marriage, but "Mothers who loved in loving union, and obeyed the health-laws which I taught them, obtained immunity from suffering," and were delivered of radiantly healthy babes. To become a physician, and to teach other women to become physicians, became a sacred duty.

> It was like rolling the stone away from the door of the tomb of Love incarnated in woman. It was the last atonement that I had to make in the world of duty, and the opening up of a way for me, and for many of my sisters, to come into a world of attraction—

that new heaven and new earth wherein dwelleth righteousness.

There was, moreover, as Mrs. Gove pointed out in a more sober moment, a certain delicacy and decency in women doctors for their own sex; many women were not willing to expose themselves to examination by a male practitioner. This fact alone, considering the general prevalence of women's diseases, opened up a broad field of usefulness for the sex.[36]

Deep devotion and self-education were necessary: there were no schools to teach women to be physicians. She herself, wrote Mrs. Gove, had met much opposition, both to water cure as a system of practice and to herself as a woman. But she had an important truth to tell and she would be heard. She decided to take pupils willing to "grapple with iron prejudice," and before long several "brave and true women" had determined to follow in her footsteps and qualify themselves as water cure physicians.[37]

Mrs. Gove, as we have seen, had long since joined the circle of reformists, through her lecture tours and her alliance with Henry Wright. Moreover, she had never completely given up her taste for purely literary composition. Her first desperately needed income after reaching New York was fifteen dollars for some stories previously published in *Godey's Lady's Book*, under the pseudonym, "Miss Mary Orme." These betray a certain repetitive quality: in each the ultimate degradation of the beautiful but vain female who marries for wealth or social position or the joy of conquest is contrasted with a true-love marriage between usually poor but invariably honest hearts.[38] Soon after, she sold an article to the *Democratic Review* and then, for the grand sum of one hundred dollars, a novel, *Uncle John; or, "It Is Too Much Trouble,"* which Harper published in April 1846. Its theme differs little from the stories she had written before.[39] She also republished her *Lectures to Ladies* with an appendix on water cure and began contributing to the *Water-Cure Journal* and other magazines. The editor of *Godey's*, Mrs. Sarah J. Hale, did not pay as much or as promptly as Mrs. Gove would have liked, but she noticed *Uncle John* as "a very entertaining and well-written story" and supported the *Lectures* as "a work which cannot be too earnestly commended to the attention of the mothers of America." Such praise from the arbiter of correct taste and fashion was worth more to a "compromised" woman than a few additional dollars. In 1849 she published two more novels. *Agnes Morris; or, The Heroine of Domestic Life,* and *The Two Loves; or, Eros and Anteros.*[40]

Under the spell of Mrs. Gove's literary reputation, reformist sympathies, and evident charm, her water cure house soon became "a general depot of Ultraisms in thought." A variety of writers, philosophers, musicians, and artists, believers all in cold bathing, exercise, and a vegetable diet, found a home there, along with her pupils and patients. Regular Saturday evening gatherings attracted additional talent, ranging from Edgar Allen Poe reciting "The Raven" to Albert Brisbane discoursing on Fourier. Several times during her first year in New York she visited Poe at the Fordham cottage where his wife lay dying, and she induced some friends to give him their help. Her account of these visits, published later in the *Six Penny Magazine* and reprinted in 1931, has often been quoted.[41] Poe, on his part, in his series "The Literati of New York City," in *Godey's Lady's Book* in July 1846, summed Mrs. Gove up thus:

> Mrs. Mary Gove, under the pseudonym of "Mary Orme," has written many excellent papers for the magazines. Her subjects are usually tinctured with the mysticism of the transcendentalists, but are truly imaginative. Her style is quite remarkable for its luminousness and precision—two qualities very rare with her sex. An article entitled "The Gift of Prophecy," published originally in "The Broadway Journal," is a fine specimen of her manner.
>
> Mrs. Gove, however, has acquired less notoriety by her literary compositions than by her lectures on physiology to classes of females. These lectures are said to have been instructive and useful; they certainly elicited much attention. Mrs. G. has also given public discourses on Mesmerism, I believe, and other similar themes—matters which put to the severest test the credulity or, more properly, the faith of mankind. She is, I think, a Mesmerist, a Swedenborgian, a phrenologist, a homœopathist, and a disciple of Priessnitz—what more I am not prepared to say.

> She is rather below the medium height, somewhat thin, with dark hair and keen, intelligent black eyes. She converses well and with enthusiasm. In many respects a very interesting woman.[42]

On Christmas Eve, 1847, Mary Gove met a young writer whose works she had admired, Thomas Low Nichols. She was disappointed at first sight, but soon there grew between them "a divine passion—the love of two human souls," all clearly related in Mary's autobiography. Providentially Hiram Gove, anxious to marry another, just at this time secured a divorce, leaving Mary free. On July 29, 1848, Thomas and Mary were married by a Swedenborgian clergyman.[43]

After their marriage Mrs. Nichols continued her lectures, illustrating them now by hundreds of wax and papier mâché models, which offered an opportunity "for scientific study and practical improvement" such as had "never before been opened to women." She also continued writing, including a volume, *Experience in Water-Cure* (1849), and practicing, restoring to life "a child supposed to be dead."[44] Thomas Nichols meanwhile was qualifying himself as a physician. Some fifteen years earlier he had studied medicine at Dartmouth, without completing the course. Moving west, he had then edited a newspaper in Buffalo and been thrown in jail for his frank appraisal of the local boss. Continuing his journalistic career, he had moved to New York City, where his advanced views on women's rights had attracted the attention of Mary Gove. Inspired by her "thorough understanding . . . remarkable philosophic powers . . . clear judgment . . . [and] remarkable intuition" as well as her miraculous cures, he took up the serious study of hydropathy. For a basic scientific education—and to learn from "the very errors and absurdities" of regular medicine—he returned to medical school, graduating from New York University with a medical degree in 1850. In the spring of that year Dr. and Mrs. Nichols opened a new and more elaborate water cure establishment at 87 West 22d Street, near Sixth Avenue.[45] With his long experience as a writer and editor, Nicholas quickly blossomed as a leading contributor to the *Water-Cure Journal*. In November 1850 was born their first (and only) child, Mary Wilhelmina, who died of bronchitis at the age of thirteen. In contrast to her experience as

Hiram's wife, Mary suffered only slightly, her labor being "a labor of love for a beautiful daughter." She was confined to her room one day and after the fourth was again seeing patients. Natural childbirth and early ambulation were cardinal points of Mrs. Nichols's obstetric practice.[46]

While Mary sought the salvation of her sex, Thomas from the beginning of their joint career went after higher stakes. He would be satisfied with nothing less than the salvation of all mankind. Water cure, in Dr. Nichols's view, was "the foundation of reforms." Like the sick man, the "sick world" must first regain its health, and with it "vigor, clear-sightedness, and a capacity for all other reforms." Just as the water cure washed out a man's "moral ailments" along with the physical diseases on which they depended, so health reform was "the best means for the renovation of human society."[47]

Ever an active and ardent advocate, Nichols reported favorably on the declaration of the American Vegetarian Convention in May 1850, that vegetarianism "unfolds the universal law of man's being . . . and . . . is the inlet to a new and holier life." A month later he was elected secretary of the newly formed American Hygienic and Hydropathic Association of Physicians and Surgeons. In July 1850, he appointed himself general agent and permanent secretary of the Society of Public Health, which he had established to arouse the public to the need for health reform, and invited contributions. In September, the American Vegetarian Society at its first annual meeting elected Nichols one of nine vice-presidents.[48] As another way to free women, dress reform also claimed the Nicholses' attention, Mrs. Nichols advocating the "American Costume"—bloomers—in public lectures as well as in print. Not unreasonably she argued that restrictive and hampering fashions marked woman "as a thing owned, . . . for the avenues of self-support are closed against a being so manacled."[49] Mrs. Nichols was well aware of woman's need for economic independence.

Starting out as a teacher, Mrs. Gove, after moving to New York in 1845, had gained increasing reputation as a physician for her own sex. Thomas Nichols, on the other hand, seems never to have cared for medical practice. He much preferred to educate the world. Since regular medicine, or "allopathy" as all the sectarians called it, "grovelling in the dust of ignorance and mercenary motives,"

failed with rare exceptions to teach the laws of health or to prevent disease, water cure physicians must point the way.[50] Later in 1850 Dr. Nichols announced a year's course in water cure, to supplement the regular courses obtainable at medical schools in New York.[51] This evidently fell through, one reason, no doubt, being the incompatibility of "allopathic" and "hydropathic" schools, so the following year Mrs. Nichols joined her husband in establishing their own American Hydropathic Institute, which they billed as the first medical school in the world on water cure principles. The faculty consisted of Mrs. Nichols, who lectured on midwifery, the diseases of women and children, and special topics in physiology; and Dr. Nichols, who modestly covered chemistry, anatomy, physiology, pathology, theory and practice of medicine, and surgery. They presented three to four lectures a day, with clinics in their own water cure establishment. The first term opened in September 1851, with twenty-six students from as far as Alabama and Ohio, including several with previous experience in the health and temperance crusades. In contrast to the usual medical students of that day, they engaged in "no brandy drinking, tobacco chewing, dissipation, or rowdyism of any description."[52] The students, most of whom boarded with the Nicholses, were expected to live the laws of health as well as to study them, and to attend lectures and debates on moral as well as medical and scientific questions. After three months twenty students—including nine women—were awarded diplomas. The pain of parting was eased for Mary Nichols only by her confidence that they went forth a "band of apostles" prepared to teach the "life-giving knowledge of the laws of health, thus giving the people God's regenerating truth. . . ."[53] A second term beginning January 1852 appears to have been equally successful, and plans were soon laid for a third term the following fall.[54]

Despite the apparent success of the Hydropathic Institute's first season, the Nicholses were soon turning their thoughts in another direction. "To establish an educational institute where a true life can be lived, where labor can be united with learning, and where men and women can be fitted to do a more extensive good than has yet been accomplished," was now their ultimate aim, the healing of the sick but incidental and preferably limited hereafter to "worthy workers in their Lord's Vineyard." In May 1852, they had moved to a new water cure establishment in Port Chester, New York, and here the new ideas were first tried out during the summer in a School of Integral Education for young ladies who learned and lived health while receiving instruction in academic subjects as well.[55]

In the meanwhile, Thomas Nichols was also engaged in writing *Esoteric Anthropology*, which would explain fully and frankly his ideas—and also Mary's, although her name is not on the title page—on anatomy, physiology, water-cure, and the preservation of health. In her lectures and writings, Mary Gove had long emphasized the importance of diseased or perverted "amativeness" as a source of ill health in women, the sin of marriage without love, and the viciousness of marriage laws that denied to women any property rights or semblance of freedom. Taking a slightly different view in his book *Woman, in All Ages and Nations*, first published in 1849, Thomas Nichols had praised American customs, compared to those of other times and places, for the comparative freedom given to women to accept or reject suitors and thus to control, to some extent, the choice of their husbands. Yet even here, because of an imperfect social system, economic, social, and other extraneous considerations intervened to prevent that complete freedom of choice necessary to insure true marriage, the union of the two sexes in "pure and exalted mutual love." A confidently expectant reformer, Nichols looked forward to the inevitable day when this would be the universal experience.[56]

Fortified in her opinions, if such were possible, by those of her husband, Mrs. Nichols turned increasingly from palliative treatment of her female patients' ills to a more radical attack on the ultimate sources of their troubles. As to the confessional—or as to the psychoanalyst—women came to this sympathetic woman and, with proper prompting, poured out their troubles. To women who were the victims of their husbands' lusts—as many, in Mary's opinion, were—she preached the gospel of freedom. Union without love, Mary proclaimed, whether in or out of legal marriage, was prostitution. Union with love was true marriage, whatever the legal form. The woman who was truly free and healthy in body and soul had no need for human laws to protect her virtue. Hers was the "Heaven conferred right to choose the father of her babe."[57] In his new textbook, *Esoteric Anthropol-ogy*, Thomas Nichols enshrined these views and much more in print.

While it covered a number of topics in physiology and water cure, Nichols's text concentrated on subjects that most books for laymen, in that prudish day, did not dream of mentioning. Nichols not only described fully—if not always accurately—the anatomical and physiological facts of sexual intercourse; he explicitly proclaimed it to be "the last, fullest, and most perfect action of the amative passion; that which consummates the life and happiness of the individual, and governs the destiny of the race." With Mary he agreed that "every child should be a love-child," this being "the only legitimacy that nature knows."[58] Although less explicit and detailed about sex than books available in eminently respectable shops today, in 1853 *Esoteric Anthropology* was a real shocker. Denounced wherever it was noticed at all, it sold by the thousands.[59]

The publication of *Esoteric Anthropology* undoubtedly drove Dr. and Mrs. Nichols farther away from the main current of health reform, for the editor of the *Water-Cure Journal*, Dr. R. T. Trall, probably the nation's leading hydropathist, refused to print any mention of the book, even in a paid advertisement. The Nicholses consequently stopped contributing and in April 1853 established their own organ, *Nichols' Journal of Health, Water-Cure, and Human Progress*.[60] Most other water-cure physicians undoubtedly found the Nicholses' ideas on marriage no more acceptable than did Trall, who apparently felt that they were blackening the reputation of water cure by tying it up, for their own immoral purposes, with licentious free love. According to Nichols, Trall fostered dissension at Port Chester and joined the *New York Tribune* in propagating false and scandalous reports that they were teaching "the philosophy of the brothel." In the fall of 1853 Trall established a Hydropathic and Physiological School in New York as a rival to the Nicholses' institute, an action well calculated to make their break irreparable.[61]

Although *Nichols' Journal* continued to promote water cure as the road to universal health, educational reform, "social science," and free love were clearly claiming the editors' increasing and more devoted attention. For some years before meeting Dr. Nichols, Mary had been an enthusiast for the social principles of Fourier as expounded by Albert Brisbane. Her second husband believed even more devoutly in the necessity of a complete re- form of the basis of society. In 1850 Josiah Warren, America's original native-born philosophical anar- chist, appeared from the West in New York City to dispute the associationist views of the phalanxes. Warren held a number of revolutionary economic and social ideas summed up in the slogans "Cost the Limit of Price" and "Individual Sovereignty." As an illustration of the value of equity and justice in human relations, he established a community, Modern Times, on Long Island, where the Indi- vidual Sovereigns, in accord with the founder's principles, were free to act as they wished, so long as they accepted the consequences of their own actions and did not interfere with the rights of others. It quickly became a haven for "ultras" of every description, including one gentleman who believed in dress reform to the point of removing all dress.[62] The Nicholses no doubt became ac- quainted with Warren through the "parlor conver- sations" in which he spread his ideas through re- form circles: they certainly knew his chief supporter and popular interpreter, Stephen Pearl Andrews, who was their patient and a prominent advocate of ideas about marriage similar to their own.

Attracted by the freedoms of "Individual Sov- ereignty" and increasingly anxious to move for- ward with their educational ideas, the Nicholses were overjoyed when Andrews in the summer of 1853 gave them one hundred acres of land at Mod- ern Times to establish a School of Life for true education in health, science, industry, and art. Grand plans for the Institute of Desarrollo, as they named the school, were soon announced. By Oc- tober the Nicholses expected to have completed a four-story building, forty by one hundred and twenty feet, with a lecture room, study rooms, and sixty private lodgings. Wings for a gymnasium, art galleries and studios, and a dining hall would fol- low, along with a printing office, kitchen, laundry, and power house. The pupils, awakened by sere- nades, were to engage in parades, songs, and cheerful labor before breakfast, which would be followed by lectures, reading, discussion, music, study, and baths. After dinner, "a feast of reason and a flow of soul," would come poetry and danc- ing, more study and work. A sunset parade, sup- per, lectures, and a social assembly would complete the day in time for lights out at ten. There would of course be no disorder in this harmonious home,

for, with everyone completely free and a law to himself, each would soon see that what was best for one was best for all. Naturally anyone so "diseased, perverted, and insane, as to be unfit for such a home," would have to be dismissed.[63]

Selling their Port Chester home, the Nicholses prepared to move to Modern Times for the fall opening of the fourth session of the American Hy- dropathic Institute. They soon encountered de- lays—caused chiefly by lack of money—and in September 1853 perforce moved to New York City instead, where Dr. Nichols opened a reform book store and inaugurated a lecture series, "Principles and Ultimations of Physiological and Social Sci- ence."[64]

Pending the establishment of their school, Ni- chols published a new edition of *Woman, in All Ages and Nations*, with a preface by Stephen Pearl An- drews, and, jointly with his wife, *Marriage: Its His- tory, Character, and Results; Its Sanctities, and Its Pro- fanities; Its Science and Its Facts*. Building on the ideas of Josiah Warren and Andrews, T. L. Nichols proclaimed that freedom in love would be "the last and highest achievement of Individual Sov- ereignty." Marriage was "the center and the soul" of "that system of superstition, bigotry, oppression, and plunder, which we call civilization," and the chief cause of drunkenness, poverty, slums, pros- titution, disease, and crime. True morality, he ar- gued, was to live in accordance with Nature. If Nature had made man with certain passions and faculties, they were made for use, and efforts to repress, thwart, control, or taboo the passions were in fact one of the chief causes of disease. When a free man and a free woman were drawn together by mutual attraction and love, true marriage ex- isted. But it need not exist forever or be limited to one: "some like a single flower, or a single dish— others will have a bouquet or a feast."[65] While Dr. Nichols spoke and wrote in theoretical terms of the abolition of marriage and the reconstruction of so- ciety, Mrs. Nichols brought these ideas down to earth in plain unvarnished counsel to her patients to be, if the occasion demanded, what the common world called adulterous.[66]

Mrs. Nichols's tendency to write in more per- sonal terms than her husband is epitomized in *Mary Lyndon*, first published in *Nichols' Journal* in 1854. An autobiography with changed names and a chal- lenging vagueness about dates, it was a soul-baring revelation of Mary's loveless marriage with Hiram Gove, a damning indictment of contemporary marriage laws and customs which subjected women to the complete control of their husbands, and a fervent plea for freedom and love. Physiological teaching and water cure were presented as fundamental aspects of freeing women from the physical miseries rendered widespread by prevailing ignorance and marriage practices.

As might be expected, *Mary Lyndon,* appearing in book form in 1855, made a "considerable sensation." The *New York Times* took nearly a page to denounce it. A typical review, in *Norton's Literary Gazette,* while commending its literary merit, regretted that it might become an evil influence because of its "extreme and loose positions . . . , especially in reference to the sacredness of marriage and religious truth."[67] For the modern reader, *Mary Lyndon,* written with the burning intensity of searing personal experience, speaks most strongly of all Mrs. Nichols's works as a passionate plea for the individuality and freedom of women.

As the months went by without the needed funds for Desarrollo forthcoming, the Nicholses' affairs seemed to be approaching a crisis. Fortunately, just at that moment the spirits intervened, showing them how inadequate their old plan was. Brought to the fore by the "Rochester rappings" of the Fox sisters in 1848 and bolstered by the mesmeric lecturer Andrew Jackson Davis, spiritualism had early attracted the attention of Mary Gove Nichols. Though at first she would rather have been called a sheep thief than a medium, by the spring of 1854 she too was receiving messages from the departed and thus found a new "holy and beautiful work to do."[68] From a particular group of spirits—including, incidentally, the same Henry G. Wright who had once taught her the meaning of love—Mrs. Nichols learned that men and women should live in harmonic societies. Individual Sovereignty was now seen as merely a step in progress, necessary to destroy the existing evil social organization preparatory to the construction of the new, in which the personal will of the individual would be submerged in the harmonized will of all. To create the new heaven on earth, the Nicholses formed the Progressive Union, a Society for Mutual Protection in Right, inviting all who agreed with their principles to join, and to send their contributions to the secretary of the Central Bureau, Dr. Nichols him-

self. Giving up the idea of settling in proximity to Modern Times, the Nicholses went west to seek a larger and more suitable domain.[69]

In the fall of 1855 Dr. and Mrs. Nichols settled in Cincinnati.[70] After some months of publishing and lecturing to spiritualist groups—"Free-Love, a Doctrine of Spiritualism" was a sensation—and gathering converts to the Progressive Union, they discovered an old water cure establishment at Yellow Springs, Ohio, which seemed like a perfect setting for their new School of Life, or, as they now called it, Memnonia Institute. They looked forward to friendly association with Antioch College, newly founded on liberal principles, and mutual intellectual stimulation. President Horace Mann had read *Marriage,* however, and wanted no truck with a free love, spiritualist colony. The "Calvin of that modern Geneva," as Nichols called him,[71] did his best to prevent the establishment of Memnonia, and he almost succeeded; he made it quite clear that any student associating with this "superfoetation of diabolism upon polygamy"[72] might consider himself as resigning from the college.

President Mann's fears concerning Memnonia Institute failed to take into account the fundamental law of progression in harmony more recently revealed through Mrs. Nichols which enjoined material union only when the wisdom of the harmony demanded a child. Far from being a hotbed of licentiousness, Memnonia proved to demand in fact a life of asceticism. Only the pure in spirit, person, and diet; the chaste in thought, word, and deed; the consecrated, harmonious, and economically self-sustaining, could be accepted. No "discordant individualism" was permitted. Daily confessions and penances were required. The right to do right was the only freedom that could be allowed, if the Nicholses were to lead their followers into the "new social order wherein dwelleth righteousness."

Memnonia, which opened in July 1856, is reminiscent of Fruitlands not only in regimen—for the Nicholses still favored the vegetarian diet and cold bathing—but also in its complete collapse during the first winter. Like Fruitlands, Memnonia, which never numbered more than about twenty inmates, was an economic failure. The primary cause of its dissolution, however, was the conversion of Mrs. Nichols, her husband, and most of their immediate followers to the Roman Catholic faith following instruction from the spirit of Loyola himself. That

Mrs. Nichols should have turned Catholic is not, perhaps, inexplicable. "In that church," wrote her husband, "we see the order, the devotion, the consecration, the faith and obedience necessary for the great work of human redemption. . . . I have found already unexpressible peace."[73] But in view of Dr. Nichols's earlier statement that "spiritualism meets, neutralizes, and destroys Christianity,"[74] the alleged method of conversion is surely one of the strangest on record. Mrs. Nichols remained a devoted adherent until her death.[75]

The conversion of Dr. and Mrs. Nichols, and most of their followers as well, marked the end of Memnonia, and a return to more prosaic aspects of health reform. For several years they visited Catholic institutions in the Mississippi Valley, teaching nuns and priests the lessons in health and offering hydropathic treatment of their pupils' ills. Early in 1861 the Nicholses moved to New York to establish a weekly newspaper. They found themselves out of sympathy with Lincoln's effort to coerce the South after Fort Sumter, and in 1861 sailed to England.[76]

Arriving in London with a letter of introduction to Cardinal Wiseman and little else, Dr. and Mrs. Nichols soon were writing for a variety of editors and publishers. Dr. Nichols worked on *Chambers' Encyclopedia*—from Fourier to Z—and wrote *Forty Years of American Life* (2 volumes, London, 1864), a delightful account of nineteenth-century America republished as recently as 1937, while Mrs. Nichols turned out reviews and stories for the *Athenaeum, All the Year Round, Frazer's,* and other journals. In 1864 she also published *Uncle Angus,* a two-volume novel (which, wrote Dr. Nichols in 1887, "may probably still be found at the larger libraries"),[77] and in 1872, *Jerry; a Novel of Yankee American Life.* Among their literary correspondents, friends, and acquaintances, the Nicholses numbered William and Mary Howitt and their daughter Anna Mary Watts, Robert Chambers, Charles Dickens, Charles Kingsley, and John Ruskin.

After several years of a rather precarious literary career in London, Dr. and Mrs. Nichols returned again to the cause of health reform—no longer, however with overtones of free love. In 1867 they leased a large house at Malvern, a health resort, which soon was filled with patients and pupils. Here Dr. Nichols established a new journal,

the *Herald of Health,* edited an English edition of *Esoteric Anthropology,* and wrote tracts like "How to Live on Six-pence a Day," and "How to Behave: a Manual of Manners and Morals." (Here, too, Mary's first daughter, Elma, met and married Thomas Letchworth of Apsley Guise, Woburn, Bedfordshire.) Mary, hoping still to establish a "School of Life," indefatigably gave medical advice by correspondence, and with her husband's help—for cataracts had made her nearly blind—she published in 1874 *A Woman's Work in Water Cure and Sanitary Education.* Increasingly given to mysticism, she claimed in her later years a "gift of healing" by laying on of hands. In 1875 Dr. Nichols found the necessity of traveling frequently between London and Malvern too trying and they returned to the metropolis to live. An operation by Dr. Charles Bell Taylor of Nottingham had restored Mary's sight, but a cancer of the breast growing progressively worse, to which was added a very painful neuralgia from an improperly healed fracture of the left femur, at last wore out her mortal body. Mary S. Gove Nichols died on May 30, 1884, and was buried in Kensal Green Cemetery. Dr. Nichols continued the *Herald of Health* and his health food store in London for some years, retiring eventually to the Continent, where he died in obscurity in 1902.[78]

Mary Gove Nichols had two intertwined careers, in literature and reform. As a literary figure, her contributions were voluminous but slight. She wrote several novels and unnumbered stories, reviews, and articles, all of which are now virtually unknown. Although *Uncle John* was sufficiently popular to go to a second edition nine years after the first, even the Library of Congress contains only one of her novels today. To historians of American literature she is known chiefly for her descriptions of Poe at his Fordham cottage in 1846.[79] Her husband, perhaps her most candid literary critic, pointing out that her novels expounded a cause instead of portraying life, conceded that lengthy conversations between precocious pupils and accomplished nursery maids were a dreary mistake. All her novels, he remarked, were "sanitary."[80]

Far more significant was her contribution to health reform. Literature on personal hygiene was certainly nothing new in the 1830s, but to endow it with all the fervor of a moral crusade was. This was the contribution, first and foremost, of Sylvester Graham. Mary Gove was one of his early converts and the first to address herself specifically to the female sex. Moreover, she went much further than Graham and presented a much broader program. By combining hydropathy with health reform, she helped give the latter a therapeutic content that undoubtedly strengthened and prolonged its existence.[81] Through Harriet K. Austin, a graduate of the Hydropathic Institute and physician at the Glen Haven Water-Cure, there is a direct connection between Mary Gove Nichols and Mrs. Ellen G. White, prophetess of the Seventh-day Adventists and founder of their special interest in personal health reform and medical missionary endeavor. As a church historian writes, referring specifically to the Nicholses and other hydropathists, "With such a background of reform, and with able exponents of health principles, the way was prepared in the providence of God for impressing upon the minds of Seventh-day Adventists the importance of physical reform as an adjunct to their message setting forth the need for the restoration of Bible truths and the keeping of God's commandments." Today the globe-circling medical activities of the Adventists include 115 hospitals and sanitariums, an even larger number of clinics, and the schools of medicine, dentistry, and related professions at Loma Linda, California. On a more mundane level there is also a direct connection between the health reformers of the 1840s and the vast prepared-cold-cereal empires of Kellogg and Post today.[82]

Mary Gove was also one of the first American women to practice medicine as a profession, albeit without a license (which was not required at the time) or a medical degree (which no school would have permitted her to obtain). "Mrs. Gove Nichols merits and will receive exalted praise," wrote a contemporary,

> as being the first woman of the age to throw off the thralldom of Conventionalism—to burst the fetters of custom—to step out, in all the pride of genius, in all the true dignity of woman, to grasp a diploma from nature in the highest and most useful department of Art and Science, and to teach her sex and the world, that the sufferings of human na-

ture may be lessened—that the sorrows of women may be lightened, and that females are competent to rank with the most intelligent and most successful in alleviating the physical and mental miseries of mankind.[83]

Her practice was "sectarian" and therefore suspect in the regular medical profession; the standard histories of women in medicine do not recognize her influence or her career. But her training through reading and apprenticeship was at least as thorough as that of many practitioners of her day, and it is not inconceivable that her water cure treatments were more effectual—because less harmful—than the calomel and opium dear to the hearts of innumerable "allopaths." Her advocacy of prepartum care for pregnant women, of proper mental and physical preparation, of "natural" childbirth and early ambulation strikes a modern—and still controversial—note.

Indeed, Mary Gove Nichols's frankness on the physiology of marriage and the role of sex in mental and physical health and disease is a refreshing contrast to the excessive prudery of mid-nineteenth-century America. She was only one of many writers, and by no means the most significant, who condemned existing marriage institutions and advocated property rights for married women; she was only one of several who advocated free love. But where most advocates of marriage reform talked in legal and political or economic and sociological terms, Mary Nichols pioneered in emphasizing a hygienic outlook through her repeated emphasis on unhappy, indissoluble marriages as a cause of mental and physical disease in women and of weak, unhealthy children.

Mary Gove Nichols played a vigorous role in marriage reform, dress reform, and diet reform, before she was carried away, during the 1850s, by spiritualism and her husband's all-embracing educational views. Very few Americans today are vegetarians, marriage laws still exist, and Amelia Bloomer's costume would arouse as much comment on Fifth Avenue today as it did in 1850. But married women are no longer without legal recourse if their husbands abuse them, our diet is far more temperate, and it is the old-fashioned conservatism of the radical dress of 1850, not its daring, that would cause remark today. It is easy to poke fun at the "ultra" reformers like Mary Gove Nichols, but many of the things they fought for are in essence the commonplace conditions of life today.

Only the most rash of biographers could suggest that these changes have occurred because Mary Gove Nichols lived. Others could have and did work for these changes more effectively than she. But she is worth remembering for the insight her ca-

reer can give us into the reform spirit of nineteenth-century America and also into the medicine of the time. Mary's autobiography, despite many tendentious passages, is still a compelling indictment of contemporary marital institutions, and with her other works, it reveals a vivid and fascinating personality.

NOTES

This article is an outgrowth of one prepared for *Notable American Women, 1607–1950: A Biographical Dictionary*, eds. Edward T. James, Janet Wilson James, and Paul S. Boyer (Cambridge: The Belknap Press of Harvard University Press, 1971).

1 Robert Latou Dickinson and Lura Beam, *A Thousand Marriages: A Medical Study of Sex Adjustment* (Baltimore, 1932), 203, quoted by Bruno Gebhart, in "Robert Latou Dickinson, 1861–1950: a nonconformist studies marriage and sex," annual meeting American Association for the History of Medicine, May 20, 1961.

2 Mary Sargeant (Neal) Gove Nichols, *Mary Lyndon: or, Revelations of a Life: An Autobiography* (New York, 1855), 9.

3 This account of Mary's childhood is based primarily on her *Mary Lyndon*, 5–116, passim, and Thomas Low Nichols, *Nichols' Health Manual, Being Also a Memorial of the Life and Work of Mrs. Mary S. Gove Nichols* (London, 1887), 1–20 (microfilm from British Museum). See also T. L. Nichols, "A brief record of a well-spent life," *Herald of Health* (London), no. 79 (July 1884), 78–80. The principal accounts of her career are: Bertha-Monica Stearns, "Two forgotten New England reformers," *New England Quarterly*, 1933, 6:59–84; Helen Beal Woodward, *The Bold Women* (New York, 1953), 149–80; Grace Adams and Edward Hutter, *The Mad Forties* (New York, 1942).

4 M. S. G. Nichols, *Mary Lyndon*, 117–47.

5 M. S. G. Nichols, *Experience in Water-Cure: A Familiar Exposition of the Principles and Results of Water Treatment, in the Cure of Acute and Chronic Diseases . . .* (New York, 1849), 22–23.

6 Ibid., 23; M. S. G. Nichols, *Lectures to Ladies on Anatomy and Physiology* (Boston, 1842), vi; I. T. Richards, "Mary Gove Nichols and John Neal," *New England Quarterly*, 1934, 7:340–41; M. S. G. Nichols, *A Woman's Work in Water Cure and Sanitary Education* (London, 1874), 11; *Graham Journal of Health and Longevity*, 1838, 2:128. On Graham, see Mildred V. Naylor, "Sylvester Graham, 1794–1851," *Annals of*

Medical History, 1942, ser. 3, 4: 236–40; R. H. Shryock, "Sylvester Graham and the popular health movement, 1830–1870," *Mississippi Valley Historical Review*, 1931–32, 18: 172–83.

7 Hebbel E. Hoff and John F. Fulton, "The centenary of the first American Physiological Society founded at Boston by William A. Alcott and Sylvester Graham," *Bulletin of the History of Medicine*, 1937, 5: 687–734; M. S. G. Nichols, *A Woman's Work*, 11–12; *Graham Journal of Health and Longevity*, 1838, 2: 248, 272, 303, 304. On later lecturers, see, for example, "Medical miscellany," *Boston Medical and Surgical Journal*, 1849, 40:107; M. A. Sawin, "Physiological introduction to women," ibid., 1849–50, 41:201–3; "Ladies Physiological Institute," ibid., 1853, 48: 443–44; Marianne Finch, *An Englishwoman's Experience in America* (London, 1853), 85–88.

8 *Graham Journal of Health and Longevity*, 1838, 2: 325–30, 337–42, 345, 357–59, 373–75, 385; 1839, 3: 20, 37, 69; *Library of Health and Teacher on the Human Constitution*, 1838, 2: 357–58; M. S. G. Nichols, *Mary Lyndon*, 155, 159.

9 "Lectures in Boston," *Boston Medical and Surgical Journal*, 1829–30, 2: 638; James Silk Buckingham, *America: Historical, Statistic, and Descriptive* (London, 1841), 3: 229–33, 313–15, 319–20; John Robert Godley, *Letters from America* (London, 1844), 2: 48–49; Lemuel Shattuck, *Report to the Committee of the City Council Appointed to Obtain the Census of Boston for the Year 1845* (Boston, 1846), 74.

10 Besides the material on Graham cited above (note 6), see, for example, M. L. North, "On the expediency of popular lectures on health by physicians," *Boston Medical and Surgical Journal*, 1835, 12: 365–70; "Medical miscellany," ibid., 1837–38, 17: 195.

11 Oliver Wendell Holmes, *Medical Essays, 1842–1882* (Boston, 1891), 203.

12 M. S. G. Nichols, *Mary Lyndon*, 65.

13 Many historians have written of the pre–Civil War reform movements. See, for example, Carl Russell Fish, *The Rise of the Common Man, 1830–1850* (New York, 1927), 256–90; Merle Curti, *The Growth of*

American Thought (New York, 1943), 368–96; Allan Nevins, *Ordeal of the Union* (New York, 1947), 1: 113–51; Alice F. Tyler, *Freedom's Ferment* (Minneapolis, 1944). For the status of American medicine and the influence of European thought, see, for example, R. H. Shryock, *The Development of Modern Medicine: An Interpretation of the Social and Scientific Factors Involved*, rev. ed. (New York, 1947), 248–72; R. H. Shryock, *Medicine and Society in America, 1660–1860* (New York, 1960), 117–66; James Harvey Young, *The Toadstool Millionaires: A Social History of Patent Medicines in America before Federal Regulation* (Princeton, 1961), 48–89.

14 M. S. G. Nichols, "To the friends of truth," *Nichols' Journal*, 1853, *1:* 45–46.

15 Quoted in *Graham Journal of Health and Longevity*, 1839, *3:* 181.

16 M. S. G. Nichols, *Experience in Water-Cure*, 20; M. S. G. Nichols, letter to John Neal, December 1839, quoted in Richards, "Mary Gove Nichols and John Neal," 341.

17 M. S. G. Nichols, "Solitary vice: an address to parents and those who have the care of children," Portland, 1839 (copy in Boston Medical Library).

18 *Health Journal and Advocate of Physiological Reform*, 1840, *1:* 3, 14, 110; Richards, "Mary Gove Nichols and John Neal," 344–52; T. L. Nichols, *Nichols' Health Manual*, 24.

19 *Library of Health and Teacher on the Human Constitution*, 1842, *6:* 136; "'Lectures to ladies on anatomy and physiology,' by Mary S. Gove," *Boston Medical and Surgical Journal*, 1841–42, *25:* 374; "'Lectures to ladies on anatomy and physiology,'" ibid., 1842, *26:* 97–98.

20 M. S. G. Nichols, *Lectures to Ladies on Anatomy and Physiology* (Boston, 1842), 97. Like many vegetarians, Mrs. Gove ate milk, cheese, butter, and eggs, which saved her from the deficiencies of a strictly vegetarian diet.

21 M. S. G. Nichols, "Solitary vice"; M. S. G. Nichols, *Lectures to Ladies*, 220–37.

22 M. S. G. Nichols, *Lectures to Ladies*, 53–54.

23 Richards, "Mary Gove Nichols and John Neal," 349.

24 M. S. G. Nichols, *Mary Lyndon*, 148–60. This apparently occurred some time after February 1, 1842, when Mary wrote John Neal of her desire for a separation (Richards, "Mary Gove Nichols and John Neal," 352–55), but before Mary met Henry Gardiner Wright, late the same year (Franklin B. Sanborn, *Bronson Alcott at Alcott House, England, and Fruitlands, New England, 1842–1844* [Cedar Rapids, 1908], 48).

25 M. S. G. Nichols, *Mary Lyndon*, 227–72; Richards, "Mary Gove Nichols and John Neal," 336; Lynn (Mass.) *Vital Records* (Salem, 1906), 2: 544; T. L. Ni-

chols, *Nichols' Health Manual*, 88; M. S. G. Nichols, "To the friends of truth."

26 Sanborn, *Bronson Alcott at Alcott House*, 13–18; Odell Shepard, *Pedlar's Progress: The Life of Bronson Alcott* (Boston, 1937), 335–36.

27 Sanborn, *Bronson Alcott at Alcott House*, 48–50; Shepard, *Pedlar's Progress*, 341–44, 350–51.

28 M. S. G. Nichols, *Mary Lyndon*, 178–226; Sanborn, *Bronson Alcott at Alcott House*, 22–24.

29 *Health Journal and Independent Magazine* 1, no. 1 (February 1843), esp. "Editorial sanctum: the times," 11–14, and prospectus on outside back cover; Sanborn, *Bronson Alcott at Alcott House*, 49.

30 M. S. G. Nichols, *Mary Lyndon*, 197.

31 *Water-Cure Journal*, 1845–46, *1:* 14–15, 38–39, 93; 1846, *2:* 16; M. S. G. Nichols, *Experience in Water-Cure*, 29–30; M. S. G. Nichols, *Lectures to Women on Anatomy and Physiology, with an Appendix on Water Cure* (New York, 1846), 248–49. Dr. Wesselhoeft's water cure house opened May 29, 1845; for its history, see Mary R. Cabot, *Annals of Brattleboro, 1681–1895* (Brattleboro, 1921), 2: 563–75. Mary Gove Nichols evidently was in error in saying she went to New York in the fall of 1844.

32 R. H. Shryock, *The Development of Modern Medicine*, 163–64, 252.

33 M. S. G. Nichols, *Lectures to Women*, 224–38.

34 Ibid., 239–43; M. S. G. Nichols, *Experience in Water-Cure*, 7–17.

35 M. S. G. Nichols, *Experience in Water-Cure*, 30–32; Sarah Josepha Hale, *Woman's Record; or, Sketches of All Distinguished Women, from "the Beginning" till A.D. 1850* (New York, 1853), 756–61.

36 M. S. G. Nichols, *Experience in Water-Cure*, 17–18; M. S. G. Nichols, *Mary Lyndon*, 317–18.

37 M. S. G. Nichols, *Lectures to Women*, iii–iv; M. S. G. Nichols, *Experience in Water-Cure*, 18–19.

38 "Marrying a genius," *Godey's Magazine and Lady's Book*, 1844, *29:* 104–7; "The artist," ibid., 1845, *30:* 154–56; "The evil and the good, " ibid., 1845, *31:* 36–38. Later stories include: "Mary Pierson," ibid., 1846, *32:* 39–41; "Minna Harmon; or, the ideal and the practical," ibid., 1848, *37:* 335–38.

39 The preface is dated March 20, 1846. Harper & Bros. also published a second edition in 1855 (copy in library of Western Reserve University).

40 "Editor's table," *Godey's Magazine and Lady's Book*, 1846, *32:* 287, *33:* 239. *Uncle John* also received a laudatory review in *American Review*, 1846, *3:* 562–63. A copy of *Agnes Morris* is in the Library of Congress. Bibliographical data for *The Two Loves* are from Lyle H. Wright, *American Fiction, 1774–1850: A Contribution toward a Bibliography*, rev. ed. (San Marino, 1948), 208.

41 M. S. G. Nichols, *Mary Lyndon*, 273–344, passim;

M. S. G. Nichols, *Reminiscences of Edgar Allan Poe* (New York, 1931).

42 *Godey's Magazine and Lady's Book*, 1946, *33:* 16.

43 M. S. G. Nichols, *Mary Lyndon*, 331–86. Gove married Mary Ann Thurber of Farmington, New Hampshire, September 3, 1848. He was then practicing homeopathy in Rochester, New Hampshire, having earlier been put through Washington University School of Medicine in Baltimore by his first wife. Later he practiced in Salem and East Boston. According to the Gove family history, "He gained a large practice,—his genial good nature, dignified personal appearance and gentle manners inspiring confidence in the sick room." He died February 13, 1871, and was buried in Lynn. William Henry Gove, *The Gove Book* (Salem, 1922), 204–5.

44 *Water-Cure Journal*, 1849, *8:* 123; 1850, *9:* 55.

45 T. L. Nichols, "A position defined, or reasons for becoming a water-cure physician," *Water-Cure Journal*, 1850, *9:* 100–103; ibid., 1850, *9:* 157; Stearns, "Two forgotten New England reformers."

46 M. S. G. Nichols, "Maternity and the water-cure of infants," *Water-Cure Journal*, 1851, *11:* 57–59; T. L. Nichols, "The curse removed," *Water-Cure Journal*, 1850, *10:* 167–73; T. L. Nichols, *Nichols' Health Manual*, 90, 105–8.

47 T. L. Nichols, "The progress of water-cure," *Water-Cure Journal*, 1850, *9:* 153–54.

48 T. L. Nichols, "American Vegetarian Convention," *Water-Cure Journal*, 1850, *10:* 5–6; "American Hydropathic Convention," ibid., 1850, *10:* 14–15; "Society of Public Health," ibid., 1850, *10:* 27–28 (the society died a-borning); "American Vegetarian Society," ibid., 1850, *10:* 157–58.

49 M. S. G. Nichols, "A lecture on woman's dresses," *Water-Cure Journal*, 1851, *12:* 34–36; "A word to water-cure people," ibid., 1852, *13:* 8; "Letter from Mrs. Gove Nichols," ibid., 1853, *15:* 10–11; "A letter to women," *Nichols' Journal*, 1853, *1:* 6.

50 T. L. Nichols, in *Water-Cure Journal*, 1850–52, passim. The quotation is from T. L. Nichols, "Medical education: the American Hydropathic Institute," ibid., 1851, *12:* 65–66.

51 T. L. Nichols, "Medical education," *Water-Cure Journal*, 1850, *10:* 119–20, 235–36.

52 "American Hydropathic Institute," *Water-Cure Journal*, 1851, *12:* 114.

53 M. S. G. Nichols, "A word to water-cure people."

54 The progress of the American Hydropathic Institute may be followed in the pages of the *Water-Cure Journal*. See especially articles and advertisements by T. L. and M. S. G. Nichols in 1851, *11:* 91, 129–30, 157, *12:* 10–11, 65–66, 73–75, 97–100, 114, 115; 1852, *13:* 8, 19–20 40–41, 64–65, *14:* 13, 14, 75, 80.

55 T. L. Nichols, "Water-cure movements," *Water-Cure Journal*, 1852, *13:* 64–65; T. L. Nichols, "Physiology the basis of education," ibid., 1852, *13:* 78; M. S. G. Nichols, "Education," ibid., 1852, *14:* 13–14; "Letter from Mrs. Gove Nichols," ibid., 1852, *14:* 67–68; "Port Chester, New York," *Nichols' Journal*, 1853, *1:* 7.

56 T. L. Nichols, *Woman, in All Ages and Nations: A Complete and Authentic History of the Manners and Customs, Character and Condition of the Female Sex, in Civilized and Savage Countries, from the Earliest Ages to the Present Time*, [2d ed.?] (New York, 1854). In the preface this printing is called a "new edition"; the work was copyrighted in 1849.

57 T. L. Nichols and M. S. G. Nichols, *Marriage: Its History, Character, and Results; Its Sanctities and Its Profanities; Its Science and Its Facts; Demonstrating Its Influence, as a Civilized Institution, on the Happiness of the Individual, and the Progress of the Race*, [rev. ed.] (Cincinnati, [1855]), 205.

58 T. L. Nichols, *Esoteric Anthropology* (Port Chester, N.Y., 1853), 142, 172.

59 T. L. Nichols and M. S. G. Nichols, *Nichols' Medical Miscellanies: A Familiar Guide to the Preservation of Health, and the Hydropathic Home Treatment of the Most Formidable Diseases* (Cincinnati, 1856), 5; *Nichols' Journal*, 1853, passim.

60 "The reason why," *Nichols' Journal*, 1853, *1:* 5. The bibliography of this journal is rather complex; so far as I have been able to trace it, the publishing history is:

1. *Nichols' Journal of Health, Water-Cure, and Human Progress* (New York) 1, nos. 1–8 (Apr.–Nov. 1853).

2. *Nichols' Journal: A Weekly Newspaper, Devoted to Health, Intelligence, Freedom, Individual Sovereignty and Social Harmony* (New York) 2, nos. 1–31 (Jan. 7–Aug. 12, 1854); 3, nos. [1]–2 (Aug. [?] and Sept. 2, 1854). No copy of vol. 3, no. 1, was seen. Vol. 2 is not paginated. Vol. 3 was intended to be issued initially as a weekly, but each four issues were to be sold together as *Nichols' Monthly*, and three monthly issues together as *Nichols' Quarterly*. So far as I know, the weekly did not last beyond September 1854.

3. *Nichols Monthly* (New York) [3], no. [2?] (November 1854): 65–134, plus five unnumbered leaves (97–112 missing in copy seen). "This Monthly, intended to be issued permanently in its present form . . . takes the place of Nichols' Journal, of which there has been a weekly issue during the present year" (65).

4. *Nichols' Monthly*, new ser. 1, nos. [1–4] (June, [July], Aug.–Sept., Oct.–Nov. 1855). The June and Aug.–Sept. issues were published in New York, the Oct.–Nov. in Cincinnati. No copy of no. 2 was seen.

5. *Nichols' Monthly: A Magazine of Social Science and Progressive Literature* (Cincinnati), new ser. 2–3 (1856).

I am indebted to the American Antiquarian Society for a microfilm of *Nichols' Journal;* to the Stanford University library for the loan of *Nichols' Monthly,* 1854–55; and to the University of Illinois library for a microfilm of *Nichols' Monthly,* 1856.

61 T. L. Nichols, "Calumny," *Nichols' Journal,* 1853, *1:* 44–45; "Hydropathic colleges," ibid., 1853, *1:* 46–47; M. S. G. Nichols, "To the friends of truth." An announcement of Trall's school is in *Water-Cure Journal,* 1853, *16:* 45.

62 William Bailie, *Josiah Warren: The First American Anarchist* (Boston, 1906), 57–64.

63 M. S. G. Nichols, "A word to the believers in the sovereignty of the individual," *Nichols' Journal,* 1853, *1:* 21; "Human culture," ibid., 1853, *1:* 29; "To the world's reformers," ibid., 1853, *1:* 31; "American Hydropathic Institute," ibid., 1853, *1:* 38; "Institute of Desarrollo: a school of life," ibid., 1853, *1:* 49–50; T. L. Nichols and M. S. G. Nichols, *Marriage,* 427–37.

64 T. L. Nichols, "Hydropathic colleges," *Nichols' Journal,* 1853, *1:* 46; "Reform book store," ibid., 1853, *1:* 47; "The world's conventions," ibid., 1853, *1:* 55; "The ways and means to build the Institute of Desarrollo," ibid., 1853, *1:* 57–58.

65 T. L. Nichols and M. S. G. Nichols, *Marriage,* 9–18, 96–105, 289–98 (quotations 15, 96, 295).

66 Ibid., 189–268, passim.

67 T. L. Nichols, *Nichols' Health Manual,* 428–32; *Nichols' Monthly,* Aug.–Sept. 1855, 198–200; 1856, *new ser. 2:* 314.

68 M. S. G. Nichols, "Narrative of spiritual experiences," *Nichols Journal,* 2, no. 10; "A letter from Mrs. Gove Nichols to her friends," *Nichols' Monthly,* November 1854, 67.

69 T. L. Nichols, "The Progressive Union: a society for mutual protection in right; first report of the Central Bureau," *Nichols' Monthly,* June 1855, 53–60; ibid., Aug.–Sept. 1855, 145. See also T. L. Nichols, *Nichols' Health Manual,* 91–97; T. L. Nichols and M. S. G. Nichols, *Marriage,* 407–26; *Nichols' Monthly,* 1856, new ser. 2 and 3, passim.

70 *Nichols' Monthly,* Oct.–Nov. 1855, 217.

71 Ibid., 1856, *new ser. 2:* 385.

72 *Dial,* 1860, *1:* 326.

73 *New England Spiritualist,* April 25, 1857, quoted in Bertha-Monica Stearns, "Memnonia: the launching of a utopia," *New England Quarterly,* 1942, *15:* 294.

74 *Nichols' Monthly,* Nov. 1854, 66.

75 T. L. Nichols, *Nichols' Health Manual,* 97–98. This history of Memnonia is based primarily on: *Nichols' Monthly,* passim; *Dial,* 1860, *1:* 325–26; and Moncure D. Conway, *Autobiography, Memories, and Experiences* (London, 1904), 1: 231–33. Detailed accounts may be found in Stearns, "Memnonia," and Philip Gleason, "From free-love to Catholicism: Dr. and Mrs. Thomas L. Nichols at Yellow Springs," *Ohio Historical Quarterly,* 1961, *70:* 283–307.

76 T. L. Nichols, *Nichols' Health Manual,* 99–103; M. S. G. Nichols, *A Woman's Work,* 138–47; T. L. Nichols, *Forty Years of American Life* (London, 1864), 1: 1–12, 2: 96, 118, 348–68.

77 T. L. Nichols, *Nichols' Health Manual,* 432.

78 Ibid., vi, 103–11, 172–222, 262–74, 425–28, 439–40, 444–46; M. S. G. Nichols, *A Woman's Work,* 3–6; M. S. G. Nichols, "Cataract: remarkable cases of cure," *Herald of Health* (London), 1875, *[1]:* 21–22; M. S. G. Nichols, "The education of women," ibid., 1875, *[1]:* 36–38; T. L. Nichols, "A brief record of a well-spent life"; "Death of Mrs. Nichols," *Dietic Reformer and Vegetarian Messenger,* 1884, new *[3d] ser. 11:* 205–7; Stearns, "Two forgotten New England reformers."

79 M. S. G. Nichols, *Reminiscences of Edgar Allan Poe.* See, for example, Hervey Allen, *Israfel: The Life and Times of Edgar Allan Poe* (New York, 1926), 712–15, 722–23.

80 T. L. Nichols, *Nichols' Health Manual,* 115–16, 432–33.

81 William B. Walker, "The health reform movement in the United States, 1830–1870," Ph.D. diss., Johns Hopkins University, 1955, 148.

82 Dores Eugene Robinson, *The Story of Our Health Message: The Origin, Character, and Development of Health Education in the Seventh-day Adventist Church* (Nashville, 1943), 25–33; *Modern Medicine,* March 20, 1961, 14, 18; Gerald Carson, *Cornflake Crusade* (New York, 1957).

83 Alonzo Lewis, quoted in T. L. Nichols, *Nichols' Health Manual,* 425n. Mrs. Gove was preceded by Harriot K. and Sarah Hunt, who began practice in Boston in 1835. Harriot received an honorary M.D. in 1853. Kate Campbell Hurd-Mead, *Medical Women of America* (New York, 1933), 20–21.

26

Ministries of Healing:
Mary Baker Eddy, Ellen G. White, and the Religion of Health

RONALD L. NUMBERS AND RENNIE B. SCHOEPFLIN

During the nineteenth century medicine and religion appeared to be headed in divergent directions. Supernatural explanations of disease, even of epidemics and insanity, fell into disrepute, and the once-common practice of combining physical and spiritual healing—called the "angelical conjunction" by the Puritan cleric-physician Cotton Mather—became anachronistic. But despite the secularization of medical theory and the professionalization of medical practice, religiomedical activities continued to flourish. Church-sponsored hospitals grew at an unprecedented rate, medical missionaries circled the globe, and faith healing experienced a late-century revival. Equally indicative of the continuing interaction between religion and medicine was the appearance of two new churches, Christian Science and Seventh-day Adventist, that actively integrated physical and spiritual concerns.[1] This essay focuses on the lives of the women who founded these sects, Mary Baker Eddy and Ellen G. White, and explores the ways in which their strikingly similar personal experiences influenced their unique healing ministries.[2]

RELIGIOUS AND MEDICAL REFORM

The formative years of Mary Baker Eddy and Ellen G. White coincided with a period of intense cultural ferment, during which Jacksonian democrats challenged the hegemony of elites, fire-and-brimstone revivalists awakened the churches, and

unorthodox healers split medicine into competing sects. During the first half of the nineteenth century the leading churches of the colonial period (Episcopalian, Presbyterian, and Congregational), which supported an educated clergy, gave way to evangelistic Methodists and Baptists, who prized personal experience over theological expertise. Within the various denominations charismatic men and women, each claiming "new light," broke off to form their own movements. It was a time, writes Sydney E. Ahlstrom, in which "farmers became theologians, offbeat village youths became bishops, odd girls became prophets."[3] Each decade seemed to feature a new religious attraction: Mormonism in the 1830s, Millerism in the 1840s, and spiritualism in the 1850s.

Spiritualism, a bane of both Eddy's and White's, prospered in part because of its apparent connection with mesmerism (or hypnotism, as it would be called today). Although mesmerism, also known as animal magnetism, originated in Europe in the 1770s, it failed to attract much American attention until the 1830s, when a young French practitioner arrived in White's hometown of Portland, Maine, and began demonstrating his talents. Before long mesmeric displays became a favorite American pastime. "Animal Magnetism," recalled one observer, "soon became the fashion, in the principal towns and villages of the Eastern and Middle States. Old men and women, young men and maidens, boys and girls, of all classes and sizes, were engaged in studying the mesmeric phenomena, and mesmerizing or being mesmerized."[4] In this way Americans gained a familiarity with trances and, in some instances, with spirit communication during these states. Thus when the notorious Fox sisters of Hydesville, New York, introduced the country to spirit rapping in the 1850s, they found a

RONALD L. NUMBERS is Professor of History of Medicine and History of Science at the University of Wisconsin, Madison, Wisconsin.
RENNIE B. SCHOEPFLIN is Assistant Professor of History at Loma Linda University, Riverside, California.

well-prepared audience. In fact, so many mesmerists embraced spiritualism that it became virtually impossible for the uninitiated to differentiate between the two. As R. Laurence Moore has noted, "Mesmerized persons, especially those who attributed their powers to the inspiration of guardian spirits, were indistinguishable in their actions from many of the later trance mediums of the spiritualist movement."[5] The same was true of Eddy and White.

The medical, like the religious, world of antebellum America produced numerous reformers.[6] Despite the nation's apparent vitality, sickness abounded, and Americans grew increasingly skeptical about the efficacy of regular physicians, who, in the absence of specific remedies, often bled, puked, and purged their patients. This unhappy state of affairs gave rise in the 1830s to a popular health crusade led by Sylvester Graham, an evangelist and temperance lecturer, who promised health to all who would obtain adequate rest and exercise, control their sexual passions, dress sensibly, avoid all stimulating and unnatural foods, and subsist "entirely on the products of the vegetable kingdom and pure water." He especially touted the benefits of homemade whole wheat bread (which bore little resemblance to the commercially made graham crackers of today). In the unlikely event of illness, Graham recommended letting nature take its own beneficent course. "ALL MEDICINE, AS SUCH, IS ITSELF AN EVIL," he declared.

Many Americans who shared Graham's antipathy toward traditional medicine nevertheless lacked his faith in the healing power of nature alone. Thus when sick they turned for therapeutic assistance to one of the many sectarian healers—most notably, botanics, homeopaths, and hydropaths—who arose in competition with regular physicians. Not surprisingly, health reformers displayed a particular fondness for the one medical sect that offered healing without drugs of any kind: hydropathy or the water cure.

Hydropathy originated with a European peasant, Vincent Priessnitz, who employed an array of water treatments—baths, packs, and wet bandages—to promote healing. When news of his methods reached the United States in the mid-1840s, it touched off a "water-cure craze" that continued unabated until the outbreak of the Civil War. Part of the popularity of hydropathy un-

doubtedly stemmed from the inadequacies of nineteenth-century medicine, but equally significant was its harmony with the democratic spirit of the times. "The water treatment of disease may fairly be said to originate with an un-titled man," wrote one devotee. "This is the people's reform. It does not belong to M.D.'s of any school." Before long, however, enterprising hydropaths began opening schools to train professional hydropathic physicians, roughly one-fifth of whom were women.

Homeopathy, the invention of a German physician, Samuel Hahnemann, enjoyed even greater and longer lasting popularity. During the last decade of the eighteenth century Hahnemann, dissatisfied with the heroics of orthodox medicine, began constructing an alternate system based in large part upon the healing power of nature and two fundamental principles: the law of similars and the law of infinitesimals. According to the former, diseases are cured by medicines having the property of producing in healthy persons symptoms similar to those of the disease. The latter held that medicines are more efficacious the smaller the dose, even as minute as one-millionth of a gram. Following its appearance in the United States in 1825, homeopathy rapidly grew into a major medical sect. By the outbreak of the Civil War there were nearly twenty-five hundred homeopathic physicians and a multitude of devoted patients. Its appeal is not difficult to understand. Instead of the harsh purgatives and emetics prescribed by regular physicians, homeopaths dispensed pleasant-tasting pills that produced no discomforting side effects. In part because of its suitability for children, homeopathy won the loyalty of large numbers of American women, who constituted an estimated two-thirds of its patrons and who were among its most active propagators.

In a society that offered women few opportunities outside the home, that kept them out of the pulpit and in the pew, that allowed them to be patients but rarely physicians, medical and religious reform provided a possible way of escape. If women could not be theologians and evangelists, they could at least claim spiritual insight and, if particularly talented, perhaps found their own cult or sect. And if they could not enter regular medical schools and practice orthodox medicine, they could lecture on health reform and practice heterodox healing. Thus it is not coincidental that two of the most influential women in Victorian America found their social niche at the intersection of medical and religious reform.

MARY BAKER EDDY

On a cold evening in February 1866 Mary Baker Patterson, the forty-four-year-old wife of an itinerant dentist, slipped on the icy streets of Lynn, Massachusetts. Friends carried the stricken woman to a nearby house and summoned a local homeopathic physician and surgeon, Dr. Alvin M. Cushing, to treat the semiconscious woman for severe head, neck, and back pains. By morning she had recovered sufficiently to endure the sleigh ride to her home in adjacent Swampscott, but when she showed no sign of improvement the following day, her friends feared the worst. Some time during the afternoon of 6 February 1866, while her friends attended Sunday services, Mrs. Patterson opened her Bible to read about the healing ministry of Jesus; "the healing Truth dawned upon my sense," she later recalled, "and the result was that I rose, dressed myself, and ever after was in better health than I had before enjoyed."[7] For the rest of her life she celebrated those moments of visionary insight as the birth pangs of a new age for Christianity.

Abigail Ambrose Baker gave birth to her sixth and last child, a girl named Mary, on 16 July 1821. For the first fourteen years of Mary's life, the Baker family farmed a homestead near Concord in the township of Bow, New Hampshire; in 1836 they resettled near Sanbornton Bridge. From childhood on, religious anxiety and physical sickness plagued Mary and prevented her from obtaining more than a smattering of formal education. However, she did receive a little training from her oldest brother, Albert, who instructed her by mail and during visits home. Later in life Mary fostered an image of her youthful self as a budding litterateur, who wrote simple verse, short articles, and letters for newspapers.

Although Mary's parents were both long-standing Congregationalists, their theological orientations differed considerably. Abigail rooted her religious faith in a loving God who eagerly seeks to relieve the trials of his children, while her husband, Mark, measured true belief by adherence to theological

tenets and strict moral behavior. Mary welcomed her mother's advice to take her troubles to God in prayer, which often provided relief from her mental and physical torment. During a period of about twelve months around her eighth birthday, Mary often heard voices calling her name. Her mother, initially confused, soon directed her to respond as Eli had instructed the child Samuel under similar circumstances: "Speak, Lord; for thy servant heareth" (1 Samuel 3:9).[8] Such advice encouraged Mary to infuse spiritual meaning into the experiences of everyday life.

Mary often discussed religion with her father, who enjoyed engaging friends and acquaintances in religious debate. On one occasion, when she questioned the fairness of divine predestination, the discussion drove her into a fevered state that demanded the soothings of her mother and the attention of a doctor. She stumbled over the same doctrine just after her seventeenth birthday, while she was preparing for membership in her parents' church. Her father struggled to convince her of the fairness of the doctrine by emphasizing the evil of sin, the reality of eternal hell, and the justice of God, but this only made Mary ill; so the pastor accepted her despite her doubts.[9] Mary's inability to love a God who damns some persons to eternal hell later played an important role in the development of Christian Science theology.

Not all of Mary's sicknesses, however, stemmed from intense religious turmoil. Colds, fevers, chronic dyspepsia, lung and liver ailments, backache, and nervousness plagued her youth, and throughout her adult life she suffered from gastric attacks, severe depression, and short episodes of incoherent babbling or foaming at the mouth. In 1843 she married George Washington Glover, a successful builder in Charleston, South Carolina, who died seven months later, leaving her pregnant. This traumatic experience plunged her into a deep depression, and for several months she remained physically and mentally unable to care for her infant son, George. Upon temporarily recovering, she refused to be tied down by routine child care and sought instead to find fulfillment in a literary career. In 1851 young George moved in permanently with his nurse and her husband, thus freeing his mother from her maternal obligations. Desirous of a man's companionship, Mary married a ne'er-do-well dentist, Daniel Patterson, in the summer of 1853, but their marriage foundered when Mary's recurring maladies confined her to bed for long periods and her wandering husband intermittently deserted her. After 1866 they no longer lived together, and the marriage legally ended in divorce in 1873.

In her prolonged battle against physical and mental illness, Mary tried practically every therapy available to the chronically ill of the nineteenth century. In 1837 she briefly adopted Graham's vegetarian regimen, but, although she returned to it off and on through the next twenty-five years, it brought little relief. In the 1840s she experimented with mesmerism and learned about the possibilities of mental healing. At times she consulted homeopathic physicians, and for a while in the 1850s she herself practiced homeopathy on neighbors and friends, in the process discovering the therapeutic power of positive thinking. In 1862 she visited the Vail Hydropathic Institute in Hill, New Hampshire, but the water treatments she received did little to improve her deteriorating health. Disillusioned with the water cure, she turned her hopes toward the healing hands of the famous mentalist of Portland, Maine, Phineas Parkhurst Quimby.

Quimby, an early convert to mesmerism, had carefully studied the principles of mesmeric healing and transformed them, believing that if a healer simply helped patients to create a positive mental attitude toward their illnesses, their bodies would heal themselves. The healer vicariously assumed the patients' symptoms, discussed their problems with them to instill a positive attitude, and occasionally manipulated their injured limbs or rubbed their heads. Mary Patterson flourished in Quimby's hands, and when she fell ill again in 1863 she returned to the Portland therapist and remained as his student during the following winter. With near adoration she served as his pupil, disciple, evangelist—and patient, whenever her maladies reoccurred. Several times she attempted to practice Quimbyism on her own, but she repeatedly encountered difficulty ridding herself of her patients' symptoms, vicariously acquired, and returned to Quimby for release. When she learned of his death on 16 January 1866 she felt a severe loss. Less than a month later she discovered "the healing Truth."

For the next four years Mary Patterson bounced from one boardinghouse to another as she struggled to write down the views of humans, God, sickness, and sin that she believed God had revealed to her. She continued to fight occasional relapses and the symptoms she acquired from her practice of Quimby-like healing and occasionally dabbled in spiritualism. Impressed that she could financially support herself by instructing others in her healing methods, she first advertised classes in the 4 July 1868 issue of the spiritualist journal *Banner of Light*. Her literary efforts resulted in notes for a commentary on Genesis and a pamphlet entitled *The Science of Man, By Which the Sick are Healed*, which she first used in 1870 to instruct students in "Moral Science," an early form of her teachings that she later called Christian Science.[10] In the spring of 1870, she moved to Lynn, Massachusetts, established a partnership with Richard Kennedy, an early student whose healing practice helped support her teaching, and began to write the textbook of Christian Science, *Science and Health* (1875).

At the basis of Eddy's doctrine lay a radical idealism that denied the existence of anything but God and the ideas that generate from his being.[11] As she stated in the last edition of *Science and Health* to appear before her death, "God is incorporeal, divine, supreme, infinite Mind, Spirit, Soul, Principle, Life, Truth, Love."[12] God is one, and humans and the universe are his reflections (ideas). Since only God and synonyms for him, such as Mind, Life, Truth, and Good, exist, it follows that matter, death, error, and evil do not exist. On such grounds Eddy proclaimed a theodicy that erased all her anxieties about her father's doctrine of predestination and created a universe infused with the spirituality of her mother's proddings.

Drawing upon the language of religious contemporaries who believed that Christianity should be updated or reformed by scientific principles, Eddy called her religion Christian Science. She believed that her doctrines contained a kind of mathematical certainty that followed from their syllogistic form. To illustrate: God is All; God is Good; therefore, evil (sin) does not exist. Or God is All; God is Spirit; therefore, matter (sickness and death) does not exist. Or God is All; God is Truth; therefore, error does not exist. Furthermore, Christian Science doctrine could be tested just like scientific knowledge. Eddy believed that healings and victories over sin and death demonstrated the truth of her claims for the Allness of God and the unreality of disease, sin, and death. By demonstrate she meant that one could test her teachings in the laboratory of life just as scientists test their theories by observing nature and experimenting in their laboratories. If one overcame sickness or sin by studying and practicing Eddy's teachings, then one had proven their truth.

To give demonstration a fair chance, however, the prospective practitioner of Christian Science needed to receive proper instruction, theoretically obtained by the careful study of *Science and Health,* but preferably acquired by attending a course of instruction directed by Eddy or one of her appointed teachers. Since healing provided the ultimate proof of Eddy's teachings, she filled her writings with practical instructions, which changed over time to meet different situations, resulting in various sets of instructions and three basic types of practice. The first type of practice, commonly known as "audible treatment," closely followed the methods of Quimby. Since sickness was an erroneous belief, the practitioner corrected the belief of the patient through verbal argument. Using the second method, "mental argument," the practitioner aimed to correct the thought of the patient not by verbal instruction but by thought alone. The third and most esoteric level of treatment, "impersonal treatment," was based on Eddy's view that "if the *healer realizes* the truth, it will free his patient."[13] Therefore, practitioners directed their attention toward correcting their own thoughts and argued with their own error-filled minds.[14]

The 1870s were filled with turmoil for Eddy as she met challenges to the uniqueness of her teachings. Tensions with Kennedy over her insistence that he reduce the amount of rubbing and manipulating in his practice led to a separation in 1872; that same year a former student, Wallace W. Wright, charged in a Lynn newspaper that Moral Science was nothing more than mesmerism. In the face of such criticism, Mrs. Patterson ceased all manipulation and labeled it a sign of mesmerism, a term she used to describe all forms of mental healing that did not coincide with her practices. Suspicious that certain students stole spiritual energy from her while others directed magnetic forces against her, she denounced such "malicious animal magnetism" and gathered her closest followers around her to ward off its evil influences. Buoyed by faith-

ful supporters, and later encouraged by her new husband, Asa Gilbert Eddy, a converted sewing machine salesman whom she married in 1877, Eddy refused to allow anyone to wrest control of the movement from her hands.

From 1872 to 1875 Eddy industriously wrote and rewrote drafts of *Science and Health,* based on what she claimed to be divine insights gained through study of the Bible and early morning visions, which usually occurred at times of severe stress and anxiety and which provided supernatural answers to problems encountered in her work. Adamantly rejecting the claims of critics who found similarities between her writings and those of mental healers or idealist philosophers, Eddy asserted that she had "consulted no other authors and read no other book but the Bible for about three years," adding that "it was not myself, but the divine power of Truth and Love, infinitely above me, which dictated 'Science and Health with Key to the Scriptures.'"[15] Using an allegorical hermeneutic, which she generously applied to the Bible, she interpreted her visions and dreams in terms of her developing doctrines and metaphysical principles. At times when former students opposed her teachings or leadership, her visions featured apocalyptic images of cosmic struggle that revealed her human antagonists and identified her movement with the male child of Revelation 12, which the great red dragon sought to devour.[16] Although Eddy's basic views on sickness and health and her understanding of reality remained fairly stable, she believed that inspiration guided her continual revision of *Science and Health,* and she adapted her beliefs to a growing movement and a changing world.

Eddy's attitudes toward nineteenth-century physicians verged on outright derision, as, for example, when she claimed that "when there were fewer doctors and less thought bestowed on sanitary subjects there were better constitutions and less disease."[17] In addition to denouncing the drugging of allopaths, the bathing of hydropaths, and the eating habits of Grahamites, she saved a special dose of invective for all mentalists and mind curists, whom she regarded as at best frauds and at worst criminals. Homeopathy, she believed, stood midway between the darkness of allopathy and the radiance of Christian Science, but since the truth of Science had dawned, homeopathy too must be put aside. At times she acknowledged that many physicians possessed "great philanthropy of purpose," but she urged them to "make their endeavors more effectual by changing their basis of action" to the metaphysics of Christian Science.[18] Confronted by the concrete realities of medical licensing laws and public health ordinances requiring vaccination and quarantine, Eddy and her followers moderated their radicalism with some practical compromise. She instructed Christian Scientists to submit to vaccination and to report contagious cases to the proper authorities when the laws demanded, but her lieutenants continued to lobby to exclude religious healing from state regulation. Problems with metaphysical obstetrics, the application of Christian Science to childbirth, provide the best illustration of Eddy's adaptive ability.

In an attempt to add prestige to her movement and to garner the respect of the medical profession, Eddy chartered the Massachusetts Metaphysical College in 1881 and in 1882 published a prospectus that carried the names of cooperating physicians in the Boston area. Although she advertised herself as "Profesor of Obstetrics, Metaphysics, and Christian Science," she did not offer a course in obstetrics for five years; nevertheless, many women found the principles of Christian Science especially attractive during childbirth, when their beliefs removed or lessened pain.[19] Testimonies praising the methods of painless childbirth often appeared in the monthly *Christian Science Journal,* and Eddy capitalized on this application of her doctrines by instructing students during 1887 in the mental control of the errors of childbirth— belief in anatomy, physiology, physical intercourse, and pain. However, the tragic death three years later of a mother and her newborn during a mentally assisted childbirth led to an indictment of manslaughter against a Christian Science practitioner, Abby H. Corner. The case ended in acquittal, but in view of the harmful impact such incidents could have on her movement, Eddy instructed her followers to cooperate with physicians in cases of childbirth. Although she discouraged mixing the material with the spiritual as a general policy, she gave her blessing to a group of associates who enrolled in medical school with the purpose of uniting physical obstetrics with the metaphysical techniques of Christian Science, including pain control.[20]

Eddy best displayed her talents through the or-

ganization and administration of her movement. Whenever ambitious lieutenants or popular healers threatened to usurp her authority or infringe upon her popularity, she skillfully maneuvered them from positions of leadership or declared their beliefs unorthodox. When disaffection and dissent decimated the movement's leadership and decreased its membership by one third during 1888, Eddy took the drastic measure of dissolving all of her existing church organizations. She withdrew from Boston, which had been the center of her activities for the past ten years, to Concord, New Hampshire, where she reflected, wrote, and reorganized her movement. From this distance she directed the construction of the Mother Church in Boston and formalized regulations for instruction in Christian Science. These two efforts centralized control of the church and placed it firmly within the hands of boards of directors appointed and controlled by Eddy. She devoted special attention to the publication of Christian Science literature, establishing the Christian Science Publishing Society in 1898 to spearhead a strong program of world evangelism. The society published numerous editions of Eddy's writings, as well as weekly, monthly, and quarterly journals; in 1908 it began publishing the *Christian Science Monitor.*

During this period of reorganization and consolidation, Christian Science membership exploded. Numbering only 8,724 in 1890, by 1906 the church had grown to 47,083, 72.4 percent of whom were women.[21] These years of growth coincided with the expansion of leadership roles for women in the movement. The Christian Science doctrine of a bisexual God, Eddy's own influence as a role model, and the career opportunities open to Christian Science healers had always attracted women, but before the mid-1880s they occupied few important positions of leadership in the movement. After the defection of many of Eddy's male leaders, she came to recognize the talents of female practitioners, who outnumbered males five to one by the 1890s, and appointed them as journal editors, lecturers, and teachers.[22] However, most key positions of administration, such as board directorships, remained in the hands of men. Through the evangelistic efforts of public lectures, urban dispensaries, and reading rooms, Christian Scientists disseminated their doctrines and distributed their literature throughout America, and foreign evangelism soon transformed the church into a worldwide movement with major centers of activity in Germany and England.

Assailed by physical pains and mental anxieties that mirrored her fears for the future of her movement, Eddy struggled during her final years to direct the affairs of the church through subtle adjustments of the church manual and public defenses of her mental stability. Finally her constitution, weakened by old age, succumbed to pneumonia, and she "passed on" in December 1910, leaving a movement best known for its striking physical healings to search for a new identity in a world increasingly devoted to the therapies of scientific medicine.

ELLEN G. WHITE

Ellen Gould Harmon was born 26 November 1827 in the village of Gorham, Maine, less than a hundred miles from where six-year-old Mary Baker lived in New Hampshire.[23] A few years after her birth her father, a self-employed hatter of modest means, moved his family to nearby Portland, where Ellen subsequently enrolled in school. After completing only three grades or so, she nearly lost her life when an angry schoolmate hit her in the face with a rock, knocking her to the ground unconscious. For three weeks Ellen lay in a stupor, while friends and relatives waited for her to die. She survived, but her injuries continued to plague her for years, and her facial disfigurement—initially so bad that her own father could scarcely recognize her—caused frequent embarrassment and prevented breathing through her nostrils. Frayed nerves rebelled at simple assignments such as reading and writing. Her hands shook so severely she could not write, and words appeared to be mere blurs on a page. Try as she might, she could not continue her studies. Thus frustrated, she resigned herself to the life of a semi-invalid, passing the time of day propped up in bed knitting or helping her father make hats.

In March 1840 a touring farmer-preacher named William Miller visited Portland and aroused the citizens with his prediction, based on biblical prophecies, that Christ would return to earth "about the year 1843." Ellen, who had been raised a Methodist, joined the crowds who turned out to hear Miller and became convinced that indeed the world would soon end—and that she would probably be lost. At times she sank into deep despair and spent sleepless nights bowed in prayer, "groaning and trembling with inexpressible anguish, and a hopelessness that passes all description." Sermons vividly depicting the red-hot flames of hell intensified her torment and pushed her to the verge of a mental breakdown.

While in this state of mind Ellen began having religious dreams. At her mother's urging, she consulted her minister, who interpreted this development as a sign that God had chosen her for "some special work." Her mother agreed, on one occasion insisting that her daughter's fainting during an emotional prayer meeting was not a cause for concern but merely a manifestation of "the wondrous power of God." Reinforced by the views of her minister and mother, Ellen began speaking at public meetings and holding private prayer sessions for her teenaged friends.

As the months of 1843 slipped by, Millerite leaders began to suspect an error in their calculations; Christ's second coming, they finally decided, would actually occur on 22 October 1844. Ellen, by now convinced that she would be among the saints, eagerly awaited this date—only to have her hopes dashed when Christ failed to appear. Confused and disappointed, she sought divine guidance. One day in December, while praying with a few women friends, seventeen-year-old Ellen felt the "Holy Spirit" resting upon her in a new and dramatic way. Bathed in light, she seemed to be "rising higher and higher, far above the dark world." In this trancelike state, the first of her many visions, she received reassurance that her faith in Christ's return had not been misplaced. In a subsequent vision an angel guide explained that Christ could not come to earth until the Millerites began keeping Saturday instead of Sunday as the sabbath.

Ellen's visions followed no set pattern; she might be praying, addressing a congregation, or lying sick in bed, when suddenly she would be off on "a deep plunge in the glory." During these episodes, which lasted from a few minutes to several hours, she frequently described the colorful scenes—past and future, celestial and terrestrial—she was seeing. According to the testimony of numerous physicians and curiosity seekers, her vital functions slowed alarmingly, her heart beating sluggishly and respiration becoming imperceptible. Although she was able to move with complete freedom, strong men could not budge her limbs. Until the 1870s, when nighttime dreams gradually replaced daytime trances, Ellen averaged five to ten visions a year.

As both Ellen and skeptics recognized, her visionary experiences differed little from the trances of countless mesmerists, spiritualists, and religious enthusiasts. In fact, she herself for a time suspected that her visions might be only a mesmeric delusion. As divine punishment for questioning her gift, she was temporarily struck dumb and forced to communicate by means of a pencil and slate— the first time since her accident that she could write without shaking. Like Eddy, she greatly feared coming under the influence of unscrupulous mesmerists, whom she regarded as being "channels for Satan's electric currents."[24] When threatened by such a force, she requested an extra angel God had promised to send to protect her.

In one of her early visions Ellen received directions to travel among the scattered flock of Millerites, relating what she had seen and heard. Shy but ambitious, she worried that her new role as God's messenger might make her proud. But after an angel assured her that the Lord would preserve her humility, she determined to carry out his will. Only one obstacle stood in her way: the need for a traveling companion. At five feet, two inches, and barely eighty pounds, she was little more than skin and bones. Fatigue from long trips on steamboats and railway cars brought on dangerous fainting spells, during which she sometimes remained breathless for minutes. Obviously she could not travel alone.

The solution to her problem appeared in the form of a twenty-three-year-old Millerite minister and erstwhile teacher, James White. Soon after meeting Ellen in 1845, James accepted her claim to be a latter-day prophet and volunteered to serve as her escort. Over the objections of Mrs. Harmon, who feared for her daughter's good reputation, the couple began contacting Millerites in New England. Because of James's conviction that marriage was inconsistent with belief in the imminent return of Christ, he and Ellen postponed marriage—until ugly rumors about them began to circulate. It was clear, said James one day, that "something had got to be done." So on 30 August 1846 they became husband and wife.

Married life for the Whites was far from glamorous. For years they worked as itinerant preachers, barely surviving on the meager contributions of their supporters. When their first child, born in 1847, was only one, they reluctantly left him with friends. The separation nearly broke Ellen's heart, but she vowed not to let her motherly affection keep her "from the path of duty." The arrival of a second son, in 1849, brought only a brief interruption to their nomadic life. He, too, was soon left with a kind Adventist sister in New York.

In 1852 the impoverished couple, worn out by years on the road, settled down to a semipermanent home in Rochester, New York, and collected their children about them. In 1854 Ellen gave birth to a third boy, and the following year she and James moved on to Battle Creek, Michigan, which remained their home until the 1880s. Here they established institutional headquarters for their fledgling church, which by the early 1860s numbered thirty-five hundred members who called themselves Seventh-day Adventists. These people believed in the imminent return of Christ, observed the seventh-day sabbath, and regarded Ellen White as a divinely inspired prophet. They also provided financial support for the Whites, allowing them for the first time to enjoy a relatively comfortable existence. During these years Ellen not only served as wife and mother to a growing family—a fourth baby boy arrived in 1860—but continued to fill speaking engagements and to publish her "testimonies" and other writings.

Her health, however, remained precarious. Sprinkled liberally throughout her various writings are complaints of lung, heart, and stomach disorders, frequent "fainting fits," paralytic attacks (at least five by her mid-forties), pressure on the brain, and breathing difficulties. At least once a decade from her teens through her fifties she expected imminent death from disease. She frequently suffered from anxiety and depression and at times wanted to die. On one occasion her "mind wandered" for two weeks; on another it became "strangely confused." Although she commonly ascribed the illnesses of others to intemperate living, she tended to attribute her own mental and physical ailments to the machinations of Satan and his evil angels, who had made her and her husband "the special objects" of their attention and who had caused several near-fatal accidents.[25]

On the evening of 5 June 1863 Ellen White, now thirty-five, joined friends in rural Michigan for vespers. Lately her mind had often turned to matters of health. Her sons had recently been threatened by diphtheria, James appeared to be on the verge of a physical and mental breakdown, and she herself was, in her own words, "weak and feeble, fainting once or twice a day." While praying, she went into a trance and began receiving instructions from heaven on preserving and restoring health. God's people, she learned, were to give up eating meat and other stimulating foods, shun alcohol and tobacco, and avoid drug-dispensing doctors. When sick, they were to rely solely on nature's remedies: fresh air, sunshine, rest, exercise, proper diet, and—above all—water. Adventist sisters were to abandon their fashionable, floor-length dresses for "short" skirts and pantaloons, and all believers were to curb their sexual passions. As a result of this vision, health reform for Ellen White and her followers became a religious obligation, essential to salvation. It is, she declared, "as truly a sin to violate the laws of our being as it is to break the ten commandments."

The horrible consequences of self-abuse or masturbation especially impressed her. "Everywhere I looked," she later recalled in describing her vision, "I saw imbecility, dwarfed forms, crippled limbs, misshapen heads, and deformity of every description." Her first book on health reform consisted of *An Appeal to Mothers: The Great Cause of the Physical, Mental and Moral Ruin of Many of the Children of Our Time* (1864), a work designed to strike fear in the most hardened of hearts. Graphically describing the effects of masturbation among girls, particularly vulnerable because they possessed less "vital force" than boys, she wrote: "The head often decays inwardly. Cancerous humor, which would lay [*sic*] dormant in the system their life-time, is inflamed, and commences its eating, destructive work. The mind is often utterly ruined, and insanity takes place."[26] For the first time she appreciated her childhood accident: it had allowed her to grow up in "blissful ignorance of the secret vices of the young." Only after her marriage to James, she insisted, had she learned about masturbation from "the private deathbed confessions of some females."

For several years most of White's sexual advice focused on self-abuse. In 1868, however, she received a second revelation on sex, in which she was shown that even married persons were accountable to God "for the expenditure of vital energy, which weakens their hold on life and enervates the entire system." After this vision, she began counseling Christian wives not to "gratify the animal propensities" of their husbands, but to seek instead to divert their minds "from the gratification of lustful passions to high and spiritual themes by dwelling upon interesting spiritual subjects." Husbands who desired "excessive" sex she described as "worse than brutes" and "demons in human form." Although she never defined exactly what she meant by excessive, some evidence suggests that she frowned on having intercourse more than once a month.

From 1863 until her death in 1915 White, with varying degrees of zeal and success, proclaimed the gospel of health. Largely as a result of her crusade, many Adventists adopted a twice-a-day diet of fruits, vegetables, grains, and nuts and gave up tea, coffee, meat, butter, eggs, cheese, rich desserts, and "all exciting substances," which, she argued, not only caused disease but stimulated unholy sexual desires. Although she at first reported great progress in changing the eating habits of her followers, there soon appeared signs of "a universal backsliding." Fish and flesh reappeared on Adventist tables, and even among ministers vegetarianism became the exception rather than the rule. By the mid-1870s White herself was indulging her fondness for flesh foods, to the chagrin of disciples who remained true to her health reform message. It was not until the 1890s that she finally gained a permanent victory over meat and began leading her church back into the vegetarian fold.

Dress reform proved equally frustrating. During the 1850s a number of prominent feminists, including Elizabeth Cady Stanton, Susan B. Anthony, and Amelia Bloomer, briefly abandoned their corsets and long skirts for an outfit consisting of a short skirt over pantaloons. Although these women soon discarded the Bloomer costume, it remained popular attire at some water cures and among certain spiritualists. At first—even after her 1863 vision—White damned the reform dress and the political goals of its advocates. "Those who feel called out to join the movement in favor of women's rights and the so-called dress reform," she declared, "might as well sever all connection with the third angel's message," as she called her theology. Not only was it wrong for women to wear men's clothing, she explained, but the practice might lead nonmembers to confuse Adventists with spiritualists, a likelihood increased by White's claim that she, too, communicated with celestial beings.

Within two years of her vision, however, White changed her mind and began advocating a skirt-and-pants costume she claimed to have seen in her vision. She further confused her followers by first saying that God wanted skirts to clear the ground by "an inch or two," then declaring that they should reach "somewhat below the top of the boot," and finally settling on nine inches from the floor. Her version of the Bloomer—called a "woman-disfigurer" by her own niece—never caught on. It was, complained the prophetess in 1873, "treated by some with great indifference, and by others with contempt." Two years later God mercifully granted her permission to discard her pantaloons and end her divisive dress reform campaign.

During her seminal 1863 vision White, who had long held doctors in low esteem—in fact, she had once condemned the use of "earthly physicians," only to reverse herself after being accused of contributing to the death of a follower who failed to seek medical help—learned that God shared her suspicions about the medical profession. "I was shown that more deaths have been caused by drug-taking than from all other causes combined," she wrote. "If there was in the land one physician in the place of thousands, a vast amount of premature mortality would be prevented." All drugs, vegetable as well as mineral, were proscribed; of the various medical sects, only hydropathy received divine sanction. This is not surprising, since White had discovered the water cure only a few months earlier and had employed it successfully to save two of her sons from possible diphtheria. Before the Adventists built their own water cure, White frequently gave hydropathic treatments to her neighbors in Battle Creek.

In 1864 and again the next year Ellen and James White visited one of the most successful water cure establishments in America, operated by Dr. James Caleb Jackson in Dansville, New York, and returned home to set up a similar operation in Battle Creek. Their Western Health Reform Institute, staffed by both male and female "doctors," experi-

enced a rocky first decade. Then a young protegé of the Whites, Dr. John Harvey Kellogg, took over and turned the ailing institute into a world-famous sanitarium with branches from coast to coast. In his spare time he invented cornflakes and other health foods, from which his brother W. K. Kellogg made a fortune.

In 1907 a cabal of Adventist ministers excommunicated the imperialistic Kellogg, ostensibly for questioning the supernatural origin of White's visions. In departing the doctor took the Battle Creek Sanitarium and the church's only medical school, American Medical Missionary College, with him. To compensate for this loss, White loyalists two years later converted a sanitarium in Loma Linda, California, into the College of Medical Evangelists (now Loma Linda University), which accepted both male and female students. According to White, it was "the Lord's plan" that women be treated by members of their own sex; ignoring such distinctions offended God and led to "much evil." Of the six M.D.'s on the original C.M.E. faculty, two were women: Julia A. White, professor of obstetrics and gynecology, and Lucinda A. Marsh, who taught pediatrics. Both had received their medical degrees from A.M.M.C., which, like C.M.E., taught a mixture of regular and hydropathic medicine.[27]

Over the years Ellen White wrote hundreds, perhaps thousands, of pages on health-related subjects. Although she repeatedly stressed the divine origin of her "testimonies" and denied acquaintance with earthly sources—"My views were written independent of books or of the opinion of others"—a comparison of her writings with those of other nineteenth-century health reformers reveals close parallels in both content and language, a problem discovered by Kellogg and other contemporaries.

For years Ellen relied on James to correct her grammar, polish her style, and publish her work. All that ended in 1881, when James died. Their marriage had not been without its trials. James was an impetuous man who easily took offense. He was excessively jealous of his wife's friendship with real or imagined rivals in the church hierarchy and during the last decades of his life suffered from long bouts of mental illness. At times he resented his wife's superior position and on occasion refused to sleep in the same house with her. Nevertheless, he was a man quick to forgive and to make amends, and, whatever his failings, Ellen loved and respected him and leaned on him in her hours of need. Without him, her career as a prophetess would probably have never gotten off the ground. Since the 1840s, publishing had been his passion—and the key to her success. In those early days it was he who insisted on printing her visions and on creating a strong church organization, over which for ten years he presided as president. Seventh-day Adventism would not have been the same without Ellen White; it would not have existed without James.

After her husband's death, the grief-stricken widow sank into a yearlong depression. Then one night the Lord appeared to her in a dream and said: "LIVE. I have put My Spirit upon your son, W. C. White, that he may be your counselor. I have given him the spirit of wisdom, and a discerning, perceptive mind." Comforted by these words and the knowledge that her favorite son would remain by her side, she resumed her ministry with renewed zeal, spending two years in the mid-1880s in Europe and most of the 1890s in Australia and New Zealand. In 1900 she returned to the United States and settled on a comfortable farm in northern California, from which she continued to guide her growing church. Five years later she published her last major work on health, *The Ministry of Healing*.

On 16 July 1915, five months after a broken thighbone confined her to a wheelchair, Ellen White, aged eighty-seven, died. After a lifetime of illness and frequent brushes with death, she finally succumbed to chronic myocarditis, complicated by arteriosclerosis and asthenia resulting from her hip injury. In a fundamental way, her life had been a paradox. Consumed with making preparations for the next world, she nevertheless devoted much of her energy toward improving life and health in this one. At the time of her death thirty-three Adventist sanitariums and countless treatment rooms spanned six continents. Although she had never received the national attention given to Mary Baker Eddy, whom she regarded as a satanically inspired spiritualist, over 136,000 devoted followers mourned her passing. By the early 1980s her church had grown to 3.5 million members, many of whom enjoyed healthier and longer lives for having adopted White's advice.

PARALLEL AND DIVERGENT CAREERS

The striking parallels between Eddy and White, from their births in New England in the 1820s to their creation of health-conscious churches, are more than historical curiosities; they illuminate the relationship between health and religion and the role of women in Victorian America. As youths, both rebelled against orthodox theology, much as they would later reject orthodox medicine. Eddy's struggles against her "father's relentless theology" were so intense they occasionally precipitated spells of sickness, while White became so agitated by theological issues, she nearly went insane. As she herself surmised, "many inmates of insane asylums were brought there by experiences similar to my own."[28] Both women also suffered intensely from physical complaints, which restricted their activities and impelled them on a lifelong quest for health. Of course, nineteenth-century America abounded with physical invalids and religious rebels, but few turned their afflictions to such advantage as Eddy and White, who proudly displayed their sufferings as badges of divine calling.

Both women struggled to make their mark, to escape from the anonymity of domestic life and fulfill ambitious dreams. Eddy, who believed that her "mission was to write poetry," aspired to a literary career; White, who described herself as "naturally proud and ambitious," aimed "to become a scholar."[29] Above all, Eddy and White sought control: over sin, sickness, and society. For ambitious Victorian women, moral reform offered one of the few avenues to power. Since the beginning of the century women had outnumbered men as churchgoers, and, as long as they submitted to male authority, ministers encouraged them to engage in religious education and moral uplift. This arrangement, writes Nancy F. Cott, "enabled them to rely on an authority beyond the world of men and provided a crucial support to those who stepped beyond accepted bounds."[30]

Both Eddy and White went out of their way to attribute their activities to divine selection rather than personal ambition, having been told since childhood that God had chosen them for a special mission. Both of their mothers, who no doubt viewed their daughters in the context of the biblical prophecy about the "last days"—"your sons and your daughters shall prophesy, and your young men shall see visions, and your old men shall dream dreams" (Acts 2:17)—attached religious significance to unusual dreams, hallucinations, and fainting spells.

Many nineteenth-century visionaries and mystics claimed divine inspiration for their teachings, but success depended as much upon organization as upon inspiration. Within Adventism, James White, who "discovered" Ellen and orchestrated her early career, was the organizational genius. While his wife provided spiritual guidance and theological validation, James ran the printing presses, built the institutions, and fought the political battles. Eddy, who seemed to prefer weaker men, tended to rely on her own formidable administrative skills, although she often delegated responsibilities to male subordinates.

An essential element behind Eddy's and White's achievement was their ability to combine pragmatism with dogmatism as the situation demanded. Both of them repeatedly adapted their teachings to meet the needs of the time. Eddy, for example, abandoned metaphysical midwifery when the costs became too great and, despite her conviction that Christian Science could cure all ills, allowed her followers to seek surgical assistance for such conditions as broken bones, reasoning that "in the present infancy of this Truth so new to the world, let us act consistent with its small foothold on the mind."[31] Over the years White lifted her ban on the use of physicians, discarded her reform dress, and moderated her dietary advice, especially with regard to the use of dairy products. Although such shifts led to criticism and charges of inconsistency, both women executed them with a deft timing that left their authority intact, if not untarnished. Against serious challenges to their authority, however, both Eddy and White stood firm. When evidence came to light of troublesome similarities between the views of Eddy and Quimby and between those of White and other health reformers, each insisted, with an intensity that betrayed their anxiety, that they depended solely on divine revelation.

Eddy and White attracted followers in part because their systems met real medical and religious needs, but also because of the magnetic personalities they both possessed. Their styles, however, differed considerably. Eddy's piercing blue eyes, attractive countenance, and fashionable attire revealed a contagious self-assurance. White, a plain woman

in both appearance and dress, felt less secure in public, but her personal piety inspired emulation and her clear, forceful sermons could bring hardened sinners to their knees.

Such differences are important in understanding their respective teachings. Although both viewed illness in a moral light, as resulting from sin, the metaphysically inclined Eddy followed Quimby in identifying illness with wrong belief, while the practical White followed Graham and other health reformers in viewing sickness as resulting from wrong practices, violations of divinely ordained laws of physiology. Not surprisingly, both claimed divine endorsement for the type of therapy each had found most efficacious in her own life. Eddy benefited little from hydropathy and Grahamism but obtained at least occasional relief from homeopathy and Quimbyism, the influence of which is readily apparent in Christian Science. White's vision on the merits of health reform and hydropathy came within months after she had discovered the water cure and employed it to save the lives of her children.

Although both women might be called visionaries, visions played substantially different roles in their ministries. For White and her followers, the visions validated her claim to divine inspiration. Often occurring in public and accompanied by dramatic physical signs, her visions induced a sense of awe and reverence and provided theological direction for the Adventist church. Eddy's visions, in contrast, occurred in private and served primarily a rhetorical function, guiding her writing and uplifting her spirits. Rather than looking to her visions for validation of her claims, Christian Scientists examined the internal logic of her doctrines and the evidence of healed bodies and changed lives.

Whatever their respective motivations and teachings, Eddy and White exerted a marked influence on nineteenth-century American culture: on religion, medicine, and women. They founded two of the largest churches of American origin, which ultimately touched millions of lives. The therapeutic success of Christian Science helped to promote a renaissance of faith healing in Protestant churches and provided physicians with compelling evidence of the relationship between mind and body. Adventist medical workers helped to transform sectarian hydropathy into the hydrotherapy of scientific medicine, and the health principles taught by White aided her followers in living healthier and longer lives. Through her influence on Kellogg, she revolutionized the breakfast habits of a nation. Eddy and, to a lesser extent, White also expanded the opportunities for women interested in health-related careers. From the early days of Christian Science female practitioners far outnumbered males. Although White displayed little

sympathy for feminism and discouraged Adventist sisters from following in her footsteps, she urged the creation of nursing schools and, by insisting on the immorality of men treating women, encouraged at least a few Adventist women to take up the practice of medicine, especially obstetrics. Few of their contemporaries—male or female—accomplished more.[32]

NOTES

1 Ronald L. Numbers and Ronald C. Sawyer, "Medicine and Christianity in the modern world," in *Health/Medicine and the Faith Traditions: An Inquiry into Religion and Medicine,* ed. Martin E. Marty and Kenneth L. Vaux (Philadelphia: Fortress Press, 1982), 133–60.

2 Born Ellen Gould Harmon, White used her married name, Mrs. White or Ellen G. White, for most of her professional career. Her followers often referred to her as Sister White. Eddy was known by many names over her lifetime. Born Mary Morse Baker, she became Mary Baker Glover after her first marriage in 1843. Usually called Mrs. Patterson or Mary M. Patterson after her second marriage in 1853, she returned to the use of Mary Baker Glover after a prolonged estrangement from her husband and her "discovery" in 1866. After her marriage to Asa Gilbert Eddy in 1877, she used Mary Baker Glover Eddy, Mary Baker Eddy, or simply Mrs. Eddy. Her followers often referred to her as Mother.

3 Sydney E. Ahlstrom, *A Religious History of the American People* (New Haven: Yale University Press, 1972), 475.

4 John D. Davies, *Phrenology—Fad and Science: A 19th-Century American Crusade* (New Haven: Yale University Press, 1955), 126–27. See also Eric T. Carlson, "Charles Poyen brings mesmerism to America," *Journal of the History of Medicine and Allied Sciences,* 1960, *15:* 121–32; and Robert C. Fuller, *Mesmerism and the American Cure of Souls* (Philadelphia: University of Pennsylvania Press, 1982).

5 R. Laurence Moore, *In Search of White Crows: Spiritualism, Parapsychology, and American Culture* (New York: Oxford University Press, 1977), 9.

6 The following paragraphs on medical reform are extracted from Ronald L. Numbers, *Prophetess of Health: A Study of Ellen G. White* (New York: Harper and Row, 1976), chap. 3.

7 Mary Baker Eddy, *Miscellaneous Writings, 1883–1896* (Boston: The Trustees under the Will of Mary Baker G. Eddy, 1924), 24. Eddy sometimes recalled Mark

3 and sometimes Matthew 9:2 as the passage of healing.

8 Mary Baker Eddy, *Retrospection and Introspection* (Boston: Allison V. Stewart, 1916), 8–9.

9 Eddy, *Retrospection,* 13; Robert Peel, *Mary Baker Eddy: The Years of Discovery* (Boston: Christian Science Publishing Society, 1966), 23, 50–51.

10 Eddy first called her teachings Moral Science, later Metaphysical Science or simply Metaphysics, and finally Christian Science.

11 Although Eddy believed God exhibited both masculine and feminine characteristics, except in the third edition of *Science and Health* (1881) she regularly used the masculine pronouns.

12 Mary Baker Eddy, *Science and Health with Key to the Scriptures* (Boston: First Church of Christ, Scientist, 1971), 465.

13 Mary Baker Eddy, *Rudimental Divine Science* (Boston: Allison V. Stewart, 1915), 13.

14 For this categorization of healing practices, we acknowledge Charles S. Braden, *Christian Science Today: Power, Policy, Practice* (Dallas: Southern Methodist University Press, 1958), 336–49.

15 Mary Baker Eddy, *The First Church of Christ Scientist and Miscellany* (Boston: Allison V. Stewart, 1916), 114. *Science and Health* included *Key to the Scriptures,* a glossary containing allegorical meanings for key biblical words, after the sixth edition of 1883.

16 Robert Peel, *Mary Baker Eddy: The Years of Trial* (Boston: Christian Science Publishing Society, 1971), 25–28, 75, 135.

17 Mary Baker Eddy, *Science and Health* (Boston: Christian Science Publishing Company, 1875), 341.

18 Ibid., 365.

19 Peel, *Years of Trial,* 80–82, 111.

20 Ibid., 236–40.

21 Henry King Carroll, *The Religious Forces of the United States Enumerated, Classified, and Described* (New York: Charles Scribner's Sons, 1912); A. J. Lamme III, "Christian Science in the U.S.A., 1900–1910: a distributional study," Discussion Paper Series, Depart-

ment of Geography, Syracuse University, no. 3, April 1975.

22 Stephen Gottschalk, *The Emergence of Christian Science in American Religious Life* (Berkeley: University of California Press, 1973), 244.

23 Except where otherwise indicated, the discussion of Ellen White is based on Numbers, *Prophetess of Health*.

24 *Early Writings of Ellen G. White* (Washington: Review and Herald Publishing Association, 1945), 21.

25 Ronald L. Numbers and Janet S. Numbers, "The psychological world of Ellen White," *Spectrum*, no. 1, 1983, *14:* 21–31.

26 Ellen G. White, *An Appeal to Mothers: The Great Cause of the Physical, Mental, and Moral Ruin of Many of the Children of Our Time* (Battle Creek, Mich.: SDA Publishing Association, 1864), 27.

27 College of Medical Evangelists, Calendar, 1909–1910.

28 Eddy, *Retrospection*, 13; Mrs. E. G. White, *Testimonies for the Church, with a Biographical Sketch of the Author,* 9 vols. (Mountain View, Calif.: Pacific Press Publishing Association, n.d.), *1:*25.

29 Peel, *Years of Discovery*, 27; *Life Sketches of Ellen G. White* (Mountain View, Calif.: Pacific Press Publishing Association, 1915), 39; White, *Testimonies*, 1:13.

30 Nancy F. Cott, *The Bonds of Womanhood: "Woman's Sphere" in New England, 1780–1835* (New Haven, Conn.: Yale University Press, 1977), 140. On the role played by women in Victorian religious life, see also Ann Douglas, *The Feminization of American Culture* (New York: Alfred A. Knopf, 1977).

31 Eddy, *Science and Health*, 1875, 400.

32 A fuller development of the healing aspects of Christian Science will appear in Schoepflin's forthcoming dissertation, "Christian Science healing in America: theory and practice from 1865 to 1910."

PHYSICIANS

In the middle of the nineteenth century, when women sought medical education within male institutions, they met rejection more often than admission. Although Elizabeth Blackwell received her medical education and degree from the all-male Geneva Medical College in 1849, most women were frustrated when trying to follow in her footsteps. The women's response to the repeated rebuffs from the male schools was to open their own medical colleges: seventeen all-female medical schools were founded in the United States in the nineteenth century. Practical clinical experience was also scarce for women learning medicine, and in response to this need Dr. Marie Zakrzewska opened the New England Hospital for Women and Children, here described by Mary Roth Walsh. Walsh emphasizes the importance of the moral and financial support of the women's movement for this hospital as for women's medical education in general. In contradistinction to the next article by Regina Morantz and Sue Zschoche, Walsh posits that the practice of the women doctors differed qualitatively from that offered at male-run hospitals. Morantz and Zschoche closely examine the therapeutic regimens of male and female doctors at two Boston hospitals and conclude that the doctor's medical training made them more alike than their sex-role training made them different.

Because of the success of female medical education during the second half of the nineteenth century, many male schools began to admit women students, the largest breakthrough coming in 1893 when Johns Hopkins accepted $500,000 in contributions from the women's community with its stipulation that women students be admitted equally with men. Sectarian medical schools more readily admitted women than did the regular schools. Yet William Barlow and David Powell relate the controversy over coeducation at one homeopathic medical school in the 1870s and remind us of the deep and widespread societal prejudice against women in the professions. Cora Marrett describes the trials and successes of women physicians within their own professional societies, and Constance McGovern analyzes the tensions that women doctors endured in psychiatric institutions.

Despite all the difficulties, women achieved significant successes in medicine. By 1910 over nine thousand women practiced medicine in the United States (6 percent of the total), and in some cities, like Boston and Minneapolis, almost 20 percent of practitioners were women. But in the twentieth century women lost ground within the medical profession. All but one of the women's medical schools closed when male colleges in their areas admitted women students, and the remaining Woman's Medical College of Pennsylvania (which became coeducational in the 1970s) itself trained one-third of the women medical graduates during the first half of the twentieth century. Women found limited welcomes in the male schools and discovered that their minority status compromised their educational experiences. Only since the 1970s, under strict federal guidelines and with the full support of the new women's movement, have women in medicine again found as supportive an environment within medicine as they enjoyed at the height of their successes in the nineteenth century.

27

Feminist Showplace

MARY ROTH WALSH

Historians, by concentrating on the political side of feminism, have largely ignored the material and psychological support that the movement offered.[1] Nowhere is this better illustrated than in the case of the New England Hospital for Women and Children, established by Dr. Marie Zakrzewska.

Zakrzewska has attracted relatively little attention from historians, although she was one of the most influential female physicians of the nineteenth century. In many ways she played a greater role in developing careers for women in American medicine than the more famous Blackwell sisters.[2] Born in Berlin in 1829, her childhood experiences had a great deal to do with shaping her career. When Zakrzewska was ten, her father was dismissed from the Prussian army, forcing her mother to become a midwife and the family breadwinner. That same year Zakrzewska contracted an eye infection and was placed under the care of a physician who took a liking to her, allowed her to follow him on his hospital rounds, and loaned her medical books from his personal library. She quickly developed a keen interest in medicine and, as soon as she was old enough, began assisting in her mother's midwifery practice. At age twenty, after two years of petitioning the state authorities for a position in the government-sponsored midwifery school, Zakrzewska finally succeeded in gaining admission to the school at Charité Hospital, the largest hospital in Prussia. The fact that Zak-

rzewska was the youngest woman to have entered the school made her highly visible. In a short time, her medical aptitude and outstanding performance as a student won the admiration of Dr. Joseph Schmidt, the director of the hospital. A French midwife, Madame La Chapelle, had won international fame in obstetrics; Schmidt, in a burst of patriotic pride, predicted that Prussia, as well as France, might boast of "a La Chapelle" and, before Zakrzewska ever had an opportunity to earn the title, dubbed her "La Chapelle the Second." The name stuck and, like a self-fulfilling prophecy, Zakrzewska became his star pupil.

In 1852, a year after Zakrzewska's graduation, Schmidt, although critically ill, was able to overcome strong internal opposition against the appointment of a woman as his successor. Zakrzewska became the chief midwife and professor in the hospital's school for midwives with responsibility for more than two hundred students, including men in the medical school. Unfortunately, the announcement of the appointment came only a few hours before Schmidt's death, and Zakrzewska was unprepared for the jealousy and hospital politics that followed. Schmidt's protective sponsorship for three years had eliminated the necessity of her learning strategies for coping with competition in the hospital. Within six months, she found the job to be too burdensome and resigned, attempting for a time to establish a private midwifery practice. But an early taste of success in her field made it difficult for her to practice quietly and forget about assuming a larger role in medicine beyond that of an anonymous midwife. She recalled later: "my education and aspirations demanded more than this." Not surprisingly, in view of the recent tide of emigration, her search for expanded opportunities turned to America. She remembered the positive reaction of Schmidt to the news of the establishment of the Female Med-

MARY ROTH WALSH is Professor of Psychology and American Studies at the University of Lowell, Lowell, Massachusetts and a Visiting Scholar in the Psychology Department at Harvard University, Cambridge, Massachusetts.

Reprinted with permission from "*Doctors Wanted: No Women Need Apply:*" *Sexual Barriers in the Medical Profession 1835–1975* by Mary Roth Walsh (New Haven: Yale University Press, 1977), pp. 76–105. Copyright © 1977 by Mary Roth Walsh.

ical College in Philadelphia: "In America, women will now become physicians like the men: it shows that only in a republic can it be proved that science has no sex."[3]

Convinced that she would find greater freedom to practice medicine in the United States, she sailed with her younger sister to New York in 1853. There she contacted a family friend, a German-American doctor, who quickly dispelled her illusions about American medicine. Pointing out that female physicians were of the lowest rank, even below that of a good nurse, he offered Zakrzewska a position as his own nurse, which she politely but firmly refused, unwilling "to be patronized in this way."[4] Handicapped by her difficulty in learning English and unsuccessful in attracting midwifery cases, she was soon forced to turn to the establishment of a cottage industry in her tenement apartment in New York. She and her sister began the production of worsted materials, employing as many as thirty employees at one time.

The success of her business in no way diverted Zakrzewska from her goal of pursuing a medical degree, but her lack of contacts and difficulty in communicating made progress in this direction slow. Finally, a year after she had arrived in New York, she visited a Home for the Friendless and was able to describe her frustrated attempts to learn more about the Female Medical College in Philadelphia. The woman in charge introduced her to Dr. Elizabeth Blackwell, who, in addition to her regular medical practice, had opened a one-room dispensary on the East Side of New York for poor women and children. Blackwell not only offered to tutor the young immigrant in English in return for her aid at the dispensary, but also promised to help her gain admission to a medical college. Through Elizabeth Blackwell's efforts, Zakrzewska was accepted by the medical department of Cleveland Medical College (Ohio) from which Emily Blackwell had recently graduated. Up to this point, Zakrzewska had no sympathy for the woman's rights movement. The demands raised at one New York convention seemed so ridiculous that she found the caption in one newspaper, "The Hens Which Want to Crow," as "quite appropriate." However, when she received the news that ways and means had been found for her to attend medical school, she realized that she had been trying to crow as hard as any of the women without realizing it.[5]

A combination of Zakrzewska's neglect of her knitting business and changes in the fashions of the worsted industry had left her with little money for her education. Fortunately, Dr. Harriot Hunt had recently toured Ohio raising funds for female medical education in that state.[6] As a result of scholarship aid from this source, Zakrzewska's lecture fees were waived for an indefinite period, and since Elizabeth Blackwell supplied all the necessary medical textbooks, Zakrzewska had to pay only the twenty-dollar matriculation fee. Furthermore, Caroline Severance, a friend of Blackwell's and president of a ladies physiological society near Cleveland, agreed to pay for her board out of a fund established by the society to assist needy women medical students.[7] If one had attempted to construct a story revolving around the tangible benefit of sisterhood, one could hardly improve upon the example of Zakrzewska's early career.

It is impossible to exaggerate the importance of this web of feminist friendship. One of only four women out of two hundred students at the college, Zakrzewska encountered obstacles unknown to her male colleagues. It took several weeks for her, even with the aid of a society woman's sponsorship (in this case Caroline Severance), to locate a boarding-house that would accept a female medical student. Even here, the other boarders would quickly leave when Zakrzewska and her roommate, another female medical student, entered the room.[8] Upon completion of her medical education, Zakrzewska returned to New York ready to hang out her shingle and begin private practice. Once again, however, she encountered resistance unknown to a male physician. The ordinarily simple task of securing an office elicited three types of negative response, all pointing out the stigma attached to being a female physician in the 1850s. One group of landlords could not accept the notion of a female physician and refused to rent space to her on the grounds that she was probably masking her real identity as a spiritualist or clairvoyant. The second group accepted her credentials, but doubted that she would be able to support herself and pay the rent. The third group asked no questions, but demanded such expensive rents that she could not afford to lease their quarters. After a month of fruitless searching, Elizabeth Blackwell allowed her to open an office in her back parlor.[9]

The burden of locating an office paled in comparison with the difficulty of finding patients to develop a medical practice. Rothstein has described the necessary elements for success in the nineteenth-century medical world: "Family background and wealth, social standing and friendship were paramount in gaining admission to a medical school, setting up a practice, obtaining appointments to hospitals, medical schools, and elite medical societies, and attracting a wealthy clientele."[10] A female physician began her pursuit of a career severely stigmatized because of her sex, and this fact hindered her in every step she took in establishing herself as a professional. Elizabeth Blackwell had already experienced every possible discouragement in her five years in New York. She was barred from practice in the city hospitals and dispensaries, ignored by her medical colleagues, and was the target of anonymous hate mail. She had solved the problem of office space by buying her own home, and she had dealt with the loneliness by adopting a seven-year-old orphan in 1854. By the time Zakrzewska joined Blackwell, she was eagerly awaiting the return of her sister Emily who had been studying medicine for two years in Edinburgh.

In numbers there was strength as well as sociability. Both Zakrzewska and Elizabeth Blackwell were eager to reestablish the dispensary in which Zakrzewska had first assisted Blackwell and which failed for lack of funds. Zakrzewska, drawing on her business experience, drew up an operating budget for the proposed hospital. She then threw herself into fund raising and traveled to Boston to meet with Harriot Hunt, Caroline Severance (who had moved to that city), and a number of other local women interested in woman's rights. She was able to extract a promise of $650 to be paid over a three-year period to the new hospital. This promise stimulated donors in New York to raise an additional $1,000, enough to open New York Infirmary for Women and Children on May 1, 1857; it was the first hospital staffed by women in the United States.[11]

For two years Zakrzewska served without salary as resident physician and general manager of the hospital, sharing with the Blackwell sisters the responsibilities connected with a growing institution. By 1859, with the infirmary firmly established, Zakrzewska felt that she had fulfilled her debt to the Blackwells. Moreover, her own financial situation had improved as a result of her private prac-

tice. In March of that year she accepted an offer from Samuel Gregory's New England Female Medical College to be professor of obstetrics and resident physician of the proposed hospital. At least three factors appear to have influenced her decision: the conviction that achievement would add to a woman's personal happiness; a desire for greater independence and leadership; and a conviction that the women of Boston were intent in "their desire to elevate the education of womankind in general and in medicine especially." In a letter to Harriot Hunt, Zakrzewska revealed how depressing she found working with the Blackwell sisters, especially after opening New York Infirmary. The two women had such gloomy outlooks on life that Zakrzewska found them bewildering: "these two women for instance have all right to be satisfied with their efforts as it resulted . . . but they won't acknowledge it either to each other or to themselves. . . . I feel sad that nothing can cheer them up . . . they do wrong not to reward their friends by showing them a pleased countenance." Zakrzewska's letter was filled with good wishes for all her friends in Boston, especially Hunt, whose pleasure in personal achievement was uninhibited and who had been hostess to Zakrzewska for several of her visits.[12]

Zakrzewska failed to realize her second objective in coming to Boston and resigned in 1862 after repeated clashes over school policy with Gregory. Yet, despite the problems connected with the Female Medical College, her experience there only reinforced her original convictions that a supportive body of women shared her belief in medical education for women: "I decided to work again on the old plan, namely to establish the education of female students on sound principles, that is to educate them in hospitals."[13] Hospital training was increasingly becoming recognized as an essential ingredient in a complete medical education,[14] yet the only American hospital open to women was the New York Infirmary. Fundamental to Zakrzewska's plans for a training hospital was her conviction that medical colleges such as Harvard would accept women students once pioneers like herself had demonstrated that women could perform a meaningful role in medicine.

Sound principles for Zakrzewska also meant uniting with the regular physicians and avoiding any association with the irregulars, particularly the homeopaths. In an effort to counter the conventional medical histories which dismiss the irregulars as quacks, recent historians have supplied us with a useful reinterpretation by focusing on the positive contributions of the irregulars. No doubt a thorough analysis of the irregulars will contribute to a new understanding of one particular strand of feminist ideology. Similarly, in order to understand the difficulties that have beset women seeking professional medical careers, we must study the pioneer women (such as Zakrzewska) with a view of understanding why they chose not to identify with the irregulars.

From both a political and a medicoscientific point of view, Zakrzewska was convinced that women must follow the regular medical path. Formally trained as both a midwife and a physician, she had little patience with those whose remedies verged more on mind cure than body cure. Her experience with the male-dominated medical world of Europe coupled with her initial experiences as a struggling immigrant made her a realist about the significance of professional power. For her, the only solution for medical women was to force men to deal with them as equals.

Accordingly, New England Hospital for Women and Children, a "sunny, airy house" at 60 Pleasant Street in Boston's South End, was rented for $600 and opened July 1, 1862. When it was incorporated the following March, its charter spelled out the two primary goals of the hospital: to furnish women with medical aid from competent physicians of their own sex, and to provide educated women with an opportunity for practical study in medicine. Significantly, two-thirds of the first board of directors were the same women who had served on the board of lady managers of the New England Female Medical College.[15] There was no qualified woman surgeon available, so Zakrzewska was forced to employ a leading male gynecologist, Dr. Horatio Storer, in 1863; when he resigned three years later, he was replaced by a female specialist, making the hospital the first in New England to be entirely staffed by women physicians.

In the first few years these women physicians were a union of the weak, rather than a combination of the strong. For example, Zakrzewska recalled how she felt in 1863: "My co-workers were young and inexperienced, looking up to me for wisdom and instruction while the public in general

watched with scrupulous zeal in order to stand ready for condemnation." Fortunately, there were a few male physicians who were willing to cross the sexual boundary. Samuel Cabot and Henry I. Bowditch, both Harvard educated, had told her they would "refuse all aid" so long as she remained at Gregory's school; they readily came to her assistance when she left.[16]

Cabot became the first consulting physician at the hospital, offering his advice in difficult cases. He also provided Zakrzewska with important psychological support. She recounted in a letter to Dr. Lucy Sewall that Cabot did not feel it necessary for her to call him for forceps deliveries. "You see," she wrote proudly, "he rightly supposes we use the forceps *skillfully*." Bowditch had initially befriended Zakrzewska when she came to Boston in 1856 to solicit funds for New York Infirmary. She later recalled: "He remained the steadfast champion of medical women and continued as consulting physician to the New England Hospital until his death in 1892." Another physician, Benjamin Cotting, was especially helpful in sending both rich and poor patients to the hospital. Both were welcome: one group contributed much-needed fees as private patients; students treated the others in the dispensary. Such gestures, infrequent as they were, were a welcome tonic to someone generally treated as a pariah by the city's medical establishment. As Zakrzewska noted: "Every slight word or act of endorsement, even though with reservations, was like a ray of hope that at last the dawn was breaking. . . . Such consolations helped to uphold me."[17]

Although Zakrzewska praised the early male consultants, except for Henry Bowditch they were for the most part fair-weather friends who withdrew support temporarily whenever there was too much pressure from the Boston medical establishment. Thus, when Zakrzewska took their advice and applied for membership in the Massachusetts Medical Society and was turned down because of her sex, Cabot and Cotting severed their ties with the hospital until the issue faded. Nevertheless, Zakrzewska felt their presence served to quiet those in the profession "who wanted to find fault but did not dare to do so openly so long as the two or three professional men stood as a moral force behind me."[18]

Finances were a problem of another dimension

and, in the early years at least, were a major difficulty, even threatening the hospital's existence. The combined assets of the new institution in 1862 consisted of some $150 worth of hospital furniture brought from New England Female Medical College after Gregory evicted the lady managers and Zakrzewska. As the secretary of the board described the situation: "Our possessions were a few iron bedsteads, a few chairs, and bookcases, some straw, etc., our earnest purpose and our admirable Dr. Zakrzewska."[19] No gifts, however small, were refused, and the early annual reports are filled with lists of donations ranging from scissors and bandages to tea and cornstarch.

An important source of income during the hospital's first decade was an annual grant of $1,000 for maternity patients from the trustees of Boston Lying-In Hospital Corporation, which did not operate from 1856 to 1873 because it could not obtain patients.[20] In 1864, supported by a $5,000 grant from the Massachusetts legislature and matched by a number of donors, the hospital moved to larger quarters at 14 Warren Street. The state also offered additional assistance in the form of $1,000 each year for four years beginning in 1868. Fairs were also important sources of revenue; in 1871, $12,000 was realized in this fashion. Sizable donations from women during these formative years played a crucial role in the hospital's development. Zakrzewska's reputation inspired confidence as evidenced by a $2,000 bequest from the estate of Mrs. Robert G. Shaw that same year "to be used by Dr. Zakrzewska in aid of any Hospital or Infirmary . . . which may be under her superintendence in the City of Boston at the time of my decease." This money, coupled with other gifts (notably a $5,000 bequest from Miss Nabby Joy), enabled the hospital to move again in 1872 to what was to become its permanent location in the highlands section of Roxbury. By 1872 New England Hospital for Women and Children had become, in just ten years, one of the largest hospitals in Boston.[21]

The financial situation was further aided by the fact that a number of the staff, including Zakrzewska, donated their services. Driven by her desire to improve the cause of women in medicine, Dr. Lucy Sewall, for example, served as resident physician of the hospital for three years beginning in 1863 without salary or vacation.[22] Zakrzewska supported herself through her private practice and

by renting rooms in her home in Roxbury to invalid boarders. Even in her personal practice, Zakrzewska sought to expand the role of women. Thus, she regularly walked to night calls in any type of weather to prove "that a woman has not only the same (if not more) physical endurance as a man." Women physicians were handicapped by more than inclement weather in their pursuit of night calls. Zakrzewska always went with the messenger who called her. If he was unable to accompany her on her return home, she walked with the local policeman to the limit of his beat and traveled in similar fashion from one beat to another until she arrived home. This problem was solved in 1865 when she bought a horse and a secondhand buggy, which also enabled her to "uphold the professional etiquette and dignity of a woman physician on equality with men."[23]

Nevertheless, it is doubtful that Zakrzewska and her hospital could have succeeded without the support of the feminist movement. During its first fifty years, the hospital had only three presidents; Lucy Goddard, Ednah Cheney, and Mrs. Helen F. Kimball. Ednah Cheney exemplifies the close bond between feminism and the hospital. One of the lady managers of the Female Medical College, Cheney was active at every stage of the hospital's development, beginning with her pledge along with three other women in 1862 to pay the first year's rent on the first building on Pleasant Street. A close friend and later neighbor of Zakrzewska, she served on the board of directors of the hospital for forty-eight years—including fifteen as president. In addition to her hospital activities, Cheney helped found the New England Women's Club, served on the executive committee of the New England Woman Suffrage Association, and actively campaigned for women's right to vote in school committee elections. Cheney was not unique, and an analysis of the early bequest lists shows that the hospital donors often left funds to suffrage associations. In 1887 over 80 percent of the donors to a $10,000 hospital fund were women.[24]

To view feminism as simply a struggle for woman's rights and the vote is to ignore the support and companionship it offered those women who broke with their prescribed roles. It is clear that a female physician could not have functioned autonomously in nineteenth-century America. Zakrzewska's dependence on the woman's movement was

total: she needed female supporters to help finance her education, to raise money, to promote
the hospital, to help administer it, to serve as patients, and—probably most critically—to proffer
their friendship during difficult times. It was Zakrzewska herself who had originally suggested an
association of women which was translated into the
New England Women's Club and which met initially in the home of Harriot Hunt. For many
women, it was the first time they came together not
because of family, neighborhood, or church, but as
women. The club regularly supported the women
doctors; for instance, it sponsored a "social levee"
when Dr. Lucy Sewall went to Europe to study.
The members also were active in running fairs to
raise money for the hospital. In turn, female doctors regularly gave lectures to the women at the
club and sponsored discussion groups.[25]

One of the most openly militant supporters of
the woman physician was the *Woman's Journal,* which
was edited by Lucy Stone and began publication in
Boston in 1870. Zakrzewska had called for such a
journal as early as 1862 when she and another
woman doctor, Mary Breed, inserted a notice for a
Woman's Journal in the *Liberator,* but at that date
they were unable to secure enough support.[26] Lucy
Stone's *Woman's Journal* championed the cause of
women doctors and challenged the right of society
to erect barriers to stand in their way. The editors
encouraged reader response to this problem and
published in full the letters of angry women doctors who felt blocked in their careers. An 1871
letter to the paper cautioned: "Let [men] not feel
too sure that they alone hold the key that unlocks
the door to medical science. They bar and bolt the
doors of their hospitals in Boston against all women
medical students. They heap upon them undeserved ridicule. They hold up to the world their
constitutional weaknesses in a manner to lead one
to suppose that they possess no such weaknesses
themselves. They scorn the very idea of holding a
consultation with a woman physician. . . . True
women physicians would be glad to have the men
in the profession see the mistake they are making
and become their friends as they ought, in this
manner. They would be glad to see the city hospitals and dispensaries opened to women medical
students. They blush for the city of Boston that
this is not done." The writer concluded by warning: "But, aided or unaided, the day is not far dis-

tant when women will compel medical men to know
that as physicians they are their equals, whether
they have the magnanimity to acknowledge it or
not."[27]

Each act of exclusion by the medical establishment brought the wrath of the journal down on
the heads of the perpetrators. Pointing out that
Boston's Free Hospital for Women was served entirely by male physicians, the editor noted: "This is
a shame in a city where there are competent women
physicians. It is a poor, empty and prating pretense, that of indelicacy of common study, by those
men who clutch at and crowd for medical practice
among women."[28] The journal also did a great deal
in advertising the success of women in medicine. It
was happy to report that a research article of Dr.
Sara E. Brown, which had been refused by the
Boston Medical and Surgical Journal "on account of
her sex," was published by the *Archives of Ophthal-
mology and Otology* and reproduced in a number of
international medical periodicals, thus gaining wider
publicity than it would have received from the Boston publication.[29]

New England Hospital gained a great deal of
free publicity in the pages of the *Woman's Journal.*
Each year it published a lengthy report on the hospital's progress. Readers were reminded of their
obligation to support this feminist project and urged
to attend each fund-raising fair. Women doctors
were especially hard hit by the medical strictures
against advertising in the public press while at the
same time their professional brethren refused to
recognize their existence and include them in the
directories put out by doctors themselves. For example, the *Medical Register of Boston* refused to list
the names of the women physicians even after it
began to include all manner of peripheral practitioners such as artificial limb makers, collectors,
makers of optical instruments, vendors of patent
medicines, and female nurses. In order to fight the
prejudice confronting them, the women physicians
had to advertise. Here the *Woman's Journal* was a
valuable ally. It did all it could to right the balance
by publishing testimonials about the competence
of women physicians such as one from "M. W.," a
schoolteacher, who described how she had been
restored to health by Dr. Zakrzewska's "skill and
kindness, a debt that words are feeble to portray."
Similarly, the journal publicized each addition to
the hospital staff. Thus, Dr. Fanny Berlinerblau

was introduced in a typical report that told the story of her difficulties in securing a medical education, extolled her "admirable scientific training," and informed the readers that she had abbreviated her name to Dr. Fanny Berlin "to suit the American tongue."[30] But the *Journal's* public relations efforts on behalf of the hospital could do only so much; in the final analysis, the hospital's performance would be the ultimate arbiter of its fate.

The two primary objectives of the New England Hospital were to provide women with medical aid from doctors of their own sex and to contribute to the supply of competent women doctors by providing them with an opportunity for practical clinical experience. While specializing in obstetrics, gynecology, and pediatrics, the hospital also offered a full range of medical treatment, including surgery on a bed-patient as well as a dispensary basis. Zakrzewska's hospital filled an important void in Boston medicine. Boston City Hospital, which opened two years after Zakrzewska's institution, did not provide gynecological treatment until 1873, and then only on an outpatient basis. It did not create a gynecological department until 1892. Massachusetts General Hospital, which had been operating since 1822, did not provide obstetrical services until the twentieth century. At the time of its inception, New England Hospital was unique in its provision for both obstetrical and gynecological treatment of patients. The only other hospital in the city to have specialized in obstetrics, Boston Lying-In Hospital, had closed its doors in 1856, "a white elephant of mastodonic proportions." Every effort had been made to attract patients, including a massive advertising campaign in eighty-five newspapers, but women, if they had any choice in the matter, avoided using Boston Lying-In.[31]

The unwillingness of such women reflected an accurate assessment of the dangers connected with most maternity hospitals. Puerperal disease, which frequently resulted in death, stemmed from the unsanitary techniques that were characteristic of midcentury hospitals. There were a few physicians early in the nineteenth century who had suspected the cause of the high mortality rates of women in childbirth. Dr. Oliver Wendell Holmes, for example, had attended a lecture in Paris in 1833 which suggested that doctors themselves may have played a role in communicating the disease. In 1843 he read a paper on his research findings to his Boston

medical colleagues and published an article which demonstrated that the obstetrician, midwife, and nurse were active agents in transmitting the infection from one mother to another. He was promptly rebutted by Dr. Walter Channing who delivered a paper on the noncontagious nature of the disease, although Channing later reversed his position.[32]

Zakrzewska's work in the large Charité Hospital in Berlin had given her far more opportunity than most American physicians to observe the unsanitary conditions which were conducive to spreading puerperal disease. Her experience confirmed Holmes's theory. She had observed that when the medical students appeared in the Berlin hospitals with their forceps, "untimely rupturing the membranes or by other meddlesome interference with nature," the cases of the disease soared. During her appointment as chief midwife in Berlin in 1852, not a single case of the disease occurred because of the precautions that she took in the administration of the hospital. Zakrzewska's scientific acumen and her experience with the advantages of cleanliness were enormous assets to the hospital in its early years when bacteriology and asepsis were still matters of debate. A number of leading Boston physicians, including Walter Channing, C. P. Putnam, Henry I. Bowditch, and Samuel Cabot, signed an 1864 circular attesting to the hospital's success in preventing various contagious fevers, so impressed were these men with Zakrzewska's leadership in this matter.[33]

By contrast, Boston Lying-In Hospital, reopened in 1873, was forced to close three times in the next thirteen years because of puerperal epidemics within its wards. In 1883, at the height of a puerperal disease epidemic in Boston, only one of the patients in New England Hospital died from the fever. In contrast, over five hundred women contracted the disease and fifty died from it at Boston Lying-In Hospital from 1878 to 1883. Whether women physicians offered medical care superior to their male counterparts remains speculative, especially in view of the dearth of evidence related to treatment and the difficulties connected with comparing different patient populations. One researcher, whose pioneering investigation of this question involved an examination of doctors' comments on patient records at four different nineteenth-century Boston hospitals, concluded that the male practitioners reflected a negative or even hostile attitude toward their female patients. Complaints that the maternity patients were too lazy to "work" in delivering their babies or that their infections were their own fault were quite common. On the other hand, she found that these remarks were absent from the patient records at New England Hospital.[34] While it is difficult to assess the effect of physicians' attitudes on their patients, it would be wrong to underestimate it.

One can make a strong case that a good deal of New England Hospital's success can be attributed to the fact that the physicians there were also women with special insights and sensitivity toward the medical problem of their own sex. In an age when medical techniques were generally undeveloped and often unsafe, the women physicians' restraint, coupled with compassion, may have done much to effect a healthier hospital environment. For example, unlike many male doctors, the women seem to have been more willing to let nature take its course in childbirth. Avoiding the temptation to demonstrate their virtuosity with scalpel and forceps, the female physicians also avoided the medical dangers these instruments caused to both mother and child.[35]

Much of the work of the hospital in the nineteenth century was given over to charity cases. A number of "Free Hospital Beds" were donated by friends of the hospital. The dispensary charged ten cents a visit and twenty-five cents to fill a prescription at the hospital pharmacy, but those who could not afford these modest fees were treated without charge. Zakrzewska, who supervised the dispensary during the early years, noted: "A crowd of women, some from towns miles distant, came every morning."[36] One of her difficulties was to persuade wealthy women not to use the dispensary but rather to visit staff members who maintained a private practice. In one letter, she urged a friend of the hospital to recommend the services of two women physicians on the staff who were just starting their private practices: "Be sure to send them all the rich patients by telling [the patients] plainly that I don't want them."[37] In fact, charity cases became such an important part of the hospital case load that Lucy Sewall complained that many of the sick poor supposed the physicians were paid by the city, "and that they had a legal right to their services."[38]

The large number of charity and obstetrical patients in the early years led the hospital to establish the first social service department in an American hospital. Each patient was interviewed; for those women who had no family, places were found for them to board both prenatally and postnatally. Jobs were also found for those women who were the sole support of their children. The women who provided these counseling services were the same lady managers whom Samuel Gregory found so annoying at Female Medical College. At the hospital, Zakrzewska used their desire to serve in a way which she described as mutually enriching: "It is thus the privilege of the [lady manager] to round off and finish the large charity done by the physicians, while she herself has her sympathies quickened and her experiences enlarged by intimate acquaintances with life flowing in different channels from her own."[39] The number of patients serviced by the hospital grew steadily throughout the century. During its first sixteen months, the hospital treated 1,507 individuals; by the end of the century more than 19,000 patients annually passed through the dispensary doors. There were now specialized clinics for eye, ear, nose, and throat; maternity; and child health. The sophisticated turn-of-the-century hospital was a far cry from the single room that Zakrzewska supervised in 1862.[40]

By 1900 the hospital had made a great deal of progress. Most important, it had at least convinced its patients that women could be successful physicians. Far better than statistics in showing how far the hospital had come was Zakrzewska's encounter at the end of the century with an Irish immigrant, whose wife had been a charity case at the original Pleasant Street location. He wanted to arrange an operation for one of his family, and he insisted on having one of the woman physicians at New England Hospital. When he noticed Zakrzewska's surprise, he explained: "Well, Doctor, when I came to this country with my wife, we were very poor and knew nothing. The good women of the Pleasant Street Dispensary attended to us and taught us to take care of ourselves. All our children were born under their care and they watched that we did right by them, all without any charge. Now that we can afford good pay, I am sure we want the same, for I swear by the woman doctors."[41]

The second objective of the hospital was to provide educated women with an opportunity for practical study in medicine. One of the most difficult obstacles to the advance of women in medicine during the latter half of the nineteenth century was the lack of adequate facilities for clinical instruction. When women sought to gain this practical experience to supplement their classroom education, they were rebuffed because of the alleged indecency of observing cases in the presence of men—despite the fact that very frequently the patients themselves were females. The existence of this deep-seated opposition to the participation of women in clinical situations is dramatically illustrated by the experience of women at Philadelphia's Pennsylvania Hospital in 1869. Some thirty female medical students were invited to clinical lectures, but the male students objected "with insolent and offensive language." During the last hour, despite the efforts of members of the faculty, the men showered the women with "missiles of paper, tinfoil, and tobacco quids." Thus ended the effort at coeducation at the Pennsylvania Hospital.[42] It was obvious that with the exclusion of women from existing hospitals, they needed their own institutions in order to obtain clinical instruction.

Zakrzewska's hospital anticipated a need that was only surfacing in 1862. Luckily, only a small number of women doctors applied to the hospital in the 1860s, for the staff was inadequate and the facilities severely limited. Of the twenty-seven interns in the first ten years of the hospital's existence, twelve were graduates of a medical college before coming to the hospital and the other fifteen were stimulated by their experience to complete the academic requirements for the degree shortly after leaving the hospital. While it was fairly commonplace for Boston hospitals to accept male "House Pupils" who had not yet earned their M.D. degree, what was unusual about New England Hospital interns was the distance they had to travel to finish a degree or to obtain advanced training. Five young women went to Europe for medical study, two of whom were pursuing postdoctoral training; seven went to the University of Michigan; four to the Woman's Medical College of Pennsylvania; one to Howard University. The reason, of course, was that in the early years, there were few medical schools open to women students. Zakrzewska was never enthusiastic about Gregory's school when he was alive, and after the merger with Boston University she refused to recommend students to or accept applications from what was in its early years the city's only coeducational medical school, because of its irregular curriculum.[43]

The actual training that the hospital provided appears to have consisted of a minimum of formal instruction and a maximum of practical experience. The overtaxed staff had little time to devote exclusively to the students, and the education itself was on a learn-as-you-go basis. The hospital kept no intern records, and the only picture of the training is based on the variegated reactions of the students themselves. While some found all they had hoped for and others were disappointed, one is struck by how many influential women doctors passed through the hospital during its first decade.

Most notable of the hospital's "alumnae" of the 1860s was Dr. Mary Putnam Jacobi who, although twenty-one years old when she arrived, was a graduate of both New York College of Pharmacy and Woman's Medical College of Pennsylvania. She entered New England Hospital in 1864 but instead of the specialized training she expected, Jacobi found herself thrown into the work of the dispensary where close to two thousand women were treated during the year. No bed remained empty and many patients had to be treated in their homes. During one two-week period, Jacobi counted eleven nights when Zakrzewska was called out on emergencies. Seeing so many patients suffering from such a variety of ailments day after day temporarily persuaded Jacobi that she was not cut out for a regular medical practice. Convinced that she was destined for a career in medical research, she went to Paris, where in 1868 she became the first woman to be admitted to the Ecole de Medicine. After her return to America, she embarked on a career of research and medical school teaching which made her the leading woman physician in America in the late nineteenth century.[44]

Unlike Jacobi, Susan Dimock entered New England Hospital as the very first step in her medical career. Although only eighteen years old when she arrived in January 1866, her ability and prodigous capacity for work attracted the special attention of Zakrzewska and Sewall. With their encouragement, she and another student at the hospital, Sophia Jex-Blake, applied to Harvard Medical School the following year and were both turned down. Despite their rejection, New England Hospital was able to temporarily arrange for a limited amount of clinical instruction for the two at Massachusetts General Hospital when the Harvard students were not at the hospital. The 1867 Annual Report of the New England Hospital proudly announced: "They have availed themselves of all the opportunities offered them."[45]

Meanwhile Zakrzewska and Sewall persuaded Dimock to apply to the University of Zurich, which had been accepting female medical students since 1864. Two Boston women paid Dimock's expenses with the only stipulation that she return to New England Hospital for three years and assist some other struggling women medical students in the future. After graduating with high honors from Zurich and then spending an additional year in Paris and Vienna, Dimock returned in 1872 to become the most skilled surgeon on the staff.[46]

Sophia Jex-Blake, Dimock's companion in the attempt to enter Harvard in 1867, first exhibited at the hospital the spirit that would eventually make her the spokeswoman for a woman's right to a medical education in her native Great Britain. Unwilling to accept Harvard's refusal, she embarked on a personal campaign while at the hospital to build up support to break this barrier. She arranged interviews with each member of the Harvard faculty and the Massachusetts General staff. Some, like Oliver Wendell Holmes, expressed a willingness to lecture to women "always provided that any special subject which seemed not adapted to an audience of both sexes, should be delivered to male students alone." A more representative response was recorded in Jex-Blake's diary: "Dr. A. 'not afraid of responsibility, of course'—only—he'd rather not admit us till other people do!"[47]

Georgia Sturtevant, an assistant nurse at the time the young women medical students were being permitted at Massachusetts General Hospital, noted in her memoirs that Dimock and Jex-Blake, "though championed by some of the most popular of the visiting staff, were really allowed this privilege under protest, and were under many restrictions, and were only allowed to visit in certain wards."[48] Jex-Blake, particularly, felt a constant sense of insecurity as one member of the staff was bitterly opposed to the presence of women and constantly searched for mistakes to bolster his prejudices. Such tensions took their toll as Jex-Blake wrote in her diary:

"July 5th. Rest yesterday, but altogether weighed down yesterday and today with the fear and horror of this irritability which seems so fatally unconquerable." Dissatisfied with the situation at Massachusetts General and convinced that she had received enough practical experience, Jex-Blake went to New York where she was able to obtain private lessons in anatomy from the head demonstrator at Bellevue Hospital. A month later she left for home where she won fame as the leader of the movement to admit women to the medical profession in Great Britain and the founder of the London School of Medicine for Women.[49]

Elizabeth Mosher, whose only previous medical experience involved nursing her tubercular brother, entered New England Hospital in 1869. After a successful internship and a year of assisting Lucy Sewall in her private practice, Mosher left for the University of Michigan where she received her M.D. degree in 1875. She went on to a number of important medical posts which culminated in her appointment as the first dean of students and professor of physiology at the University of Michigan. She later credited her year at New England Hospital as the turning point in her career: "I believe I voice all of the women ... when I say I feel I largely owe to the teaching, the spirit of devotion, and the high standard maintained by this hospital whatever of success I may have been able to achieve in medicine."[50]

With each year the hospital raised the quality of its training. By the mid-1870s the staff of the hospital began debating the problems of selecting from the large number of qualified applicants for the internship positions and by 1879 they accepted, with reluctance, the solution of taking only those women who already possessed the M.D. degree.[51] Increasing numbers of women were also coming to the hospital for experience after having attended a liberal arts college as well as receiving the medical degree. This was the case with Dr. Minerva Walker, who attended Cornell University before receiving the M.D. from the Woman's Medical College of Pennsylvania in 1879.[52] The larger, more specialized staff of the last decades of the nineteenth century provided a far more intensive training period than had been possible in the 1860s. Dr. Kate Hurd-Mead, who interned at the hospital in the 1880s, described her experience there as highly structured: "Life was indeed serious to the young doctors under the watchful eye of resident and visiting physicians. If, in an unguarded moment, the intern was heard humming a little air or whistling softly at her work, or even if her shoes squeaked a trifle, she was taken to task by one of these dignified censors and questioned as to her reasons for studying medicine and for her unseemly deportment."[53]

By 1887, on the twenty-fifth anniversary of New England Hospital, Zakrzewska's original goal of a hospital run by women for women had been realized. From the board of directors to the delivery of health care to patients, women held full responsibility and authority, though, as the anniversary report pointed out, "the counsel and help of the other sex is gladly welcomed." This was especially true in regard to the consulting physicians, men who were selected not as mere status symbols but because "they have taken an active interest in the Hospital, and have been chosen for special eminence in some department."[54] As a result of the vision of Zakrzewska, an increasing number of trained doctors were being turned out to meet the rising patient demand. But the hospital was more than an institution where women absorbed the technical knowledge and skills of their profession. Equally necessary in the sexually polarized world of the late nineteenth century was the psychic support and energy which they needed to enable them to practice a profession that did everything it could to discourage them. Herein lies the significance of the hospital. It was not only a showcase in which women physicians could prove themselves; it was also an island of feminist strength and sisterhood in a society only familiar with brotherhood.

Consequently, when a group of twelve Greater Boston women physicians, ten of whom had been associated with the hospital, gathered in 1878 to form the first female medical society in the United States, they named the organization the New England Hospital Medical Society. At a time when the Massachusetts Medical Society was closed to women, this separate group offered its members both a sense of colleagueship and a common voice. One of its first steps was to pressure the editors of the *Boston City Directory* to list its members under the heading of the society, a service which the directory had always rendered to the members of the Massachu-

setts Medical Society and any other local male medical group. The separate listing was important, for while the Massachusetts Medical Society members had been divorced from the other sectarian and irregular physicians, including patent medicine promoters, the women physicians had been indiscriminately lumped under the heading of "female physicians," which included phrenologists, magnetists, Christian Scientists, and electricians, as well as midwives and nurses. Zakrzewska was particularly eager to dissociate her hospital from any taint of homeopathy and sectarianism. Graduates of Boston University Medical School as well as other irregular schools were excluded from the New England Hospital Medical Society, and interns from such schools were likewise barred from the hospital. The women hoped that by not confusing the issue of women's competence in regular medicine with the sectarian controversies in the profession at large, they would advance the cause of women more directly.[55]

Thus, New England Hospital fought for the causes of medical women and, indirectly, feminists, on a variety of fronts. Its separatism was a means to an end; ironically, that end was the elimination of separatism and the movement of women into the mainstream of medicine. Whenever Zakrzewska spoke publicly about women physicians and particularly when she addressed her student interns, she always expressed the hope that the hospital would convince the medical profession of the ability of women physicians, "and shall thus force them to open Harvard College to such women as desire entrance there."[56] She believed that the presence of male consultants on the staff would demonstrate that men and women physicians could work side by side to the advantage of both sexes and society as a whole. In this spirit, the New England Hospital Medical Society even invited male physicians to membership, an invitation that the men chose to ignore, though a few did toy with the idea briefly.[57]

Quite clearly, many female physicians believed that as women they brought a much-needed dimension to the practice of medicine. But it was equally obvious that these benefits would not accrue to the profession as long as women were isolated.

NOTES

1 Books on political feminism include: Eleanor Flexner, *Century of Struggle: The Woman's Rights Movement in the United States* (Cambridge, Mass., 1959); Andrew Sinclair, *The Better Half: The Emancipation of the American Woman* (New York, 1965); Robert Riegel, *American Feminism* (Lawrence, Kans., 1963); Aileen Kraditor, *The Ideas of the Woman Suffrage Movement, 1890–1920* (New York, 1965); William O'Neill, *Everyone Was Brave: The Rise and Fall of Feminism in America* (Chicago, 1969); Anne F. Scott and Andrew M. Scott, *One Half of the People: The Fight for Woman Suffrage* (Philadelphia, 1975).

2 Elizabeth Blackwell left America in 1869, spent most of her life in England, and died there in 1910. A recent, well-documented study is: Nancy Sahli, "Elizabeth Blackwell, M.D. (1821–1910): a biography," Ph.D. diss., University of Pennsylvania, 1974. Emily Blackwell, who also died in 1910, was in many ways overshadowed by the fame of her older sister though she devoted her life to the practice of medicine in America. Both women have been the subject of many popular articles and biographies. Zakrzewska's life, on the other hand, has gone relatively unnoticed except for two autobiographical memoirs cited in n. 3 below. Bibliographies of all three women are in Edward James, ed., *Notable American Women* (Cambridge, Mass., 1971).

3 Caroline Dall, ed., *A Practical Illustration of Woman's Right to Labor or a Letter from Marie Elizabeth Zakrzewska* (Boston, 1869), 60, 85; Agnes Vietor, *A Woman's Quest: The Life of Marie E. Zakrzewska* (New York, 1924), 84–85.

4 Dall, *Practical Illustration*, 105.

5 Vietor, *Woman's Quest*, 134.

6 Ibid., 485.

7 Ibid., 119–21.

8 Ibid., 131.

9 Ibid., 179–81.

10 William G. Rothstein, *American Physicians in the Nineteenth Century: From Sects to Science* (Baltimore, 1972), 206–7. Although there were important differences in the social stratification systems of England and America in the mid-nineteenth century, it is interesting to note how similar the plight of the beginning physician was in both countries—even without the added difficulty of sex discrimination. For an analysis of the problems of the male physician who started out alone in London, see M. Jeanne Peterson, "Kinship, status, and social mobility in the mid-Victorian medical profession," Ph.D. diss., University of California, Berkeley, June 1972, 153:

"for all the growth in medical education and licensing and the advancement of medical science, the basis on which Victorian medical men built their careers was not primarily that of expertise. Family, friends, connections, and new variations of these traditional forms of social relationships and social evaluation were the crux of a man's ability to establish himself in medical practice." Peterson uses statistical and biographical materials to substantiate this thesis.

11 Vietor, *Woman's Quest*, 211.

12 Ibid., 237–39, 149, 186, 192, 197; Marie Zakrzewska to Harriot Hunt, May 14, 1857, Caroline Dall Collection, (Massachusetts Historical Society).

13 Vietor, *Woman's Quest*, 292.

14 Rosemary Stevens notes that the first use of the term "intern" in American hospital records was apparently in the Boston City Hospital Board of Trustees Report for 1865 (*American Medicine and the Public Interest* [New Haven, 1971], 116–17). See also "Background and development of residency review and conference committees," *Journal of the American Medical Association*, 1957, *165:* 60–64. By 1904 the AMA Council on Medical Education found that as many as 50 percent of new medical graduates went on to hospital training; by 1914 it was estimated that 75 or 80 percent of graduates were taking an internship (see Stevens, 118). Rothstein claims that by 1865 about two-thirds of medical schools made arrangements for some hospital and clinical instruction of students—see 282.

15 Vietor, *Woman's Quest*, 486–87. See also the "Records of the lady managers of the New England Female Medical College," (Boston University Archives), and the first Annual Report of the New England Hospital (1864).

16 Vietor, *Woman's Quest*, 330, 256.

17 Ibid., 301, 336, 256, 332, 330–31.

18 Ibid., 277–78, 330.

19 Cited by Alice B. Crosby, *The Fiftieth Anniversary of the New England Hospital for Women and Children, October 29, 1912* (Boston, 1913), 17.

20 See the annual reports of the New England Hospital for Women and Children (AR-NEH) from 1863 to 1871; the 1871 report indicates final payment from the Lying-In Hospital Corporation, November 7, 1871.

21 AR-NEH (1871), 17; Vietor, *Woman's Quest*, 353. Francis H. Brown, M.D., *The Medical Register for the Cities of Boston, Cambridge, and Chelsea* (Boston, 1873) deliberately downplayed the importance of New

England Hospital by omitting it from its otherwise comprehensive listing of Boston hospitals. The judgment of the comparative size of New England Hospital is based on 1872 statistics given for the other Boston hospitals listed in the directory. Significantly, New England Hospital is the only "hospital" listed in the "Other Institutions and Societies" category of both directories.

22 Vietor, *Woman's Quest*, 348; *Woman's Journal*, February 22, 1890, p. 61.

23 Marie Zakrzewska to Paulina Pope, October 28, 1901, New England Hospital Papers, (Sophia Smith Collection, Smith College).

24 Vietor, *Woman's Quest*, 335; Ednah Dow Cheney, *Transcript of the Memorial Meeting of the New England Women's Club* (Boston, 1905), (Schlesinger Archives, Radcliffe College); bequest lists appear in the annual reports of the New England Hospital.

25 Mrs. Walter A. Hall, Mrs. Joseph S. Leach, and Mrs. Frederick G. Smith, *Progress and Achievement: A History of the Massachusetts State Federation of Women's Clubs, 1893–1962* (Lexington, Mass., 1962), 16; Julia A. Sprague, *History of the New England Women's Club from 1868 to 1893* (Boston, 1894), 3; "Record book of the weekly social meetings, New England Women's Club, 1869–1871," and records of discussion groups for entire period of its history, New England Women's Club Collection, Schlesinger Archives, Radcliffe College.

26 *Liberator,* June 27, 1862.

27 *Woman's Journal,* July 29, 1871.

28 Ibid., November 8, 1879.

29 Ibid., December 12, 1874.

30 Ibid., April 14, 1877; May 26, 1883; December 3, 1887.

31 Frederick C. Irving, *Safe Deliverance* (Boston, 1942), 122–23; Frederic A. Washburn, *The Massachusetts General Hospital: Its Development, 1900–1935* (Boston, 1939), 364–65; Committee of the Hospital Staff, *A History of the Boston City Hospital from Its Foundation until 1904* (Boston, 1906), 157–58.

32 Irving, *Safe Deliverance*, 145–59; Eleanor M. Tilton, *Amiable Autocrat: A Biography of Dr. Oliver Wendell Holmes* (New York, 1947), 169–76, 366, 409–10.

33 Marie E. Zakrzewska, "Report of one hundred and eighty-seven cases of midwifery in private practice," *Boston Medical and Surgical Journal*, 1889, *121:* 557–58; ibid., "Report of the attending physician," AR-NEH (1868), 9–21. An excellent source of information on maternity practices in the New England Hospital is Emma L. Call, "The evolution of modern maternity technic," *American Journal of Obstetrics and Diseases of Women and Children*, 1908, *58 no. 3:* 392–404. Call, whose association with the hospital began in 1868, documents and analyzes the puer-

peral disease statistics of the hospital from 1862 to 1907. Her article is an invaluable source of information on the hospital procedures of this period and it quotes from internal reports of the New England Hospital. For the earliest period there is a printed circular, 1864, with letter from John H. Stephenson endorsed by Drs. Horatio Storer, Walter Channing, C. P. Putnam, S. Cabot, and Henry Bowditch in New England Hospital Collection, Schlesinger Archives, Radcliffe College; Irving, *Safe Deliverance*, 143, and annual reports of Boston Lying-In Hospital.

34 Laurie Crumpacker, "Female patients in four Boston hospitals of the 1890's," Paper delivered at the Berkshire Conference on the History of Women, October 26, 1974; on file in Schlesinger Archives, Radcliffe College.

35 Ibid. See also Virginia G. Drachman, "Women's health through case records," Paper delivered at the Third Berkshire Conference on the History of Women, Bryn Mawr College, June 10, 1976.

36 Alice B. Crosby, *The Story of New England Hospital for Women and Children through Seventy-five Years, 1862–1937* (Boston, December 10, 1937), 4 and 13.

37 Marie Zakrzewska to Caroline Dall, March 6, 1869; ibid., March 26, 1869, Caroline Dall Collection, Massachusetts Historical Society.

38 Crosby, *Story of New England Hospital*, 11.

39 Vietor, *Woman's Quest*, 497–98; Grace E. Rochford, M.D., "The New England Hospital for Women and Children," *Journal of the American Medical Women's Association* 5 (1950), p. 497; Felicia A. Banas, M.D., "The History of the New England Hospital," 1955, *10:* 199; AR-NEH (1864), 4, and succeeding reports which annotate the social services rendered patients. A similar service was not established at Massachusetts General Hospital until 1905 and at Boston City Hospital until 1918. See Washburn, *Massachusetts General Hospital*, 570, and John J. Byrne, ed., *A History of the Boston City Hospital, 1905–1964* (Boston, 1964), 372.

40 Crosby, *Story of New England Hospital*, 13; AR-NEH (1863), 11; AR-NEH (1900), 23.

41 Vietor, *Woman's Quest*, 469; AR-NEH (1911), 10.

42 *Evening Bulletin* (Philadelphia), November 15, 1869. Cited by Clara Marshall, M.D., *The Woman's Medical College of Pennsylvania: An Historical Outline* (Philadelphia, 1897), 20.

43 AR-NEH (1863). Statistics on the early graduates, even names and dates, are extremely unreliable if one uses the compilations in the New England Hospital "fact sheets" published in the twentieth century, for example, one entitled "Former interns of the New England Hospital for Women and Children," c. 1934, New England Hospital Collection,

Sophia Smith Collection, Smith College. To insure an accurate portrait of the 1862–72 interns, I cross-checked information and verified it in a number of sources: New England Female Medical College graduate list; *Medical and Surgical Register of the United States* (Polk's) beginning with the first edition in 1886; *Woman's Medical College Graduates List;* and several listings in the AR-NEH to eliminate printing errors. There are eight women for whom information could not be obtained because they either died, left no forwarding addresses, or were of foreign birth and could not be traced in U.S. sources. The total of interns from 1862–72 was twenty-seven.

44 Jacobi was at New England Hospital for a few months during the summer of 1864. Neither her personal papers, her two-volume edited autobiography and articles, nor her later published works refer to her internship at New England Hospital. The reference to the busy schedule of Zakrzewska is taken from Rhoda Truax, *The Doctors Jacobi* (Boston, 1952), 36. Truax refers to private Putnam collections in writing her popular biography of Jacobi. See the complete bibliography on Jacobi in James, *Notable American Women.*

45 AR-NEH (1867), 7; their letter of application to Harvard is in the Harvard Medical School Dean's Records, 1867, and in Chadwick Scrapbook (Harvard Countway Library Archives).

46 Dimock's correspondence with Samuel Cabot about her Zurich experience is in the New England Hospital Collection, Sophia Smith Collection, Smith College. *Notable American Women* contains a complete bibliography on Dimock. Dimock's reputation as a surgeon is demonstrated in a research article and obituary published simultaneously in "The death of Dr. Dimock," *Medical Record* (1875), x, 357–58.

47 Margaret Todd, *The Life of Sophia Jex-Blake* (New York, 1918), 192.

48 Sara E. Parsons, *History of the Massachusetts General*

Hospital Training School for Nurses (Boston, 1922), 15. Sturtevant's memoirs are reproduced on 4–18 of Parsons; they originally appeared in "Personal recollections of hospital life before the days of training schools," *The Trained Nurse* (Boston, 1895).

49 Todd, *Life of Sophia Jex-Blake,* 201. See also Edythe Lutzker's pioneering studies: "Medical education for women in Great Britain," M.A. thesis, Columbia University, 1959; and *Women Gain a Place in Medicine* (New York, 1969).

50 *The Fiftieth Anniversary of the New England Hospital for Women and Children, October 29, 1912* (Boston, 1913), 11.

51 AR-NEH (1880), 13; Marie Zakrzewska, address to students (April 1, 1876), 3, New England Hospital Collection; Sophia Smith Collection, Smith College.

52 Frances Willard and Mary Livermore, eds., *American Women* (Buffalo, 1897), 2: 741.

53 Kate Campbell Hurd-Mead, *Medical Women of America* (New York, 1933), 34.

54 AR-NEH (1887), 9–11.

55 Margaret Noyes Kleinert, "Medical women in New England: history of the New England Women's Medical Society," *Journal of the American Medical Women's Association,* 1856, *11:* 63–64, 67; "Memoirs of Dr. Emma Call, June, 1928," Schlesinger Archives, Radcliffe College; *New England Women's Medical Society Directory of Members 1878–1928,* Sophia Smith Collection, Smith College, *Boston Directory* (1846–1910, annual editions).

56 Marie Zakrzewska, address to students (April 1, 1876), 7; Marie Zakrzewska, address to students (October 30, 1891), New England Hospital Collection, Sophia Smith Collection, Smith College.

57 Vietor, *Woman's Quest,* 336; *Woman's Journal,* January 6, 1872; for a discussion by a male physician (Dr. Derby) of whether or not the men should accept the women's invitation, see H. Derby to Dr. J. R. Chadwick, June 14, 1882, Chadwick Scrapbook.

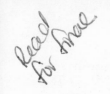

28

Professionalism, Feminism, and Gender Roles: A Comparative Study of Nineteenth-Century Medical Therapeutics

REGINA MARKELL MORANTZ AND SUE ZSCHOCHE

Some historians have argued that nineteenth-century medicine reflected a belief system that oppressed women and that doctors' cultural prejudices biased both treatment and the doctor-patient relationship. Nineteenth-century physicians have been accused of administering harsh and painful therapies to punish and control female patients who were unresponsive to the dictates of "true womanhood." Doctors allegedly practiced a form of medicine that attempted to reinforce childlike dependency in women, defined females as inherently weak and sickly, and discouraged excessive mental or physical exertion which might have turned a woman's attention to pursuits beyond her sphere.

This interesting thesis, which has caught the imagination of many contemporary critics of the present-day medical establishment, deserves careful examination. Medical practice does reflect and has in the past mirrored larger cultural and social ideologies.[1] We know, for example, that many standard nineteenth-century medical texts described puberty, menstruation, menopause, and pregnancy as critical periods in women's health when innate physiological weaknesses involving the reproductive system could cause permanent and serious damage if not properly managed. Many male physicians vociferously opposed the higher education of women on the grounds that it threatened female health. Indeed, the confluence of medical opinion and cultural attitudes concerning woman's role has been one of the most intriguing aspects of

REGINA MARKELL MORANTZ is Associate Professor of History at the University of Kansas, Lawrence, Kansas.
SUE ZSCHOCHE is an instructor at Kansas State University and is finishing her dissertation at the University of Kansas.
Reprinted with permission from *Journal of American History*, 67 (Dec., 1980), 568–588.

recent investigations into the social history of nineteenth-century medicine.[2]

Although nineteenth-century women physicians rarely criticized their male colleagues for overt oppression of female patients, they did believe themselves far more capable of treating women and children than their male colleagues. They took particular pride in their attention to preventive medicine, a concern that they often chided the men for neglecting. The medical literature reveals that most women physicians viewed women and children as their primary constituency, and they busied themselves in teaching and in practice primarily with definitions of female health and disease. Ella Ridgeway wrote in her 1873 thesis at the Woman's Medical College of Pennsylvania that women had been called upon to "supply a deficiency" in medicine "in regard to the diseases of women." There were many questions about the subject that "no doubt" have arisen in the "mind of every woman student which are not answered either by our professors or the books. One of these is why do women generally suffer so much more from ill health than men?"[3] Anna Longshore-Potts displayed pique at her male colleagues when she wrote that their opinions about women were "cut and dried" and if women had pursued medicine earlier, "today women would have had more healthy bodies."[4] Female medical educators spoke constantly of medical women's humanizing effect on medical practice. "Educated medical women," observed Eliza Mosher, "touch humanity in a manner different from men; by virtue of their womanhood, their interest in girls and young women, both moral and otherwise; in homes and in society."[5]

The effect of such attitudes on actual therapeutic practice has been hotly contested by historians. Some have argued that in this realm women physicians made a wholesale ideological attack against male-defined and male-dominated medicine, unanimously rebelling against the contention that women were innately weak and sickly. The medicine that women physicians practiced has been pictured as deliberately and consciously feminist, concerned less with "restoring" women to good health (the shortsighted goal of their male colleagues) than with controlling future definitions of female health and reworking the medical ideology that kept women sequestered by attributing the cause of female ill health to the inherent defects in female physiology.[6]

Because many nineteenth-century women physicians expected their own practice to differ from that of their male teachers and colleagues, it is hardly surprising that historians have actually believed this to have been the case. Yet taking the statements of women physicians at face value may be naive. What women physicians thought to be true need not have actually reflected reality. Such claims must be verified. How accurately did women physicians' pronouncements reflect accounts of their own behavior, and how much did they reflect ideology or merely wishful thinking? How close was their self-image to the reality of their daily care? Did the majority practice a different kind of medicine, and if so, how different, and in what ways?

In this study we propose to examine the hypothesis that female physicians practiced medicine differently from their medical brethren. We have compared late-nineteenth-century records of obstetrical cases at two Boston hospitals, one male staffed and one female staffed, in an attempt to examine several historical issues. First, we hope to clarify the relationship between women physicians and the medical profession as a whole. Second, we will seek to obtain further insight into the complex process of patient-physician interaction. Finally, underlying these two problems is a more basic question: when they received similar professional training and education, did women generally behave like men, or were their responses more often shaped by considerations of gender?

Historians have often depicted the views of nineteenth-century male and female physicians toward childbirth as polarized. On the one hand, male physicians treated pregnancy as a disease and therefore tended to be interventionist. Female physicians, on the other hand, supposedly ac-

cepted birth as a natural physiological process and remained cautious in the use of instruments.[7] One comparative study of the management of obstetrical cases at the female-run New England Hospital for Women and Children and the male-run Boston Lying-In Hospital found male physicians more careless about infection, more eager to use forceps and other types of intervention procedures, and more callous toward patients.[8] We attempted to test this hypothesis in two ways. First, we examined the medical literature for evidence of differences in theoretical approach between male and female doctors. Second, we made a statistical comparison of obstetrical cases at the aforementioned Boston hospitals in order to compare ideology with actual practice.

Any extensive examination of nineteenth-century medical literature reveals that the historian's assumption of medical unanimity on any subject is risky. Neither male nor female physicians exhibited a consensus on any of the crucial topics regarding female health. Women internalized many "male" values, and men were sometimes advocates of "female" positions.

An excellent example of such diversity may be drawn from the obstetrical literature. The persistent reader of medical journals appearing in the last third of the nineteenth century will likely discover that a debate raged among obstetricians over whether childbirth was a natural event requiring the obstetrician to "wait on nature" or a pathological crisis demanding active and vigorous intervention. Prominent male physicians distributed themselves on both sides of the issue. The debate crystallized in the pages of the *American Journal of Obstetrics and Diseases of Women and Children* for 1888, where Henry T. Byford, esteemed teacher in Rush Medical College and president of the Chicago Gynecological Society, and A. F. A. King, president of the Washington, D.C., Obstetrical and Gynecological Society, warmly contested "The Physiological Argument in Obstetric Studies and Practice." King's article had a familiar ring. Though childbirth perhaps should be natural, "in the present age, and among civilized communities," he wrote, a case of natural labor can be only "hypothetical." The bad habits of modern life had exacted their toll on parturient women. Byford, on the other hand, scorned King's distorted picture of American womanhood. The doctor's patients were not representative: "Let the author look elsewhere than in Washington and in large cities and he will find plenty of healthy women in physiological labor—he might indeed have found plenty in Washington." Byford's positive approach to female health led him to decry passionately the "meddlesome practices" of some of his colleagues.[9]

Just as male physicians lacked unanimity on many medical issues, women physicians also differed significantly among themselves. As females struggling to strike a balance between science, professionalism, and their own womanhood, they were bound to develop individual solutions to the problems of female health. There was no "party line" among these women on how to treat, diagnose, or prevent illness. Yet they did share a common approach. What drew them together was the conviction that women had a right to good health, that their own role should facilitate that right, and that better health among their contemporaries and future generations of women was indeed possible. Even when a woman physician advised caution during the physiological crises of puberty, childbirth, and menopause, her own concern was to determine the reasons for ill health during these times and develop fresh methods for managing female problems. The female doctor who believed it was woman's fate to suffer because of her physiology was a rare exception. Nevertheless, a careful study of journal articles and medical school theses by women suggests that in theory female physicians approached childbirth much as their male colleagues did. That is to say, their overall opinions reflected professional and scientific trends, and their divergences among themselves were similar to those of male doctors.

The theses on childbirth at the Woman's Medical College of Pennsylvania, for example, reflected the thinking of the medical profession at large. In the early decades, from the 1850s to the 1870s, the theme was deference to nature, limited interference, and patience in delivery.[10] By the end of the century, however, when doctors began to worry that excessive civilization had complicated delivery for middle-class women, the women's theses reflected this change. Pregnancy, wrote Phoebe Oliver in 1869, though a physiological condition, "has the peculiarity of being in some susceptible constitutions, pathological." She recommended moderate interference, including some drugging, rather than

"waiting on nature," especially when there were spasms. Other students noted the dire effects of advancing civilization on the ability of women to give birth easily.[11] Lucy R. Weaver believed that the way in which the physical system changes during pregnancy "may easily become pathological, for it borders so closely on disease." Mary Jordan Finley chided old-fashioned obstetricians reluctant to use forceps. She warned that much serious damage could be prevented by "timely" use of both forceps and ergot to ease pain, secure the child, and conserve the strength of the mother. "A timid or incompetent practitioner," she complained, "sits by the patient waiting for nature to accomplish the delivery until the life has been crushed out of some point in the soft tissues." The result: vesico-vaginal fistula, caused not by the forceps, but by the hesitation of the physician to use them.[12]

Articles on childbirth in the *Woman's Medical Journal,* established in 1893, also reflected prevailing wisdom. While old-timers such as Marie Zakrzewska reminded young practitioners that childbirth was "the most natural process in a woman's life" and decried "meddlesome interference," other women physicians shared the attitude of Agnes Eichelberger. Childbirth may be a physiological function, she conceded, but "from the moment of conception to the end of the lying in state, our patient is in danger and it is our duty to protect her."[13]

Eliza Root recommended wide experience in the use of forceps in teaching obstetrics because of the frequency of faulty development of the reproductive system caused by modern civilization. Other women doctors were actually innovative with certain surgical procedures. Anna E. Broomall, who ran the obstetrical service at the Woman's Hospital of the Woman's Medical College of Pennsylvania, was one of the first surgeons of either sex to recommend episiotomy as a safe and justifiable procedure. When she presented her findings to the Philadelphia Obstetrical Society in 1878, she was criticized by the men for too much interference and for needlessly exposing the patient to septic poisoning.[14]

It is important to point out here, however, that both the "natural" and the "medicalized" view of childbirth could be and in fact were used to justify both feminist and antifeminist positions. For example, the women who advocated certain types of interference did so on the grounds that such interference could be liberating—either from pain itself or from male incompetence. The twilight sleep movement in the early part of the twentieth century presents an excellent case in point. In this instance women physicians and other feminists campaigning for woman's relief from birth pain pressured the medical profession into using a technique of anesthesia which at the turn of the century had been rejected by male doctors as unreliable and unsafe. In contrast, antifeminist physicians often used intervention as a means of asserting control over the birth process and keeping women in their places.[15]

Even when women physicians remained critical of accepted therapies, they were occasionally confronted with demands from female patients who expected the same heroic dosing performed by the most respected male practitioners. Although the following example does not involve the management of childbirth, it eloquently illustrates this larger point. Soon after she set up practice in New York City in the 1850s, Elizabeth Blackwell wrote to her sister Emily, who was then studying medicine in Europe:

> a lady called on me today three weeks returned [from Paris]. . . . This lady had had the red hot iron applied to the uterus by Jobert, for ulceration, [so she said] and felt so much better that she thinks there is nothing like it, and means to advise all her friends to be scorched—she came to me hoping that I would apply it to a sister-in-law! So Milly you must be prepared to cut and burn, and practice every conceivable abomination, for it is perfectly evident to me that the more unnatural the application, the more the women like it. This lady was frizzled twice, the smoke filled the room and she is only desirous now to find some one who will practice as Jobert did.

Though historians have accused nineteenth-century surgeons of performing gynecological surgery unnecessarily, there is occasional evidence to suggest that surgeons were often pressured by female patients. Zakrzewska, writing to Elizabeth Blackwell in 1891, noted that women came to the New England Hospital begging for operations "on the slightest cause." Married women "between 28

& 40 years" came in asking for ovariotomies "because causing [*sic*] dismenorrhea & children were not desired." When surgeons were thus tempted, she mused, "do you wonder . . . [that they] go the whole length of disregard for Nature?"[16]

Lay pressure notwithstanding, our study of the medical literature on childbirth suggests that men and women physicians showed no significant theoretical differences in their approach to parturition. Though women physicians expected to take an especial interest in female health, and though this interest led them to reject the most extreme positions on woman's innate physiological infirmity, they nevertheless reflected in their thinking the influence of professional trends and shifts of opinion in generally the same degree as their medical brethren.

Though gender played a small and relatively insignificant part in the theoretical approach of men and women physicians to treatment, it is now necessary to turn to the actual clinical records. Nineteenth-century Boston offers a unique opportunity for the study of the treatment of women. Many hospital records have been preserved and are still available for study. Boston also boasted one of the first hospitals for women and children staffed by women physicians. The New England Hospital, founded by Zakrzewska in 1862, became a showplace for quality medical care in the latter third of the nineteenth century. Ambitious women doctors longed to receive clinical training there, and its teaching program was rigorous and demanding. Standards reflected the very highest of the day. Fortunately, medical, surgical, and obstetrical records for this institution are virtually intact, and if used along with comparable records for the Massachusetts General Hospital and the Boston Lying-In—both teaching facilities for Harvard Medical School—some interesting comparisons can be made.

Although case histories vary in completeness from hospital to hospital, even carelessly marked records allow the researcher to ask three basic questions. How frequently were certain medical procedures used; did the patients' medical histories dictate any specific treatments, and what was the social profile of the patients receiving such treatment? Without evidence to the contrary, we must assume that the use of any medical procedure was predicated on the patients' medical history. The patients' condition was surely also affected by environmental factors such as housing or diet. This information can be at least partially inferred from the social data available on case records. Data pertaining to the patients' condition and social situation are an invaluable source of control variables.

Our objective was to determine whether women in childbirth were likely to receive treatment from women physicians different from that given by men and to test in as statistically sophisticated a manner as possible the thesis that childbearing women received better care from female physicians. A systematic sequential sample was drawn from maternity cases at the female-run New England Hospital for the period 1873–99 and Harvard's Boston Lying-In for the period 1887–99.[17] Three broad areas of medical treatment and outcome were recorded: the incidence of complications among patients, the use of drugs, and the use of physical intervention techniques, particularly forceps. We assumed that any significant differences between hospitals in these areas could be attributed to the sex of the physicians involved if inherent differences in patient population and other non-gender-related institutional differences could be statistically controlled.

This qualification is critical. Nineteenth-century hospitals were institutions of the urban poor, who were by no means a homogeneous group. Nor did nineteenth-century sensibilities perceive the poor as such. This distinction in perception was reflected in the development of two different types of hospitals. On the one hand stood the free municipal hospital, a medical almshouse which represented a refuge of last resort for the chronically ill and indigent. The private or "voluntary" hospital, in contrast, ministered to a paying clientele or the "industrious and worthy" poor who came to fill its endowed beds.[18] Though Boston Lying-In and New England Hospital were both voluntary institutions, evidence reveals that there were important differences in their clienteles.

Hospital records and annual reports indicate that the "worthiness" of patients was an appreciably more significant factor in New England Hospital admissions policy than at Boston Lying-In. New England Hospital patients generally paid at least a nominal fee for the medical services they received. At Boston Lying-In, only 23 percent were paying patients. Like the male-run Boston Lying-In, the female-run New England Hospital normally refused

obstetric service to unwed mothers bearing their second illegitimate child. Unlike Boston Lying-In, the proportion of single mothers at New England Hospital declined throughout the time period studied. One of the hospital's senior physicians, Emma Call, referred to this trend when she noted that after the hospital moved to surburban Roxbury in 1871, "the class of patients was . . . a much better one, and we have never had any number of the most undesirable cases, which inevitably gravitate to an institution located in the midst of a dense population."[19]

This concern with the "worthiness" of patients corroborates impressionistic evidence gathered from other sources that women physicians showed a greater interest than the male physicians at Boston Lying-In in moral reform and in providing a Christian atmosphere for erring patients. These women preferred to treat the respectable poor because they were amenable to change. One is tempted to speculate that the male physicians viewed their role in the hospital from a narrower perspective. As Charles Rosenberg has recently pointed out, hospital internships were plums for the ambitious and economically secure and were procured only with difficulty. Young men of good family and appropriate social connections vied for the opportunity to gain prestige and essential clinical experience.[20] Though women physicians also came to the New England Hospital to gain needed clinical experience internship was not for them a ticket to a prestigious medical practice. In fact, they realized that their scope and power within the larger profession would always be circumscribed. Perhaps such circumstances freed them to view patients as more than just clinical material and to seek personal fulfillment in a more holistic approach.

Whatever the explanation for these differences, clearly discernible here is a conflict between old and new concepts of professionalism. In the middle of the nineteenth century, doctors of both sexes believed in the medically curative powers of morality and natural living—a belief that technocratic male physicians increasingly abandoned after the 1880s. The differences in approach suggest that male doctors surrendered their concern with morality more quickly than did the women. One can only speculate why female physicians clung to traditional values, although we strongly suspect that it had much to do with Victorian culture's identification of women as the moral guardians of society.[21]

Whatever the reasons, the patient selectivity on the part of the New England Hospital means that other differences between the hospitals will be partially obscured by inherent differences in the patient populations. Both groups of patients were undoubtedly poor, but Boston Lying-In's were poorer. There was a substantial social distance between doctor and patient at both hospitals, but probably less of one at a hospital staffed by women physicians, many of whom were upwardly mobile and of a lower status than the elite physicians of Boston Lying-In.

This socioeconomic difference in patient populations also indicated that New England Hospital patients should have had an advantage, however slight, in their general medical condition. The sex of the physician in this case has introduced something of a tautological pattern into the data. That is, women physicians attracted a somewhat different type of patient, with somewhat different medical and social problems, which in turn affected the type of medicine women doctors practiced.

The sheer amount of information on the hospital records implies another broad difference between Boston Lying-In and New England Hospital. The latter's records appeared consistently more complete. In addition to the record of actual treatment, they provided a greater amount of information regarding patients' medical backgrounds (for example, general physical condition, number of prior miscarriages) and more complete information regarding social status.

This relatively meticulous record keeping reveals the self-conscious professionalism typical of women physicians, but it also indicates a "leveling" process at work in the Boston Lying-In. The women doctors at New England Hospital made an attempt to know whom they were treating and distinguished, at least in their records, between various levels of poverty. The lack of similar distinctions at Boston Lying-In implies that poor women treated in an often overcrowded teaching facility may very well have presented a single category to the male physicians. Interestingly enough, case records were scrupulously complete when male Boston Lying-In physicians presided at the home deliveries of middle-class women.[22]

The impression that male physicians lumped the poor together finds support in the fact that the maternal recuperative period at the Boston Lying-In was a standard two weeks with very little variation. The hospital's annual reports indicate regret that overcrowding made this policy necessary. However unavoidable, it stands in marked contrast to New England Hospital practice. New England Hospital patients remained under care for from four days to three months and were, on the average, under medical supervision over one week longer than their Boston Lying-In counterparts, even during the identical time period (1887–99). Perhaps this variation can be attributed to a greater sensitivity to individual physical considerations coupled with the availability of space. But the evidence also suggests social considerations. Single mothers normally remained under medical care longer, perhaps because they had nowhere else to go or because the women doctors of New England Hospital felt such patients required more of the hospital's meliorative moral influence. Bits and pieces of evidence suggest that we must consider the medical variables with the recognition that women physicians were concerned with their patients' social situations. This factor alone implies a very different subjective experience for each group of patients.

We may assume that a parturient woman's concerns centered on the medical outcome for herself and her child. Regarding infant mortality, the rates at the two hospitals are roughly comparable: 6 percent at the women-run New England Hospital and 8.5 percent at the male Boston Lying-In. This slight difference is not significant, though there is an idiosyncratic, and presently inexplicable, pattern at Boston Lying-In. Over three-quarters of the infant deaths in the sample occurred in 1895 or later.

As far as maternal outcome is concerned, only two deaths were reported in each hospital's sample. Of greater interest was the relative incidence of delivery-related complications. For the purposes of comparison, we divided maternal complications into types: those labeled infection or systemic complications such as fever, pain, general infection, and puerperal infection, and those categorized as traumas or injuries such as ruptured perineums, fistulas, or lacerations. When the complications for hospitals are compared for the identical time period, there is no statistical difference in the success of each hospital's therapeutics. (See appendix, Table 1.) The state of the medical art, rather than the sex of the physicians, seems to be the logical determinant of the outcome for the obstetric patient.

This analysis, however, confronts the issue of complications only in general terms. We next asked whether any particular group of women was more likely to suffer. In particular, we were concerned with the impact of nationality and marital status on the patient's care. Accordingly, we compared the complication rates among American single, American married, foreign single, and foreign married women (Table 2). Analyzed in this fashion, a distinctive pattern emerges. At Boston Lying-In, we found no significantly higher complication patterns among any of the four groups of women. This information appears consistent with either the observation that Boston Lying-In doctors recognized no particular nuance of social status among their patients or the possibility that there was objectively little difference in the patients' social circumstances. For patients at New England Hospital, however, the complication rate among foreign single women is nearly double that of any other group.

The explanation for this pattern is more likely to be found in social than in medical factors. Single foreign women were twice as likely to be admitted in the New England Hospital's earlier period—that is, prior to 1887— than later. Furthermore, these women suffered a disproportionate number of systemic or infection types of complications. Such complications are as likely to be caused by the patient's prior state of health as by medical treatment per se. Given the fact that over 90 percent of these women worked at menial tasks, the probability exists that environmental factors such as diet and cleanliness were of significance in their medical outcomes. It should be noted that this group of women fared considerably better in the second half of the time period when the state of medical art had improved. But significantly, they and working women in general were a smaller proportion of the hospital's population at the end of the century. We are left with the conclusion that the New England Hospital was indeed drawing, if not a "better," at least a healthier class of women—that is, more homemakers of any nationality and fewer domestics and factory operatives.

Did the sex of the physicians have any bearing on the medical outcome for their patients? The answer is that it did, but only to a small extent and only in an indirect manner. On the issue of complications, the difference between male and female physicans lies less in their medical practice than in the types of hospital and patient populations with which they worked.

A second concern was the treatment offered patients after delivery, particularly prescriptions for relief. In this instance, a strong pattern of differences emerged which can be more directly related to medical policy within the two hospitals.

By the 1870s heroic medicine was on the decline. Large doses of painful and life-threatening therapies were generally avoided by the physician conscious of changing medical trends. Nevertheless, drugs were often deemed necessary. We surmised the drugs would be given in direct proportion of the severity of the complaint, and that women physicians, who had often decried heroic procedures, would be more conservative in their prescriptions. The hospital records revealed precisely the opposite pattern.

We calculated the proportion of women at each hospital receiving certain types of medication, ranging from supportive types such as beef tea to strong and "heroic" types of medication.[23] (Table 3). Nearly two-thirds of all Boston Lying-In patients received no medication whatsoever from their male physicians, and the statistical correlations revealed that the use of drugs was strongly predicated on the occurrence and severity of complications. At the New England Hospital, every patient was given some form of medication by the women doctors, usually in the range of what was classified as mild to strong pharmaceuticals. Moreover, the prescription of drugs at the New England Hospital did not correlate decisively with any discernible medical factors, meaning that drug prescriptions for postdelivery women were simply standard procedure among women physicians. In short, the male Boston Lying-In physicians followed an objective model: drug prescription was dependent on the physical symptoms. The implied corollary here is that women physicians dispensed medication for less codifiable and nonphysical reasons.

However, an alternative explanation is also possible. While it may be that most of the Boston Lying-In patients were protected from needless medication, it is also possible that they were virtually ignored after delivery. The scanty medical charts certainly suggest that to be the case. At the least, New England Hospital's medication policy implies an alternative ethos concerning the needs of post-delivery women, and the greater prescription of medication by women doctors may be the objective indicator of more patient-doctor contact. If this speculation is correct, then the female physicians were exhibiting a concept of professionalism which deemed supportive therapy as important to the patient as purely technical concerns.

The third factor under consideration was the relative use of intervention techniques, particularly forceps, upon parturient women. This area is easily the most controversial since it is one of the main issues on which recent historians have based their case that male physicians were arrogantly insensitive to the needs of maternity patients. In particular, the use of forceps is symbolic of the definition of childbirth as a doctor-controlled medical crisis. Hypothetically, women physicians, because they were women, were more sympathetic to the concept of childbirth as a natural process and hence were less prone to resort to instrumental interference in delivery.

Examined over the entire time period, the data revealed no dramatic difference in the relative willingness of doctors at either hospital to resort to intervention techniques. At New England Hospital roughly 18 percent of the patients received anesthetic, forceps, or both. The comparable figure for Boston Lying-In is 20 percent. When we consider only forceps, the rate at New England Hospital is 9.5 percent; at Boston Lying-In it is 13.5 percent. Neither difference is statistically significant.[24]

In addition, medical criteria for forceps use were similar at both hospitals. The labors of those women involved in forceps deliveries were significantly longer than the average, probably because most were bearing their first child. Moreover, these women tended to receive stronger medication in the recuperative period. Finally, the use of forceps increased gradually at both hospitals in the last decade of the nineteenth century. This fact suggests that once sepsis could be controlled forceps deliveries became more likely.

There is, however, a notable difference in the two hospitals' relative success with the forceps. While both institutions resorted to instrumental deliveries with roughly the same frequency, the forceps patients at Boston Lying-In experienced a higher complication rate than did other women at the hospital. No such differential pattern emerged at New England Hospital (Tables 4 and 5). There are at least two possible explanations for this situation. The New England Hospital doctors may have handled forceps cases more carefully than their male counterparts. Or the Boston Lying-In forceps patients might have been in relatively poorer health than their New England Hospital counterparts.

On the issue of puerperal fever, several historians have charged male physicians with negligence in correcting their role in transmitting the dreaded disease. It is true that Boston Lying-In had more difficulty controlling puerperal infection than did New England Hospital. Before the introduction of successful antiseptic techniques there in 1886, the hospital had been forced to close three times because of epidemics, in contrast to once at New England Hospital. More lives were lost at the male-run hospital. Why did this occur, and can it in any way be attributed to differences in approach by male and female physicians? One researcher claimed that Boston Lying-In's comparatively poorer record in preventing sepsis stemmed from the staff's stubborn reluctance to accept the nurses' and physicians' role as possible sources of infection, whereas women physicians at New England Hospital were more willing to "view themselves as fallible."[25]

An examination of the annual reports of the two hospitals suggests that their divergent records on the fever may not be directly related to the sex of the physicians in charge, but rather may originate in complex causes relating to hospital architecture and finances, the personalities and experience of the resident physicians, and blind luck. Although New England Hospital did not institute successful antisepsis until 1884 and Boston Lying-In until 1886, the doctors at both hospitals experimented vigorously with different methods for several years prior to those dates. The annual reports of Boston Lying-In make it clear that sepsis remained a grave problem which was dealt with vigorously, if not always effectively.[26] W. L. Richardson, chief of obstetrics, outlined the hospital's frustrating search for an effective method in an article published in 1887. The procedures used at New England Hospital paralleled those at the other hospital, except that New England Hospital instituted the use of bichloride of mercury, which ultimately proved the most effective, two years before Boston Lying-In. This method, ironically enough, probably came to the attention of the women physicians earlier because many were forced, because of discrimination, to seek postgraduate training in Europe, where more advanced opinions regarding the bacterial nature of infection prevailed.[27]

Yet before 1884 the New England Hospital had a demonstrably superior mortality rate from puerperal sepsis. Why? The answer seems to lie primarily with both Zakrzewska's ideas about maternity care and her greater power to implement them. Before coming to America, Zakrzewska studied clinical midwifery with J. H. Schmidt at the Royal Charité, Berlin's largest and most prestigious lying-in hospital. In 1853, her outstanding work led to her appointment as accoucheuse-en-chef, a position that required teaching both midwifery candidates and medical students. Here she had an opportunity to develop strong opinions regarding proper delivery and efficient means of avoiding sepsis. Thus, although the woman's hospital was no more enlightened on the actual source of infection in the years before the discoveries of bacteriologists, it implemented Zakrzewska's prejudices, which happened to be empirically, if not necessarily scientifically, sound.[28]

In the annual report for 1868, she discussed her ideas concerning the proper organization of lying-in hospitals. Experiments had been conducted in Europe, she wrote, but so far no one knew exactly how to avoid the fever. She advised caution. Lying-in institutions should be small, spread throughout the city, and retain separate wards for isolation cases. She then detailed the ideal set-up—a room for women in labor, two rooms for delivery used alternatively, and still another for convalescents—thus keeping women at different stages of childbirth separated from each other. She also proposed isolation procedures, including requiring nurses and physicans treating fever cases to be disqualified from the normal deliveries.[29] Zakrzewska may have been ignorant of germ theory, but she did everything she could think of in the area of prevention. When the new hospital buildings were completed in Roxbury at the end of 1872, the lying-in facilities followed her plan.

In practice these procedures could not consistently be followed to the letter. Demand for space usually exceeded the supply, partly because New England Hospital, in contrast to Boston Lying-In, did not always release patients after the standard two weeks. And even with all their precautions, New England Hospital was not immune from epidemics of puerperal fever. In 1872 the lying-in wards temporarily closed because of a scourge which killed four patients.[30] Yet for severe problems New England Hospital at least owned an isolation cottage, something Boston Lying-In never had.

The trustees of Boston Lying-In wrote in 1874 of the desirability of small contiguous dwellings and isolation wards. Yet their cautious financial policies, which probably derived from the fact that the hospital had been forced to close in the 1860s because the trustees had overextended themselves financially with an ambitious building program, never allowed them to implement these goals.[31] Boston Lying-In functioned primarily on income from investments, whereas New England Hospital depended mostly on donations. Although their budgets were roughly comparable, New England Hospital exhibited a boldness in management which reflected more active and more consistent support from wealthy subscribers. At the very least, the two hospitals' funding practices represented entirely different philosophies regarding financial management.[32]

Boston Lying-In's failure to implement in practice what its medical staff recognized in theory was suggested by Zakrzewska in her autobiography. She claimed that the women physicians were given much more power to carry out policy decisions:

> Our Hospital is utterly different from all hospitals carried on by the City or the State or by private individuals and endowments.
>
> In these latter there exists either a need to provide for the helpless who are dependent on the Commonwealth, or benevolent persons wish to provide a charity and so they establish hospitals. In both conditions, the staff of physicians is employed by those who manage the institutions and, consequently, either money or thanks are due to such physicians as serve.
>
> With us, it is entirely different. None of our original directors wanted a hospital; none of them was inspired by charity or had the means to provide such charity. I, the representative of an idea in its earliest evolution—

I sought those Directors that they might serve the purpose of carrying out that idea.

They served then and in the future the women physicians connected with the Hospital. They never dictated as to the number of physicians or internes; they never proposed to enlarge the work; this has always been done by the professional staff. *We* thank *them* for their generous aid, but they cannot thank us for doing much or little.

Of course, the Directors are the corporate body, and they represent us legally before the public; but they carry out our ideas, not we theirs. They simply stand ready to support the principle of giving to women physicians full opportunity to manifest their skill and judgment.[33]

Thus, although sources indicate that physicians at Boston Lying-In made every attempt within the limitations of their knowledge to control infection, their success was hampered by financial burdens and a decentralized system of authority on policy decisions such as hospital structure that may have been crucial before antisepsis. Perhaps if the male physicians had taken the problem more to heart, they would have been better able to assert pressure on the trustees successfully. In contrast, it seems likely from the history of New England Hospital that the degree of control exercised by the women physicians there derived at least in part from a shared feminist ideology, which of course was conspicuously absent at Boston Lying-In.

This comparative study of male and female physicians' clinical behavior has revealed that as far as the mechanics of obstetric practice are concerned, the complication rates and frequency of forceps use within each hospital indicate a rough parity between the therapeutics of male and female physicians. Drug prescription, in fact, represented the only discernible difference between the two hospitals that can be directly attributed to the sex of the physicians.

Physicians' social attitudes also influenced their medical practice. Our findings suggest that male and female physicians' attitudes toward their professional roles may well have been diverging.

As men embraced a more modern, technocratic approach to their patients, women physicians continued to cling to traditional holistic orientations. Thus New England Hospital sought a different type of patient from the Boston Lying-In: the "worthy poor." Its annual reports consistently emphasized the women's concern with the hospital's Christian atmosphere. That the obstetric care at the two hospitals was therapeutically similar suggests that the impact of such attitudes remained indirect.

Letters, diaries, written literature, and hospital records have served to illuminate the differences between male and female physicians in their approach to medical care. We see a picture certainly more penetrating than that revealed by what women physicians said and wrote about themselves. The therapeutic similarities remind us that the staff members of New England Hospital were not only women, but doctors as well. As doctors, the New England Hospital staff operated under the dictates of their profession: they viewed themselves as full-fledged health professionals, they read the same journals as the men, and they subscribed to theories that represented the collective wisdom of their group.

Nevertheless, the gender of the physician may well have mattered in more subtle ways. One wishes to believe that some, perhaps most, parturient women were comforted by the attendance of a professional physician of their own sex. Certainly women physicians never forgot that they were women, and it is clear that their interests within medicine as well as their affective behavior as doctors were influenced by that fact. Our study suggests that women physicians probably exhibited a different orientation toward patient care. Thus men and women doctors acted alike in most therapeutic situations, but for very different reasons and with meanings different both to themselves and to their patients. The hospital records offer a final valuable insight into this complex and as yet dimly understood relationship between attitudes and therapeutic behavior. Such evidence suggests that future researchers would do well to at least modify the polarized perspective with which they have hitherto approached the subject of medical treatment for women.

APPENDIX: NOTES ON METHODOLOGY

Our sample of the case records of the two hospitals is best described as a systematic sequential sample; that is, we drew a random sample of the case records from alternate years. For New England Hospital, this included a sample from the odd-numbered years, 1873–99, with a total n of 171. For Boston Lying-In, the sample included the alternate years of 1887–99, with a total n of 305. We attempted to codify virtually every piece of information that was available from the case records. One group of variables may be said to be related to the patient's social position and included: marital status, nationality, race, place of residence, and kind of employment (if any). The second group of variables provided the patient's medical profile and included: age, number of living children, miscarriages, stillbirths and/or abortions, general physical condition, the birth presentation of the fetus, length of labor, use of anesthetics or forceps, type of postpartum complication, drugs used after delivery, length of hospital stay, and maternal and infant mortality. We also noted whether the woman paid for hospital services. We attempted to codify the type of comments that the physicians occasionally wrote on the charts, but there were too few to be of any use.

As reported in note 24, our ability to analyze the hospital data using multiple regression was hindered by the fact that Boston Lying-In case records were relatively less complete. In particular, we had to exclude from comparison the impact of a woman's prior health condition and the impact, if any, of the patient's employment status, since Boston Lying-In did not usually include such data on their records.

The most obvious discrepancy in our samples is the difference in the time period studied. As we have noted, data from Boston Lying-In were available beginning with the year 1887. We were concerned whether the New England Hospital data remained consistent throughout the time period or whether we could legitimately use the data only after 1887. Accordingly, we compared the New England Hospital data before 1887 with those from 1887 and later. With two important exceptions, both discussed in the text, the data remained consistent, and we therefore concluded that we could appro-

priately use the entire sample. The first exception was the aggregate change in the patients' employment status. The number of employed women treated at the New England Hospital declined dramatically from the first half of the sample to the second. In 1873, only 11 percent of the maternity cases in our sample were listed as housewives; by 1899, 63 percent were so listed. Supporting our conclusion that the condition of the patients did improve at the New England Hospital toward century's end, 44 percent were listed in poor condition in 1873; by 1899 only 12 percent were so listed.

The second change over time was the decline in the complication rate at the New England Hospital from 1887 on. This decline is most dramatically shown by comparing the first year of our sample with the last. In our 1873 sample, all patients are listed as having some type of postpartum complication; in 1899, 87 percent are complication-free. Although our decision to compare complication rates from 1887 on was dictated by the availability of Boston Lying-In case records, we feel that the time demarcation is less arbitrary than it first appears. Since successful antisepsis was instituted at both hospitals in the mid-1880s, we were able to compare directly the complication rates during a period immediately after a significant improvement had just been made in obstetrical therapeutics.

Tables 1, 2, and 3 compare the complication rates and drug usage at the two hospitals. To analyze the differences in frequencies we used a chi square test of independence which has the advantage of correcting for an unequal number of cases.

In order to analyze the relationship between complications and drugs within each hospital, we computed the correlation between the two. We scaled the complications from least to most severe. In ascending order of severity they were: (0) no complications; (1) pain in groin; (2) fever and chills; (3) lacerations of vulva; (4) other–constipation, ulcerations; (5) ruptured perineum; (6) hemorrhaging; (7) vaginal fistula; (8) puerperal fever. In similar fashion, drugs were scaled from mildest to strongest prescription: (0) no drugs; (1) general supportive (teas, rubs); (2) mild pharmaceutical; (3) strong; (4) heroic; (5) combination of the pre-

Table 1
Proportion of Patients Suffering Complications, Boston Lying-In versus New England Hospital

	Boston Lying-In Hospital 1887–1899 (n = 305)	New England Hospital 1873–1899 (n = 171)	New England Hospital 1873–1885 (n = 72)	New England Hospital 1887–1899 (n = 99)
Proportion of patients with no complications	73.4%	68.4%	59.7%	74.7%
Proportion of patients with complications	26.6%	31.6%	40.3%	25.3%
(Proportion with injuries)	(7.5%)	(12.3%)	(16.7%)	(9.1%)
(Proportion with infections)	(19.0%)	(19.3%)	(23.6%)	(16.2%)

Comparison of Boston Lying-In with New England Hospital for the years 1887–1899:

chi square = .066   degrees of freedom = 1   no significant difference

Table 2
Proportion of Patients Suffering Complications by Marital Status/Nationality Groups

	New England Hospital 1873–1899		Boston Lying-in 1887–1899	
	Number of Women in Group	Proportion with Complications	Number of Women in Group	Proportion with Complications
Single American patients	18	27.8%	55	36.4%
Married American patients	54	24.1%	58	25.9%
Single foreign patients	29	55.2%	80	26.2%
Married foreign patients	65	27.7%	107	21.0%
Total cases	166	—	300	—
Aggregate complication rate	—	31.3%	—	26.7%

Comparison of differences in the frequency of complications among groups within each hospital:

New England Hospital	*Boston Lying-in*
chi square = 9.39	chi square = 3.59
degrees of freedom = 3	degrees of freedom = 3
probability <.05	no significant difference

Table 3
Postdelivery Drug Prescription: New England Hospital versus Boston Lying-In

	New England Hospital 1873–1899		Boston Lying-In 1887–1899	
	Number of Patients	Proportion of Patients	Number of Patients	Proportion of Patients
No medication prescribed	0	0%	194	63.6%
General supportive treatments	1	.6%	5	1.6%
Mild pharmaceuticals	89	52.0%	60	19.7%
Strong medication	74	43.3%	42	13.8%
Heroic medication	6	3.5%	4	1.3%
Combination of above	1	.6%	0	0%
Total cases	171	100.0%	305	100.0%

Comparison of the frequency of drug prescription at the New England Hospital and Boston Lying-In:

chi square = 189.86   degrees of freedom = 5   probability <.05

ceding. We admit that the scaling is open to debate. However, the scaled variables did in fact correlate significantly at both hospitals though there was an enormous difference in the relative predictive values of the correlations. When we attempted a multiple regression on drug usage at New England Hospital, we could explain only 4.5 percent of the variance in drug prescription on the basis of complications (multiple R = .21375). In comparison, the same regression performed on the Boston Lying-In data revealed that 38 percent of the variance could be explained solely on the severity of the complication (multiple R = .61691). In neither regression did any other variable add much to the explanation of the variance in a direct—that is, logically causal—way. In this regard, we would have liked to pursue the question of whether complications were related to the patient's prior medical history and/or her socioeconomic status; the gaps in the Boston Lying-In data precluded this line of analysis.

Tables 4 and 5 analyze the differences in complication rates between the group at each hospital that received neither forceps nor anesthetics and

Table 4

Frequency of Complications among Patients
with Different Intervention Treatments,
New England Hospital, 1873–1899

	Number of Patients	Number Suffering Complications	Proportion with Complications
Patients with no intervention treatment	139	45	32.4%
Patients with intervention treatment	31	8	25.8%
(anesthetic only)	(15)	(4)	(26.7%)
(forceps only)	(5)	(1)	(20.0%)
(both)	(11)	(3)	(27.3%)

Comparison of the frequency of complications between the group of patients with no intervention treatment and the group with one or both types of intervention:

chi square = .51
degrees of freedom = 1
no significant difference

Table 5

Frequency of Complications among Patients
with Different Intervention Treatments,
Boston Lying-In Hospital, 1887–1899

	Number of Patients	Number Suffering Complications	Proportion with Complications
Patients with no intervention treatment	244	58	23.8%
Patients with intervention treatment	61	23	37.7%
(anesthetic only)	(20)	(7)	(35.0%)
(forceps only)	(20)	(8)	(40.0%)
(both)	(21)	(8)	(38.1%)

Comparison of frequency of complications between the group of patients with no intervention treatment and the group with one or both types of intervention:

chi square = 4.86
degrees of freedom = 1
probability <.05

the group that received one or both intervention treatments. Once again, a chi square test of independence was used to test for significant differences in frequency of complications.

Finally, by using the scaled complications and a t-test for differences in means, we were also able to calculate whether any intervention group suffered more severe complications than those patients that received neither anesthetic nor forceps.

At New England Hospital there was no significant difference in mean complication severity among the intervention groups. At Boston Lying-In the mean complication for the groups that received forceps or both forceps and anesthetic was significantly higher. For the group labeled "no intervention," the mean on the severity scale was .9. For "anesthetic only," "forceps only," and "both," the means were 1.2, 1.7, and 1.8 respectively. The latter two means are significantly higher at the .05 level. Thus we concluded that at Boston Lying-In, patients who were delivered by forceps were more likely to experience complications and, moreover, were likely to have more severe complications than other patients.

NOTES

1 Probably no single example better illustrates the cultural dimension of nineteenth-century medicine than physicians' attitudes toward masturbation. Because Victorian culture disapproved of any form of sexuality divorced from reproduction, doctors, who were representative Victorians, took to defining masturbation as a disease, complete with specific etiology and a catalogue of symptoms. Physicians, however unwittingly, thus used science to create rewards and sanctions for a sexually repressive ideology. See H. Tristram Englehardt, Jr., "The disease of masturbation: values and the concept of disease," *Bulletin of the History of Medicine* 48 (Summer 1974): 234–48.

2 See Ann Douglas Wood, "'The fashionable diseases': women's complaints and their treatment in nineteenth-century America," in this volume; Charles Rosenberg and Carroll Smith-Rosenberg, "The female animal: medical and biological views of woman and her role in nineteenth-century America," in this volume; Carroll Smith-Rosenberg, "The cycle of femininity: puberty and menopause in 19th century America," *Feminist Studies* 1 (Winter 1973), 58–72; Carroll Smith-Rosenberg, "The hysterical woman: sex roles and role conflict in 19th-century America," *Social Research* 39 (Winter 1972): 652–78.

3 Ella Ridgeway, "The causes of uterine diseases," M.D. thesis, Woman's Medical College of Pennsylvania, 1873. All Woman's Medical College theses may be found in the Medical College of Pennsylvania Archives, Philadelphia.

4 Anna Longshore-Potts, *Discourses to Women on Medical Subjects* (San Diego, 1897), 122.

5 Eliza Mosher, "The value of organization—what has it done for women?" *Woman's Medical Journal* 26 (June 1916):1–4.

6 See Virginia Drachman, "Women doctors and the women's medical movement: feminism and medi-

cine, 1850–1895," Ph.D. diss., State University of New York at Buffalo, 1976.

7 For the medicalization of childbirth, see Jane Bauer Donegan, "Midwifery in America, 1760–1860: a study in medicine and morality," Ph.D. diss., Syracuse University, 1972; Catherine Scholten, "'On the importance of the obstetrick art': changing customs of childbirth in America, 1760–1825," in this volume; Richard W. Wertz and Dorothy C. Wertz, *Lying-in: A History of Childbirth in America* (New York, 1977). For a more extreme view of doctors' culpability, see Mary Roth Walsh, *"Doctors Wanted: No Women Need Apply": Sexual Barriers in the Medical Profession, 1835–1975* (New Haven, 1977), 76–105; Drachman, "Women doctors," 121–26; and Patricia Branca, *Silent Sisterhood: Middle Class Women in the Victorian Home* (London, 1975), 62–73.

8 This was the contention of Laurie Crumpacker, "Female patients in four Boston hospitals of the 1890s," a paper delivered at the Berkshire Conference on the History of Women, Oct. 1974 (copy on deposit at the Schlesinger Library, Cambridge, Mass.). In some cases historians have merely assumed the accuracy of nineteenth-century statements when critics of male midwifery insisted that women were more willing to "wait on nature." For an example of the contention that men interfered more than women, see Samuel Gregory, *Man-Midwifery Exposed and Corrected* (Boston, 1848), 12–13. Occasionally even physicians deplored the enthusiasm of their colleagues for instruments. G. S. Bedford, professor of midwifery at the New York University, warned his class not to take part in the "indiscriminate and unpardonable use of instruments" which he believed "generally prevailed." Ibid., 31. Because midwives did not use instruments and rarely administered drugs, contemporaries mistakenly assumed that women physicians

would follow suit. Here they underestimated the impact of professional training, a matter about which historians of female professionalism are still in conflict. For the differences in practice between physicians and midwives at parturition see Janet Bogdan, "Care or cure? childbirth practices in nineteenth century America," *Feminist Studies* 4 (June 1978): 92–99.

9   A. F. A. King, "The physiological argument in obstetric studies and practice," *American Journal of Obstetrics and Diseases of Women and Children* 21 (April 1888): 372; Henry T. Byford, "The so-called physiological argument in obstetrics," ibid. 21 (Sept. 1888): 899. See also H. M. Cutts, "The necessity of preparatory treatment for child-bed," ibid. 19 (Aug. 1886): 796–801; T. P. White, "The normal puerperal state," ibid., 19 (Nov. 1886): 1191–1205; Thomas Opie, "Is the frequent use of forceps abusive?" ibid. 21 (Oct. 1888): 1088–92.

10 Jane S. Heald, "Obstetrics," M.D. thesis, Woman's Medical College of Pennsylvania, 1855; Phoebe Wilson, "Disquisition on parturition," M.D. thesis, Woman's Medical College of Pennsylvania, 1857. For a general overview, see Wertz and Wertz, *Lying-In*.

11 Phoebe Oliver, "Eclampsia," M.D. thesis, Woman's Medical College of Pennsylvania, 1869; Katharine D. Perry, "Puerperal troubles," M.D. thesis, Woman's Medical College of Pennsylvania, 1887; Louise Schneider, "Anaesthesia in natural labor," M.D. thesis, Woman's Medical College of Pennsylvania, 1859.

12 Lucy R. Weaver, "Symptoms of puerperal peritonitis," M.D. thesis, Woman's Medical College of Pennsylvania, 1879; Mary Jordan Finley, "On vesico vaginal fistula," M.D. thesis, Woman's Medical College of Pennsylvania, 1880. See also Margaret Hoeflich, "Eclampsia," M.D. thesis, Woman's Medical College of Pennsylvania, 1872–1873; Laura V. Gustin, "A thesis on interference in natural labor," M.D. thesis, Woman's Medical College of Pennsylvania, 1873.

13 Marie E. Zakrzewska, "Report of one hundred and eighty-seven cases of midwifery in private practice," *Boston Medical and Surgical Journal*, 121 (Dec. 1889): 557–60. See also Frances Rutherford, "The perineum and its care during parturition," *Woman's Medical Journal*, 2 (Feb. 1894): 29–33; Mary Whery, "The prevention of lacerations of the perineum," ibid. 13 (Jan. 1903): 5–6; Agnes Eichelberger, "Prophylaxis in obstetrics," ibid. 11 (July 1901): 255–58; Eliza Root, "The study and teaching of obstetrics," ibid. 9 (Oct. 1899): 324–28; Prudence Saur, *Maternity: A Book for Every Wife and Mother* (Chicago, 1889), 218–20; Sarah Hackett Stevenson, *The Physiology of Woman* (Chicago, 1882), 91.

14 Root, "Study and teaching of obstetrics," 324–28.

Anna E. Broomall, "The operation of episiotomy as a prevention of perineal ruptures during labor" *American Journal of Obstetrics and Diseases of Women and Children* 11 (July 1878): 517–27.

15 See Wertz and Wertz, *Lying-In*, 150–54, 164–73.

16 Elizabeth Blackwell to Emily Blackwell, Nov. 27, 1854, Blackwell Manuscripts (Library of Congress, Washington); Maria Zakrzewska to Elizabeth Blackwell, March 21, 1891, Blackwell Manuscripts (Schlesinger Library).

17 Case records are available only after 1887 for Boston Lying-In Hospital.

18 Charles E. Rosenberg, "And heal the sick: the hospital and the patient in 19th century America," *Journal of Social History* 19 (June 1977): 428–47.

19 Emma L. Call, "The evolution of modern maternity technic," *American Journal of Obstetrics and Diseases of Women and Children* 58 (Sept. 1908): 392–404. For an explicit statement of Marie Zakrzewska's philosophy concerning the hospital's admission practices, see her comments in New England Hospital, Annual Report (1868), 9–21, Sophia Smith Collection, Smith College Archives, Northampton, Mass. Virtually every New England Hospital annual report contains rather self-conscious testimony concerning the advantages of the hospital's Christian atmosphere. For examples, see New England Hospital, Annual Report (1873) 5–7; ibid. (1880), 5–9.

20 Rosenberg, "And heal the sick," 488.

21 See Regina Markell Morantz, "'The connecting link': the case for the woman doctor in 19th century America," in *Sickness and Health in America: Readings in the History of Medicine and Public Health*, ed. Judith Walzer Leavitt and Ronald Numbers (Madison, Wisc., 1978), 117–28.

22 See Boston Lying-In Hospital, outpatient records, Countway Library, Harvard Medical School, Boston.

23 In this sample, "heroic" medicine was defined as any dosage of extremely harsh remedies, such as calomel or opium.

24 Our choice of statistical methods was dictated to some degree by the relative paucity of data on the Boston Lying-In case records. We limited our direct comparisons between hospitals to tests for signficant differences in the frequency of occurrence for which chi square tests of independence were used. For analyses of data within each hospital, we used a variety of methods. In all instances where a significant difference is either claimed or rejected, a probability level of .05 was the minimum level accepted.

25 This argument was made by Crumpacker, "Female patients." See also Branca, *Silent Sisterhood*, 86–90, Walsh, *Doctors Wanted*, 93–95.

26 See New England Hospital Annual Report (1879),

8–9; ibid. (1880), 7–13; ibid. (1885), 7; ibid. (1886), 7–8; ibid. (1888), 8–9; W. L. Richardson, "The use of antiseptics in obstetric practice," *Boston Medical and Surgical Journal* 116 (Jan. 1887): 73–79; Boston Lying-In Hospital Annual Report (1874) Countway Library, 5–6; ibid. (1879), 7–8; ibid. (1881), 7.

27 Call, "Evolution of modern maternity technic," 392–404. Zakrzewska wrote, "Our best women physicians have been educated there [Switzerland] as well as in Germany and in France—for even these two latter countries have received women into their schools more on an equality with men than has America." She said they returned "with a higher standard of scientific learning" than in America. See Agnes C. Vietor, ed., *A Woman's Quest: The Life of Marie E. Zakrzewska, M.D.* (New York, 1924), 359.

28 For an account of the staff's ignorance of theory and the hit-and-miss approach before bacteriology, see Call, "Evolution of modern maternity technic," 392–404.

29 New England Hospital, Annual Report (1868), 12, 18.

30 Ibid. (1872), 11.

31 Boston Lying-In Hospital, Annual Report (1874), 5–6.

32 New England Hospital, Annual Report (1879), 19–23; Boston Lying-In Hospital, Annual Report (1879), 13.

33 Vietor, ed., *A Woman's Quest*, 449–50.

29

Homeopathy and Sexual Equality:
The Controversy over Coeducation
at Cincinnati's Pulte Medical College, 1873–1879

WILLIAM BARLOW AND DAVID O. POWELL

The number of women physicians in the United States increased dramatically during the late nineteenth century. From a mere 200 or less in 1860, their ranks swelled to over 7,000 by 1900.[1] In Ohio, the number of female doctors grew from 42 to 451 in the last three decades of the century.[2] Although reliable statistics are not available, it has been estimated that a majority of these women in Ohio and elsewhere were trained in schools sponsored by groups of physicians who dissented from orthodox medical therapy and were branded as irregular sects by the American Medical Association.[3] Homeopathy, a major dissenting sect which advocated extremely small doses of medication, provided much of this early educational opportunity.[4] In Ohio, for example, the second woman to receive an M.D. degree, Helen Cook, was graduated from Cleveland Homeopathic College in 1852. From that date until 1914, 260 women earned homeopathic degrees in Cleveland compared to only 64 regulars. Nationally, by 1880 nine of the eleven homeopathic schools admitted women.[5]

Explanations of the apparent absence of sexual barriers in homeopathy range from the noble to the crass. They vary from the sect's genuine dedication to a variety of nineteenth-century reforms including women's rights, through a desire to spread its creed by any means, including using women, to a crude entrepreneurial attempt to make money by expanding enrollments in its educational insti-

tutions.[6] Whatever the reason, historians have assumed that in contrast to orthodox centers of medical education, homeopathic colleges eagerly welcomed women. This assumption has never been examined in detail. Moreover, since homeopathic medical schools either disappeared or converted to regular therapeutics in the twentieth century, few materials remain for a thorough and systematic investigation. Fortunately, the records of Pulte Medical College of Cincinnati are extant and provide the basis of this study.[7]

If Pulte was typical of her sister colleges, the belief that homeopathic schools ardently espoused sexual equality must be reexamined. From its founding in 1872 until 1879, coeducation was hotly debated and proved so divisive that it almost destroyed the school. The wrangling reached a fever pitch in 1878 when it was taken up by the press and aptly headlined "Homeopathic War." Before the issue was resolved, it produced mass resignations from the board of trustees and faculty, vitriolic personal attacks on professors, and lawsuits charging libel and slander.[8]

The dispute over female students at Pulte did not occur in a vacuum. It coincided with a national debate concerning coeducation prompted by the well-publicized views of Dr. Edward H. Clarke, a Harvard Medical School professor. Dr. Clarke argued that although capable women had a right to study medicine, they must be segregated from male students and would be hampered professionally by their periodicity. His *Sex in Education; or, A Fair Chance for Girls*, published in 1873, extended his argument against mixed classes to include all female education beyond puberty. Concentrated study would divert "force to the brain" which was neces-

WILLIAM BARLOW is Professor of History at Seton Hall University, South Orange, New Jersey.
DAVID O. POWELL is Professor of History at C. W. Post Center of Long Island University, Greenvale, New York.

Reprinted with permission from *Ohio History* 90 (1981): 101–113.

sary in the "manufacture of blood, muscle, and nerve, that is, in growth." The result would be women with "monstrous brains and puny bodies . . . weak digestion . . . and constipated bowels."[9] The feminist counterattack was immediate. Articles, books, and investigations quickly appeared which concentrated on proving that menstruation did not impair women's ability to study or work.[10] The champions of women, however, did not deal specifically with the question of medical coeducation.

That issue was at the time, however, in contention at a number of academic institutions. The University of Michigan and several other schools opened their doors to women medical students early in the 1870s. In 1878, the same year that the Cincinnati squabble reached a climax, even Harvard considered coeducation. Conceding that there was "a legitimate demand for, and an important place to be filled by, well-educated women as physicians," the professors nevertheless voted against their admission. It is significant that what was given at Michigan and denied at Harvard was equal but separate education. At Michigan the only course in which the sexes were integrated was chemistry. At Harvard the rejected plan provided for "complete separation" in laboratories and most lectures.[11] At irregular institutions from 1869 to 1877, six homeopathic schools opted for coeducation, although several restricted women to segregated classes. By 1878, only Pulte and two other homeopathic colleges remained exclusively male.[12]

At the center of the protracted confrontation over women at Pulte stood four prominent faculty members: Drs. Thomas P. Wilson, M. H. Slosson, Seth R. Beckwith, and John D. Buck. They were all among the founders of the school, were graduates of Cleveland Homeopathic College, and, with the exception of Dr. Slosson, had taught there before coming to Cincinnati. Drs. Beckwith and Slosson emerged as opponents of coeducation, with Drs. Buck and Wilson as proponents. Other faculty members took less consistent or conspicuous stands during the controversy.[13]

Either by intent or neglect, Pulte's original by-laws and announcements left the status of women undefined.[14] Consequently, at "every session of lectures a number" of women applied for admittance "but were turned away."[15] Such was the fate of Frances Janney of Columbus, Ohio. In 1874 her preceptor wrote "to Cincinnati to see if they would admit me this fall." Denied acceptance, she entered Boston University where she received her M.D. degree in 1877. During the spring of 1876, however, she studied in Cincinnati at Dr. Wilson's Ophthalmalic Clinic, which was housed in the same building as Pulte. After Dr. Wilson persuaded some of Pulte's teachers to permit her to attend their classes unofficially, she proudly informed her mother that she would "be the *first lady student* to attend lectures at Pulte College after all." But other professors, she complained, "Beckwith among the number, say they *will not* lecture to ladies." They were "not true gentlemen," she felt, "& want to say things they ought not to, & do not want the restraint of the presence of ladies."[16] Thus, despite Frances Janney's attendance at a few classes, Pulte's doors remained formally closed to women.

On four occasions from 1873 to 1878, coeducation was debated and voted on by Pulte's faculty. In 1873, spurning the idea of mixed classes, "a Spring Term for women only" was approved. A circular advertising the course was issued, but since "not a single woman applied for admission," segregationist Dr. Beckwith concluded that women did not want to become physicians. Coeducationist Dr. Buck, however, exclaimed "Good for them," elated that women had repudiated sexual segregation in favor of full equality with men. Again in 1875 the question of admitting women was raised and "promptly voted down." Three years later on February 5, 1878, Dr. Buck introduced a resolution approving matriculants "without distinction of sex" which was passed, only to be rescinded four days later. Thereupon, Drs. Buck and Wilson angrily submitted their resignations to the board of trustees and demanded an "investigation of the lying & bullying by which women were excluded."[17] When reconciliation efforts failed, the trustees requested that the two antagonistic factions present their ideas in writing in order to provide a basis for discussion and decision.[18]

The arguments for and against the entrance of women to Pulte were presented to the board of trustees at a meeting on May 28, 1878.[19] Speaking for a majority of the faculty, Dr. Beckwith was supported by Dr. Slosson and three other professors. A longtime foe of female physicians, Dr. Beckwith had earlier fought unsuccessfully to exclude them from local, state, and national homeopathic organizations. By the 1870s, however, with increasing numbers entering the profession, he grudgingly admitted that "no one denies her right" and capability of "practicing medicine." Even so, he doubted if they could succeed as general practitioners. "Nature" had adapted women only for the "treatment of disease peculiar to her own sex." Furthermore, they must be trained in "Colleges established for them, or in entirely separate departments" and only "for the very limited sphere . . . in which they can reasonably hope to succeed"—obstetrics, gynecology, and diseases of children.[20]

But Pulte, Dr. Beckwith proclaimed, must remain a male bastion. It was "organized for the medical education of men," and the "large and intelligent" male student body "almost to a man" opposed female students. More importantly, mixed classes would attract immoral women who would corrupt the "clinical instruction given to male students." A separate department for women was "utterly impracticable" at Pulte. Moreover, lecturing to women separately on surgery, anatomy, and obstetrics "would be obviously improper and embarrassing to all parties." Adjunct female professors in these sensitive chairs, Dr. Beckwith continued, likewise would be unacceptable "to the gentlemen occupying them." In addition, even if women were admitted to Pulte, they could not fulfill the graduation requirement of clinical observation and lectures because the Cincinnati Hospital barred them from its teaching facilities. In short, Dr. Beckwith concluded, female students would destroy "the harmony and increasing popularity, usefulness and prosperity of the College." There the opponents rested their case.[21]

The arguments for coeducation were contained in an eleven-page printed brief signed by Drs. Buck and Wilson and part-time professor Dr. William Owens. A wide-ranging document, it criticized the organization of the board, attributed the school's unstable finances to Dr. Beckwith's antifeminism, and mustered evidence from home and abroad supporting coeducational classes. Charging that Dr. Beckwith had manipulated the members of the board of trustees to his will, the brief demanded that he be removed as its president. In that position, he had alienated "a great and growing portion of influential and cultured society." More specifically, he was guilty of the "slanderous assertion, broadly and loudly advocated that no respectable

women will attend a Medical College with men, and that the College which admits them is but another name for a Whore House," thus casting "offensive and indecent asperities on women and sister Colleges" which accept them.[22]

The brief went on to link certain financial "failures and shortcomings" to Dr. Beckwith's refusal to sanction coeducation. Dr. Joseph H. Pulte, after whom the school was named, originally promised a handsome endowment but after women were excluded changed his mind, stating that "his wife, as his apothecary, had done as much to establish Homeopathy in Cincinnati as he had, and he did not propose to take her money as well as his own, to endow a college that refused to her sex equal rights and opportunities." In addition, Dr. Beckwith's "out spoken and violent opposition" to women "greatly reduced the number of our students" and thus "most seriously affected our financial revenues."[23]

In a more positive vein, the brief argued that coeducation was in keeping with the "spirit of the present age, the progress of time, and the course of medical education." Even in "conservative Europe the barriers" to women had crumbled at the Universities of Paris, London, Upsala, and Zurich, along with other prestigious schools in Italy, Russia, and Austria. On the domestic scene, the recent May 1878 Homeopathic Inter-Collegiate Conference declared unanimously that "our" colleges should be opened "to all . . . without distinction of sex."[24] While attending that conference, Dr. Wilson had solicited the candid evaluations of coeducation from representatives of the seven institutions where it existed. Six replied in lengthy letters which were included in the brief. Eschewing all theoretical speculations, the respondents, some of whom were formerly hostile to female students, detailed the actual results of mixed classes in their institutions and thus provided a thoroughly practical refutation of Drs. Beckwith's and Clarke's tirades against coeducation.[25]

Women, observed Dr. J. G. Gilchrist of the University of Michigan Homeopathic Medical College, were intellectually "equal to the men in exact knowledge . . . and class standing." Dr. J. R. Sanders of Cleveland Homeopathic College, on the basis of "near twenty years" experience, even felt that women acquired "this knowledge with greater rapidity" than men and held "it with equal tenacity." During "the last year . . . the *best* paper" in Dr. Charles Adams's surgical examination at Chicago Homeopathic College "was from a woman." Women also possessed special healing talents which "naturally endowed" them for medicine, declared Dr. A. C. Cowperthwait of the Homeopathic Medical Department of the University of Iowa. "For the more delicate ministry of the art," Dr. Sanders insisted, they had "qualities prominent above man."[26]

Although women were decorous creatures, Dr. David Thayer of Boston University had "no trouble" instructing "both sexes together on all subjects, even those of the greatest delicacy." Dr. Adams had "no more trouble with the cases in my cliniques on account of their presence than the gynecologist has with his on the men's account." Nothing had ever occurred in Dr. T. S. Hoyne's lectures at Hahnemann Medical College of Chicago "to offend even the most modest woman in the land." Dr. Sanders never had "any difficulty or embarrassment by reason of women's presence, or . . . any evidence of any lady student suffering any offense, or wound of delicacy, or tarnish or true womanly modesty. If this is possible in Obstetricy," he emphasized, "it surely must be in every other department of medical teaching."[27]

The attendance of such superior moral beings in classes with men in fact "had a *silently* beneficial effect on the sterner sex," reported Dr. Gilchrist. Their presence at Cleveland was a "perpetual challenge" to "boorishness and vulgarity." The faculty there would never "forget the experience of lawlessness, rudeness, unmannerly and unmanly demeanor" of male students at one session when women were excluded. After women restrained the animalistic male, however, he exerted an "inevitable challenge" to her "high endeavor and rivalry of success." In short, Dr. Thayer was convinced that coeducation allowed a "healthy emulation between the sexes which contributes to the mutual advantage of both."[28]

Finally, menstruation may account for woman's "emotional nature," wrote Dr. Gilchrist, but rather than proving debilitating it produced in female students an "esprit de corps" which men lacked. At the University of Michigan "in not a single instance has a case of break-down occurred among them, that cannot be matched by enough, yes, *more* than enough cases among the men." Women were "equally enduring in the strain incident to pro-

longed and somewhat severe mental application." "Dr. Clarke would find a most overwhelming defeat of his system, if he were here." Dr. Cowperthwait summarized the views of his colleagues: "The day for ladies to either starve or else be wash and sewing ladies is past."[29]

Armed with these findings, the petitioners requested not only the admission of women but their full equality as students, arguing that "our College building is peculiarly adapted to the wants of a mixed class." They indicated, however, they would settle for less by acknowledging, "we have large unoccupied rooms for separate classes when so desired." But for their overall case, it could be "further substantiated, if need be, by 'a cloud of witnesses.'"[30]

Both factions of the faculty asked the board of trustees for a speedy resolution of the "vexing question." Initially, by removing Dr. Beckwith as its president and forcing him and three other faculty members to resign as trustees, the board appeared ready to accept women. However, the resignation of eight additional trustees left the remaining twelve divided and uncertain as to how to proceed. Therefore, at a series of meetings in May and June of 1878, the board procrastinated.[31]

Deliberations were further complicated when the imbroglio erupted in the public press. On June 13, the *Cincinnati Times* published segments of the "serious charges against Dr. Beckwith" made by Drs. Buck and Wilson. The following day the *Times* joined by the *Enquirer* and *Commercial* featured Dr. Beckwith's denouncements of the "libelous and slanderous" accusations. These exchanges and other newspaper reports centered on the possibility of financial irregularities and added little to the women's question. On June 15, Dr. Beckwith instituted a $10,000 libel suit against Drs. Buck, Wilson, and Owens.[32]

Under such emotional circumstances, the board met on June 18. Conflicting resolutions were presented. One stated that it would be "detrimental . . . to admit females." A substitute resolution asserted that matriculants "be admitted . . . without distinction of sex" but with separate lectures on certain "delicate" topics. Unable or unwilling to support either position, the board after much maneuvering deferred a decision until March 1879. While the substantive question was sidestepped, procedural votes suggest that the board was evenly divided.[33] A trustee later confessed that they "were in doubt as to the wisdom and propriety" of which course to follow. As "business men," they were "generally unacquainted with the real merits of such questions" and "hesitated when disaster and ruin were predicted."[34]

Having postponed a verdict on coeducation until the following year, the board next considered the seething hostility among the professors. As with the women's issue, they followed an erratic and contradictory course. On July 1, Dr. Slosson, spokesman for the Beckwith group, introduced a plan removing Drs. Buck and Wilson from the faculty and adding five new professors. In response to this opportunity to clear the air, the board temporized and inexplicably accepted Dr. Wilson's resignation but refused Dr. Buck's.[35] A Cincinnati paper interpreted these actions as a "triumph for Dr. Beckwith and his party" and concluded that the "question of the admission of women . . . is now practically decided in the negative." Dr. Buck retorted that such an assessment was "rather premature" because the "whole matter" was still "in the hands of the trustees."[36]

Dr. Buck's prophecy proved partially accurate. Within a month and without explanation, Dr. Slosson resigned and Dr. Buck's allies Drs. Wilson and Owens were reappointed by the board. In addition, two of Dr. Beckwith's former supporters now joined the Buck faction to form a pro-women faculty majority. Disappointed at his sudden loss of power and peeved by the board's probing into his financial conduct, Dr. Beckwith indignantly resigned. Therefore, by the fall term of 1878 professors supporting coeducation appeared triumphant, and a favorable ruling on women by the trustees seemed assured.[37]

Such, however, was not the case. The board proved as incapable of resolving the quandary in 1879 as in 1878. On March 17, they decided to postpone "indefinitely" the "subject of the admission of women."[38] Frustrated by this delaying tactic, the faculty took matters into its own hands and published the annual announcement for 1879–80 which proclaimed that "hereafter all properly qualified matriculants, without distinction of sex, will be admitted."[39]

Presented with this fait accompli, the board met on July 22 "for the purpose of considering the action of the faculty relative to the admission of Fe-males" but again was hopelessly divided and unable to assert control. After several unsuccessful attempts to censure the faculty for "infringement of the privileges and duties" of the trustees, the board appointed a special investigating committee. After deliberating for a week, the committeee submitted two conflicting reports—one harshly criticizing the professors, demanding a faculty reorganization, and recommending that the annual announcements be destroyed, and the other upholding the faculty and asserting that in the absence of bylaws to the contrary the admission of students was a prerogative of the professors. The board divided evenly on both reports, and as a result neither was adopted.[40] Thus, women were admitted to Pulte by the faculty without sanction of the board of trustees. In this unusual and perhaps unprecedented fashion, the controversy was finally resolved.

The victory for the supporters of women was less than complete. In order to gain the necessary faculty support and the reluctant acquiescence of the trustees, Drs. Buck and Wilson had compromised the principle for which they had so long fought. Coeducation would not mean total integration of all classes at Pulte. While promising "women advantages equal, in every respect, to those enjoyed by men," the new announcement added vaguely that "instruction will be given in some departments separately, whenever desirable or necessary."[41] In actual practice, the sexes would attend segregated classes in anatomy, obstetrics, and gynecology as well as some of the clinics.[42]

In the fall of 1879 seven women were enrolled at Pulte. Observing that three were college graduates and two public school teachers, the *Cincinnati Enquirer* proclaimed extravagantly that their qualifications were better than "any class of male students in any medical college."[43] The following year, 1880–81, saw eight female matriculants, three of whom received M.D. degrees. Dr. Buck announced with satisfaction: "The joint medical education of men and women . . . is no longer an experiment."[44] By 1883–84 women comprised 31 percent of the students and 19 percent of the graduates.[45] While women reported that they were welcomed with "courtesy and respect," the faculty asserted that their presence had improved "general deportment" and that they had displayed a "high degree of scholarship."[46] As evidence, in 1880 Miss

Stella Hunt received the "prize for the best examination in physiology," thus casting doubt on a famous obstetrician's comment that woman "has a head almost too small for intellect but just big enough to love."[47]

Although the controversy over the admission of women to Pulte was eventually settled in favor of common sense and justice, the evidence suggests that sexual barriers at irregular medical institutions could be much more rigid than scholars have assumed. A majority of the faculty and trustees at a homeopathic college were as reluctant to embrace sexual equality as were their counterparts at most orthodox schools. Pulte's Dr. Beckwith was as adamant in his antifeminist stance as was Harvard's Dr. Clarke. Moreover, even when coeducation was adopted, it involved, as elsewhere, equal but separate instruction. Before generalizing about the medical education of women in nineteenth-century America, historians must research more completely homeopathic and other irregular medical schools. In fact, a thorough reexamination of medical coeducation seems necessary.

NOTES

The authors wish to acknowledge the support of the American Philosophical Society, Penrose Fund, Grant Number 8438. A shortened version of the paper was read at a joint meeting of the Ohio Medical Association and the Ohio Academy of Medical History, Columbus, Ohio, May 15, 1979.

1 Mary Roth Walsh, *"Doctors Wanted: No Women Need Apply": Sexual Barriers in the Medical Profession, 1835–1975* (New Haven, 1977), 186.

2 Frederick C. Waite, "Ohio physicians in the nineteenth century: a statistical study," *Ohio State Medical Journal* 40 (August 1950): 791–92.

3 Carol Lopate, *Women in Medicine* (Baltimore, 1968), 6.

4 Homeopathy was one of several medical sects which emerged in the first half of the nineteenth century and were considered irregular because of their rejection of the heroic therapy then practiced by most orthodox physicians. Heroic medicine consisted of extensive bleeding, blistering, and sweating, together with drastic purging and puking induced by massive doses of calomel and other toxic substances. In contrast, homeopathy was based on the law of infinitesimals—the smaller the dose the more effective the result—and provided welcome relief to many patients formerly subjected to the heroic regimen. Becoming popular and somewhat fashionable in the middle and late nineteenth century, homeopathy established its own medical societies and schools and was a major source of competition to the regular profession. After the rise of scientific medicine, homeopathy and its medical institutions largely died out in the early twentieth century. See Martin Kaufman, *Homeopathy in America: The Rise and Fall of a Medical Heresy* (Baltimore, 1971).

5 Frederick C. Waite, *Western Reserve University Centennial History of the School of Medicine* (Cleveland, 1946), 328, 330.

6 John B. Blake, "Women and medicine in ante-bellum America," *Bulletin of the History of Medicine* 39 (Spring, 1965): 99–123; Waite, "Ohio physicians," 792; John Duffy, *The Healers: The Rise of the Medical Establishment* (New York, 1976), 271.

7 Pulte Medical College Papers, Cincinnati Historical Society, Cincinnati, Ohio.

8 *Cincinnati Daily Times*, June 13, 1878.

9 Walsh, *"Doctors Wanted,"* 119–27; Edward H. Clarke, *Sex in Education; or, A Fair Chance for Girls* (Boston, 1873), 41.

10 Walsh, *"Doctors Wanted,"* 127–32; Julia W. Howe, ed., *Sex and Education: A Reply to Dr. E. H. Clarke's "Sex in Education"* (Boston, 1874).

11 Bertha Selmon, "Early development of medical opportunity for women in the United States," *Medical Woman's Journal* 54 (January 1947): 25–28, 60; Thomas F. Harrington, *The Harvard Medical School: A History, Narrative and Documentary, 1782–1905*, 3 vols. (New York, 1905), 3: 1223–34.

12 William H. King, *History of Homeopathy and Its Institutions in America*, 4 vols. (New York, 1905), 2: 211–14, 380–95, 410; 3: 106–7. For examples of equal but separate instruction at homeopathic schools, see University of Michigan, Ann Arbor, The Homeopathic Medical School, *Second Annual Announcement, 1876–77* (Ann Arbor, 1876), 3, and *Tenth Annual Announcement of Hahnemann Medical College, Chicago, Illinois, Session of 1869–70* (Chicago, 1869), 8–9.

13 *Cleave's Biographical Cyclopaedia of Homeopathic Physicians and Surgeons* (Philadelphia, 1873), 53, 319–20; King, *History of Homeopathy*, 2: 221–23, 36–61, 384–85.

14 *Articles of Incorporation of By-Laws of the Pulte Medical College, Cincinnati, Ohio* (Cincinnati, 1881); *First Annual Announcement of Pulte Medical College . . . Session of 1872–73* (Cincinnati, 1872).

15 Letter, John D. Buck, William Owens, Thomas P. Wilson to Board of Trustees of Pulte College, June 11, 1878, Pulte Medical College Papers (hereafter cited as Buck et al. to Board of Trustees).

16 Letters, Frances Janney to Rebecca A. S. Janney, August 7, 1874, May 3, 4, 1876, Janney Family Papers, Ohio Historical Society, Columbus, Ohio.

17 Letter, Seth R. Beckwith, M. H. Slosson, C. C. Bronson, D. W. Hartshorn, W. H. Hunt to Board of Trustees of Pulte College, June 11, 1879, Pulte Medical College Papers (hereafter cited as Beckwith et al. to Board of Trustees)

18 Pulte College Board of Trustees Minutes, 1872–1889 (handwritten copy), May 28, 1878, 72–74, Pulte Medical College Papers (hereafter cited as Board of Trustees Minutes).

19 Ibid.

20 Seth R. Beckwith, "Medical education of women," *Cincinnati Medical Advance* 1 (July 1973): 304–6; Beckwith et al. to Board of Trustees.

21 Ibid.

22 Buck et al. to Board of Trustees.

23 Ibid.; *Cincinnati Daily Times*, June 13, 1878.

24 Buck et al. to Board of Trustees.

25 Letters, David Thayer to Thomas P. Wilson, February 26, 1878; J. C. Sanders to Wilson, February 26, 1878; J. G. Gilchrist to Wilson, February 25, 1878; T. S. Hoyne to Wilson, February 25, 1878; Charles Adams to Wilson, February 25, 1878; A. C. Cowperthwait to Wilson, Feburary 26, 1878, Pulte Medical College Papers.

26 Letters, Gilchrist to Wilson, Sanders to Wilson, Adams to Wilson, Cowperthwait to Wilson.

27 Letters, Thayer to Wilson, Adams to Wilson, Hoyne to Wilson, Sanders to Wilson.

28 Letters, Gilchrist to Wilson, Thayer to Wilson, Sanders to Wilson.

29 Letters, Gilchrist to Wilson, Cowperthwait to Wilson.

30 Buck et al. to Board of Trustees.

31 Board of Trustees Minutes, May 28, June 3, June 11, 1878, 72–77.

32 *Cincinnati Daily Times*, June 13, 14, 1878; *Cincinnati Enquirer*, June 14, 1878; *Cincinnati Commercial*, June 14, 16, 1878.

33 Board of Trustees Minutes, June 18, 1878, 78–80.

34 *Cincinnati Commercial*, March 3, 1881.

35 Board of Trustees Minutes, July 1, 1878, 81–83.

36 *Cincinnati Commercial*, July 3, 5, 1878.

37 Board of Trustees Minutes, July 31, August 2, November 23, 1878, 83–87. A special announcement dated August 1, 1878, was issued to clarify the various changes in the faculty during the hectic months of June and July. *Pulte Medical College . . . Session 1878–79* (Cincinnati, 1878).

38 Board of Trustees Minutes, March 17, 1879, 94–95.

39 *Annual Announcement of Pulte Medical College . . . Session of 1879–80* (Cincinnati, 1879), 13–14.

40 Board of Trustees Minutes, July 22, 29, 1879, 95–108.

41 *Annual Announcement of Pulte Medical College . . . Session of 1879–80* (Cincinnati, 1879), 17.

42 *Annual Announcement of Pulte Medical College . . . Session of 1880–81* (Cincinnati, 1880), 13.

43 Ibid., 18–21; *Cincinnati Enquirer*, March 24, 1880.

44 *Annual Announcement of Pulte Medical College . . . Session of 1881–82* (Cincinnati, 1881), 20–23; *Cincinnati Commercial*, March 3, 1881.

45 *Annual Announcement of Pulte Medical College . . . Session of 1884–85* (Cincinnati, 1884), 18–21.

46 *Cincinnati Enquirer*, March 21, 1880.

47 Ibid., March 5, 1880; C.D. Meigs, *Lecture on Some of the Distinctive Characteristics of the Female, Delivered before the Class of the Jefferson Medical College, January, 1847* (Philadelphia, 1847), 62. For examples of examinations written by one woman graduate of Pulte, see *Examination Papers of Mary Wolfe, Pulte Medical College, Class of 1883* (Cincinnati, 1883).

(30)

On the Evolution of Women's Medical Societies

CORA BAGLEY MARRETT

Toward the end of the nineteenth century a new type of organization emerged within the American medical profession: the women's medical society. This organization sought to bring the women physicians in a community, who were usually few in number, into a closer fellowship. The idea of cooperation among women interested in health matters had antecedents in the nineteenth century. The Ladies Physiological Institute of Boston had been founded in 1848, and a few years later a small number of hospitals, dispensaries, and medical schools operated by women appeared. But the formation of the New England Hospital Medical Society in 1878 ushered in the era of the professional association of women physicians.[1]

This new type of organization developed only gradually. Although a few associations of female homeopaths were organized in the 1880s, only one society for allopathic women doctors—the Practitioner's Society of Rochester, New York, (1887)—seems to have been founded in this period.[2] During the 1890s the situation changed, and the following medical groups for allopathic women were established:[3]

Woman's Medical Club of Portland (Oregon)	1891
Physicians' League of Buffalo	1892
Woman's Medical Club of San Francisco	1893
Puget Sound Woman's Medical Club (Tacoma)	1894
Medical Women's Club of Chicago	1894
Denver Clinical Society	1895
Woman's Medical Club of Cincinnati	1896
Woman's Medical Club of Minneapolis	1898
State Society of Iowa Medical Women	1898

Despite this flurry of activity, by 1900 there were still communities with several women physicians practising but no separate female medical society. Why did such an organization emerge in some communities and not in others? This is the central question of this study. In an attempt to determine the factors governing the development of such medical societies, I selected five communities where an organization of regular medical women was formed between 1890 and 1899; namely Buffalo, San Francisco, Denver, Cincinnati, and Minneapolis.[4] I then matched each city with another which had a comparable number of regular women physicians but had no women's medical society prior to 1900. The comparison cities were Brooklyn, Detroit, Los Angeles, Washington, and Indianapolis (see Table 1).

Investigation showed that two conditions seemed to distinguish the cities with organizations from those without. First, in those cities where women's societies developed, a host of male medical associations already existed. These seem to have been communities with a highly organized medical profession. Second, the women physicians who began the early medical groups usually shared certain institutional ties. In contrast to their counterparts elsewhere, these women often had attended the same medical schools or had joined together to operate such service agencies as hospitals or dispensaries.

Women first entered the regular medical profession near the middle of the nineteenth century and throughout the century represented only a fraction of the total number of physicians. The 1880 census—the second one to identify physicians by sex—listed 2,423 women. This represented 3 percent of all medical professionals. By 1890 the count

CORA BAGLEY MARRETT is Professor of Sociology and Afro-American Studies at the University of Wisconsin, Madison, Wisconsin.

Reprinted with permission from *Bulletin of the History of Medicine* 53 (1979): 434–448.

Table 1
Female Physician Population in the Selected Cities

City	Year	All Women Physicians		Regular Women Physicians	
		Total Women	Women as Percent of all Physicians	Total Women	Women as Percent of all Regular Physicians
Buffalo	1892	25	5	18	5
Brooklyn	1892	60	5	15	2
San Francisco	1893	64	9	35	7
Detroit	1893	38	8	25	7
Denver	1895	28	8	21	7
Los Angeles	1895	28	8	20	7
Cincinnati	1896	58	8	24	5
Washington	1896	41	5	25	4
Minneapolis	1898	32	9	18[a]	7
Indianapolis	1898	40	8	18	5

Source: Figures are based on a count of names as given in various issues of *Polks' Medical Register of the United States and Canada*

[a]This underestimates the pool available for membership in the Minneapolis association, as that group admitted homeopaths as well as regulars.

for women physicians had nearly doubled (4,557), yet they were still only a small proportion (4.3 percent) of American physicians.

In keeping with the national pattern, Brooklyn, Detroit, and the other cities without an early medical association had relatively few women physicians and even fewer allopathic female doctors. Of the sixty medical women in Brooklyn during 1892 only fifteen, or one-fourth, were allopaths. Similarly, there were only eighteen allopathic medical women in Indianapolis near the end of the century. Yet the paucity of numbers did not explain the absence of a women physicians' association in these cities. Women were greatly outnumbered as well in Buffalo, San Francisco, and the other cities with organizations. In 1892 Buffalo had twenty-five women physicians, seven of whom were in sectarian medicine. The Denver roster of twenty-eight (1895) included six homeopaths and two eclectics. The societies established were small because of the small numbers of women physicians and the non-participation of some who were eligible. In San Francisco, for example, the organizers sent invitations to one hundred and nineteen women, but only twenty-nine joined during the first year of the association.[5] The charter membership was even

smaller in Buffalo (five), Denver (fifteen), and Cincinnati (eighteen). Since the formation of a women's medical society did not depend on there being a substantial number of women physicians in the community, this was not the reason which precluded the formation of a society in Brooklyn and the four other comparison cities.

Although the female physician population was small in both the cities with societies and those without, the possibility existed that they had different patterns of growth. The pattern might have been steady in one group and more sudden in the other. The investigation showed no such difference. In all the cities the number of women doctors did continue to increase, but the changes were small and rather similar across the locales. During the five years preceding the organization of a given club, the number of regular women in the city with the club and in the city with which it is being compared increased as follows:

Buffalo—9	Brooklyn—4
San Francisco—18	Detroit—19
Denver—12	Los Angeles—10
Cincinnati—18	Washington—15
Minneapolis—9	Indianapolis—9

Thus, the way in which the female medical force expanded was not distinctive in the five communities where the separate societies emerged. Instead, it was the actual growth of medical societies that was different in Buffalo, San Francisco, and their counterparts.

In the late nineteenth century, medical societies multiplied rapidly. According to one source, these societies "formed in such profusion, at all population levels, encountered such vicissitudes, and often such oblivion that no one has yet ventured an attempt to render an orderly, comprehensive account of this particular movement."[6]

Such profusion characterized the cities where women's societies were formed. Buffalo, for instance, had more regular medical societies though fewer physicians than had Brooklyn. In fact, eight local societies of regular doctors were already active in Buffalo when the women set up the Physicians' League in 1892. That activity was comparatively recent: five years earlier only three local associations had existed. Likewise, San Francisco medical men showed great interest in organizing medical societies. In 1893 the city had twice the number of societies to be found in Detroit.

Usually, the city where a women's society developed had more medical groups than had the one with which I have chosen to compare it. This was not true for the Washington-Cincinnati pair, however. Washington had considerably more associations than Cincinnati in 1896. Nonetheless, in proportion to physician population, the Washington profession was substantially less organized than the medical group in Buffalo, San Francisco, or Denver. In general, then, those locales where a woman's society appeared were rich in medical associations.

Apparently, the level of activity among the male physicians influenced the evolution of the women's societies. Through what process might this have occurred? Did women organize because they were excluded from this expanding network of doctors? The results do not indicate this. In those cities where the late-nineteenth-century groups developed, women had already gained admission to the larger associations.

By 1890 most medical societies admitted women members, usually after a bitter and protracted battle. The San Francisco Medical Society, for example, in 1874 had soundly rejected an application from a woman physician, Charlotte Blake Brown. Reportedly, some members "felt very strongly that the female of the species was mentally, physically, and morally unfitted to study medicine."[7] The group finally relented in 1877, one year after the state medical society had admitted its first women members. The struggle was even more prolonged in Washington. There, Mary Parsons (Howard University, 1873) first applied to the medical society in 1876. She failed to gain admission and reapplied in 1878, 1879, and 1888. Her application was finally accepted, but it would be another three years before a second woman won admittance.[8]

In spite of these difficulties, by the last decade of the century, in San Francisco and Detroit, in Cincinnati as well as Washington, women were able to join the general medical societies. And some usually did. In fact, the women's group often counted among its members an officer from an established medical society. Consider both the Minneapolis and Denver associations. In Minneapolis, Bessie Haines was treasurer of the state medical society at the same time as she helped organize the women's club. In Denver, Mae Cardwell was serving as secretary of the Colorado Medical Society when she participated in the creation of the Clinical Society.

Women had gained entry into the general societies, and at least some were active participants. But overall few of the female doctors joined the wider associations. Of the 18 regular female physicians in Buffalo during 1892, only 4 held membership in the Medical Society of the County of Erie and only 2 in the state society. There were only 3 women, one of whom was from Cincinnati, among the 550 members of the Ohio State Medical Society in 1891. However, in that year Cincinnati had only 6 allopathic women physicians in practice. The participation of women physicians in general medical societies was even more limited in Detroit. Only 6 Detroit women were members of the Michigan State Medical Society in 1893, although the city had six times that number of women eligible for membership.

In 1900 the editor of the *Colorado Medical Journal* censured the women in his region for their lack of participation in society activities. He reported that a mere fourteen women belonged to the Colorado State Medical Society and fewer still, only ten, to the Denver and Arapahoe Medical Society. He continued:

They may urge in their defense that they have their own women's medical society, the Denver Clinical Society, and do their duty in that. Let us see. In the first place, that society is properly classed with the special and restricted societies, membership in which should supplement and not supplant that in the general societies. . . . Again, its membership is but twenty-five, with an average attendance of six or eight, and during the past year they have read nine papers. Truly they are doing nobly by their profession.[9]

The women physicians in Buffalo and Denver were neither more nor less involved in the general societies than were women in the other cities. Nor were they necessarily less active than were their male colleagues. In 1891 only 6 percent of the allopathic male doctors in Cincinnati held membership in the state association. Similarly, although 75 percent of the Buffalo medical men were members of the county society in 1892, only 3 percent belonged to the state organization. Thus, while the general medical associations did not include all of the female medical force, neither did they incorporate the male profession in its entirety.

Women formed their own groups in communities where medical societies abounded, societies which accepted female members. It might have been their involvement in the larger societies which prompted these women to organize independently. They saw their male associates in the general organizations generate countless societies of distinct categories of physicians and for limited purposes. In San Francisco, for example, a Society of German Physicians and a Medical Benevolent Society sprang up alongside specialty groups for gynecologists, bacteriologists, and eye, ear, nose, and throat surgeons. This would again suggest that the drive to develop professional organizations in the late nineteenth century played a crucial role in the evolution of women's medical societies.

Women doctors seemingly were influenced not only by the number of medical societies developed by male physicians but also by their stated goals. Concretely, the women adopted for their organizations the types of goals which the other societies assumed.

In general, the women's medical society could take one of three forms. First, it might stress com-panionship among medical women. In this case, the group would function as a social club. Second, an association could serve as a means through which scientific and professional information would be exchanged. Finally, the group might decide to undertake a program of social action. The members would use their medical skills for public service.

Although a group could have pursued all three objectives simultaneously, this rarely occurred. The Cincinnati group was organized to encourage "mutual benefit and to cultivate a closer acquaintanceship among the medical women" of the city. Thirty years later the club still emphasized social activities, as this statement from a member illustrates: "We very rarely have a scientific paper, but we do have roll call response limited to three to five minutes and this is very entertaining and profitable."[10]

The Buffalo association also sought to acquaint women physicians with one another, but its program was more professional. According to a charter member, the group "was founded upon the feeling of good fellowship, kindred ambition and the desire as associates in the great workshop to join in the emulation of each other's attainments, enjoy our grand delusions, criticize each other's ideals, and compare results."[11] To further these aims—as in many of the existing male associations—the Buffalo league met to discuss cases and to hear lectures. Similarly the members of the Denver Clinical Society met to discuss reports of medical cases. An officer of the association held that these types of activities were especially needed in Denver, because of the lack of other women's medical institutions in the city. The Clinical Society would provide examples against which women could measure their reports and cases and thereby improve their work.[12]

The Minneapolis association apparently was more concerned with social action than were the groups in Cincinnati, Buffalo, and Denver. In 1898 it took credit for the appointment of a woman to the health board of the city as a sanitary inspector. Of more significance was the launching by the club in that year of a course of lectures on health care to be presented before mothers' clubs at missions and in settlements. Later in 1901 the same organization founded the first emergency hospital at the state fair.[13] The San Francisco organization also displayed a commitment to community issues. It set up a committee on the quality of food in the city and seems to have scheduled rather regular reports on the Children's Home and other local institutions.

If other pre-1900 groups are considered in addition to the five focal associations then it becomes obvious that such programs for social action were not common. Few of the other associations systematically engaged in community service or political action. The Iowa society was founded to bring medical women into closer contact with one another, and it usually scheduled medical papers and scientific discussions for its annual meeting. The Rochester organization had mutual helpfulness, the discussion of medical questions, and the promotion of sociability as its objectives.

In contrast to these medical societies, the general women's clubs of the era were turning increasingly to social and welfare matters. By the later nineteenth century, the number of action groups belonging to the General Federation of Women's Clubs had increased and the number of cultural or literary societies had declined.[14] Yet, the women's medical societies did not generally show a greater concern for public service. At least three explanations can be offered for the failure of these associations to replace social interaction with political action. First, women physicians often had other channels for community involvement available to them. One of the founders of the Portland association, for example, served on numerous boards and commissions designed to improve health care, especially for women and children. A charter member of the Denver society was active in local associations concerned with the humane treatment of animals. Sometimes such activity was undertaken collectively rather than individually. The Woman's Homeopathic Medical Association of Chicago, founded in 1879, joined the other groups in 1886 to establish the Protective Agency for Women and Children, known later as Legal Aid. Moreover, the free dispensary could be regarded as a collective effort to render service. Thus, the women's medical society might have been somewhat inactive politically because there were other organizations in which women doctors could pursue political objectives.

Second, the shift to political action had only recently occurred among the general women's clubs: it did not become evident in the General Federation until the 1896 biennial meeting. Perhaps it was of too recent vintage to be reflected in the nineteenth-century medical clubs. But even the groups founded later showed no notable change in outlook. The societies formed after the turn of the century placed no more emphasis on social activism than their predecessors. This suggests a third explanation for the programmatic choices the women physicians made. They had used the predominantly male medical societies, not the general women's clubs, as their models. In the local medical associations of the nineteenth century, a program which combined discussions of cases, lectures or essays, and dinners or banquets was the usual fare. The women's medical societies were set up as institutions which would parallel the other medical groups of the period.

Conditions within the medical profession at large seem to have affected the societies of women physicians. But in addition certain circumstances relating to the activities of women physicians facilitated their organization. In particular, the women's medical societies were established in those cities where women physicians were already linked by several ties.

The women who set up the medical societies had often cooperated in the operation of a hospital or dispensary.[15] The founders of the Minnesota club, for example, were associated with one of the two hospitals managed by women in that city—either the Northwestern Hospital for Women and Children, which had opened in 1882, or the Maternity Hospital, founded in 1888. Those who organized the Buffalo association worked together at the Ingleside Home, an affiliate of the Woman's Hospital. The Pacific Hospital for Children, which Charlotte Brown had opened in 1875, was the primary employer for the charter members of the San Francisco club.

Except for Washington, the cities I have matched with those above appear to have had no similar institutions. In Washington women physicians operated a clinic and a dispensary in 1896 and much earlier had run two other dispensaries. One of these, the Woman's Hospital and Dispensary of 1881, had dissolved by 1896 and the second, the Woman's Dispensary founded in 1885, was by then under male control. Nevertheless, Washington—unlike Brooklyn, Los Angeles, and Indianapolis—was a base for a health care agency under the auspices of medical women.[16]

The organizers of the women's groups usually were linked in another way: through having attended common educational institutions (see Table 2). Four of the six original officers for the Buffalo association had been classmates at the University of Buffalo. The first leaders of the Cincinnati organization included three recent graduates from the women's medical college in that city. The situation in Washington, Detroit, and the other paired cities was different. Most of the Detroit doctors practising in 1896 had graduated from one of three schools: Howard University (seven); Columbian College (six); National University (five). But they had graduated over a wide period: from 1872 to 1892 for the Howard group. The Columbian cohort clustered somewhat more (1886–94), as that school was coeducational for only a few years. Nevertheless, the overlap in educational experience among women physicians in Cincinnati (Laura

Memorial College) and Buffalo was not typical in Washington.

Graduates from the University of Michigan predominated in Detroit, but as in the District of Columbia they spanned a twenty-year interval. No specific educational links united most of the Los Angeles women. Except for Minneapolis and Denver, in the cities where women's societies developed, many of the female physicians had known one another since medical school days.

Another factor governing whether separate women's medical societies developed was the existence of alternatives in a number of communities. These would include the medical school alumnae associations, the societies attached to hospitals for women, and female-dominated general medical societies.

Among the postgraduate organizations, the Alumnae Association of the Woman's Medical Col-

Table 2
Institution Graduating Largest Number of Women Physicians in Each City

City	Year	Total Women Graduates	Total, Single Institution	Institution	Total, Five Year Period[a]
Buffalo	1892	18	11	University of Buffalo	9 (1887–92)
Brooklyn	1892	15	7	Woman's Medical College of the New York Infirmary	2 (1887–92)
San Francisco	1893	35	10	(1) Cooper Medical College	5 (1888–93)
			10	(2) University of California Medical Department	3 (1888–93)
Detroit	1893	23[b]	12	University of Michigan	5 (1888–93)
Denver	1895	20	6	Northwestern University Women's Medical School	3 (1890–95)
Los Angeles	1895	20	4	Women's Medical College of Pennsylvania	3 (1890–95)
Cincinnati	1896	24	14	Laura Memorial College	12 (1891–96)
Washington	1896	25	7	(1) Howard University	1 (1891–96)
				(2) Columbian University	4 (1891–96)
Minneapolis	1898	17	3	Northwestern University Women's Medical School	3 (1893–98)
Indianapolis	1898	18	4	(1) Medical College of Indiana	3 (1893–98)
			4	(2) Central College of Physicians and Surgeons	2 (1893–98)

[a]This column indicates the number of graduates from the institution during the five-year period leading up to the time the relevant club was formed. Thus, nine of the eighteen graduates from the University of Buffalo who were residing in that city during 1892 had received diplomas between 1887 and 1892. The column shows the overlap among graduates.
[b]No institution given for two of the women listed as regulars.

lege of the New York Infirmary for Women and Children deserves mention. This association, established in 1873, had functions which paralleled those of a medical society. In fact, when the college closed in 1899, the alumnae group was transformed into the Women's Medical Association of New York City. Graduates of the Northwestern University Women's Medical School (which was known earlier as the Woman's Medical College of Chicago) could belong to their alumnae association, reorganized in 1882. Finally, the Alumnae Association of the Woman's Medical College of Pennsylvania served to forge and maintain links among the women who had attended that institution. Throughout the late nineteenth century this association, established in 1875, was highly active.

In a few instances, women physicians gained control of what had been male associations. One of these, the Philadelphia Clinical Society, evolved from the Northern Medical Association. The Northern society had begun in 1846 as an all-male group. It admitted women during the 1880s and by 1887–88 had become "an unusual coalition of medical women and liberal medical men." The conservatives in the group withdrew to reorganize the Northern Association and left the changed association, renamed the Clinical Society in 1884, primarily to women. Apparently, the Clinical club had dissolved by 1890, for in that year Philadelphia women started the Alumnae Medical Association. The bylaws of this group required that each member take an active part in the presentation and discussion of papers.[17]

The situation in Adams County, Illinois, was not nearly so complex, but just as in Philadelphia women were able to govern for a while an association started by males. A member of the Adams County Medical Society reported in 1895 that although there were too few women to justify a separate society, female doctors held all of the principal offices in the county association.[18]

In Baltimore, students, faculty, and other local physicians organized the Medical Society of the Women's Medical College in 1885. One account describes the officers as "ladies who had already graduated or were still students at the college."[19] But the membership of the organization was not exclusively female.

The existence of an association composed primarily or exclusively of medical women did not invariably rule out a separate women's medical society. The Chicago situation underscores this point. Members of the Northwestern Alumnae Association joined with women from the Women's Homeopathic Medical Association to establish the Medical Women's Club of Chicago in 1894. Although the homeopathic group appears to have then dissolved, the alumnae association continued. Thus, near the turn of the century, a women's medical society, an alumnae association, and miscellaneous service agencies staffed by women physicians all operated in Chicago. Likewise, the staff of the Woman's Hospital in Philadelphia organized a medical society in 1904 even though the alumnae association still functioned. Persons affiliated with the medical school there founded the Anna Broomall Society about the same time to honor a teacher who had established an outpatient maternity department.[20]

Not infrequently, the women who belonged to the separate medical societies also held membership in the ever-widening array of alumnae associations, medical sororities, and associations for the promotion of women's medical education.[21] This lends further support to the argument that as a rule a society of medical women did not evolve in an organizational vacuum.

The expansion during the late nineteenth century of physicians' associations and the presence of strong ties among women doctors probably both jointly influenced the development of women's medical societies. The founders of these groups often attributed their decision to organize to the discomfort they felt in the mainstream associations. According to a charter member of the Rochester group:

> We are members of a learned profession of which the opposite sex are as sands of the sea compared with us in number. . . . The medical societies are under their control: we have been admitted to these after the persistent knocking of the pioneer women of the profession, but we are not at home there as in our own circles. We need the general societies to broaden our minds and give us lines of thought but our work and growth should be free where we are without embarrassment or restraint.[22]

It seems unlikely that in Los Angeles, Detroit,

and Indianapolis, the male associations were more cordial to women than were the societies in Denver, San Francisco, and Minneapolis. Given this, why did the separate women's groups develop in the latter but not the former cities? The level of physician activity might have been the key. Where the medical men somewhat routinely started new associations, medical women, when disenchanted with the larger groups, perceived an alternative. The fact that other bonds connected them made the decision to organize even easier for these women. In contrast, the separate society would have been a curiosity in those communities where physicians rarely set up new professional organizations and would have been difficult where women physicians were not interconnected.

The women's medical societies commonly evolved out of existing associations of female doctors. The pattern is even clearer for some of the groups omitted from the analysis. The year before they began the Practitioner's Society, the Rochester women had organized the Provident Dispensary. The board of the dispensary and the membership of the medical society differed in only one way: the former included nonmedical women. But only the physicians associated with the dispensary belonged to the society. To what extent, then, was this a "new" organization?

The predominantly male associations often had a similar history. Generally, the medical societies emerged out of extant scientific organizations. These later groups usually accepted a more limited membership and were more specialized than were their predecessors. What this suggests is that for both men and women physicians, their medical societies often have been variations on existing models.

After the turn of the century women's medical societies developed in several other cities, including Detroit (Blackwell Medical Society, 1906), Washington (Women's Medical Society of the District of Columbia, 1909), Indianapolis (Women Physicians' Club, 1915), and Los Angeles (Medical Women's Clinical Club, 1919). By that time the rise of such groups was not so obviously connected with conditions in local communities. Instead, the development of national networks among women physicians became more significant. The *Woman's Medical Journal,* founded in 1893 and well established by the end of the century, served as an important medium for reporting on medical women's groups and encouraging their activities. In addition, some group members who moved to new locations carried a zeal for organizing associations with them. Consequently, more and more groups were organized in areas which had relatively few societies of medical men and no existing alliances among medical women. This suggests that purely local circumstances may be most significant when a new type of organization first appears. Once the mode has been tested and proven, it may be adopted in communities far different from those in which it originally developed.

NOTES

This is a revised version of a paper read before the 51st annual meeting of the American Association for the History of Medicine, Kansas City, Missouri, May 12, 1978.

1 Several sources cite the New England Society as the first professional women's medical society. See especially Kate C. Hurd-Mead, *Medical Women of America* (New York: Froben, 1933), 43; and Bertha Selmon, "Early history of women in medicine," *Medical Woman's Journal,* 1946, *53:* 44–48. But in 1870 women in Detroit organized the Woman's State Medical Association, *(Woman's Journal,* January 29, 1870, 27). A few years later (about 1876–77) a group of faculty and recent graduates from the Woman's Medical College of Pennsylvania formed the Preston Medical Society in Philadelphia. (I wish to thank Dr. Steven Peitzman for bringing this group to my attention.) Both the Michigan and the Philadelphia groups appear to have been short lived.

2 During the nineteenth century several medical therapies or schools of practice prevailed. The allopathic or "regular" doctors were those who pursued conventional therapies. The allopaths referred to other practitioners, homeopaths and eclectics, for example, as sectarians or irregulars.

3 This list omits societies attached to other institutions, such as the alumnae associations.

4 I omitted the other four societies for various reasons. For two of them—the Portland Society and the Puget Sound club—I found only fragmentary information. I excluded the Iowa association because it was the only non-city-based group. Finally,

no city without a women's society had a female physician population equal to that of Chicago in 1894. For additional information on the organizational drive before the twentieth century, see Cora Bagley Marrett, "Nineteenth-century associations of medical women: the beginning of a movement," *Journal of the American Medical Women's Association,* 1977, *32:* 469–74.

5 Invitations were sent to women throughout the Bay Area, including the city of Oakland.

6 W. B. McDaniel, "A brief sketch of the rise of American medical societies," *International Record of Medicine,* 1958, *171:* 489. On the expansion of medical societies, also see James Burrow, *AMA: Voice of American Medicine* (Baltimore: Johns Hopkins Press, 1963).

7 J. Marion Read and Mary E. Mathes, *History of the San Francisco Medical Society,* vol. 1: 1850–1900 (San Francisco: San Francisco Medical Society, 1958).

8 See the *History of the Medical Society of the District of Columbia, 1817–1909* (Washington, D.C.: The Society, 1909). For more information on women and the larger associations, see Martin Kaufman, "The admission of women to nineteenth-century American medical societies," *Bulletin of the History of Medicine,* 1976, *50:* 251–60; Catharine MacFarlane, "Women physicians and the medical societies," *Transactions of the College of Physicians of Philadelphia,* 1958, *26:* 80–83; and Phoebe Peck, "Women physicians and their state medical societies," *Journal of the American Medical Women's Association,* 1965, 20: 351–53.

9 "The women physicians of the West," *Colorado Medical Journal,* 1900, *6:* 302. The Denver Clinical Society protested and withdrew its reports from the journal. The editor responded: "The real spirit and purpose of the editorial seem to have escaped the members of the Clinical Society. They should remember that bitter tonics often are beneficial." *Colorado Medical Journal,* 1900, *6:* 409.

10 On the organization of the club see *Cincinnati Lancet-Clinic,* 1896, *36:* 580. The later account appeared in *Bulletin of the Medical Women's National Association,* 1926, *13:* 29.

11 Electa Whipple, "A résumé of the work of the Physician's League during its first decade," *Woman's Medical Journal,* 1902, *12:* 232.

12 Josephine Peavy, "Woman's clinical society," *Colorado Medical Journal,* 1897, *3:* 195–198.

13 See Nellie Barsness, "History of branch twenty-six (Minnesota)," *Journal of the American Medical Women's Association* 1955, *10:* 20–21.

14 The information on trends in the women's club movement comes primarily from Sophonisba Breckinridge, *Women of the Twentieth Century: A Study of Their Political, Social and Economic Activities* (New York: McGraw Hill, 1933); Thomas Woody, *A History of Women's Education in the United States,* vol. 2 (New York: Octagon Books, 1974); and Jennie C. Croly, *The History of the Woman's Club Movement in America* (New York: Henry G. Allan, 1898).

15 I have included only those institutions operated by women physicians. This excludes several of the hospitals for women run by male doctors. Omitted, too, are the institutions under the aegis of Catholic sisters' orders and those with a single woman physician in a key post. As examples of the latter, a woman doctor supervised the Protestant Episcopal Free Hospital for Children in Cincinnati in 1896. And in Minneapolis a female physician was in charge of a private nursing home in 1898. But these would not represent joint ventures by medical women.

16 Detroit women organized a dispensary in 1893 and a women's medical society thirteen years later. In addition, the Denver group established a hospital in 1901.

17 I am indebted to Dr. Steven Peitzman for the information on the Clinical Society. A short publication by Marshall lists some of the papers presented before that group and mentions the formation of the alumnae association. See Clara Marshall, *The Woman's Medical College of Pennsylvania: An Historical Outline* (Philadelphia: P. Blakiston, 1897).

18 *Woman's Medical Journal,* 1895, *4:* 172.

19 Harold Abrahams, *The Extinct Medical Schools of Baltimore, Maryland* (Baltimore: Historical Society, 1969), 71.

20 I found very little information on the Anna Broomall Club. An item in the *Bulletin of the Medical Women's National Association* in 1927 (*17:* 30) indicates that the group had held its twenty-seventh annual meeting that year. A later obituary for Broomall gives more detail: "[the] Anna E. Broomall Medical Club was started as a slight evidence of the respect, reverence and affection for their teacher and friend by her students. . . . She insisted it be useful educationally, and for years medical papers were read" (*Medical Woman's Journal,* 1931, *38:* 184–85).

21 In 1874 Mary Putnam Jacobi founded the Association for the Medical Education of Women. The group voted in 1900 to terminate and to turn its funds over to the Hospital Association, which by then had become an affiliate of the Women's Medical Association of New York City. See minutes of the Women's Medical Association for February 18, 1903; March 31, 1903; and March 21, 1906 on file at the New York Academy of Medicine.

22 Mary Stark, quoted in Florence Cooksley, "History of medicine in Monroe County," *New York State Journal of Medicine,* 1937, *37:* 88.

31

Doctors or Ladies?
Women Physicians in Psychiatric Institutions, 1872–1900

CONSTANCE M. McGOVERN

In the early 1890s at the Norristown State Hospital for the Insane in Pennsylvania, Dr. Lilian Welsh, then a member of the medical staff, invited a woman doctor friend to accompany her on weekly rounds. As they reached the last ward housing the most excitable patients, one of the more troubled inmates "planted herself firmly" in their way and inquired of the visiting doctor, "Say, are you a doctor or a lady?" Thus, mused Dr. Welsh, "out of the mouths of babes and defectives" come "current social opinions."[1]

Lilian Welsh was only one of the nearly two hundred women physicians who had decided to serve in psychiatric institutions in the last three decades of the nineteenth century. The experiences of these women who chose to take on two male-dominated professions simultaneously are worthy of exploration for these doctors did not correspond to Victorian expectations about the ideal woman and did not even adhere to the much-debated virtues of the "new woman."

Expected to be the preserver of culture and the mother of civilization according to the prescriptive literature, the ideal nineteenth-century woman could best perform these duties by maintaining a submissive and controlled demeanor. Rightfully and properly in her place in the home, she could influence moral attitudes and behavior in her roles as wife and mother. Commentators noted that woman's "chief work" was related to the "future of the world," and facetiously asked, "why should we spoil a good mother by making an ordinary grammarian?" But not everyone, especially in the latter part of the century, adhered to such a conservative view.

Some could, and did, acknowledge a new sphere for women; but they were no revolutionaries. If women emerged from the home and participated in volunteer and professional activities, they must still act "in a feminine manner." There was room for the "new woman," but she must acquiesce to a male colleague's advice, rely on his strength and expertise, and always conduct herself in a properly demure manner. Thus, at best, these doctors, as professional women, could expect a reserved tolerance, at worst, hostility and the label of "mannish maidens."[2]

The difficulties which beset the paths of women entering medicine in the late Victorian era are well documented. The mere logistics of obtaining a medical education raised barriers which were nearly insurmountable for all but the most stouthearted. Women's medical schools came in and out of existence with great frequency; nineteen schools for women had been founded in the nineteenth century, but by 1895 eleven had already disbanded and even those which survived offered little opportunity for any significant clinical practice. Most general hospitals did not accept female interns. Only three coeducational medical schools existed and the finest of these, Johns Hopkins, required a B.A. for admission—another difficulty to be overcome by the would-be woman doctor.[3]

The public was equally unfriendly. Women doctors were deemed "unsexed" or at least believed to have some "peculiar underlying reasons" for entering the professions. Gossip usually had it that any woman who took up medicine "must have done so from some profound emotional disturbance, some secret grief, presumably a disappointment in love." Attempts to rent office space met with cries of "no women doctors" and "no signs," even if the sign were "no bigger than a postage stamp." Own-

CONSTANCE M. McGOVERN is Assistant Professor of History at the University of Vermont, Burlington, Vermont.

Reprinted with permission from *Bulletin of the History of Medicine* 55 (1981): 88–107.

ers expressed fears that renting to a doctor would place "such a stigma on the house that they could never rent it again." Success at establishing an office usually meant renting on "Scab Row" or in "bachelors' apartments" and leaving one's self open to ridicule, laughter, and remarks about "bachelors' apartments and old maids livin' in them!" Always considered "somewhat of a curiosity," even professional acknowledgment of women physicians did not necessarily result in social acceptance. For instance, the "Ladies' Committee" of the American Medical Association meeting in Baltimore in 1895 questioned whether the women doctors should be invited to their reception and "finally decided with great reluctance to include them."[4]

Attitudes of fellow medical students were no better. For the groundbreaking women students some form of hazing seemed to be the normal, although not always expected, experience. Mary Bates who, in 1881, became the first Cook County Hospital female intern, was carried off in the midst of the night, mattress and bedding and all, to the gynecological ward "to be entered as an interesting case" by the male interns. Other women, as medical students, had to put up with being "hen-medics" or being "clucked at, bombarded with paper wads and thrown kisses."[5]

Heckling and ridicule did not stop even with the attainment of the medical degree. Almost every novice female physician met with expressions of disbelief and periods of testing from her male colleagues. These ranged from relatively harmless practical jokes and medical students boycotting clinical classes taught by women to incidents bordering on sexual harassment. Bertha Van Hoosen, while working in a Chicago clinic, described her feelings in an encounter with a "short, dapper young physician," who walked in, locked the door, and pocketed the key, as those of an "old bay mare moving slowly from side to side in the pasture lot to avoid the advances of the jumping stallion." Van Hoosen was given to barnyard descriptions; nevertheless she was probably more frank about her experiences than most women.[6]

Even salaried positions had limitations. Both Goucher College and Bryn Mawr, for instance, allowed women doctors to practice only preventive medicine. If a student became ill, a male doctor treated her because her "parents might not be satisfied to feel" that she was in the care of a woman physician. Further, when women finally started out on their own voluntary projects, such as evening dispensaries for the poor, these were usually the first to have funds rescinded, sometimes under the guise that "women physicians for women patients represented a specialty" and were therefore not eligible for public support. The problems seemed endless, but they were minimal compared to the additional difficulties met by those women who chose to serve in psychiatric institutions.[7]

Removed from the protection of all those images placing the woman on a pedestal and confronted with questions about their respectability and their physical and intellectual stamina, some women doctors still took on this double burden of proving their worth to both the medical and psychiatric professions. The more difficult to convince would prove to be psychiatry because, with few exceptions, psychiatry in the nineteenth century was still practiced within the asylum walls and stringently controlled by one of the most long-standing professional organizations—the Association of Medical Superintendents of American Institutions for the Insane (later renamed the American Psychiatric Association). Breaking down brick and mortar walls, as well as emotional and professional ones, proved to be a formidable task.[8]

In only one respect did the would-be woman psychiatrist have an advantage over her sister general practitioner—public opposition was minimal. Treatment of the mentally ill was not an issue of prime public attention in the late nineteenth century. Earlier in the century, some had crusaded for the humane treatment of all types of downtrodden and unfortunate people. But the general postwar cynicism arising from disillusionment with humanitarianism and the growing pessimism of the psychiatric profession itself left few outraged at the mere custodial care of the insane. Many were grateful to have those felt to be defective removed from their view, and most were simply indifferent or uninformed about what occurred in public institutions. Thus, although the women did not enjoy the support of the public, neither did they have to brook its opposition.[9]

Within the psychiatric profession, the prospect of women physicians in mental institutions generated intense discussion. At least one asylum superintendent and his board of trustees welcomed the appointment of a woman and, without hesitation, awaited the "result with confidence," fully expecting that her work would "increase the usefulness of the asylum." Those who favored this innovation stressed the issue of modesty, the modesty of the patients. The theory that women would be more open about their problems and more willing to agree to treatment, either local or surgical, from a doctor of their own sex was constantly discussed in the late nineteenth century and provided a persuasive argument.[10]

Another even more effective argument concerned the sexual behavior of the female patients. The pervading sexual mores, according to the normative literature of the period, and the frequent remarks about the sexual behavior of their female patients seem to indicate on the part of some psychiatrists both a fascination with and an unspoken fear of female sexuality, at least as expressed through the uninhibited actions of mentally ill women. Unlike the rest of society, which believed masturbation to be fairly common (although not acceptable) in single men but rare in women, the hospital doctors daily faced the manifestations of this "perversion," this "secret" cause of insanity, in their encounters with women patients. Moreover, despite the general belief that women seldom experienced sexual pleasure, these doctors recorded the remarks of women who reported that they felt "very erotic," that "sexual matters chiefly occupied" their thoughts, and they noted patients whose behavior they attributed to "an infatuation for the male sex" or "strongly developed" amativeness.

Particularly unsettling were the sexual delusions of female patients. A number of medical superintendents had observed that insanity in these patients was "tinctured" by sexual delusions about the male physicians, the examining doctors. Some seemed to need a "manifestation of affection" from the doctor, and others, in a disturbed state, would recite accounts of "immoral relations" between hospital employees, were willing themselves to go off on an escapade of carnal pleasure, and even accused the officers of attempting to rape them. The situation was often uncomfortable, and thus some doctors were quick to advocate the appointment of women assistant physicians because the "female insane," they believed, were "peculiarly susceptible" to any influence which might weaken the "restraints" which society had developed "around the passions." Many responded readily to this argument.[11]

Other doctors, in response to changes in medical theory, attributed women's emotional and mental illness to their reproductive system and became convinced that either local treatment or, especially, the surgical removal of uteri and ovaries would restore mental health to some suffering women. In the 1870s and early 1880s this was a convincing argument with the rise of both gynecology and surgery as specialties, and in the wake of the publicity accruing around Battey's "normal ovariotomy." Robert Battey, an obscure Georgia physician, had added the surgical technique and rationalization whereby nondiseased ovaries also might be removed in order to relieve purely neurotic conditions. The vogue for ovariotomy and the resultant optimism did not last long, but the initial fervor, coupled with the growing idea that women doctors could more properly treat female patients both psychologically and surgically, was enough to help break down the first barriers to women physicians in psychiatric institutions.[12]

A few superintendents, moreover, had hired women doctors for their staffs in the 1870s. Merrick Bemis of the Worcester (Massachusetts) Asylum, "having comprehended the difficulties insuperable by men physicians in the care and treatment of insane women patients," was the first and, in 1869, he employed Mary Stinson as assistant physician in the department for women. Others, like the administrators of the hospitals at Augusta, Maine, and at Kalamazoo and Pontiac, Michigan, also considered women's "services beneficial to patients." As these individual efforts became known, some realized that the "limited avenues for women physicians" made it "easy to get a woman" and "easier to keep her" and that she could be of "great help to the morale of the hospital" because she could more comfortably treat the "special illnesses of female employees." But these were only individual appointments and subject to change with the end of the term of office of each superintendent. Most hospital administrators remained adamantly opposed to the employment of women doctors in public institutions until their presence was required by statute.[13]

The first successful struggle for obligatory staff appointments for women doctors took place in Pennsylvania in 1878–79. Dr. Hiram Corson, who earlier had waged a campaign in the Pennsylvania State Medical Society for more than a decade to gain recognition for graduates and faculty of female medical schools, now launched a fight for that society to petition the legislature to assure that every psychiatric institution in the state of Pennsylvania would have a woman physician in charge of the care of incarcerated females. A dedicated crusader for justice for women in medicine (some would say a fanatic), Corson could be persuasive and rational, although sometimes overbearing, and was not above using emotionalism. Thus, in 1878, he asked the members to "fancy, if you can, your own mother or daughter taken to a hospital for the insane . . . are these sad mothers, these loved sisters, these unhappy daughters likely to reveal aught of their condition" to an inexperienced male staff doctor? The appeal was a standard one by now and Corson cited all the usual arguments: women's reluctance to reveal gynecological infirmities, doctors' aversions to pursuing such questions, "moral and mental delusions" produced by the peculiar female organic susceptibility, and women doctors' innate "devotion and self-sacrifice" and "gentleness and care."[14]

Positions as staff doctors were one thing, but Corson also urged the placement of women as superintendents in complete charge of all the business of the female wards. He scoffed at the objection that it had never been done before and dismissed physical weakness and inexperience as straw-man arguments: male superintendents were not chosen for their strength, and male staff doctors (the ones who dealt with patients on a daily basis) were equally unqualified when hired. The only objection to which Corson gave credence was that of the untested managerial skill of women. Did they have executive talent? Never one to be unprepared, in reply Corson cited at length the organizational abilities and dedicated work on behalf of the insane of Elizabeth Fry in England and Dorothea Dix in America, threw in a few remarks about the stamina of Elizabeth Blackwell, and then plunged into his most convincing evidence. At that moment, he reported, Sarah J. Smith was heading the Indiana Reformatory for Women and Girls which housed 184 "fallen, vicious, and criminal females," and Eudora Atkinson was directing the Massachusetts Reformatory Prison for Women (416 women and 45 children as inmates), and both had

received testimonials from all parts of the country hailing their rehabilitative work and administrative skill. Thus Corson tapped every responsive chord in his audience. Ill women needed understanding, they would respond with confidentiality, and their natural timidity would disappear in the face of the talented, "kind, consoling, sympathizing" women doctors who could alleviate, even possibly eliminate, their sufferings and the cause of their illnesses.[15]

Despite having the support of some hospital doctors, Corson was aware of the possibility that "great opposition" might arise from others. It was not long before his suspicions were verified. His report had passed the medical society and the House of Representatives at the state capital. To almost everyone's surprise, however, the Senate committee brought it out with a negative recommendation. The superintendents of hospitals had indeed been at work. Thomas Kirkbride, head of the Pennsylvania Hospital for the Insane for thirty-nine years, and original founder and "grand old man" of the American Psychiatric Association, had written to the governor, lieutenant governor, and members of the House and Senate and had circulated his own petition in the Philadelphia area (garnering sixty signatures of doctors and hospital administrators) in opposition to the proposed law. John Curwen, superintendent of the Harrisburg Hospital, who had earlier supported Corson in his struggle to gain recognition for women doctors, now viewed Corson as a troublemaker and ungentlemanly adversary. Even John Gray, the editor of the prestigious and powerful *American Journal of Insanity* and administrator of the Utica (New York) Hospital, denigrated Corson and his followers, calling Corson "malicious and blackhearted" for his criticism of the psychiatrists' resistance to women doctors as administrators of female wards.[16]

The opposition of the superintendents was not an across-the-board disagreement with the idea of women doctors on staffs, but an objection to the placing of women in offices of independent authority within the institutions, thus creating two separate positions of control. Corson had already illustrated that the male and female wards were run quite separately anyway and that a steward as business manager and a male doctor in charge of the medical care of men and a female one for women would be an even more efficient arrangement. Unsympathetic to psychiatrists' worries about divided authority and loss of power, Corson mounted a countercampaign in the Senate and succeeded in having his bill passed. The only drawback was that the wording had been changed and the law, instead of *requiring* the appointment of women physicians, merely suggested that state institutions "may" appoint a woman. Undeterred, the trustees of the state hospitals at Harrisburg and Norristown immediately established women doctors as the heads of their female departments. In the 1880s, a few other states besides Pennsylvania passed more limited legislation (requiring women as assistant physicians but not as autonomous heads of departments) and opened doors to women doctors.[17]

The women did not receive a wholehearted welcome. Initial reactions within the profession ranged from strong and friendly encouragement through mild surprise at the women doctors' competency to cool disregard and outright hostility. Some superintendents made clear that in hiring women doctors they were merely complying with the decisions of their boards—decisions with which they did not agree. (One of these superintendents, however, did express some satisfaction that the woman physician would relieve him from the burden of conducting the training school for attendants.) Other superintendents, at least in their official reports, simply ignored the first appointees, mentioning everyone on the staff by name except the woman physician. One of the more extreme reactions was that of John Chapin, who resigned the superintendency of the Willard Asylum in New York in 1884 just as its trustees appointed a woman, and took over the administration of the Insane Department of the Pennsylvania Hospital—where no woman physician was appointed until he retired in 1912![18]

Once ensconced in hospital positions, women faced the further obstacles of the ambiguous expectations others had both about their behavior and about their work within the institutions. Clearly, these were professional women and did not fit the Victorian mold of submissiveness and domesticity, yet they were expected to "keep their place." One superintendent remarked that he was satisfied with the way in which the "first incumbent" had performed her duties under the "requirement of the statute" because among her virtues, she exhibited

"feminine self-adjustment" and was always "in the right place at the right time." This practice she "maintained" as a "sensible habit," although, he warned, this was "by no means invariably the case in practice elsewhere." Let the woman who could not adjust to the demands and expectations of the male-dominated institutions beware.[19]

Devotion, fidelity, earnestness, and service were other preferred qualities, and not unlike the desirable characteristics expected in the male assistants. Crossing these lines, however, and asserting one's self, even for the sake of the patients, brought only personal discomfort and possible dismissal for a woman physician. For example, one of the Illinois Commissioners on Charities asked for the resignation of Harriet C. B. Alexander in 1885 when she complained about the quality of the institutional food at the Chicago State Hospital. The commissioner had asked the cook if the food was always good. Hearing the cook's affirmative answer, Alexander had "held up an iron-ringed, unwashed snout of a pig suffering from catarrh, and asked if that was a specimen of the good food." Apparently the superintendent was equally taken aback by Alexander's outspokenness, for he later described her as having a "bad moral influence on the discipline of the institution." Although he acknowledged that she was perhaps "conscientiously unselfish," that made her even more of a "danger" because she might become involved with "some association of determined advocates of feminine ascendancy." He was right: Harriet Alexander stayed at the hospital for only one year and then pursued a highly successful practice in Chicago, regularly publishing articles illustrating her ongoing concern with the care of mentally ill women, and becoming a strong supporter of and active worker for the Medical Women's National Association.[20]

Other women exhibited more perseverance on the institutional scene, but many of them eventually gave up and entered private practice or pursued their interests in psychiatry by establishing their own sanitaria. A woman like Margaret Cleaves, at the Harrisburg Hospital in Pennsylvania, seemed to be in an ideal position with full autonomy over the women's wards. One of the early women graduates of the medical school of Iowa State University (1873), Cleaves had been assistant physician at the Mt. Pleasant State Hospital in Iowa, a member of the board of trustees of that institution after she resigned her staff appointment, and was practicing in Davenport, Iowa, when the Harrisburg trustees recruited her for their new position. But Cleaves lasted only three years, 1880–83, at Harrisburg. Although her male counterpart believed that it was the "inalienable right of women" to do the work among insane women, it is clear that some resentment about the reorganization remained. Each of her annual reports made specific reference to this problem.[21]

Cleaves encountered other difficulties as well, some of her own making. She was too optimistic. She entered upon her duties with such "intense interest," "conviction," and "love for the work" that she promptly set out to establish a new program of treatment which in turn led her to radical speculation as to the causes of insanity in women. As her theories evolved, even in those three short years, she challenged a number of long-held beliefs. Using her annual reports as her forum, she questioned the relationship of utero-ovarian disease to insanity. At first, in 1881, she believed that such disease "may sustain the relation of cause to effect." But within a year, Cleaves felt that mental and physical improvement after local treatment was perhaps only coincidental and, after a "certain point," further gains were impossible, although patients could at least be made "more comfortable." This uncertainty about causal relationships loomed large in her last report. Acknowledging that in a very small proportion of cases diseased reproductive organs did act as a "causative influence," Cleaves quickly pointed out that the "undermining effect upon the general health" was the real culprit. Finally, she stated flatly that her experience convinced her that the percentage of recoveries would not increase as a result of "such special treatment." Women would remain insane, but they would do so in greater physical comfort.[22]

Her discussion of other issues also reflected her growing pessimism. Stressing heredity factors in the causality of insanity, Cleaves suggested that the formerly insane should "cease to assume the responsibilities of father or motherhood"; otherwise the "grand work of prevention" would never begin. Deciding that the circumscribed social roles of women contributed to their mental illness, Cleaves decried the "endless monotony of the lives of the majority of women," the "never ceasing routine of work," and the "too frequent child bearing." Thus

Cleaves weakened the rationale which underlay her appointment. Gynecological treatment she deemed ineffective in lessening the causality of mental illness in women; she raised the controversial issue of sterilization; and attacked the very warp and woof of the social fabric—the role of women. There was little she could do about the propensity of her patients to have too many children too close together, except lament the unhappy circumstances. Cleaves had other reasons for giving up as well and, in 1883, she left the asylum and returned to private practice concentrating on the treatment of neurasthenic women. Private practice would free her from institutional constraints and, at least with these women, of a different class from that of her patients at the state hospital, she might have some success in convincing them that their ways of "social dissipation" had led them into illness. They might listen and reform their way of living.[23]

Shortly after Cleaves resigned, the trustees changed the administrative structure of the institution "because of friction between the superintendent and the women physicians." Cleaves's successor, Jane Garver, no longer had control over personnel in the women's wards and had to report directly to the superintendent, as did the first assistant in the men's wards. Garver took the hint and her reports were short, without personal comment or innovative professional suggestions. Although she continued the gynecological work, she turned over much of the follow-up care to nurses and, after more than a decade of service, referred to the patients as a "stagnant mass of humanity" and made remarks about their "obstreperous character." When Garver died in 1902, the trustees under the guise of "greater efficiency" once more tightened up the administrative structure so that the formerly autonomous and theoretically powerful "woman physician" at Harrisburg became nothing more than a second or third assistant with at least two male doctors always outranking her in authority. The same two women doctors served until the 1920s, and their therapeutics slipped into regular sedation of patients and routine medical care without any gynecological specialization.[24]

Alice Bennett of the Norristown Hospital in Pennsylvania was of a different character. A woman of incredible energy, she had earned the tuition for her medical education at the Woman's Medical College of Pennsylvania by teaching school. Receiving her degree in the spring of 1876, she worked in a Philadelphia dispensary for the poor until her appointment as demonstrator of anatomy at her alma mater that fall. For the next four years she taught anatomy and other courses, maintained a private practice, and worked toward her Ph.D. degree at the University of Pennsylvania. In 1880, when the trustees of the Norristown Hospital were searching for their first woman doctor-administrator, Alice Bennett was one of the most likely candidates. Unlike Margaret Cleaves who had taken an original approach and ended up, through her own actions, questioning therapeutic procedures and social mores, Bennett almost immediately fitted into many of the male patterns of professional behavior and conformity. She took up all the causes of her male colleagues: expressing dissatisfaction with the classification of the causes of insanity, noting the effects of heredity, and complaining of overcrowded conditions.[25]

But because she was untouched by the pessimism of many of those who had labored in the field for years and inspired by the educational milieu of her medical training, Bennett brought a refreshing attitude to her task. She reinstituted and gave new life to the educational and occupational aspects of the traditional moral therapy regime. Not content with the idea that her responsibility ended when she discharged patients, she made regular follow-up contacts with them through visits and letters. She became worried also about the efficacy of drugs. Suggesting that work therapy was "not inferior to drugs" and urging that a "change *out* of the hospital" might be equally effective, she waged a campaign against unnecessary sedation.[26]

In keeping with the expectations of her role in the asylum, she carried on her gynecological work. Year after year, she increased the proportion of patients examined and treated for gynecological disorders, extending and systematizing the work until it became a "large and laborious part of the medical work of the department." As she proceeded, Bennett observed that since most of the conditions occurred as a result of childbirth, they were not diseases in and of themselves nor were they causal elements in insanity. Moving increasingly further from the thought of some of those who had supported the employment of women doctors in asylums, she searched for other explanations and ultimately decided that insanity itself

was not a true disease but simply a symptom of general ill health. Nevertheless, Bennett continued to relieve her patients' physical discomfort.[27]

For ten years, everything went smoothly. Then Bennett found herself under siege from the Pennsylvania press, the editors of the *American Journal of Insanity*, and the state Commissioners on Lunacy. Bennett allegedly set aside a special building in which to perform "illegal" ovariotomies on a large number of nonconsenting insane women with the misguided goal either, as her detractors claimed, of curing insanity or of moving up the "ladder of fame." Bennett did not perform the operations, however. Dr. Joseph Price and Dr. Marie B. Werner did them in the presence of at least six other doctors. The trustees, the superintendent, and Bennett as Female Physican had all concurred in the decision to carry out the gynecological surgery in the most severe cases. But only six operations were performed and in each case there were obvious pathological conditions. Furthermore, Bennett had obtained the permission of the nearest relatives.[28]

Many rallied to support Bennett. The editor of the *Philadelphia Press* praised Bennett's fine reputation and argued that the Lunacy Commission was interfering with the discretionary rights of a physician, and possibly depriving poor women of quality care. Dr. Price dismissed the charge that the operations were experimental and constituted "inhuman and brutal treatment," stating there was "no more unselfish and conscientious woman filling public place" than Alice Bennett. Despite this support, Bennett reacted with dismay at the ferocity of the attack, and withdrew from the public limelight. No longer did her annual reports contain references to gynecological work (although she continued it); instead she took up other, safer causes, such as the state's neglect of the chronic insane and the means of combating tuberculosis.[29]

Paradoxically, it was in this very same year that the American Psychiatric Association devoted a large part of its annual meeting to a discussion of the use of surgical methods in the treatment of insanity. George Rohé, superintendent of the Maryland Hospital for the Insane, led the discussion. Having polled 120 medical officers of asylums on the question of the relationship of the removal of ovaries and uterine appendages to insanity, he had difficulty tabulating the data because some doctors, he said, had performed the operations not only for mental conditions, but also for physical problems. Nevertheless, he himself had operated on fourteen women in the last ten months with some success and even delayed the discharge of four of his "cured" cases for the members to observe. His offer to perform an operation when they toured his institution met with a round of applause. Further discussion illustrated that the members generally approved of the removal of ovarian tumors for the mental welfare of the patient. Some disagreed, and Bennett later found herself the butt of those who not only opposed surgery but had also remained adamant against having women physicians in the asylums. When questions about the so-called experimental surgery arose again in an 1895 legislative investigation, Bennett finished out her last three-year contract at Norristown and in 1896 returned to her hometown.[30]

Many of the American Psychiatric Association members did remain opposed to women in the profession, especially if there was some question that these women doctors might rise to positions of authority. Already beleaguered by decades of attack for inflexibility, stiff competition from other professional groups, and rumblings of reform from within, some members were particularly sensitive about the possibility of further weakening their position by giving in to female incursions. The request from Margaret Cleaves merely to *attend* the 1881 meeting at Toronto had created such petty quibbling that Cleaves was not seated as a member although her male counterpart at Harrisburg, J. Z. Gerhard, was. The question was not brought up for another decade and a half and, by that time, the association had changed its name, its rules for membership, and most of the "old guard" had died.[31]

The passing of the founders and their protégés was crucial, for it had been they who, from the 1840s on, had determined the nature of the psychiatric profession, argued psychiatric theory, established therapeutic procedures, and wrested the control of the treatment of the mentally ill from the hands of the poorhouse steward and jail keeper. Although some dissent was tolerated, where the line was to be drawn was always uncertain. Alice Bennett, despite her attempts to remain within the boundaries of her male colleagues' expectations, crossed that line.[32]

Mechanical restraint (the use of physical means or contraptions to control patients) had long been a controversial question among the psychiatrists and the association never sanctioned total nonrestraint. Bennett did, however, justifying it in her reports, boasting annually that not a patient had been restrained, and even delivering a paper on the subject before the Medico-Legal Society of New York. For this she might have been forgiven, but she also joined the National Association for the Protection of the Insane and the Prevention of Insanity, which had the aims of scrutinizing more carefully and controlling the administration of state psychiatric institutions. Outraged by implications of incompetency, the American Psychiatric Association not only scorned, but denigrated, the new organization and helped to bring about its early demise. But Bennett (as well as Cleaves) had been one of the original members and had served on the editorial board of its journal. This was too much for many of her colleagues, and although she retained membership in the American Psychiatric Association, she never attended meetings. Indeed, few women attended and not one delivered a paper or took part in discussions. As the representative, at least in a symbolic way, of the entire profession of psychiatry, the association was on record in opposition to any significant role for women doctors.[33]

What of the other women who were in less powerful positions than either Cleaves or Bennett? By the nature of their appointments they did not run into the same kinds of difficulties and, in many ways, were little different from the male doctors in institutions who held similar subordinate positions. Like many young male doctors, the women frequently entered asylum service directly from medical school and stayed only a short time (an average of four years for both sexes). The asylum offered an opportunity to observe and treat a variety of physical and mental ailments—an experience that was not readily available elsewhere, especially for women. Economic security also played a part. The asylum provided room and board, plus a salary, and this was, at least initially, attractive to neophyte physicians. Upon leaving institutional service, many, both male and female, established practices in nearby areas—illustrating that another function of asylum service was the making of contacts or reputation in the interest of building up a future clientele. Although marriage while in service was out of the question (the bylaws of nearly every asylum required that assistant physicians remain single), social intercourse did not prove impossible. At least two dozen of these aspiring women doctors married men who were serving on the medical staffs at the same time they were.[34]

There were significant differences, however, in the professional treatment of women within the institutions. Regularly passed over for promotion, women must have felt the ramifications both in the lessening of personal and professional self-confidence and in their lower salaries. Many male assistants received superintendencies, and other men were hired as first or second assistants at salaries of $300–$700 more than the woman (as third or fourth assistant) who had served for a number of years. Some of this spilled over into quibbling about titles. One woman always designated herself as the "woman physician," while her superiors insisted on listing her as merely "second assistant physician." Some of it was immortalized in the bylaws of asylums. In most sets of regulations, among the duties of male assistants was that of taking over the administration of the hospital in the absence of the superintendent; women assistants could take over only his medical duties. Thus women tended to move from hospital to hospital more frequently than men, perhaps in search of recognition, and ultimately opted for private practices.[35]

In certain respects, women did not differ much from their male colleagues. For instance, both while at the asylums and later in private practice, their medical and psychiatric theories generally followed the same lines as those of their male contemporaries. Most had had neither the opportunity nor the authority to carry out experimental programs as Margaret Cleaves and Alice Bennett had done. When they did establish their private offices they clearly and purposely chose sites, especially in large cities, where male doctors had been successful. In Chicago, the majority of women doctors clustered in the "Loop" area and in Philadelphia most settled on Spruce, Pine, Walnut, Chestnut, and Broad Streets.[36]

Women doctors were not without their own resources, however. It seems clear that certain support systems were devised by the early practitioners and used by the younger women. One pattern which emerged was that of co-practice, that is, a

number of women doctors practicing at the same address. A closer look reveals that these women had either served in the same public institution (although not necessarily at the same time), that they had attended the same medical school, or that some were in the same graduating class as a woman who had served in an institution with one of the partners. The emotional and psychological support that this system offered is obvious, but the practice also resulted in women doctors being clustered in large cities and in particular neighborhoods—restricting themselves geographically as well as by their tendency to treat only women and children.[37]

It had taken most women only a few years to realize the intellectual and professional constrictions of institutional service. Although some, like Bertha Van Hoosen, reacted as if the whole experience had been somewhat of a lark, remarking that in a year and a half she "never made a note" on any patient; others could attribute their "tale of woe" to the blows received "at the hands of insane patients." Most, it appears, had assessed their possible professional future in the asylums and had moved on.[38]

Whether primarily motivated to alleviate the sufferings of insane women or using their institutional positions for other reasons, there is no doubt these would-be psychiatrists and women physicians faced multifarious forms of sexism. Not unlike other women entering the professions, these doctors strove to overcome barriers which emerged from deep-seated feelings about traditional sex roles and societal judgments about the intellectual and emotional limitations of women who pursued professional careers. As they circumvented each barrier, new ones appeared. By the end of the century, medical education was available, many medical societies had dropped their exclusive male membership policies, and general hospitals accepted some female interns. But individual and organizational reservations had not completely disappeared, particularly in the psychiatric profession. Thus as some of the more perceptive and innovative women proceeded they faced a dilemma of such proportions that they withdrew from institutional service rather than continue to confront the almost unabated professional hostility toward them and their work.[39]

There had originally been utopian expectations of these women. The very idea of requiring women physicians in public institutions had been promoted on the grounds that they would be the saviors of the female insane. This specialized treatment would result in lower death rates, it would eliminate all sexual delusions, and causes of insanity peculiar to women would disappear. Yet they could not singlehandedly do away with sexual delusions. They might only relieve the stress these delusions engendered among the male medical staff. They could, and did, deal effectively with some gynecological problems, but they could not eliminate them as a cause of insanity. When they attempted to, they were caught up in intraprofessional disputes about the use of surgery and, if they questioned whether reproductive organs, either diseased or healthy, actually did cause insanity, they were reprimanded professionally for undermining long-held, and cherished, beliefs.

Questions, however, remain both about these women doctors and about the nearly two hundred others who served in similar positions in other institutions in the first decades of the twentieth century. Given the paucity of internships and residencies for women, did they use these appointments as virtually their only opportunity and then perceiving the limitations, move on? Or were many of them opting for a less rigorous speciality: one which offered more regular hours? Unlike surgery, or even general medicine, a private practice in psychiatry allowed for accommodation with marriage and family life. But, at the same time, did this choice unintentionally fulfill the popular assumptions about the innate limitations of women in the professions?

What of those who stayed? Did they work out viable strategies for avoiding conflict and thereby win the confidence of their male critics and still manage to demonstrate their competency? It would seem that in many cases they did, but not without sacrifice. Pockets of sexism, not unlike that experienced by Harriet C. B. Alexander, remained. In the 1880s, Alexander's performance had illustrated the "desirability of female physicians" to one of her male superiors, but she appeared insubordinate and a "bad moral influence" to another. In the early twentieth century, administrators still referred to the "weaker side of woman's nature" as a handicap or remarked that women worked out well only when they were the "right kind of women." After 1900, the tenure of many of the women as-

sistant physicians was longer than that of their predecessors. This may be explained partially by their adjustment to the realities of institutional constrictions. They were, of course, not in positions to initiate or direct new programs of treatment and thus they were not so likely to come in conflict with traditional ideas about bureaucratic authority, psychiatric therapy, or feminine behavior and roles. The adaptation necessary for becoming the "right kind" of woman may have eased the living and working conditions of these women, but not without checking opportunity for meaningful and innovative contributions on their part.[40]

The inability to maintain and submit to discipline, a lack of executive skill, and the absence of ambition in women were other frequent complaints. One superintendent criticized women doctors because "their likes and dislikes were too pronounced" and, furthermore, their "jealous nature" frequently surfaced. Another thought that they required "more waiting on" than men, and that patients did not "consider them as real doctors." There was little realization that if women doctors were kept in subordinate positions, given no chance to exercise authority or experiment, and looked upon by their superintendents as inferior and troublesome, then the women themselves might react in such a way as to fulfill the dire prophecies about their innate unworthiness and incompetency. The lack of executive talent was a moot question. Few of these women were in situations which allowed them to exercise any authority or exhibit managerial ability. Of the approximately 270 state, county, city, corporate, and private psychiatric hospitals founded by 1914, only one-third employed women as assistant physicians. Besides the woman at Norristown, only one other headed a county hospital; three women ran their own private sanitaria.[41]

If women appeared less ambitious than men it was simply because they had little by way of reinforcement to preserve their zeal. Except in institutions like the Government Hospital for the Insane in Washington, D.C., the Kankakee (Illinois) Hospital, and the Worcester (Massachusetts) Asylum, all of which were headed by sympathetic and supportive male superintendents, there was little room for women to participate in progressive scientific work or to advance in administrative hierarchies. The Norristown Hospital was the only state hospital which left untouched the autonomous position of the "Female Physician." It took a rare soul indeed who could maintain her ambitions in the face of nonexistent opportunity. Thus the failure of an appreciable number of states to require the appointment of women, the continued resistance on the part of many institutional psychiatrists, and the plethora of dead-end positions had limited the success of women doctors in psychiatric institutions and nearly precluded them from carving out a new area of endeavor. Moreover, these trends may well have lessened the desire of others to enter the profession.[42]

It appears that, like so many other women's crusades, many of these women doctors in psychiatric institutions fell prey to the very forces which promoted their cause. In many ways the good they supposedly were to accomplish was to rise from their very femininity, from the nature of their sex, not from their professional acuity. Thus they were faced with fitting the Victorian mold of submission and quiet dedication to prescribed duties or, if innovative and truly professional, they provoked the ire of their colleagues and society in general and were labeled as "dangers" and failures, in an unfeminine manner, at adjusting to "place and time." In other words, they were "unsexed." If they were to accomplish professional miracles yet remain "ideal" women, in the eyes of Victorian society and the psychiatric profession (and, perhaps, in their own), they failed.

NOTES

Research for this paper was funded in part by a grant from the Penrose Fund of the American Philosophical Society and by a grant from the University of Arizona Foundation.

1 Lilian Welsh, *Reminiscences of Thirty Years in Baltimore* (Baltimore: Norman Remington, 1925), 44–45.

2 The virtues of the Victorian "ideal woman" have been described in the now classic article by Barbara Welter, "The cult of true womanhood," *American Quarterly*, 1966, *18:* 151–74. Although scholars have lately pointed out that much of Welter's evidence is prescriptive and normative (see especially Carl Degler, "What ought to be and what was: women's sexuality in the nineteenth century," in this volume), other scholars have applied Welter's description in their studies. For the quotation on "ruining a good mother," see T. S. Clouston, "Female education from a medical point of view," *Popular Science Monthly*, 1884, *24:* 322–33. For a discussion of the virtues of the "new woman," see John S. Haller and Robin M. Haller, *The Physician and Sexuality in Victorian America* (Champaign: University of Illinois Press, 1974), 39–40 and 77–78.

3 The most recent and definitive study of the difficulties experienced by women in their search for a medical education and the barriers raised by the profession itself is Mary Roth Walsh, *"Doctors Wanted: No Women Need Apply": Sexual Barriers in the Medical Profession, 1835–1975* (New Haven: Yale University Press, 1977). Other standard sources are Mary Putnam Jacobi's chapter, "Woman in medicine," in Annie Nathan Meyer, *Woman's Work in America* (New York: Henry Holt, 1891); Thomas Woody, *A History of Women's Education in the United States* (New York:

Science Press, 1929), especially vol. 2; and the voluminous testimony of the women themselves.

4 I have taken the illustrations of difficulties faced by women doctors from the autobiographies of both Welsh, *Reminiscences*, 43–46, and Bertha Van Hoosen, *Petticoat Surgeon* (Chicago: Pellegrini & Cudahy, 1947), 59; since both of them served as women physicians in psychiatric institutions early in their careers. Thus their accounts, besides being fairly typical, seem particularly apropos.

5 Van Hoosen, *Petticoat Surgeon*, 52 and 57–58. Also see the account of Van Hoosen in "Opportunities for medical women interns," *Medical Woman's Journal*, 1926, *33:* 282 for the "raid" on Mary Bates.

6 For instance the seven male doctors at the Kalamazoo State Hospital convinced Van Hoosen that it was her duty to extract the teeth of the patients. She went on for weeks before learning of the joke. As newly appointed professor of clinical gynecology at the Chicago College of Physicians and Surgeons, Van Hoosen also had her first lecture boycotted. See Van Hoosen, *Petticoat Surgeon*, 83, 140–43, and 127–28.

7 Welsh, *Reminiscences*, 5 and 50.

8 For a discussion of the problems facing women who entered the profession, see Barbara J. Harris, *Beyond Her Sphere: Women and the Professions in American History* (Westport, Conn.: Greenwood Press, 1978).

9 For background on the way in which this crusade, and the waning of it, applied to the psychiatric profession, see Gerald Grob, *The State and the Mentally Ill* (Chapel Hill: University of North Carolina Press, 1966) and *Mental Institutions in America* (New

York: Free Press, 1973), and David Rothman, *The Discovery of the Asylum* (Boston: Little, Brown, 1971).

10 *Sixteenth Annual Report of the Trustees of the Willard Asylum for the Insane* (Buffalo: Baker, Jones, 1885), 6. See arguments about modesty in Virginia Penny, *The Employments of Women* (Boston: Walker, Wise, 1863), 24–26; G. C. Paoli and James G. Kiernan, "Female physicians in insane hospitals," *Alienist and Neurologist* 8(Jan. 1887): 21–29; Edward N. Brush, "On the employment of women physicians in hospitals for the insane," *American Journal of Insanity* 47(Jan. 1891): 323–30; *Eighth Annual Report of the Committee on Lunacy of the Board of Public Charities of Pennsylvania* (Harrisburg: Edwin K. Meyers, 1890), 30–31; and Mary Putnam Jacobi's letter to the editor, *Medical Record*, May 10, 1890, 543–44.

11 See especially, W. B. Goldsmith, "A case of moral insanity," *American Journal of Insanity* 40(Oct. 1883): 162–77 (quotation on 171) and the discussion of this article in the "Proceedings of the thirty-ninth annual meeting of the Association of Medical Superintendents of American Institutions for the Insane," *American Journal of Insanity*, 40(Jan. 1884): 280–85; E. D. Bondurant, "Two cases of oophorectomy for insanity," *American Journal of Insanity*, 42 (Jan. 1886): 324–45, (quotations on 343 and 344); S. G. Webber, "Cases of hysteria treated by hypnotism," *Journal of Nervous and Mental Disease*, September 1890, 585–96; Allan McLane Hamilton, "The abuse of oophorectomy in diseases of the nervous system," *New York Medical Journal*, 1893, *57:* 180–85; and Paoli and Kiernan, "Female physicians," 21–22. See physician's remarks on cases in the 1882–1884 case book for the women's wards at Harrisburg State Hospital, Harrisburg, Pennsylvania (hereinafter referred to as the HSH Case Book). Refer also to John Duffy, "Masturbation and clitoridectomy," *Journal of the American Medical Association* 186 (Oct. 19, 1963): 246–48 and Charles Rosenberg, "Sexuality, Class, and Role," in *No Other Gods* (Baltimore: Johns Hopkins University Press, 1976).

12 Scores of articles appeared in a variety of professional journals in the late Victorian era which assumed this connection. See especially, W. H. Baker, "Removal of the uterine appendages for nervous disease," *Boston Medical and Surgical Journal*, March 7, 1895, 224–28; Bondurant, "Two cases of oophorectomy," 342–45; Carlos C. Booth, "Report of a few cases of laparotomy: melancholia successfully treated by the removal of the ovaries," *Cleveland Medical Gazette*, 1896, 209–11; and Joseph Meyer, "A case of insanity, caused by diseased ovaries, cured by their removal," American Association of Obstetricians and Gynecologists, *Transactions*, 1895, 503–

4. Also see Robert Battey, "Normal ovariotomy," *Atlanta Medical and Surgical Journal*, September 1872. Ben (G. J.) Barker-Benfield, in "The spermatic economy: a nineteenth-century view of sexuality," *Feminist Studies*, 1972, *1:* 45–74 and in *The Horrors of the Half-Known Life* (New York: Harper and Row, 1976), argues that "castration" of women by surgeons and gynecologists was widespread both over time and and in numbers. Hard evidence is lacking, however, and, within a very short time, the medical profession itself cried out against the abuse. Battey himself gave warning. For a more balanced view see Regina Morantz, "The lady and her physician," in *Clio's Consciousness Raised*, ed. Mary S. Hartman and Lois Banner (New York: Harper and Row, 1974), 38–53. See also Lawrence D. Longo, "The rise and fall of Battey's operation: a fashion in surgery," in this volume.

13 See biographical file of Mary Henderson Stinson at the Florence A. Moore Library, Medical College of Pennsylvania (formerly known as the Woman's Medical College of Pennsylvania and hereinafter referred to WMCP), Philadelphia, Pennsylvania. Stinson was the woman doctor Bemis hired. See also Mary M. Wolfe, "The present status of women physicians in hospitals for the insane," *Proceedings of the American Medico-Psychological Association at the Sixty-Fifth Annual Meeting*, 1909, 350 and 354–56; Eveline P. Ballintine, "Women physicians in public institutions," *Woman's Medical Journal*, April 1908, 79; and "The employment of women physicians in state hospitals," *Woman's Medical Journal*, May 1912, 116–17.

14 See the report of the committee on the "propriety of having a female physician for the female department of every hospital for the insane, which is under the control of the State" in Hiram Corson, *A Brief History of Proceedings in the Medical Society of Pennsylvania to Procure the Recognition of Women Physicians by the Medical Profession of the State* (Norristown, Pa.: Herald Printing, 1894), 27–36, for Corson's wide-ranging arguments.

15 Corson, *A Brief History*, 29–35.

16 Corson, *A Brief History*, 25 and 41–43. Thomas S. Kirkbride to Gov. Hugh (n.d.); to Lieut. Gov. Stone (n.d.); to the Senate and House of Representatives of the Commonwealth of Pennsylvania (n.d.); John Curwen to Thomas S. Kirkbride, May 12, 1881; and John P. Gray to Thomas S. Kirkbride, March 11, 1881, Thomas S. Kirkbride MSS, Pennsylvania Hospital, Philadelphia. John Curwen's votes on the issue of the Pennsylvania State Medical Society's recognition of women in medicine are cited in Corson, 14, 21, and 23.

17 Letters of Thomas S. Kirkbride cited above; Cor-

son, *A Brief History*, 40–41; Minutes of the Board of Trustees, Harrisburg State Hospital, Harrisburg, Pennsylvania (hereinafter referred to as HSH Trustee Minutes), July 10, 1879; and "By-Laws" in *The Hospital for the Insane for the South Eastern District of Pennsylvania: Acts of Assembly, By-Laws, and Rules and Regulations Governing It* (Philadelphia: Reen & Trump, 1880), 7.

18 See *Forty-Eighth Annual Report of the Managers of the Utica State Hospital at Utica* (Albany: James B. Lyon, State Printer, 1890), 56; *Friends' Asylum for the Insane, Reports, 1895* (Philadelphia: William K. Bellows, 1895), 6 and 26–27; *Fifty-Third Annual Report of the Trustees of the Worcester Lunatic Hospital* (Boston: Wright & Potter, 1886), 8 and 18; this is a clear pattern if one follows the career line of John B. Chapin, especially since Chapin was the superintendent who ignored the woman physician in his annual report.

19 *Forty-Ninth Annual Report of the Managers of the Utica State Hospital at Utica* (Albany: James B. Lyon, State Printer, 1892), 29.

20 These qualities are gleaned from the phrases used to describe both the male and female assistants in numerous reports of superintendents throughout the last three decades of the nineteenth century. Alexander's experience is cited in Paoli and Kiernan, "Female physicians," 26 and 28–29. See also Harriet C. B. Alexander, "Paranoia in the female," *Alienist and Neurologist* 8 (July 1887): 360–65.

21 Cleaves's career line is evident from the information in Polk's *Medical and Surgical Registers* (Detroit: R. L. Polk, 1890, 1898, and 1900); Henry M. Hurd, *The Institutional Care of the Insane in the United States and Canada*, 4 vols. (Baltimore: Johns Hopkins Press, 1916), 3: 434; *Biennial Reports of the Trustees, Superintendents, and Treasurers of the Iowa State Hospital for the Insane at Mt. Pleasant* (Des Moines: R. P. Clarkson, 1874–1880); and HSH Trustees Minutes, July 8, 1880 and August 5, 1880. See also "Report of physician-female department" in the 31st, 32d, and 33d annual reports of the Harrisburg Hospital.

22 "Report of physician-female department" in the 31st, 32d, and 33d annual reports of the Harrisburg Hospital.

23 See Cleaves's annual reports, 1880–1883, and HSH Case Book, 1882–1884. Two-thirds of Cleaves's patients were married (or widowed), and for the fifty on whom she recorded usable data, they averaged a childbirth every 2.1 years (and if miscarriages are included, a pregnancy every 1.9 years). The average number of children born was 6.42, and this statistic obscures even more trying individual cases like the woman who bore twelve children in twenty years or one who in seven years gave birth to three in-

fants, suffered three miscarriages, and the death of one of her children. See *Autobiography of a Neurasthene: As Told By One of Them and Recorded by Margaret A. Cleaves, M.D.* (Boston: Richard G. Badger, Gorham Press, 1910) for other reasons for Cleaves's resignation. The internal evidence makes it clear that this is the autobiography of Cleaves herself. Her long battle with neurasthenia and her frequent remarks about "blows received upon my head at the hands of insane patients" (63 and 84) indicate that the roots of her problem were existent before her actual attack. See also Cleaves's articles: "Neurasthenia and its relation to diseases of woman," *Proceedings of the Thirty-Fourth Annual Session of the Iowa State Medical Society*, May 19–21, 1886, 164–79; in the "Asylum notes" section, "Can the gynaecologist aid the alienist in institutions for the insane," *Journal of Nervous and Mental Disease*, July 1891, 472–75; and the report of her work in the "Abstracts and extracts" section of the *American Journal of Insanity*, July 1888, 163–64.

24 Hurd, *The Institutional Care of the Insane*, 3: 434–35; HSH Trustee Minutes, August 30, 1883; "Report of the physician-female department" in *Forty-Fifth Annual Report . . . Harrisburg*, 15, and *Forty-Seventh Annual Report . . . Harrisburg*, 16; HSH Trustee Minutes, October 16, 1902 (in which for the first time there is no report by a female physician; nor is there again); and HSH Case Book, 1904–1918.

25 For Bennett's early career, see Minutes of the Faculty, January 13, January 27, 1877, January 12, February 7, 1878, January 1, 1879, January 11, January 30, and July 3, 1880; Board of Corporators Minutes, September 30, 1879; and Treasurer's Report, April 27, 1879, to February 29, 1880, WMCP. Also consult biographical material in the file of Alice Bennett, Alumnae Files, WMCP, the *Philadelphia Ledger*, May 5, 1896, and biographical sketch by Stanley I. Kutler in *Notable American Women*, ed. Edward T. James (Cambridge: Belknap Press of Harvard University Press, 1971). For Bennett's years at the Norristown Hospital, see the "Department of Women-Report of the Resident Physician," first through seventeenth (1880–1896) *Annual Reports of the State Hospital for the South-Eastern District of Pennsylvania at Norristown, Pa.* (Allentown: Allen W. Haines, 1880–1896).

26 For Bennett's remarks on the follow-up of patients, see especially her 1881 annual report, and for her concern about drugs, see her 1882–1894 reports.

27 See especially Bennett's 1882, 1883, and 1884 reports on gynecological treatment.

28 See the *Philadelphia Press* of January 9, 1893; Thomas G. Morton, "Removal of the ovaries as a cure for insanity," *American Journal of Insanity* 49 (Jan. 1893):

397–401; the "Notes and comment" section, 497–99 and the "Correspondence" section, 512–15 of the same journal. Morton, and the editor of the journal (John P. Gray), were responding to an "extract in advance" from the *Tenth Annual Report of the Committee on Lunacy of the Board of Public Charities of Pennsylvania, 1892,* which supposedly stated that "several patients have already had their ovaries extirpated." After an inquiry by the board of trustees at Norristown and their wholehearted backing of Bennett, that section of the reports was withdrawn and never appeared in print. See Bennett's reports, 1893–1896; "Correspondence" section of the 1893 issue of the *American Journal of Insanity,* January 1893, 514–15; and "In the matter of certain charges against the management of the State Hospital for the Insane for the South-Eastern District of Pennsylvania," *Proceedings before the Legislative Committee* (Norristown: Hospital Press, 1895). It is fairly clear from the published transcript of the hearings that Dr. Marie Werner had brought a complaint against Bennett because Bennett refused to allow Werner to continue "experimental surgery." Werner perceived it as experimental and Bennett, worried about that aspect of it, discontinued the service of Werner although she allowed four operations by Price later.

29   See the *Philadelphia Press,* January 10 and 12, 1893. See the fourteenth through seventeenth (1893–1896) *Annual Reports.* Bennett does not mention gynecological work and her last reports are merely perfunctory.

30   See "Proceedings of the forty-eighth annual meeting of the Association of Medical Superintendents of American Institutions for the Insane," *American Journal of Insanity* 49 (July 1892): 216–306. Among the doctors who both opposed the use of surgery and the presence of women physicians in the institutions were the lukewarm superintendent of the Utica (New York) Asylum, G. Alder Blumer, and none other than John Chapin, who had moved from the Willard (New York) Asylum to the Pennsylvania Hospital in order to avoid appointing women. See "Correspondence" section of the January 1893 issue of the *American Journal of Insanity* and "Proceedings of the forty-eighth annual meeting."

31   For evidence of the precarious position of the psychiatric professional organization in the last half of the nineteenth century see Hurd, *The Institutional Care of the Insane,* especially vol. 1; Albert Deutsch, *The Mentally Ill in America* (New York: Columbia University Press, 1949); John Burnham, "Psychiatry, psychology and the Progressive movement," *American Quarterly,* 1960, *12:* 457–65; Grob, *The State and the Mentally Ill;* and Charles Rosenberg, "The crisis in psychiatric legitimacy: reflections on psy-

chiatry, medicine, and public policy," in *American Psychiatry: Past, Present, and Future,* ed. George Kriegman et al.(Charlottesville: University Press of Virginia, 1975). See "Proceedings of the thirty-seventh annual meeting of the Association of Medical Superintendents of American Institutions for the Insane," *American Journal of Insanity* 38 (Oct. 1881): 174–77.

32   That the psychiatrists themselves recognized the power of their organization is clear in John Curwen's account, *History of the Association of Medical Superintendents of American Institutions For the Insane* (Harrisburg: Theo. F. Scheffer, 1875) and in those of later historians. See Deutsch, *The Mentally Ill in America;* Hurd, *The Institutional Care of the Insane,* vol. 1; Grob, *Mental Institutions.*

33   See Alice Bennett, "Mechanical restraint in the treatment of the insane," *Medico-Legal Journal of New York,* 1884, *1:* 285–96. A possible added area of sensitivity in Bennett's case may be that she had also served on the Philadelphia committee to raise the $100,000 donation for Johns Hopkins to assure that the university would accept female medical students in their newly opened medical department. See Welsh, *Reminiscences,* 32–36. See the remarks on the history of the National Association for the Protection of the Insane and the Prevention of Insanity, in Deutsch, *The Mentally Ill in America,* 311–14, and in J. K. Hall, ed., *One Hundred Years of American Psychiatry, 1884–1944* (Columbia University Press, 1944), 351: the seven issues of the *American Psychological Journal* (Oskar Diethelm Library, New York Hospital); and such articles as Orpheus Everts, "The American system of public provision for the insane, and despotism in lunatic asylums," *American Journal of Insanity* 31 (Oct. 1881): 113–39; and "Rights of the insane," *American Journal of Insanity* 33 (Apr. 1883): 411–32. After 1885 (when women were allowed to attend because membership rules were changed to include assistant physicians) until the turn of the century only nine women made an appearance. Only one came back a second time.

34   The average tenure of both male and female assistant physicians is derived from the listings in Hurd, *The Institutional Care of the Insane,* vols. 2 and 3. The places where assistants set up private practice are sometimes listed in Hurd, vols. 2 and 3, in the narratives of each hospital. Others are traced through the various editions of *Polk's Medical and Surgical Registers* (Detroit: R. L. Polk, 1886, 1890, 1898, and 1900) (Title varies). Marital information is derived from tracing the women doctors in Hurd, vols. 2 and 3. Since many of these married women retained both their maiden and married names, they are fairly easy to trace, especially in the cases where

a future husband served in the same institution during the same time period. Some were traced back from the listings in the *Census of Women Physicians, November 11, 1918,* published by the American Women's Hospitals under the auspices of the Council of National Defense.

35 This was evident, for instance, at the Medfield (Massachusetts) Insane Asylum where the female assistant physician was regularly passed over for promotion for the first nine years. Even newly hired male assistants were listed ahead of the woman, and some men were promoted from third assistant to first with the resultant increase of salary from $800 to $1,500. The Medfield practices were not unique. See first through tenth *Annual Reports of the Medfield Insane Asylum at Medfield, Massachusetts* (Boston: Wright & Potter, 1896–1905). See particularly the experience over titles of Laura Hulme in the *Sixth Annual Report of the State Asylum for the Chronic Insane of Pennsylvania* (Lebanon, Pa.: Report Publishing, 1895), and for administrative duties, see the *Reports of the Trustees, Officers and the Visiting Committee of the Maine Insane Hospital* (Augusta: Burleigh & Flint, 1888), 11 and 12.

36 Addresses of practices were derived from the 1886, 1890, 1898, and 1900 editions of *Polk's Medical and Surgical Register* and from the 1918 *Census of Women Physicians.*

37 Information on service in psychiatric institutions is found in Hurd, *The Institutional Care of the Insane,* vols. 2 and 3, and that on medical school attendance from the 1918 *Census of Women Physicians* and *Polk's Medical and Surgical Registers.*

38 Van Hoosen, *Petticoat Surgeon,* 87, and Cleaves, *Autobiography of a Neurasthene,* 63 and 84.

39 For further discussion of the twofold type of barriers professional women faced in the Victorian era and the overcoming of barriers followed by the raising of new ones, see the essay of Richard Shryock, "Women in American medicine," in *Medicine in America* (Baltimore: Johns Hopkins Press, 1966), and Harris, *Beyond Her Sphere.* For other obstacles, see Frank Stricker, "Cookbooks and law books: the hidden history of career women in twentieth century America," *Journal of Social History,* 1976, *10:* 1–19.

40 Paoli and Kiernan, "Female physicians," 26 and 28–29. In the same article Paoli and Kiernan discussed Alexander and came to opposite conclusions about her work and effect on the institution. See also, Wolfe, "Present status," 352.

41 Wolfe, "Present status," 352 and 355–56 for complaints about women physicians, and Hurd, *Institutional Care,* vols. 2 and 3, for the assessment of the numbers of institutions by 1914 and for those which employed women doctors in any capacity.

42 Jacobi, "Female physicians for insane women," 543–44; "The reason why," *Woman's Medical Journal,* April 1896, 100; Ballintine, "Women physicians in public institutions," 79–80; Wolfe, "Present status," 352; "The employment of women physicians in State Hospitals," 116–17; and Bertha Van Hoosen, "Annual report of Committee on Medical Opportunities for Women," *Medical Woman's Journal,* August 1929, 216–17.

NURSES

Following the model established by Florence Nightingale in England, professional nursing began in this country after the middle of the nineteenth century. Before that time women, and some men too, often as patients, had provided haphazard nursing services in the few hospitals that existed. Women traditionally had also provided nursing care to their families and friends within their homes. With the new training schools for nurses and the development of organized service, however, an identifiable occupation group first emerged.

Many of the newly trained nurses found work in private homes, where they replaced family members as caretakers of the sick. Susan Reverby examines the anomalous position of these new professionals in private duty nursing, and she analyzes the tensions in their lives within the social and medical context of family health care. Nancy Tomes describes the atmosphere of one nurses' training school and explores the socioeconomic background of the new nurses. She posits that women entered nursing with educational and family experiences similar to those of contemporaries entering medical school and questions whether improving the quality of nursing education at the end of the nineteenth century might have lured women who wanted careers in the health care fields away from medicine.

Barbara Melosh writes about the hospital-based nursing experiences of the twentieth century. With the issue of autonomy as her primary analyzing focus, Melosh compares the hospital work environment with the home base of earlier private duty nursing and suggests that the divisions of labor within the hospital provided some new opportunities for nursing even within the stringent medical hierarchy. Melosh's interpretation of twentieth-century nursing leads her to the controversial conclusion that because of nursing's subordination to medicine, and, even more important, because of the sexual division between nursing and medicine, nursing should not be described as a profession. According to Melosh, nurses do not have the autonomy professionalization requires.

Darlene Clark Hine relates the struggles of Mabel K. Staupers to integrate black nurses into the armed forces during the Second World War and reminds us that race and sex produced problems of seemingly insurmountable proportions. Hine's example illustrates how much we can learn about women's positions within any of the health occupations when we add the dimensions of class and race to gender analysis.

32

"Neither for the Drawing Room nor for the Kitchen": Private Duty Nursing in Boston, 1873–1920

SUSAN REVERBY

"Neither for the drawing room nor for the kitchen" was how nursing leader Isabel Hampton Robb succinctly captured the ambiguous position of the private duty trained nurse working in a patient's home in 1900.[1] While this nurse's social standing in a household was uncertain, her particular position in the health care system was becoming clearer. At the turn of the century most Americans when ill, even seriously, took to bed at home, not in a hospital. If it appeared necessary and/or could be afforded, at the bedside stood a hired nurse. The omnipresent, harried staff nurse employed by a hospital is a figure whose vintage dates only from the World War II years. Until then, the majority of nurses we would now refer to as registered nurses worked in private duty as the employees of patients; and until the mid-1920s, most of them did this work in patients' homes.[2] This article explores the conditions and practices of this historically critical form of care giving and women's work.

To uncover the private duty world, this essay draws upon nurses' written memoirs, letters, and texts, journal articles, reports of nursing meetings, census data, and a sample of 539 nurses taken from the records of the 4,550 nurses who registered for private duty work at the Boston Medical Library (BML) Directory for Nurses, the first major registry for nurses in this country. By the last quarter of the nineteenth century, directories or registries, run by hospitals, medical and nursing societies, or private businesses, were organized to keep lists of available nurses and to match them, for a fee, to the needs of inquiring physicians or patients. Between 1880 and 1914, the BML Directory pro-

SUSAN REVERBY is Director and Assistant Professor of Women's Studies at Wellesley College, Wellesley, Massachusetts.

vided work for the majority of Boston's private duty nurses.[3]

The ubiquitous female ministering to the needs of the sick was not always a relative or an altruistic neighbor; women who were paid to nurse made their appearance in the colonies in the seventeenth century. Such "nurses" gained their label through self-proclamation coupled to some kind of experience of caring for the ill in their own families, domestic service, or hospital work.[4] In 1873, the first nursing schools were linked to hospitals and created to train women to nurse. By 1900, neither titles nor job functions clearly differentiated the "old-style" nurses from the new graduates. The label "nurse" was applied to a graduate of a two- or three-year training school, a nursing school dropout, an experienced worker with no formal education, a person who had taken a few lessons at the YWCA, or an attendant who had worked in a hospital. Lack of uniformity characterized even those who received "training" as the education was frequently haphazard and unstandardized. A nursing leader lamented in 1893 that the title "'trained nurse' may mean then anything, everything, or next to nothing."[5] The nursing associations struggled to have licensing laws enacted to differentiate the trained or graduate nurse, as she was labeled, from her many untrained competitors. But even the strongest of these generally weak registration laws could not limit which "nurses" sought work in the private duty market.

Sheer numbers were part of the problem. There were fewer than 500 graduate nurses in the United States in 1890. The numbers rose 634 percent by 1900; another 136 percent between 1900 and 1910. In Boston, the total number of nurses, both trained and nontrained, rose nearly 400 percent between

1880 and 1905.[6] By the turn of the century, the supply of nurses began to outpace the demand for their services, particularly in the urban centers. The overcrowding in nursing was a function of the limited fields of employment open to the increasing numbers of women seeking work, exacerbated by the deliberate policies of the hospital training schools.

Many hospitals, once the idea of training women to nurse was institutionalized, began to staff their wards almost entirely with nursing students and untrained nursing workers. Control over nursing education, and who was admitted to the training, was often the subject of pitched battles between nursing superintendents and hospital administrators, trustees and physicians. Under pressure from the hospitals to staff the wards as well as educate the students, nursing superintendents frequently sacrificed educational goals to the necessity of getting the work done. In many schools a two-track system developed. A few students were encouraged upon graduation to become head nurses or nursing superintendents in the hospitals while the majority were shunted into the increasingly crowded and undifferentiated private duty field.[7]

Private duty work quickly took on a peculiar, ambiguous status in the nursing and medical world. A medical student completing his training went into private *practice;* the nursing student, however, went into private *duty.* The physician was expected to apply his skills in independent action. The nurse, even without the control of the hospital and medical hierarchy, was still supposed to be submissive to higher authority and morally obligated to her work. In private duty, a nurse was working for a *doctor's* patients. Although employed by a family, she was primarily dependent on the physician to define what she did and to help her get work.

While devoted care to one private patient would seem to be the ultimate expression of a nurse's skill, the nursing superintendents expressed grave concern about the dangers of private duty and feared their students would find the work "exhausting." The exhaustion that worried them was both physical and spiritual, a loss of sheer strength and moral fiber. It was frequently assumed that a nurse could last only ten years in private duty, her collapse owing as much to the danger of "moral laxity" as to the physical labor.[8] Warnings were is-

sued about the danger of nursing single men in hotels (no respectable woman should) or the tempting advances of a patient's unscrupulous husband (to be spurned at all cost), along with admonitions to get enough rest. These warnings reflected less a fear of the vanquishing of the nurse's physical virginity than of her loss of spiritual virginity—the collapse of her moral purity, her gentleness, humanity, sympathy and tact because of the long hours and strain inherent in the work.

In private duty a nurse provided an array of services from the purely domestic to skilled nursing care. As might any domestic servant, mother, or wife, she often had to be an entertaining companion, an imaginative cook, and a competent laundress. She also had to monitor vital signs; insert catheters; prep and assist at operations and deliveries; provide cold packs, baths, and massages; even carry and decide when to give such medications as morphine. Alone with a patient, twenty-four hours a day, often weeks at a time, she crossed the ambiguous line between nursing and medical care with regularity, if trepidation. Freed from the hierarchy and controls of the hospital setting, she could practice her best skills with relative autonomy, or make terrible mistakes without supervision.[9]

The stress on the graduate nurse in private duty was due to the pressure to prove the role of the trained nurse; the ambiguity of her place in the household structure; the difficulty of the work; and the overcrowding in the field. In the 1880s and 1890s, the trained nurse was still a new creation whose necessity had to be proven to both physicians and families. Although much of what she did seemingly could be done and was done by nontrained nurses, domestic servants, or female relatives, she was somehow through her personality, bearing, and character to present herself as a new and vital creation, necessary to patient survival, worthy of being paid a high wage. Many physicians were not convinced that this kind of nurse was necessary for their patients and perceived hospital-trained nurses as a threat. Physician preference, patient income, and the nature of the illness often determined what kind of nurse was hired, and for how long.

Working in a patient's home at the time of the illness created a number of different stresses for the nurse and the family. In the patient's home, the nurse was an individual confronting a family social system. In the hospital, the patient was the lone individual, subject to a set of defined rules and a structured hierarchy. A private duty nurse warned that hard work, with many patients, "under some circumstances [may] demand much less wear and tear on the nervous system than that consequent upon the supervision of her own solitary self while engaged in nursing one patient in the bosom of that patient's family."[10]

The nurse also had to learn to make do in the home without all the equipment, supplies, and paraphernalia which even then marked hospital care. The author of one of the many manuals on "how to be a good private duty nurse" recounted the story of an overzealous private duty nurse who "thought she was distinguishing herself by extreme neatness, used to put thirty-five sheets in the wash in a week. She defeated her own end, for the laundress, naturally thought this a folly, and smoothed out those that looked clean, without washing them."[11]

The most obvious contrast between hospital and home-based care was the lack of structure in private duty. A system and schedule for performing duties was the sine qua non of the hospital training schools. But as one private duty nurse cautioned, "indeed a too loyal adherence to one certain system may prove a huge stumbling block in the way of success."[12] The very work rhythms of the home and hospital differed. In private duty, a nurse's success depended on her ability to reset her work to the demands and whims of the patient and family, not in a premeasured routine set to a rigid schedule. Private duty nursing consisted of the performance of a series of tasks whose order was determined by the ups and downs of the patient's illness and the needs of the family, as much as a farmer's work depended upon the weather and seasons. The patient and the family, not the work as in the hospital, had to be the center of the nurse's attentions.

The difficulty of private duty work was compounded by the contrast between the class of patients in the hospitals and that of the families who hired private nurses. In the hospital, the nurse confronted a patient population of primarily working-class men and women. In the home, how-

ever, most nurses were working for families whose class position was usually higher than their own. In a sample taken of the families who hired nurses through the BML Directory, more than 50 percent of the male family heads were either lawyers, owners of companies, or merchants. The others were skilled or white-collar workers and professionals. While the nurse could as easily be called to the home of a skilled bricklayer in a Dorchester triple-decker as to the bedside of a tea merchant in an elegant townhouse on Beacon Hill, few private duty nurses were hired to work in the tenements and boardinghouses to care for the majority of Boston's populace.[13]

Once in a patient's home, there were few guidelines to govern social relations for either nurses or families. Nurses, as a character in a nursing novel explained, were "always afraid of being asked to do too much. They're always afraid of being treated like ordinary servants."[14] Nurses were told during training that there was nothing which was beneath their dignity to do, but once in a patient's home a nurse had to draw the line and decide for herself what was a reasonable demand. If a nurse washed out a baby's clothes in one home because there was no laundress, should she be expected to do so in another home where such a domestic servant was employed? Should a family be subject to a nurse's wrath because she was asked to eat at a second table or in a kitchen with the servants?

The unspoken rules of class conduct between employers and servants were continually violated by private duty nurses. Clashes were inevitable between a family's expectation of servantlike behavior and the nurse's need to assert her standing above that of servants and to establish her autonomy. Patients' objections to the nurses echoed those made to servant girls unfamiliar with the furnishings of a crowded bourgeois Victorian home. Nurses were faulted for their clumsiness with precious objects, lack of knowledge of how to handle exotic pieces of furniture, and willingness to use expensive items carelessly.

At a time of illness and stress, small mistakes in social conduct by the nurse became magnified and compounded by the fears of death and disease which pervaded a household. "The families want to know 'what are the rules,'" a Philadelphia physician said. Yet, as one nursing superintendent noted, "there are no definite rules to be observed."[15] A nurse's inability to correctly judge the unwritten rules could be costly. In 1892, a Philadelphia nurse angrily reported:

> If by any chance a nurse gains the ill will of her first few patients, her career is ended. She is not told anything of this, simply waits in her boarding house until her last dollar is gone, . . . in suspense . . . and wondering why a "case don't come."[16]

The relationship of the nurse to the household's other servants was one of the problems of social conduct which caused the biggest difficulty. The dilemma centered on where the nurse would take her meals. Nurses often insisted (to make sure they were treated as ladies, not servants) that they be served their meals in the dining room with the family rather than in the kitchen with the servants. This demand was usually opposed by patients used to treating the nurse as a servant, and uncomfortable about sharing their dinner conversations with a stranger from another class. To lessen the conflict on this question, the BML Directory, for example, asked both trained and nontrained nurses on their application forms whether or not they would take their meals in the kitchen with the servants. In the sample from these records, only 40 percent of the trained nurses were willing to eat with the servants, as opposed to 74 percent of those without formal nurses' training. Of those not willing to eat with the servants, 82 percent were trained nurses, and less than 20 percent were the nontrained nurses.

Managing relationships to the family's servants required tact as the nurse had to be understanding but distant, above but not superior. A graduating nursing class at the Boston Training School for Nurses at the Massachusetts General Hospital was told by a physician: "Never assume an air of superiority when dealing with the servants; but on the other hand, never be too familiar with them. At best they recognize your superior position unwillingly, therefore do all you can to conciliate them."[17] The countless stories of the overbearing dictatorial nurse who left the household in an emotional and physical uproar suggest that finding a path to conciliation was not always easy. In desperation, families often turned to the more expensive private

room in the hospital or called for only an "old-style" nontrained nurse since in both situations the social relationships were clearer.

The letters and work records in the BML Directory suggest that the differences and difficulties in private duty existed between the trained and nontrained nurses as well. Class, age, and marital status often differentiated the two groups. Trained nurses, especially graduates of the larger and more elite schools, were likely to be middle- to lower-middle class in origin, while the nontrained nurses drew more heavily from women from the working class. However, graduates of the more numerous smaller training schools were more likely to be working class, compounding the difficulties of differentiating them on class grounds from the nontrained women. Except for large numbers of Irish and English Canadians from the Maritime Provinces, trained nurses in Boston were overwhelmingly native born. They were also much younger than the nontrained women: the graduates' average age was twenty-nine, while the nontrained average age was thirty-six. While the nature of nursing work demanded that its practitioners not be encumbered by family responsibilities, the nontrained nurses were more likely to be widowed or divorced, while 92 percent of the trained nurses had not yet married.

Few of the nurses of either type shared households with male relatives. As did other women workers, they crowded into the boardinghouse districts of Boston's South and West Ends. Many of the nontrained nurses were women already in Boston, who took up nursing as an extension of familial or domestic servant duties, while the graduates were more likely to be single women who had come to Boston or nearby towns to do their training and then stayed on in the city to work. Trained nurses, because they were younger and more often single, were twice as likely as the nontrained to leave Boston.[18]

Turnover figures had a morbid side as nursing was a dangerous occupation. Death reaped a much higher proportion of nurses than women of comparable ages in the Boston population. The BML Directory had a death rate of 16.36 per thousand, a rate greater than that for any adult age group, except those over fifty, in the general population. Even here, probably because of age and class, the nontrained nurses were twice as likely to die as the graduates.[19]

The work experiences and career patterns of the nurses varied considerably. The nontrained women had about two years more experience in nursing than the trained nurses, but both groups remained in the BML Directory on average for eight years. This figure does not measure their work commitment since dropping out of the Directory's records did not mean either giving up nursing or some other form of employment. Some nurses worked during their entire lifetimes, regardless of marital status or training. Others dropped out into related fields: to sell surgical equipment, to operate rest homes, or to work in training schools and hospitals. Some changed fields completely. Still others dropped out at marriage and never returned, while some came back to nursing when their children were older or widowhood necessitated employment.

While these nurses differed in age, morbidity, marital status, experience, and training, they competed in the same overcrowded labor market for the same jobs. It was certainly not clear to the physicians or patients who hired the nurses what skill really differentiated these women. Wage rates, specialities, and the seriousness of the patient's illness, however, were all factors in determining who was hired.

Wage rates clearly differentiated the nurses, as the graduates tended to charge the patients almost five to ten dollars a week more than the nongraduates. From the 1880s till the mid-1890s graduates received fifteen to eighteen dollars a week; by the late nineties they were commanding twenty to twenty-five dollars. But a graduate nurse just out of school and a graduate nurse with ten years experience were paid the same. Neither trained nor nontrained nurses were rewarded for their experience with a higher wage. There was clearly a "customary" wage established for each group, although there was a slightly greater dispersion in the fees asked for by the nongraduates.[20]

Nurses were allowed in most registries to state their preferences on cases. Comments such as "only surgical cases" or "no obstetrical cases" cover the application forms. Trained nurses specialized more and were less willing to care for postpartum patients, presumably because such work almost always guaranteed they would be asked to do more household labor. Nontrained nurses, in contrast, more willingly took what work they could get.[21]

The graduate nurses clearly felt their livelihood was always threatened by the nongraduates. There were frequent complaints that the nongraduates were receiving most of the work or that the directories did not apportion the work equitably.[22] But at least through the BML Directory it appears the nongraduates were the ones suffering discrimination. The graduates received consistently two or three times as much work as the nongraduates and about 20 percent more than they should have, given equal distribution.[23] Miss E. L. Blanchard, a nontrained nurse, bitter over her lack of work, wrote to the physician in charge of the BML Directory in 1895: "I feel it is a . . . way of pushing one out, for opening the way for those younger, and . . . in the training school for a few months. . . . Thus . . . experience goes for nothing." Another nontrained nurse explained the dilemma by pointing out that her costs were too high for the poor and too low for the rich who would, she believed, rather employ a graduate.[24]

Thus it appears that in the 1880s and early 1890s, the trained and nontrained nurses in Boston were competing directly with one another. By the late 1890s, the competition was caused by the enormous number of graduates entering the labor market. By 1915, in Massachusetts as a whole, the trained nurses outnumbered the nontrained two to one.[25]

Competition then developed between the graduates of the different training schools. Physicians at the BML Directory told graduates of the smaller schools that their training was not equal to that of nurses from the more prestigious hospitals.[26] Graduates of the more elite schools demanded and received higher wages than those from the smaller schools and more often demanded a wage differential to nurse male and contagious patients. The graduates of the larger schools also received slightly more cases, although the reason for this may have been that they were better known by local physicians.

Class background as much as training differences was probably the reason for this division among the graduate nurses. Graduate nurses from Long Island Hospital, the site of the city's asylum, were told they probably would not receive cases if they charged the graduate nurses' going rate.[27] One of the physicians in charge of the BML Directory bluntly wrote:

> It is preposterous to put the Long Island Hospital nurses on the same plane as those of the Mass. and City Hospitals. Certainly our patrons would not accept it. When we consider the class from which they come, their lack of education, etc. . . .the answer would seem to be obvious. The Long Island nurses are worth say from $10–15 and I could not with any feeling of fairness send them to first-class families and serious cases with a supply of the others on hand.[28]

Nursing employment in private duty for every type of nurse was sporadic, seasonal, and uncertain. The average graduate received only 3.2 cases a year from the BML Directory, the nongraduates 2.3; this multiplies out to be a work time, on average, of thirteen and nine weeks a year, respectively. In contrast, a Cleveland nurse reported that in her eleven years of private duty work from 1895 to 1906 she worked thirty-three to thirty-five weeks each year. The only time she was employed fully was the fifteen months she spent on a "luxury" case as a companion, as much as a nurse, for one wealthy patient. A comparison to other women workers in Massachusetts in 1890, however, shows nurses and midwives as sixth in unemployment frequency out of a list of twenty-five other women's occupations.[29] A nurse, trained or not, did make more money *when* she was employed than most other working women.[30] But the wait between cases was often so long that the extra wage could not make up for the unemployment.

The expense of the nurse also limited her calls. As early as 1888 nurses were aware that even what they called the "breadwinning middle class" could not afford their services. But because their own need for work made nurses feel they could not have an official sliding scale for patients, a nurse suggested that those who could not afford them should be "either taken to the hospital or put on the list of the visiting nurses."[31]

Nursing work was also seasonal, and the nurses, as much as any industrial workers, recognized that there were "slack" times. There was definitely a

higher call for nurses in the midwinter months of January through March and a slowdown between May and July caused perhaps as much by the exodus of the rich from the city during the summer as a difference in disease incidence. Similarly the demand for nurses dropped during the economic depressions.[32]

One nurse echoed a common theme while reproaching the Directory in 1895: "if I had depended entirely on the Directory for a living, of course I should have starved long ago."[33] But registering with a number of directories was still no guarantee of work. A nurse could and often did spend weeks at a time waiting at her boarding-house for cases from any source. While the nursing leadership bemoaned the nurses' increasingly "mercenary spirit," a San Francisco nurse asserted that they could not afford to be "angels of mercy."[34] Worry and anxiety over where they would get their next case dominated the thinking of many nurses. Poignantly, a California nurse warned Boston nurses not to come to the West Coast and of the danger of "the gradual fading away of resources, courage, hope—too often self-respect—and sometimes suicide. The papers here suppress all that."[35]

One solution to the difficulty of finding work was for a nurse to "attach" herself to a physician and hope he would send her all his cases. Nurses had to make the rounds of physicians' offices to announce their presence and then wait to be called. Contacts made during training were critical to a nurse launching her career. If the nurse ventured to a new city, finding work took even more time. But nurses also competed for the patient dollar with the doctors since it was not just nurses at the turn of the century who were in oversupply.[36] A New York nurse complained in 1897 that a physician had her fired from a case and then began to make more visits to the patient himself.[37] There was the danger for physicians who had taken short apprenticeships or correspondence courses that a nurse with several years of hospital training might in fact know more scientific medicine.[38] The intensity of the economic competition makes more comprehensible the constant ideological stress by physicians on the need for the nurse to know her place and remain "loyal." But physicians held the master key which opened the employment door. An informal blacklist of sorts also circulated among physicians and directories of both dropouts and troublesome nurses.[39] Despite the fact that nurses were usually employed by the patients, in actuality they had to behave as if the patient's physician was their boss.[40]

Despite the uncertainty and limits on their autonomy, nurses fashioned a variety of *individual* means for surviving, reshaping, and enjoying the work. The stories of patients who took their nurses to Europe on trips, married them, left them large sums of money, or employed them for decades, however unusual and idiosyncratic, suggest that, as with servants and governesses, the step up in nursing could mean marriage or life as the family retainer. Nurses also found ways to create alliances in the household. Reexamining the figures on eating with the servants makes clear that nearly 40 percent of the graduate nurses and 74 percent of the nontrained nurses were willing to eat in the kitchen. Nurses quickly learned that a recalcitrant servant could make their lives miserable. Letters rebuking nurses for being too friendly with the servants and gossiping with them about the patient's illness and the household life suggest that congenial working relationships frequently developed.

Nurses never lacked resourcefulness in asserting some kind of control of their work. Especially on long convalescent cases, they would sometimes leave patients to go home, to go to the theater, or to visit friends or family. Some nurses had other businesses and conducted their other work while on a case. If the job was really miserable there were ways to be relieved. One nurse was disciplined for having another nurse call and lie for her, saying an aunt was ill and she was urgently needed at home. The nurse, when discovered, said she left the case because the patient was "poor" and conditions of work were terrible. Other nurses took to sleeping while on the job, or abandoning patients, or refusing to take cases they had agreed to.[41]

These attempts to control the work were perceived by the public and many nursing superintendents, however, as counter to devotion to duty. Nurses were, after all, expected to be more like mothers than workers, forever on call, cheerful and devoted. In a 1904 editorial entitled "The Path of Duty," for example, the *American Journal of Nursing* chastised nurses for refusing to take cases: "Such failure to meet our highest obligations, such viola-tion of our common standards of right and duty, cannot be too sternly censured. The women who permit themselves to conduct their professional work in this manner are in this, at least, wrong through and through."[42]

Different kinds of organized efforts were made to introduce some rationality into the private duty labor market and to distribute the work more evenly. Those in charge of the BML Directory, for example, tried to influence the wage rate, often to the detriment of all the nurses. With nurses of equal skill, the Directory registrars would send out the nurse with the lowest fees.[43] Lavinia Dock, the outspoken socialist and feminist nursing leader, counseled nurses: "We must not undersell; that is treachery to fellow workers."[44] But Anna Maxwell, the nursing superintendent of Presbyterian Hospital in New York wrote the Directory in Boston in 1899 to ask if there would be work if more graduate nurses lowered their wage rates.[45] In *principle*, graduates tried to keep to an agreed-upon wage rate. But it was not uncommon for a nurse to lower her rates when necessary, or, more often, to overcharge the patient on items such as carriage fares and laundry bills as well as on her fees.[46]

The Directory officials also attempted to rationalize the system by grading the nurses by experience and training. This was done on a haphazard basis since they had to rely upon the nurse's self-reporting and incomplete patient and physician recommendations for their assessments. Registry officials remained uncertain, however, about their legal right to discipline nurses. All they ultimately could do was to refuse to put the nurse on their lists, but she could go elsewhere.[47]

Much of the nursing concern over the lack of work focused upon the registries. "Most graduates," a nurse reported, "do not feel that they are fairly treated by the Directory, but are afraid to complain for fear that it will be visited upon them."[48] In an attempt to equally distribute employment, when a nurse reported off a case, her name was supposed to be placed at the bottom of the rotation list. But, nurses charged, the registries played favorites, did not always follow this system, and could not control whether or not a nurse received a "good" case which guaranteed employment for a length of time in a decent home.[49]

Aware of the discontent over the registries, the extent to which both physicians' groups and commercial agencies were profiting from such services, and the necessity to control distribution, some nurses began to advocate the organization of nursing-controlled, centralized, and officially sponsored registries in each city. In Boston, for example, the BML Directory was closed as graduate nurses began to register with the nurses' officially sponsored Suffolk County Nurses' Directory. One nurse commented, however, "It is not so much a share in the government of directories, as a share in the work given out by them that is asked by the majority of nurses. . . . Each one should have a share."[50] There was no guarantee, however, that a nursing-controlled registry would mean any more work. In fact, nurses admitted that the commercial agencies often allowed the more experienced trained nurses to charge more, thus making them more attractive than the official registries, which set one rate.[51] The official agencies often enrolled only graduates from the "better schools," did not provide nontrained nurses, and were thus less able than the commercial registries to meet the varied community demand for nurses. Hospital and alumnae registries often served only to provide the institution's own graduates with positions as private duty "specials" in their hospital.

Despite the overcrowding, private duty work continued to absorb the majority of nursing graduates because there was very little else they could do to remain in nursing. Some private duty experience was considered essential for every nurse, but status in nursing quickly accrued to those in more "executive" positions within hospitals or public health nursing agencies. Private duty nursing, seen even within nursing as often no more than domestic service or a mother's work, gave those who did it little status. Furthermore, because there was no supervision, women with the weakest skills could hide in private duty. With the growth of hospital-based care in the early 1900s and the decline in the debilitating sicknesses which required more long-term nursing care, the status decline of private duty nursing increased. By the late 1920s, a major study of nursing's dilemmas could repeat the aphorism "Every nurse ought to do some private duty, but no good nurse ought to stay in the field more than a few years."[52]

Aware of the overcrowding as early as the 1890s, Lavinia Dock counseled nurses to specialize "by branching into auxiliary lines of work not strictly nursing, yet which can be better done by one having the training of nurses." Among Dock's suggestions were heading various departments in hospitals, becoming a dietician or pharmacist, directing nurseries, old people's homes, social service, settlement work, medicine and massage, or returning to nurse in small towns and the countryside. Her suggestions entailed the nurse's specializing *outside* of private duty work itself.[53] Lucy Drown, the superintendent of nurses at Boston City Hospital, was blunter in her advice. Sharing her concern over the lack of work with the physician in charge of the BML Directory she wrote:

> [there is] . . . less survival of the fittest [in nursing] than in some other walks of life. My advice to these young women would be that if they cannot make a place for themselves as nurses, to go back to the work they left when they came into the hospitals [for training], for they belong to the working class, and maintain themselves as teachers, stenographers, dressmakers, etc.[54]

But in fact, most stayed in nursing, waiting for cases, trying to find different kinds of nursing work, "making do" in an increasingly untenable form of employment.

The isolation of the work site, the severe competition for cases, and the acute divisions within the nursing ranks all worked to limit the forms of control over their labor nurses as a group could exercise. Individual nurses, sometimes with the help of others, found ways to make the work less difficult and to achieve a modicum of autonomy. But they could do little collectively to alleviate the competition and animosity between the trained and nontrained or to transform the economic structures which underlay and created the private duty system.

Sporadic efforts were made to find a more organized solution to the private duty dilemma. While waiting for a case or isolated in a patient's home, however, few nurses could attend regular meetings or put the time into the effort to sustain the few private duty leagues which briefly flourished. The professional nursing associations, dominated by nursing educators and focused on registration laws and educational reforms, often discounted the private duty nursing problems or hoped they would fade into oblivion. As women workers, providing

services in the private employ of individual patients, nurses were similarly ignored by both male
and female trade unionists.[55]

By the 1920s, private duty was increasingly becoming a nursing backwater. Home-based private
duty was relinquished to the nontrained nurses or
the older graduates as the younger nurses sought
employment in private duty as hospital "specials."
There was a brief attempt to revitalize, rationalize,
and reorganize private duty nursing at the end of
the 1920s. But economics and hospital and nursing
politics undermined these efforts. At the same time,
secluded and many times embittered by their experiences, private duty nurses became increasingly
conservative and isolated.[56]

The history of private duty nursing suggests some
insights into the broader historical concern to comprehend how different groups of workers sought
to gain individual and collective control over their
labor. Historians of male artisans and skilled workers, in particular, have often romanticized this labor and described the "degradation of work" under
monopoly capitalism in the twentieth century. As
historians of women's work, most notably Susan
Porter Benson and Barbara Melosh have argued,
however, this "lament" for the lost artisan past is a
very different tune when sung on higher notes.
The nature of the sex-segregated and overcrowded labor market for women workers, the skills
their jobs required, and the conditions under which
they labored give their history and struggles a very
different character from that of male workers.[57]

The private duty nurse cannot be equated with
the independent craftsman or the skilled worker
whose consciousness and struggles are the focus of
much historical writing today.[58] Nor, however, was
the private duty nurse in a position similar to women
who labored next to one another in factories or
department stores. The work site of private duty,
the ideology of altruism and caring which pervaded this form of service work, the competition
and lack of cases, in sum both the labor process
and the social relations of production of this form
of health care made the private duty nurse a particular kind of worker. She was indeed "neither for
the drawing room nor for the kitchen," but also
neither for the trade unions and professional associations nor for the powerful informal work
groups.

It may well be that private duty nurses were sui
generis. However, while private duty nursing was
unique in its isolation and ambiguities, other women
workers, workers of color, and the unskilled similarly faced high unemployment, competition for
jobs, and lack of collective control over their work.
Until we understand the political economy and work
cultures of these less autonomous groups, we will
have as partial an understanding of the American
working class as we have of the health work force
when we focus only on physicians.

NOTES

This is a revised version of a paper presented at the
Organization of American Historians Convention,
April 15, 1978. Research for this article was sup-
ported by Grant Number 1 RO3 HS02879–01 from
the National Center for Health Services Research,
U.S. Department of Health and Human Services.
As always, the trenchant comments of Diana Long
Hall, David Rosner, Tim Sieber, and Lise Vogel were
invaluable.

1 *Nursing Ethics: For Hospital and Private Use* (Cleveland: J. B. Savage, 1901), 32.

2 The exact date when Americans of all classes began
to use the hospital cannot, of course, be set. For a
careful analysis of this question, see both Morris
Vogel, *The Invention of the Modern Hospital* (Chicago:
University of Chicago Press, 1979), and David Rosner, *A Once Charitable Enterprise* (New York: Cambridge University Press, 1982). For a discussion of

the changes in private duty nursing in the 1920s,
see Susan Reverby, *The Nursing Disorder: A Critical
History of the Hospital-Nursing Relationship, 1860–1945*
(New York: Cambridge University Press, forthcoming), and Barbara Melosh, *"The Physician's Hand":
Work Culture and Conflict in American Nursing* (Philadelphia: Temple University Press, 1982), esp. chap. 3.

3 Boston Medical Library Directory for Nurses, vol.
A–V (vol. J is missing), 1880–1914, Rare Books
Room, Countway Medical Library, Harvard Medical School. The goodwill and support of Richard
Wolfe, Carol Pine, and the entire Rare Books Room
staff is gratefully acknowledged. The Directory
claimed to represent the majority of Boston nurses
(Boston Medical Library Association, *10th and 11th
Annual Reports*, October 1887, 23). A comparison of
the number of nurses in the Directory with the
number in the census for Boston suggests that, in

any given year (with the exception of the closing years of the Directory), anywhere from one third to three quarters of Boston's nurses could be found in these volumes. The sample included 313 graduate nurses and 226 nongraduates. The sample included only the female nurses, although the Directory did provide work for a small number of male nurses.

4   See Reverby, *Nursing Disorder*, chap. 1.

5   Isabel Hampton Robb, "Educational standards for nurses," in *Nursing the Sick 1893*, by Isabel Hampton Robb et al. (New York: McGraw Hill, 1949), 5.

6   U.S. Bureau of the Census, *Historical Statistics of the United States* (Washington; U.S. Government Printing Office, 1959), ser. B. 192–194; Carroll D. Wright, *The Social, Commercial and Manufacturing Statistics of the City of Boston* (Boston: Rockwell and Churchill, 1892), 96–98; Secretary of the Commonwealth of Massachusetts, *Census of the Commonwealth of Massachusetts, 1905*, vol. 2: *Occupations and Defective Social and Physical Conditions* (Boston: Wright and Potter, 1909), 138.

7   See Nancy Tomes, "'Little world of our own': the Pennsylvania Hospital Training School for Nurses, 1895–1907," in this volume; Jo Ann Ashley, *Hospitals, Paternalism and the Role of the Nurse* (New York: Teachers College Press, 1976); Reverby, *Nursing Disorder*, chap. 4, on the use of the student nurse in the hospital, and chap. 6 on a comparison of the career patterns of the graduates of different training schools.

8   Gertrude Harding, *The Higher Aspects of Nursing* (Philadelphia: W. B. Saunders and Co., 1919), 109; Sara E. Parsons, *Nursing Problems and Obligations* (Boston: Barrows, 1916), 115.

9   Katharine DeWitt, *Private Duty Nursing* (Philadelphia: J. P. Lippincott, 1913); Emily A. M. Stoney, *Practical Points in Nursing for Nurses in Private Practice* (Philadelphia: W. B. Saunders, 1897); Elinor Lason, "Characteristic requisites for a private duty nurse," *Report of the 18th Convention of the American Nurses Association*, June 1915, 65; E. B. M., Letter to the Editor of the *Transcript*, October 24, 1881, clipping in vol. B, Boston Medical Library Directory for Nurses.

10 Annie E. Hutchinson, "Practical nursing in private practice," *Trained Nurse and Hospital Review* 37 (August 1906): 83. "Don't imagine that you can discipline a patient in his own home as you would in a hospital ward. It can't be done," the *Trained Nurse* cautioned. "Don'ts for the Private Duty Nurse," 47 (October 1911): 202.

11 DeWitt, *Private Duty Nursing*, 70.

12 Hutchison, "Practical nursing," 84.

13 A random sample was drawn of one hundred patients who hired nurses through the Boston Medical Library Directory between 1880 and 1914. The occupations of the male patients, or males in the family of the patient, were obtained by checking names and addresses in the *Boston City Directory* for the appropriate years. The class base of those who used the services of private duty nurses continued to be an issue in nursing and health care. For further discussion of this, see Melosh *The Physician's Hand*, chap. 3, and Susan Reverby, "'Something besides waiting': the politics of private duty nursing reform in the Depression," in *Nursing History: New Perspectives, New Possibilities*, ed. Ellen Condliffe Lagemann (New York: Teachers College Press, 1983).

For quantitative evidence which suggests the changing class background of nurses, and the differences between the training schools, see Reverby, *Nursing Disorder*, chap. 5; Jane Mottus, *New York Nightingales* (Ann Arbor: University Microfilms Books, 1981); and Janet Wilson James, "Isabel Hampton and the professionalization of nursing in the 1890s," in *The Therapeutic Revolution*, ed. Morris Vogel and Charles Rosenberg (Philadelphia: University of Pennsylvania Press, 1979): 201–44.

14 Brennan Gill, *The Trouble of One House* (Garden City: Doubleday, 1950), 142. This quotation was given to me by Barbara Melosh.

15 Dr. J. Madison Taylor, Letter to the Editor, *American Journal of Nursing* 4 (May 1904): 658. Stoney, *Practical Points in Nursing*, 24.

16 Philadelphia, Letter to the Editor, *Trained Nurse and Hospital Review* 8 (September 1892):278.

17 William L. Richardson, *Address on the Duties and Conduct of Nurses in Private Nursing, June 18, 1886* (Boston: Press of George H. Ellis, 1886), 10. Richardson's address must have been very popular because it was printed and widely circulated.

18 The analysis of the nurses' class origins and migration patterns is based upon samples drawn from both nursing school student records and the records of the Home for Aged Women in Boston which admitted nontrained women nurses. Other analysis is based upon the Boston Medical Library Directory sample compared with the census and city directory evidence. The Directory does give addresses for about half the nurses. In vols. K, L, and O of the Boston Medical Library records, the hometowns for 220 nurses were given. These data were tabulated to determine where the graduates had gone to school before they came to Boston and to differentiate the nongraduates and graduates. For further discussion of class origins and migration patterns of nurses, see Reverby, *Nursing Disorder*, chap. 1, 5, and 6.

The Boston Medical Library Directory does not give ethnicity data. The migration of women from the Maritimes into nursing may be a continuation of their earlier migration into domestic service in Boston; see Alan Brookes, "Migration from the Maritime Provinces of Canada to Boston, Mass., 1860–1900," masters' thesis, University of Hull, 1974, 213–19. The role of Canadian nurses in the United States has not yet been examined, but these women were an important minority, especially in the leadership, from the 1870s through the 1930s.

Nurses were listed in the Directory either as "Miss," "Mrs." or "Mr." Marital status of the nurses given as "Mrs." was inferred by checking a subsample in the city directory and by using national census data.

19 This figure is based on all deaths *reported* to the Boston Medical Library Directory and is therefore an underestimate since not all deaths were reported. For all those who died *while registered* with the directory, the average age at death for the men was only forty-one, for the women, thirty-seven. For comparative death rates for Massachusetts, see *Historical Statistics*, Bicentennial edition, ser. B. 201–213, 63.

20 There is a statistically significant relationship between training and wages at the .00 level from 1880 till the close of the Directory in 1914, but no significant relationship between wages and years of nursing experience. On how the wages were set, see Dr. Charles Putnam to Miss Gertrude Hamilton, August 7, 1913, Directory for Nurses, *Letterbook*, vol. 1, February 11, 1891–January 7, 1914.

21 This is not to suggest that the nontrained nurses willingly did whatever the family wanted. One such nurse, for example, complained that families expected her to do the "spring housecleaning" along with the nursing. "A graduate of the training school of life," Letter to the Editor, *Trained Nurse and Hospital Review* 51 (March 1916): 369.

22 Richard Bradley, "Large part of hospital work performed in the home," *Modern Hospital* 1 (November 1913): 227–31; Charlotte Aikens, "The Committee on Grading of Nurses," *Trained Nurse and Hospital Review* 37 (March 1914): 168; Lavinia L. Dock, "Directories for nurses," *Report of the Second Annual Convention of the American Society of Superintendents of Training School for Nurses*, 1895, 59; Miss Hintze, Discussion on Dock paper, Ibid., 60.

23 There is a statistically significant relationship between training and total number of cases received throughout the Directory at the .01 level. Data on the number of nurses available to work, by type of training, were compared to the number, by type of training, who actually did the work,for the years 1889–93. The raw data for this latter calculation can be found in the *Letterbook*.

24 Miss E. L. Blanchard to Dr. Brigham, February 11, 1895, Boston Medical Library Directory, vol. E, 181; L. H., "What shall she do?" Letter to the Editor, *Trained Nurse and Hospital Review* 23 (January 1899): 42.

25 Massachusetts Bureau of Statistics, *The Decennial Census, 1915* (Boston: Wright and Potter, 1918), 510.

26 Dr. Putnam to Miss McBrien, January 20, 1894; Dr. Putnam to Dr. Brigham, September 10, 1894; Dr. Putnam to Miss Heintze, November 19, 1892, *Letterbook*.

27 Alice N. Lincoln, Secretary of the Board, Long Island Hospital, to Dr. E. W. Taylor, October 23, 1899, *Long Island Hospital Letterbook*, vol. 1, Long Island Hospital Collection, Rare Books Room, Countway Medical Library.

28 Dr. Brigham to Dr. Putnam, November 3, 1899, Boston Medical Library Directory for Nurses, *Letterbook*.

29 Case rates calculated from averages in the Boston Medical Library Directory sample. On the Cleveland nurse's experience, see James H. Rodabaugh and Mary Jane Rodabaugh, *Nursing in Ohio* (Columbus, Ohio: Ohio State Nurses' Association, 1951), 199–200. 1890 Massachusetts data were compiled from the 1890 Census and were given to me by Professor Alex Keyssar of Brandeis University from his ongoing study on unemployment in Massachusetts. Unemployment frequency was calculated by dividing the total unemployed by the total number in the occupation. Unfortunately, these numbers include both nontrained and trained nurses, as well as midwives.

30 In 1900, for example, the average weekly wage for domestic servants in Massachusetts was $3.61; in that year the nongraduates in the Directory were averaging $11.25; the graduates $20.93. For the domestic servant data, see Stanley Lebergott, *Manpower in Economic Growth* (New York: McGraw Hill, 1964), 542. For comparisons to other women workers in Boston, see Louise Marion Bosworth, *The Living Wage of Women Workers* (New York: Longmans, Green, 1911), 33–39.

31 "The social side of nursing," *Trained Nurse and Hospital Review* 2 (March 1888):95–97; Letter to the Editor, ibid. 39 (October 1916): 369.

32 Daniel Gormon to Dr. Putnam, June 14, 1894; Elizabeth Bowness to Miss McBrien, December 9, 1903, *Letterbook*. The raw data on the number of nurses requested each month for 1891 through 1914 can be found in ibid. This drop-off in demand was especially precipitous during the 1893 depression.

33 B. H. Giles to the Directory, March 10, 1895, vol. F, Boston Medical Library Directory, 176. For ex-

amples of letters which also reflect the nurses' bitterness at the lack of work, see Emilie Neale to Dr. Brigham, January 8, 1894; Dr. Putnam to Miss McBrien, February 24, 1900, *Letterbook*.

34 Stoney, *Practical Points*, 18; Henry Beates, Jr., M.D., *The Status of Nurses: A Sociologic Problem* (Philadelphia: National Board of Regents, 1909), 17.

35 Letter to the Editor, *Pacific Coast Nursing Journal* 3 (March 1914): 130.

36 Gerald Markowitz and David Rosner, "Doctors in crisis: medical education and medical reform during the Progressive Ea, 1895–1915," in *Health Care in America*, ed. Susan Reverby and David Rosner (Philadelphia: Temple University Press, 1979), 185–205.

37 "Report of the monthly meeting of the New York City Training School Alumnae, June 8, 1897," *Trained Nurse and Hospital Review* 19 (July 1897): 34.

38 "The reasons and the remedy—a training school symposium," *National Hospital Record*, 1907, *11:* 14–20; "Boston trained nurse in Chicago," *Boston Transcript*, October 24, 1881, clipping in vol. B, Boston Medical Library Directory.

39 Memo from Dr. George Rowe, superintendent of Boston City Hospital, to the Directory, no date; numerous other letters in 1892, *Letterbook*.

40 "The members of the family regard themselves as the nurse's employers. She very often does not." Editorial, "The patient's family," *Trained Nurse and Hospital Review* 46 (March 1911): 166.

41 See letters and clippings laid in the volumes of the Boston Medical Library Directory for Nurses.

42 *American Journal of Nursing*, 4 (October 1904): 2.

43 Dr. Charles Putnam to Dr. Edwin Brigham, January 31, 1894, *Letterbook*. Putnam's position was "it is but fair that a nurse who offers her services at a lower price and intrusts her engagements to us should either reap some benefit from that low price or else be informed that she will reap no such benefit." Putnam and Brigham were the physicians from the Boston Medical Library in charge of the Directory.

44 Quoted in A. S. Kavanogh, "The indispensable combination in hospital work," *Trained Nurse and Hospital Review* 37 (July 1914): 78.

45 Anna Maxwell to Miss C. C. McBrien, October 11, 1899, *Letterbook*. In his reply to Maxwell's letter, Dr. Brigham was pessimistic about how much a lowering of the rates would help the overcrowding. Brigham to Maxwell, October 16, 1899, ibid.

46 A private duty nurse who secured her own cases did not of course have to keep to an agreed-upon wage rate (see Louise Darche, "The proper organization of training schools in America," *Nursing the Sick 1893*, 106). But it was considered a "breach of faith" with the Directory for a nurse to overcharge the patients when she had agreed upon one price (see Morton Prince to Miss C. C. McBrien, February 12, 1901, *Letterbook*). However, such overcharging was not uncommon (Florence LaFleur, Boston Medical Library Directory, vol. R, 66; L. M. B. Russell, vol. I, 58; Annie Collimore to M. Adelaide Nutting, June 15, 1925, M. Adelaide Nutting Papers, Teachers College, Columbia University, File X, Folder 4, "Hours of work–domestic service."

47 Around 1904 the directory officials began to ask patients and physicians to inform them when they felt the nurse was "superior or first class." On their uncertainty about the legality of their position, see F. Morison to Dr. F. Shattuck, February 20, 1884, *Letterbook*.

48 "A graduate," Letter to the Editor, *Trained Nurse and Hospital Review* 15 (January 1895): 43.

49 On blacklists, see memo from Dr. George H. M. Rowe, Superintendent of Boston City Hospital, to the Directory, no date; numerous other letters in 1892, *Letterbook*.

50 Letter to the Editor, *Trained Nurse and Hospital Review* 23 (February 1904): 103.

51 "Private duty problems," *Trained Nurse and Hospital Review* 73 (July 1924): 57–58.

52 Committee on the Grading of Nursing Schools, *Nurses, Patients and Pocketbooks* (New York: The Committee, 1928), 361.

53 "Overcrowding in the nursing profession," *Trained Nurse and Hospital Review* 21 (July 1898): 8–13.

54 Lucy Drown to Dr. Brigham, October 18, 1899, *Letterbook*.

55 Recent historical scholarship has begun to document and analyze the divisions and conflict within American nursing. For examples, see, in addition to my previous work cited, Melosh, *The Physician's Hand;* Susan Armeny, "Resolute enthusiasts: the effort to professionalize American nursing, 1893–1923," Ph.D. diss., University of Missouri, 1983; Lagemann, ed., *Nursing History.*

56 See Reverby, "'Something besides waiting.'"

57 The historiography on workers' control and capitalist rationality is growing rapidly. For the key works and critiques, see David Montgomery, *Workers' Control in America* (New York: Cambridge University Press, 1979); Harry Braverman, *Labor and Monopoly Capital: The Degradation of Work in the Twentieth Century* (New York: Monthly Review Press, 1974); Susan Porter Benson, "The clerking sisterhood: rationalization and the work culture of saleswomen in American department stores," *Radical America* 12 (March–April 1978): 41-55; Melosh, *The Physician's*

Hand; and James Green, "Culture, politics and workers' response to industrialization in the U.S.," *Radical America* 16 (January–April 1982): 101–30.

58 For an example of an analysis of private duty work

in this mode, see David Wagner, "The proletarianization of nursing in the United States, 1932–1946," *International Journal of Health Services,* 1980, *10:* 271–90.

33

"Little World of Our Own":
The Pennsylvania Hospital Training School
for Nurses, 1895–1907

NANCY TOMES

For the daughters of the American middle class, the feminization and professionalization of nursing in the late nineteenth century meant a widening of educational and employment opportunities. Nursing promised good wages and steady work for most of those who undertook the calling. For a few, it offered more—a route to prestige and an uncommon measure of administrative power. Nursing gave highly motivated women the opportunity to create, as one nurse called it, "a little world of our own," a professional world of women centered in the nursing school. Through the new nursing education, such women generated a professional identity for the trained nurse, symbolized by the cap, pin, and uniform, and celebrated in the rituals of capping, graduation, and alumnae reunions. Historians have traced the development of this professional identity among the national leaders of nursing education, women like Isabel Hampton Robb, Adelaide Nutting, and Lavinia Dock, and have noted its expression in organizations like the National League for Nursing Education, the national and state alumnae associations, and the nurses' registries. But rarely have historians investigated the professionalization of nursing at the institutional level, as it operated in the training school, and affected the average nurse.[1]

The Pennsylvania Hospital Training School for Nurses offers the material for such an institutional case history of late-nineteenth-century nursing. Its records include not only the activities of the nursing leaders but also those of the nursing students.

From such contrasting viewpoints, we can arrive at a sense of what nursing education meant to the individuals who experienced it. This perspective is particularly useful since the socialization of nurses differed markedly from that of doctors. Historians and sociologists have used a model of professionalization based so exclusively on medicine that they have neglected the variations and alternatives evident in the development of other professions at this time. The study of nursing adds needed complexity and detail to the history of professionalization in the late nineteenth century.

This study focuses on the Pennsylvania Hospital Training School under the leadership of its superintendent, Lucy Walker. During her tenure (1895–1907), it became one of America's foremost nursing schools. Trained in England, Miss Walker brought a heritage of British nursing methods—the emphasis on rigid discipline, hierarchical authority, efficient organization, and autonomy of nursing service—which she attempted to recreate in an American hospital. Her successes and her failures are equally revealing.

An understanding of Miss Walker's career must begin with an understanding of the evolution of trained nursing in the Pennsylvania Hospital before she was appointed in 1895. In the first twenty years of the school's existence, the trained nurses made gradual gains, gains which Lucy Walker consolidated and then expanded. The process illustrates many of the familiar features of professionalization; elimination of untrained competition, constant upgrading of standards, systemization of work, consolidation of authority, and establishment of autonomy.[2]

Before the establishment of the training school

NANCY TOMES is Assistant Professor of History at the State University of New York, Stony Brook, New York.

Reprinted with permission from *Journal of the History of Medicine and Allied Sciences* 33 (1978): 507–530.

in 1876, nursing care at the Pennsylvania Hospital was performed by untrained attendants drawn from the urban working class. Convalescent patients routinely served as nurses, and some liked the work well enough to stay on after they recovered. Additional nurses were recruited from the city's servant population. A few of these early nurses achieved a certain professionalism in their skillful management of the wards and were well liked and respected by the doctors. Others exhibited less proficiency and reliability, so that the overall quality of nursing care was very uneven. Whatever their abilities, the nurses performed their duties with little supervision. In theory, the steward and matron directed their work, but in practice interfered very little in the day-to-day routine of the nurses. Each ward formed an "independent kingdom" under its own head nurse.[3]

The hospital administration lumped nurses and servants in the same category, and they performed much the same work. Nurses carted laundry and supplies to the wards, dusted the furniture, and kept the wards in order. Little labor was involved in patient care. Nurses delivered medicine to the patients' beds, but the patients were responsible for taking it themselves. (Frequently they poured it out the windows or simply ignored it.) Nurses took temperatures only in special cases. There was no night nursing; attendants made the rounds every night to see that the patients were quiet and comfortable. The low ratio of nurses to patients further illustrates the limited nature of nursing care; in the early 1870s, eleven nurses, six men and five women, cared for 160 patients.[4]

"Respectable" women of the middle classes had little place in the hospital. "Lady Visitors" came to talk and pray with the patients but had no role in the regular hospital routine. The chairwoman of the Lady Visitors' Committee chided the president of the board of managers for the "guarded manner in which we have been admitted to the institution, alluding particularly to the restriction to hours of the afternoon." And perhaps there was good reason for such caution; one hospital matron recalled that, in these years, "to go into a men's surgical ward after midnight was a risk no woman should encounter."[5]

Such was nursing care when, in 1876, the Board of Managers decided to establish a training school. Impressed with its "success in foreign institutions,"

they believed that a nursing school might be "productive of good to the hospital." They hoped that bringing "educated women" into the wards would improve the care of the patients, the cleanliness of the wards, and the hospital's general decorum.[6]

The training school staff and students began work only on the women's wards, where the untrained women nurses had never been very popular with the doctors. For the first eight years of the school's existence, its superintendent, Annie Bunting, "interfered but very little with the management of the men's wards." Not until 1885 did the president of the board of managers suggest putting trained women nurses on the men's wards as well. His suggestion shocked some. One doctor said later, "I well remember my disgust and the feeling of fear that came over me that I should live to see such a state of things." The board was determined to go through with the plan, however. At first the women's presence in the men's wards created "great difficulty and friction." When Miss Sharpless, the first woman nurse on the male surgical ward, helped a very sick man to change his "outer garments," "a cry of horror went up." According to one old employee, the nurses themselves were "soon disgusted, and said it was not fit work for women." But the women nurses stayed on the men's wards. By 1885, a new superintendent, Marion Smith, had eliminated all the male heads of wards. The remaining male nurses were called "orderlies." In 1892 the board of managers could report to the hospital's contributors, "where twenty years ago, a woman's presence would have been thought out of place, all care is now committed to her charge."[7]

Despite the gradual elimination of untrained nurses and the centralization of authority under the superintendent of nurses, the training school was far from well established in the early 1890s. A rapid turnover in superintendents had left discipline lax and the quality of nursing care uneven. A hospital committee in 1894 complained that the student nurses did not receive the "systematic, thorough and accurate instruction which they rightly expect." Their work was not well organized, and thus all the nurses overworked. The superintendent also had "failed to win the confidence and command the respect of her pupils," and the social life in the nurses' home lacked "healthful tone," the committee concluded.[8]

In 1895, the board of managers interviewed Lucy

Walker and decided to appoint her superintendent. Their choice proved wise, for the young Englishwoman possessed the "teaching experience and gift of organization" needed to upgrade the training school. Born in 1860, Miss Walker trained at St. Bartholomew's Hospital, London, in a program founded in the wake of the Nightingale reforms. She came to Philadelphia in 1892 to visit relatives and stayed on to serve as superintendent of the Presbyterian Hospital Training School. After three years at Presbyterian, Miss Walker decided to take up the challenge of reorganizing the Pennsylvania Hospital's school.[9]

During her years in Philadelphia, Lucy Walker played an important role in national organizations for nursing. She was a charter member of the American Society of Superintendents of Training Schools, founded in 1893. In 1899 she helped organize the graduate course in hospital economics for nurses offered at Teachers College, Columbia; she was the first choice of the American Society of Superintendents' Education Committee to teach the course. Although Miss Walker declined the post, citing her responsibilities to the Pennsylvania Hospital Training School as her reason, she did give a series of lectures on hospital organization. In the Philadelphia area, Miss Walker was involved in founding a nurses' registry at the Pennsylvania Hospital, a county association of training school alumnae, and a preliminary course of nursing affiliated with the Drexel Institute.[10]

While the outlines of her professional career are clear, Lucy Walker remains an enigmatic person. She was a fine administrator who inspired respect or resentment rather than affection from her students. The official documents of her superintendency clearly reveal her sternness and self-discipline, but provide few glimpses of her other characteristics. She suffered frequent attacks of ill health. In 1903 she had a nervous breakdown after the death of a favorite student. One nurse wrote of her, "Miss Walker had many ups and downs, many worries." She left the nursing profession in 1907 at the age of forty-seven, to take up a "private life." Her personal history suggests the severe emotional and physical strains that professional demands might place on a woman.[11]

Whatever her personal agonies might have been, Lucy Walker had a clear idea of administrative goals and set about achieving them from the day she came to the hospital. Her first concern was to consolidate her authority. As a condition for accepting the post, Miss Walker insisted that she act as both matron of the hospital and superintendent of the training school. Previously, the two jobs had been separate, and the matron and superintendent had numerous disputes over their areas of authority. Miss Walker wanted to avoid such conflict by assuming control over all aspects of nursing service. Thus the quality of nursing education, patient care, and the hospital environment were all her responsibilities. She supervised the housekeeping staff as well as all nursing personnel. In order to perform her new duties, Miss Walker brought two personal assistants with her to act as assistant matron and assistant superintendent.[12]

Miss Walker's next goal was to increase her control over the head nurses, who supervised patient care, housekeeping, and instruction of student nurses on each ward. She began by establishing a sense of her authority. Instead of making the rounds of the wards, Miss Walker remained in her office and had the head nurses report to her. "She came on the wards very little," remembered one head nurse. "Her assistant made the regular rounds morning and evening and made her report to Miss Walker." Then Miss Walker gradually replaced the old nurses with women she had trained. She told the hospital's board of managers in 1897 that nursing care would be unsettled "until I can secure the best of my own graduates for this work." As soon as she had suitable replacements, Miss Walker asked the resignations of the head nurses she considered inefficient or uncooperative, "for the reason that they could not or would not carry out my methods." Miss Walker also did not hesitate to ask her own graduates to resign if they refused to obey her. She fired the night superintendent Sarah McMullin "as she was not in accord with the methods of training, required by the Superintendent." Three more graduate head nurses were dismissed at the end of their first year, "as their influence over the pupils was not what was desired by their Superintendent."[13]

The transition from the old staff to the new did not proceed without tensions. One of Miss Walker's personal assistants aroused resentment because she was "inclined to criticize and make us feel they [the British nurses] were far superior nurses," wrote one head nurse. Of course, the American nurses and doctors disagreed, she observed, "and I know that there were many difficult times for her and for us to overcome." The same nurse said that once the transition was completed, the staff worked more smoothly. "As the positions were filled by our own graduates on the wards and operating room, the atmosphere became better, and we had a better understanding of Miss Walker."[14]

By 1899 Miss Walker had staffed the hospital entirely with Pennsylvania Hospital graduates.[15] The uniformity and obedience she demanded from her nursing staff aided Miss Walker in creating the educational environment she thought necessary for the student nurses. Hierarchy and discipline were the keynotes of her educational philosophy. Having established both in her staff, she now turned to the creation of them in the student body.

The student nurses ranged beneath the nursing staff in their own hierarchy of four classes; senior, intermediate, junior, and probationer. The senior or third-year students acted as assistants to the head nurse of the ward. They delegated and supervised the work of the younger nurses. The intermediate or second-year nurses received their first experience on the more demanding services such as surgery, clinic, and night duty. The junior or first-year nurses performed the basic practical nursing on the wards, such as making beds and feeding and bathing the patients. The probationers occupied the lowest position in the nursing hierarchy; they served six months to a year doing the most menial tasks—caring for the linen and bedpans—before they were "capped" and accepted as students.[16]

Distinctions among the classes of student nurses were recognized in their living arrangements as well as in their ward duties. They lived on separate floors in the nurses' home and ate their meals seated at separate tables. As they filed into the dining room, one nurse remembered, "you would note where those of higher rank took their places." Seniors naturally had the most privileges. For example, they might be invited to join the Nurses' Club or attend the alumnae association's functions.[17]

Every aspect of the student nurses' behavior was regulated by Lucy Walker's rules. All nurses lived on the hospital grounds in the nurses' home. The rules set hours for arising, eating, resting, studying, and retiring. On leaving the home in the morning, each student nurse had to have her room ready for inspection. The rules specified that "before leaving her room, each nurse must remove all bed clothing from the bed, open the window and door, and leave the room to air thoroughly." Nurses had to attend meals punctually and "remain at the table for the time allotted." One of Miss Walker's assistants presided at every meal, "to see that the nurses get their meals comfortably and that they attend regularly and punctually." After eating, the students' napkins and napkin rings had to be placed in pigeonholes outside the dining room.[18]

While on duty, student nurses had to wear a "simply made" uniform of plain blue gingham with a bibbed white apron. The style of cap worn was Lucy Walker's own, the "Sister Dora" cap used by her school in London. As for the rest of the nurse's clothing, it also had to be "simply made" if she expected to have it laundered. "No clothing will be washed that is ruffled, tucked or flounced," Walker's rules decreed.[19]

On the ward and in the classroom, more rules regulated the student nurses. They had to obey "strictly and respectfully" the orders of the nurse in charge. They could not give a patient any medicine or treatment without the order of the physician on duty. While on duty, the students had to treat patients with "the utmost gentleness." They were forbidden to bring their charges any extra food or fruit. No needlework or novel reading was allowed while a nurse was on the ward. In addition to their ward work, the students attended three hours of lectures a week. Special hours were set aside for study for the weekly quizzes given by Miss Walker and her assistants. If a student's grades fell below 75 percent she could be suspended.[20]

Even the little free time given the student nurses was regimented. The rules required them "to go out in the fresh air for at least half an hour daily in fine weather." Miss Walker had the gatekeeper note the time the students went out and came in, so that those not taking their walk might be reprimanded. On their two free afternoons a week, nurses might go out between 10 A.M. and 7 P.M. if they signed out at the gate. No visitors were allowed without Miss Walker's special permission.[21]

The discipline imposed on every aspect of the student's life seems at once trivial and overbearing, but it was not pointless. Miss Walker meant to teach the student nurses discipline and absolute obedience; the enforcement of a strict set of rules was one way to achieve such discipline. Many rules also reflected Miss Walker's concern with the students' health, that they get enough sleep, eat regularly, and get exercise in the fresh air. Since almost every student had a serious illness in her first year of training, these precautions seemed necessary indeed.[22]

Not only was Miss Walker responsible for the students' health, she had to guard their moral characters as well. The reputations of sixty young women away from their parents, many in the city for the first time in their lives, had to be guarded carefully. This was especially important since the nursing profession had a poor reputation; the old image of the female nurse as a servant with suspect morals had not entirely disappeared. The greater responsibilities assigned to the trained nurse also increased concern that she be without reproach. Thus the training school leaders felt that they had to weed out "unsuitable women" to dispel any doubts in the public mind about the morals and abilities of nurses. "We do not stand in the position of colleges and universities," wrote Adelaide Nutting in 1898. "They do not vouch for character, but only for a certain degree of schooling. We stand in a different and peculiar position. We assume a moral responsibility for the character of the nurses we send out." The Pennsylvania Hospital's managers recognized this fact in describing the training school diploma as "a certificate of efficiency and character."[23]

For these reasons, Lucy Walker worked to create an obedient, disciplined body of nurses. But hers was not an isolated, autonomous discipline; another hierarchy existed in the hospital, of which the nurses were a part. They were taught absolute obedience to the doctors as well as their nursing superiors. The doctors' authority seems to have reinforced, rather than conflicted with, that of the nursing staff, however. Although there is ample evidence of conflicts among the nurses, no problems between the nursing staff and the doctors appear in the hospital records. This does not prove that such tensions did not exist, but rather that doctor-nurse conflict was minimized. Lucy Walker undoubtedly cooperated in the effort to minimize it.

In all matters relating to patient care, the physi-

cian remained the final authority. The doctors at the Pennsylvania Hospital stated clearly, "the nurses in the various wards should be under the direction as far as the medical and surgical treatment of the patient is concerned, of the resident physician." The ritual of "rounds" reinforced the division between prescription and treatment as the basis of the doctor-nurse relationship. As the doctors examined the patients each morning, the nurse in charge of the ward followed them around with a special portfolio containing all orders for treatment. After rounds were over, she took the doctors' orders and prepared a treatment board which the other nurses consulted in caring for the patients. The doctors reported any mistakes on the nurses' part in carrying out their orders to the head nurse or Lucy Walker.[24]

The hospital staff during these years consisted of eight residents who lived in the hospital and eight attending or chief physicians, who visited the hospital a few times a week. The number of nurses averaged between sixty and eighty. The permanent nursing staff—the superintendent, her assistants, and the head nurses, all together ten or eleven in number—were undoubtedly well known to the doctors. But the average nursing student had few direct dealings with the doctors. One student remembered that a certain chief physician had the reputation for being able to diagnose a patient's illness from the foot of the bed. "I did not see him do that," she said, "for though a 'cat may look at a king,' a diet nurse could not often look at the 'Big Chief' when he was making his rounds." The same student said she "broke all the rules of the training school, by daring to exclaim out loud in the presence of the chief."[25]

The nurses knew the doctors—even if only by reputation—much better than the doctors knew them. Doctors' abilities, amusing habits, and annoying traits formed the staple of a nurses' folklore. When asked to reminisce, they told such stories at length. It was unusual, on the other hand, for a doctor to know a nurse's name. One nurse said approvingly of the chief surgeon, "He was beloved by everyone because he had such a gracious manner and was the one 'Big Chief' who always remembered a nurse's name, and addressed her by it when he had occasion to speak to her." Several other residents were praised because "they were such perfect gentlemen always, and a nurse's word was never questioned by them." Such remarks suggest that not knowing a nurse's name, questioning her word, and being less than gracious were common behavior on the part of some doctors.[26]

More frequently, however, nurses provided some doctors with the opportunity to indulge their paternal instincts. One resident recalled a representative scene between doctor and nurse: "Dr. Richard Harte's specialty was the kind of shoes the nurses wore. Many times those of us who worked with him have seen some innocent little nurse—probably a probationer—stopped in her tracks and accosted by, 'Matilda, why don't you wear sensible shoes?' She was then and there given a lecture on the proper type of footwear." (Dr. Harte does seem to have known his victim's name, unless he called all nurses "Matilda," which is a possibility.) Doctors evidently preferred such paternalism to romantic interests in the nurses. Only one romance involving a student nurse and a resident physician appeared in the disciplinary records during Miss Walker's tenure. She must have sensed some potential danger, however, for nurses were "strictly forbidden to go to the doctors' rooms for any reason."[27]

The student nurses had one other form of contact with the medical staff, their class lectures. Members of the staff gave regular courses of lectures to the nurses. This job was little sought after by the doctors, possibly because the student nurses were not always appreciative. The students had to be reprimanded for talking in lecture and copying one another's notes. Lucy Walker lamented that the younger nurses were not always able to "appreciate the good advice of the experienced members of the medical staff" given in the lectures.[28]

Most contacts between doctor and nurse reinforced the inequality of their relationship. For the most part, doctors were distant and authoritative. They delivered orders and examinations with equal decisiveness. They inspired awe when present, yet were rarely present. The real people with day-to-day power in the student nurses' lives were Lucy Walker and her staff. This may help explain the relative absence of direct conflict between nurses and doctors. The physicians left matters relating to the student nurses to Miss Walker. It was in their best interests to enforce her authority so that the hospital staff would function smoothly. In turn, Miss Walker worked well with the physicians because she put patient care—the hospital's main interest—before the interests of the students.

Yet Lucy Walker's principles and personality were only one determining factor in shaping the training school atmosphere. Having examined her principles, we must now consider the students' influence on the socialization process. They were not passive recipients of Miss Walker's educational philosophy but played a significant part in shaping the training school environment; their background and goals defined a major component of their professional experience. Fortunately, we can examine their contribution to the training school environment through the student records kept by Miss Walker. Information on 205 women entering the training school between 1898 and 1909 provides an idea of the type of women going into nursing, and their individual careers as nursing students.[29]

Applicants had to conform to certain basic requirements established by the training school. They had to be between twenty-one and thirty-five years of age, and of "at least average height and physique." They needed a "common school education," which was defined as the ability to "read aloud well, to write legibly and accurately, to understand arithmetic as far as fractions and percent, and to take notes at lectures." This amount of education was "indispensable," concluded the application form, but women "of superior education and refinement take precedence."[30]

The women accepted by the Pennsylvania Hospital Training School under these guidelines were usually young; 60 percent were between twenty-one and twenty-four years old, 88 percent were under thirty. All but two of the students were single. The exceptions were a childless doctor's widow, aged thirty-four, and a twenty-three-year-old who had "made an unfortunate marriage" and been deserted by her husband.[31] Though the application form did not specify that a woman must be single to be accepted, this must in practice have been a requirement.

Most of the student nurses had grown up in small or medium-sized towns. Only 9 percent were born in Philadelphia. Strikingly few came from other cities, probably because those cities possessed their own training schools. Of the Pennsylvania students, half were born in towns with populations under 2,500. Another third came from towns between 2,500 and 10,000 in population. The out-of-state students (29%) also came from small towns in New York, New Jersey, Maryland, Virginia, Ohio, and Indiana. Eight percent were natives of Ontario, 5 percent of the British Isles.

Not surprisingly, considering their predominantly small-town origins, the nursing students were, with the exception of one Roman Catholic, all Protestants. The majority (62%) were Presbyterians, Episcopalians, and Methodists; 8 percent each were Lutherans and Baptists; the remainder were Quakers, Congregationalists, Moravians, Reformed or United Brethren.

The students had a wide range of educational backgrounds. Forty-nine percent had at least a high school diploma. Another 17½ percent had completed eighth grade and a few years of high school. Only 16½ percent had not finished eighth grade. Seventeen percent had been educated entirely in private schools of uncertain academic level. The education of many had been piecemeal. (Requirements for postgraduate work were casual at this time; women entered colleges or normal schools who had failed to complete high school.) They also had pursued a variety of special educational programs, including business schools, art schools, conservatories of music, schools of elocution, and training schools for kindergarten or missionary work.

Half of the student nurses had had no occupation other than "home life" before entering the training school. Most of these women were under twenty-four (69%). The small number of older women who had never been employed before had all had some family obligation which prevented them from pursuing their own interests at an earlier age. Once that family obligation ended, they applied to the training school. The older women had kept house for widowed fathers and unmarried brothers, or nursed sick relatives until well past the age for marriage; then death or a male relative's marriage set them free. Margaret Derrickson's case is typical. She helped her mother run a private school for many years. When her mother became an invalid, she took over the school. After her mother's death, Margaret entered the training school.[32]

Half of the student nurses had some occupation before entering the training school. As a group they were slightly older than the never-employed students.[33] Teaching had been their most common occupation (45%). Many of the women had taught for only a short time before leaving the profession, but a few had taught as many as fifteen years before taking up nursing. The new clerical trades opening up for women in the late nineteenth century had provided jobs for 21 percent of the employed nurses. They had held positions as stenographers, clerks, and bookkeepers. Several had worked for newspapers as proofreaders and compositor-typesetters. Two women had been telephone operators. As with teaching, the length of time spent at this work before entering the training school varied greatly. Only 5 percent of the nurses had made their living by sewing, as dressmakers, milliners, or shirtwaist makers. The only two women in the group who had done factory work were involved in the needle trades. One woman had been an instructor in sewing machine operation, the other a foreman in a hosiery mill.

The nursing profession clearly attracted women with varying backgrounds and motivations. Some did not have to earn a living but were drawn by the idealism of the nursing profession. Theirs was a mission; as one alumna put it, "Never feel that your profession is necessarily for a livelihood, but reach out and attain your ideals." A nursing student from an upper-class background distinguished between the "Nurse who comes for the doubly noble reason of making her own living and doing good . . . and those like myself who come with a more sentimental idea."[34]

For the educated women, nursing was probably a respectable alternative to medical school. The number of women possessing at least a high school degree is striking. Men with similar educational backgrounds would have had no difficulty in entering medical school. As late as 1910, only two medical schools in Pennsylvania required applicants to have a high school diploma. This may reflect poorly on the status of medical education, but gives a good indication of the caliber of women going into nursing school. If they had been male, they might well have become doctors rather than nurses. This suggests that women were choosing nursing as a more fitting career than medicine.

Helen McClelland, who entered the training school in 1908, remembered that two graduates of the school told her that the "nursing profession was of more value for women than medicine unless one was going into the mission fields."[35]

For others, nursing was a livelihood rather than a profession. For many girls from small towns, nursing probably functioned as domestic service had for an earlier generation. It facilitated a rural to urban migration of women for whom there were fewer and fewer opportunities at home. It offered training in work considered natural for a woman, within a tightly structured, morally reassuring environment. Once the degree was obtained, work was plentiful and provided a chance for social mobility. The small-town girl nursing in an urban middle-class family could pick up their values and mannerisms, and perhaps enable herself to marry a more upwardly mobile man.[36]

The number of women who left another occupation for nursing suggests more concrete reasons for its popularity. In terms of wages, nursing compared favorably to teaching, clerical work, and factory work. In addition to room and board, hospital work paid an average of $35 a month for head nurses, $50 to $100 for nurse administrators. Pay for private duty work varied, but averaged between $15 and $20 a week. Teaching paid only $25 to $30 a week, clerical work, between $11 and $14 a week, and factory work $9 a week. The demand for both hospital and private duty nurses was consistently high during these decades as well.[37]

The educational and employment histories of the nursing students indicate that nursing neither attracted nor accepted urban working-class women. The predominance of Protestants from small towns shows that few recent immigrants entered the training school. The absence of women who had done factory work further supports this impression. Instead, the student biographies suggest that women came to nursing from a wide range of backgrounds within the broad category of the "middle class." A few were upper-middle-class women of "refinement" with exceptionally good educations; others were small-town girls who had failed to finish the eighth grade. Within these extremes, there were many gradations.

The biographies of four members of the class of 1904 illustrate this variety more concretely. Ella Ferguson, born in Philadelphia, age twenty-two,

had completed two years of high school and gone to business college. Since then she had worked as a clerk. Her classmate Mary Hale, born in Virginia, age thirty-two, had gone to art school. After six months in Europe, she found a position as a governess and companion. Mary Swank, born in Lancaster, Pennsylvania, age twenty-eight, had been educated in a "country school" and attended a few years of high school. Until entering the training school, she had lived with a married brother and cared for his invalid wife. Her classmate Ella Tomlinson, from Westtown, Pennsylvania, age twenty-two, graduated from Westtown Boarding School and taught three years in a private Friends' school.[38]

The mixture of motivations and backgrounds among the student nurses posed special problems for Lucy Walker. Teaching, discipline, even living arrangements were made more difficult by the disparity in education and experience. Miss Walker reminded the board of managers of this difficulty when she requested an enlargement of the nurses' home. She wrote, "It is very trying, and in some cases, a severe ordeal, for women of refinement to be obliged to share their rooms, more especially in a Training School as mixed as one of this size must necessarily be."[39] Miss Walker's strict discipline was undoubtedly aimed at controlling the potentially disruptive social differences among the student nurses. Enforcing a recognized code of discipline made up for the lack of shared, mutually understood standards of behavior. But as in any would-be "total" institution, there were cracks in the discipline, cracks which the students explored and exploited. Discipline problems did develop, and the type and pattern of infractions most frequently committed reveal important aspects of the training school regimen and the professional standards which shaped it.

The most common discipline problem was, naturally, disobedience. This term applied not only to direct defiance of the "authorities," as Miss Walker referred to herself and her staff; it also included any departure from the rules which seemed in the least deliberate. Thus if a student nurse forgot to take a patient's temperature or relabeled a bottle carelessly, she was disobedient; she had strayed from her prescribed duties.

Patterns of open disobedience reveal stresses among the nursing staff. Few students dared to be impertinent to Miss Walker or her assistants, but they were less respectful to the head nurses. Being rude, impertinent, disrespectful, or disobedient to a head nurse was a common misdemeanor. The number of staff members also opened up the possibilities for playing them off against one another. For example, Eleanor Cadbury "appeal[ed] to the night superintendent against the Head Nurse." Marianne Wood went to Lucy Walker "to make complaint of the night superintendent." Another student, Mary Groff, chose another means for annoying her nursing superior; she "made trouble by setting the patient against the head nurse of the ward."[40] The frequency of such incidents makes Miss Walker's concern with the quality of her head nurses more understandable. Any conflict of opinion among the head nurses, or with the night superintendent, could easily be used by the students to evade her strict discipline.

Relations between senior and junior nurses also developed special strains. Some senior nurses exploited their younger charges. Miss Walker noted on one nurse's record, "spends too much time on lists; younger nurses given her work to do." Other seniors were too rough or showed a "want of tact" with the younger nurses. The result was irritation between senior and junior nurses. Seniors also used their power to protect the younger nurses. Miss Walker reported to the board of managers that "some of the senior nurses placed in charge, do not realize the responsibilities of their positions, and . . . will not report irregularities to the Head Nurse." Some seniors, like Elizabeth Arnold, were guilty of "doing [the junior nurses'] work rather than seeing that it is done."[41] Neither irritation nor collusion between the senior and junior nurses made for the proper hospital discipline in Lucy Walker's estimation.

The student nurses occasionally banded together in their acts of rebellion. Miss Walker was especially wary of the influence of troublemakers in the school. For example, Marianne Wood concerned her because of her "troublesome" effect on the other nurses. Miss Walker wrote that she "stirs up the other nurses, and promised to use her influence to protect them." A full-scale defiance took place in May 1899. Fourteen students—a quarter of the student body that year—signed a petition to the board of managers protesting the dismissal of a fellow student, and asking that she be reinstated. Miss Walker acted quickly to squash that action.

She demanded an apology or threatened dismissal for every nurse who signed the petition. She received the apologies, although she felt that several did so only to save themselves from dismissal, and "did not honestly regret [their] action."[42]

Senior nurses often became unruly in more subtle ways in the last months of their terms. Since they were leaving soon, they disregarded rules without fear of serious consequence. This behavior distressed Miss Walker because it tended to unsettle all the student nurses. In 1899, she suggested to the managers that such nurses not be given the silver badge awarded to graduates of the school. Miss Walker wrote,

> Some of the nurses when within a short time of completing their term, grow careless in their work or conduct. . . . At the present time, four of those who leave very soon are setting a bad example in the school by their careless work and conduct. No one offence committed is of a very serious nature, nor such as to warrant any severe measure being taken; but all together, their actions are such as to attract the attention of the nurses, and to merit the disapproval of those in authority.[43]

Next to defiance of authority, the student nurses' work habits proved to be the most troublesome disciplinary problem. According to Lucy Walker's standards, many nurses failed to perform their duties with the proper attitude and method. They fell asleep on special duty or acted half-asleep even when awake. They were too slow or too fussy.[44]

The worst infractions of discipline involved mistakes in executing the physicians' orders. Such errors might have disastrous consequences for the patients. They were scalded with hot water bags while unconscious, blistered with burning alcohol and turpentine, and dosed with too much medicine. Patients were given medicine, douches, cuppings, and doses of salts meant for other individuals. Student nurses neglected to take temperatures or give sponge baths to the fevered. One nurse went so far as to record false temperatures to avoid giving a typhoid fever patient a sponge bath. Such actions must have done little to increase the patients' or the doctors' confidence in the student nurses' ability. Miss Walker noted in one case that a "nervous private patient was very much alarmed" when he discovered that a student had filled up his water pitcher with carbolic acid. Although errors made "rather through ignorance than actual carelessness" might merit only a reprimand, mistakes due "to carelessness and disobedience"—for example, by failing to look at a bottle's label before giving medicine—were punished severely, sometimes by dismissal.[45]

The nursing students' relationships with the patients caused recurrent discipline problems. The young women had difficulty in steering the proper line between being too "familiar" with their charges and being cruel to them. The most common infraction was being too friendly or "familiar" with patients, especially men. Frequently student nurses had to be removed from the men's wards for not maintaining the proper distance, emotionally or physically, from the patients. Walker described them as too "free and easy" and lacking "the proper dignity." One nurse was nearly suspended when she was found "dancing before the patients in the ward." Nurses were discouraged from talking too much to any of the patients, male or female, and having favorites among them. The students developed similar problems with orderlies. Emilie Cox, for example, earned Miss Walker's disapproval when she resigned from the school and "married very shortly after, one of the men employed in the hospital."[46] Such incidents suggest that since some of the students found enough in common with the male patients and orderlies to flirt with them, the two groups may have been similar in background.

Student nurses were also frequently reprimanded for roughness, rudeness, and neglect of their charges. Ida White, for example, failed to show the proper respect by "talking loudly with another nurse, on personal affairs, in a room with two dying men."[47] The dismissals of Eva Taylor and Marianne Wood for striking patients illustrate some of the personal dynamics which might lead to conflict between patient and nurse. Eva Taylor slapped a woman on her ward named Stella White. Stella White, according to the head nurse on duty, became angry at Miss Taylor for refusing to "wait on her" during the night and making her get her own breakfast tray. Miss Taylor said the patient became "impudent and rude, talking loud and noisy and in the most disrespectful manner about nurses, hospitals, *etc. etc.*" Miss Taylor lost her control and

struck Stella White on the mouth. She said, "I o ly wanted to teach her a lesson."[48]

When Eva Taylor was dismissed, another student, Marianne Wood, wrote a letter to the chairman of the board of managers defending Miss Taylor's action. Her letter reveals the kind of anger at patients which prompted student nurses' blows. She wrote:

> I can only say if you had been in her place, I think it is more than likely you would have sympathy with her as I do. The patients on "G" ward are the very lowest class of women and can frequently only be kept in order by taking extreme measures. . . . If Miss Taylor is to be expelled for this . . . in justice to yourselves and the other nurses you should go thoroughly through the training school and expel numerous other nurses who have done the same thing. . . . They are allowed to hit us and swear at us, and spit at us, not to mention calling us the most *vile* names and it is not to be wondered at if we lose our patience now and then.

Miss Wood mentioned that she herself had struck a patient who refused to lie still in her bed after an operation. The board of managers immediately dismissed Miss Wood on the basis of this statement. She brought a lawsuit protesting their action, but was never reinstated.[49]

Such incidents suggest class conflict between middle-class nurses and working-class patients. Conflict was inevitable when young women with middle-class standards of behavior were asked to supervise individuals whose action and language offended them. The nurses did not know how to manage their social inferiors with the correct combination of tact and authority advocated by Lucy Walker—and thus they resorted to force.

Other discipline problems suggest class differences of another sort. Nurses from rural and lower-middle-class backgrounds could not conform to the ideal of restraint, dignity, and ladylike behavior required by Miss Walker. From the student records, Miss Walker's preference for women of refinement is very clear. Her notion of refinement included a good education, a quiet manner, and a neat appearance. Such qualities were pleasing and attractive to her. Women who lacked refinement were equally unpleasant. She found them "loud in talk" and "loud in dress." Their manners were rough and uncouth; their appearance was untidy and undignified. They tended to be troublesome and, in Miss Walker's estimation, of doubtful trustworthiness.[50]

But the discipline problems point to another type of conflict in the training school—a conflict between levels of professional ability and consciousness. The student nurse's response to discipline— her behavior with the patients, her work habits, her attitude toward authority—all went into the training school's final evaluation of her professional ability as well as her character. In the student records, Miss Walker assessed each individual's suitability for either hospital work or private duty nursing. While social class certainly entered into her professional opinion of a nurse, Miss Walker had another standard which might conflict with her class bias. Women of refinement did not necessarily excel at the training school; they had to have more than their manners to recommend them.[51]

The real elite of the training school were the nurses deemed fit for "institutional work." The training school regimen was designed to produce nurses who were "trained to train," to go into training school work themselves.[52] Those who did not meet this high expectation became private nurses. The distinction between hospital nursing and private duty work shaped the training school's definition of a good nurse.

One aim of the training school was to produce a good private duty nurse. She needed to have a good character; she must perform her work reliably, prove herself trustworthy, and behave correctly with men. She had to have an even-tempered, cheerful disposition. She had to know the rudiments of practical nursing, which included bed making, bathing, and massaging the patient, and preparing the proper sick diet. She had to be physically strong and mentally alert. She should also be refined in manner, but refined manners were not an essential requirement. Miss Walker felt that a good, clean country girl would make a fine private duty nurse for a middle-class family. Women who met these basic requirements were given good recommendations for private duty nursing. Miss Walker's typical evaluation for this sort of student ran, "Very pleasing personality, fair average ability,

below average in class work but a good practical worker. Should make an excellent private nurse."[53]

A different set of standards applied to the woman "suited for institutional work." The requirements were far more rigorous, but the reward in terms of prestige much greater. The hallmark of the hospital nurse was her ability to manage others. She must have displayed "executive ability" and have proved herself a "good manager" on the wards. Miss Walker characterized such a student as having "special aptitude for planning work and taking responsibility . . . can do her own work and see that others work, too. If she enters a ward in an upset condition, in a short time all is quiet and peaceful."[54]

The hospital nurse had to be intelligent in order to manage the theoretical side of her work, but she also had to possess good common sense. Her work habits were very important; hospital work demanded that she be systematic, steady, and attentive to detail. Sentimentality and emotion were traits the hospital nurse could not afford to indulge. She needed to be "mentally well-balanced." Hysterical women were useless in hospital emergencies. The hospital nurse could not be too "easily excited" or "given to tears." She had to be able to manage a large number of patients and student nurses without panicking.[55]

Dedication was another requirement. In hospital work, a nurse could not be "afraid she may do more than her own share of work," or "inclined to be anxious about herself." Her mind had to be on her work; she could not "think too much of her time off duty." In personal appearance, the hospital nurse had to be "refined." Her dress had to be neat and tidy, never frivolous or "superficial." Most of all, she must have no interest in the "admiration" of men. A woman might be a good manager and an excellent nurse, but not be suited for institutional work, "as she seeks the admiration of men, first."[56]

Finally, the good hospital nurse had to have the proper respect for authority. She had to obey orders without being too "assertive." She could not be "inclined to go ahead of herself." At the same time, she could not be too timid.[57] For the hospital nurse, there was a careful line to be taken between being too respectful of authority and being too self-assertive.

The student nurses who met such difficult requirements became part of a self-conscious elite within the training school. They were highly recommended for hospital work and usually received excellent positions either within the Pennsylvania Hospital or in other hospital training schools.[58] Hospital nurses formed the Nurses' Club, the alumnae association, and the Guild of St. Bartholomew, professional organizations which served a social function as well. They kept in touch with each other through various organizations for nurses at the state and national levels.[59]

For graduates doing hospital work in Philadelphia, the Pennsylvania Hospital Nurses' Alumnae Association served as a focus for their professional and social ties with one another. The alumnae association was open to all graduates of the training school, whether doing private duty or hospital work. The graduates in hospital work dominated the leadership of the association, however; they served as its officers and faithfully attended its bimonthly business meetings. The president of the alumnae association for six of its most active years, Charlotte E. Perkins, was the head of the Maternity Hospital's training school in Philadelphia. Other particularly active members were the head nurses and the superintendent's assistants of the Pennsylvania Hospital.[60]

The purpose of the alumnae association as stated in its bylaws was "the promotion of unity and good feeling among the alumnae, the elevation of professional character, the protection of professional interests, and the establishment of a fund for the benefit of any sick among its members." To this end, the association participated in the American Nurses Association (the national organization of trained nurses), helped to found nurse registries, supported the *American Journal of Nursing*, and worked for the state registration of nurses. The meetings of the alumnae served as a forum for discussion of various professional issues. Papers were presented on such topics as "the nurse in her relation and responsibility to the patient," institutional nursing, and social service work. As might be expected, the interests of the hospital nurses predominated.[61]

Another organization within the hospital, the Guild of St. Bartholomew, promoted both religious and social aims. Under its auspices, a prayer service was held every morning for the hospital nurses. A regular monthly meeting was held "for

the reading and discussion of some article or book religious in nature." Every three months, a social meeting was held. One participant reported to the *American Journal of Nursing* that these evenings "are always enjoyable, and often novel in the nature of the entertainment." Students could join, and alumnae could retain membership after leaving the school.[62]

Pennsylvania Hospital nurses also formed social ties with nurses in other training schools in Philadelphia. With the other alumnae associations of Philadelphia schools, they formed a Nurses' Club which sponsored frequent social gatherings. The alumnae attended teas, dance and card parties, holiday celebrations, and informal social hours at the Nurses' Club. They contributed money to make the clubhouse more attractive and comfortable. Thus the hospital nurses' professional contacts furnished them with a social life as well.[63]

For those graduates doing hospital work, nursing became a true profession. Their training school experience made them conscious of a special professional identity and shaped their dedication to the upgrading of the public image of nursing. They worked to "raise the standard and establish an atmosphere that encouraged the public to consider the real trained nurse."[64] Their circle was not an all-inclusive one, however. The majority of nurses stayed outside their "little world." They passed through the training school, endured its discipline, and then went on to make their living as private duty nurses.[65] For them nursing remained a livelihood rather than a profession. They benefited from the professional activities of their fellow nurses, but did not actively work for them.

The history of late-nineteenth-century nursing, then, must be understood in terms of the *variety* of women going into the work, and the limited meaning of professionalization for the majority of nurses. The training school itself must be viewed as an institution which brought together women of diverse origin and motivation, and integrated them into a working organization. The discipline problems reveal fault lines in its organization—between nurses and their superintendent, nurses and patients, and among the nurses themselves. These same lines of conflict have persisted in varied forms to this day, and for many of the same reasons.

In one respect, however, the end of Lucy Walker's career marked the end of an era in nursing history. Having transmitted a heritage of British methods to American hospitals, she was followed by American nurses who took the lead in adapting those forms to the twentieth-century hospital. Miss Walker left behind a legacy of excellence and the example, as one nurse said, of "a person who had the ability and nursing at heart, and was doing all she could to impress the nursing world and put it on the highest level."[66]

NOTES

1 The phrase "little world of our own" comes from Mary Knabb, "Looking backward," speech, n.d., 5, School of Nursing Papers, Pennsylvania Hospital Archives. All manuscript material hereafter cited is in the Pennsylvania Hospital Archives. Standard nursing histories all concentrate on national leaders and organizations. See, for example, Lavinia Dock, *A History of Nursing,* 3 vols. (New York, 1912); Richard Shryock, *The History of Nursing* (Philadelphia, 1959); and Isabel Stewart and Anne Austin, *A History of Nursing* (New York, 1962). There are several excellent descriptive histories of individual training schools; see Ethel Johns and Blanche Pfeffercorn, *The Johns Hopkins Hospital School of Nursing, 1889– 1949* (Baltimore, 1954); Eleanor Lee, *History of the School of Nursing of the Presbyterian Hospital, 1892– 1942* (New York, 1942); Grace F. Schryver, *A History of the Illinois Training School for Nurses, 1880– 1929* (Chicago, 1930); and Mary Stephenson, *The First Fifty Years of the Training School for Nurses of the Hospital of the University of Pennsylvania* (Philadelphia, 1940)—but they too concentrate primarily on nursing leaders and advances in nursing education. Jo Ann Ashley, *Hospitals, Paternalism and the Role of the Nurse* (New York, 1976), comes closest to dealing with the professionalization of nursing as it affected the average nurse, but her book is an interpretive essay rather than a detailed history using individual training school records.

2 A brief but thoughtful discussion of the professionalization of nursing is Richard Shryock, "Nursing emerges as a profession." *Clio Medica,* 1968, 3:131– 47. See also Ashley, *Hospitals.*

3 Arthur Meigs, "The old nursing and the new," address given to the graduating class of the Pennsylvania Hospital Training School in 1897, privately printed, 4, School of Nursing Papers. The proto-professionalism of some nurses in the prereform era is discussed by Charles Rosenberg, "And heal the sick: the hospital and the patient in nineteenth century America," *Journal of Social History,* 1977, 10:434–35.

4 Meigs, "The old nursing," 4.

5 Women's Committee Minutes, 12 June 1867; Roberta West, *History of Nursing in Pennsylvania* (Harrisburg, 1939), 573.

6 Board of Managers, Annual report to contributors, 1876, 10; Board of Managers Minutes, 27 October 1879, 11:82.

7 Meigs, "The old nursing," 5, 8; "A bit of history of the Pennsylvania Hospital School of Nursing," n.d., School of Nursing Papers; Meigs, "The old nursing," 8.

8 "Report of managers Garrett, Shinn and Levis," 28 May 1895, Board of Managers, Special Committee Reports; Sarah McMullin, "Reminiscences," 3 February 1941, 4, School of Nursing Papers.

9 Board of Managers Minutes, 28 October 1895, 12: 17; West, *History,* 658, 573.

10 West, *History,* 658; Dock, *History of nursing* 3: 132; L. Walker to B. Shoemaker, 5 September 1899, School of Nursing Papers; *American Journal of Nursing,* 1900, 1: 36; Nurses' Alumnae Association Minutes, 15 June 1904, 2: 142–43; ibid., 6 December 1901, 2: 76; L. Walker to Board of Managers, 28 April 1902, School of Nursing Papers.

11 Board of Managers Minutes, 27 August 1903; 12: 247; McMullin, "Reminiscences," 9–10; West, *History,* 575; Board of Managers Minutes, 29 July 1907, 12: 473. Lucy Walker became the adopted heir and companion of a relative in Pittsburgh, taking the name Donnel. See Nurses' Alumnae Association of the Pennsylvania Hospital Training School, *Alumnae Notes,* January 1908, 11.

12 Board of Managers Minutes, 28 October 1895, 12: 17.

13 McMullin, "Reminiscences," 6; Superintendent's Report, July 1896, School of Nursing Papers; ibid., April 1900 and March 1906. It is interesting that Miss Walker, to increase her authority, distanced herself from the bedside aspects of patient care. The split between the nurse's role in administration and patient care has received considerable attention from sociologists as a major source of conflict within the modern nursing profession. See Fred Davis, "Nurses," in *The Semi-Professions and Their Organization,* ed. Amitai Etzioni (New York, 1969), 54–81.

14 McMullin, "Reminiscences," 6.

15 Superintendent's Report, October 1900.

16 This outline of the student nurses' duties was put together from the Record of the Training School, 1894–98; Superintendent's Reports; and Helen

McClelland, "Reminiscences," n.d., School of Nursing Papers.

17 McMullin, "Reminiscences," 6; McClelland, "Reminiscences," 2; Nurses' Club Minutes; Alumnae Association Minutes (such invitations were frequent).

18 "Rules for nurses," manuscript in Lucy Walker's handwriting, n.d., School of Nursing Papers; Superintendent's Report, April 1896; McClelland, "Reminiscences," 2.

19 "Rules for nurses"; Margaret Dunlop, "Speech at capping exercises," 1936, 1, School of Nursing Papers. "Rules for nurses."

20 "Rules for nurses"; Superintendent's Report, April 1901 and April 1896.

21 Superintendent's Report, April 1896; McMullin, "Reminiscences," 6–7; "Rules for nurses."

22 Health records for the students were kept in the Record of the Training School, 1894–98, the Nurses' Record no. 1, 1899–1906, and no. 2, 1906–10.

23 Helen Marshall, *Mary Adelaide Nutting* (Baltimore, 1972), 90; "Return and answer of contributors and managers to writ of alternative mandamus issued in the case of Marianne Wood," December 1900, Marianne Wood file, Board of Managers Papers.

24 "Residents' reply to Lucy Walker," 1896, School of Nursing Papers.

25 Knabb, "Looking backward," 3; Mary Knabb, "Memories of Dr. Thomas G. Morton," 18 January 1938, McClelland file no. 2, School of Nursing Papers.

26 Knabb, "Looking backward"; Knabb, "Memories"; McClelland, "Reminiscences" are good examples of this tendency.

27 Dr. Charles Mitchell, "Speech to graduating nurses," 1935, 4–5, School of Nursing Papers. Caroline Case was reprimanded for sitting in the summerhouse with a resident; see Record of the Training School, 166; "Rules for nurses."

28 Board of Managers Minutes, 29 July 1889, 11: 429; L. Walker to B. Shoemaker, July 1896, School of Nursing Papers.

29 This information was compiled from the Record of the Training and the Nurses' Records no. 1 and 2.

30 "Rules for nurses."

31 Nurses' Record no. 1, 291; Nurses' Record no. 2, 71.

32 For the life histories of the older, never-employed women, see Nurses' Record no. 1, 163, 181, 187, 225, 245, 283; Nurses' Record no. 2, 15, 21, 83. Margaret Derrickson's record is in Nurses' Record no. 1, 163.

33 The following table gives comparative ages for employed and unemployed students:

	employed	never employed
ages 21–24	56%	69%
ages 25–29	33%	22%
ages 30–35	11%	9%

34 Nurses' Alumnae Association Minutes, 19 June 1906, 1: 198–99; M. Wood to "Pupil nurses in training at the Pennsylvania Hospital," August 1900, Marianne Wood file, Board of Managers Papers.

35 Abraham Flexner, *Medical Education in the United States and Canada* (1910; reprint ed., Buffalo, N.Y., 1973), 198–99; McClelland, "Reminiscences," 1.

36 The similarities between nursing and domestic service are suggested by J. Jean Hecht, *The Domestic Servant Class in 18th Century England* (London, 1956), and Theresa McBride, *The Domestic Revolution* (Chicago, 1976).

37 Statistics on nurses' wages were taken from the Steward's Monthly Accounts, 1890–1915; see also Marshall, *Nutting*, 94; for other wage information, see United States Department of Labor, Women's Bureau Bulletin no. 225, *Handbook of Facts on Women Workers* (Washington, D.C., 1928).

38 These four student histories were taken from Nurses' Record no. 1, 189, 201, 187, 221.

39 Superintendent's Report, April 1899.

40 See, for example, the Record of the Training School, 84, 166; Nurses' Record no. 1, 173, 293; Nurses' Record no. 2, 99. Quotations come from the Record of the Training School, 176, 164, 98.

41 Nurses' Record no. 2, 49; Superintendent's Report, April 1901; Nurses' Record no.2, 49.

42 Record of the Training School, 164; Nurses' Record no. 1, 3, 5; Record of the Training School, 172, 182.

43 Superintendent's Report, October 1899.

44 This is a very common complaint. See, for example, Record of the Training School, 98, 140; Nurses' Record no. 2, 5, 29, 79.

45 For a few examples, see Record of the Training School, 78, 84, 122, 124, 126; Nurses' Record no. 1, 173. Quotations come from Record of the Training School, 394, 200; Nurses' Record no. 2, 83, 95; Record of the Training School, 96, 100, 140; Nurses' Record no. 1, 55; Nurses' Record no. 2, 57.

46 Record of the Training School, 96, 100, 140; Nurses' Record no. 1, 55; Nurses' Record no. 2, 57, 81; Record of the Training School, 84, 106; Nurses' Record no. 1, 5, 55.

47 Record of the Training School, 60.

48 "Statement of Mary E. Wittaker, Head Nurse"; and E. Taylor to L. Walker, 10 August 1900, Marianne Wood file, Board of Managers Papers.

49 M. Wood to Mr. Townsend, 11 August 1900, Board of Managers Papers.

50 See, for example, Record of the Training School, 212; Nurses' Record no. 1, 211, 253, 261, 265; Nurses' Record no. 2, 6, 109. Quotations are from Record of Training School, 397; Nurses' Record no. 1, 57, 157.

51 See Record of Training School, 182; Nurses' Record no. 1, 253.

52 Shryock, *History,* 281.

53 Nurses' Record, no. 2, 35; see also Record of the Training School, 182; Nurses' Record no. 2, 29, 53.

54 Nurses' Record no. 1, 145, Lucy Walker used the phrases "good manager" and "executive ability" frequently.

55 Record of the Training School, 148; Nurses' Record no. 1, 53, 65, 195, 197; Record of the Training School, 69; Nurses' Record no. 2, 89; Record of the Training School, 118; Nurses' Record no. 1, 9, 133; Nurses' Record no. 2, 51, 55.

56 Record of the Training School, 176; Nurses' Record no. 2, 33; Record of the Training School, 222; Nurses' Record no. 2, 17; Nurses' Record no. 1, 171, 113, 149, 199.

57 Nurses' Record no. 2, 45; Nurses' Record no. 1, 291; Record of the Training School, 56; Nurses' Record no. 2, 5.

58 See, for example, the entry for Janet McBride in Record of the Training School, 69. She became night superintendent of the Pennsylvania Hospital. Anna Groff and Emma Lindberg—Record of the Training School, 62, 130—both became head nurses.

59 Nurses' Club Minutes, 55–57; and Nurses' Alumnae Association Minutes, 1: 76–77, and 2: 68, 128.

60 Nurses' Alumnae Association Minutes, 1: 164–65, and 2: 102, 133.

61 Ibid., vol. 2, printed bylaws tipped in between 16 and 17. Sample paper topics taken from 139, 149.

62 *American Journal of Nursing,* 1900, 1:315.

63 Nurses' Alumnae Association Minutes, 1: 38, and 2: 66, 113.

64 Nurses' Alumnae Association Minutes, 15 November 1913, 2: 114.

65 In 1914, a count of Pennsylvania Hospital Training School alumnae showed that of the 105 nurses in Philadelphia, almost 60 percent were doing private duty work. Since a sizable number of women probably married and left nursing entirely, the percentage of women doing hospital work would be an even smaller number of the total alumnae. Nurses' Alumnae Association Minutes, 21 January 1914, 2: 136.

66 McMullin, "Reminiscences," 9.

34

More than "The Physician's Hand": Skill and Authority in Twentieth-Century Nursing

BARBARA MELOSH

In the complex organization of health care, nurses occupy an intermediate position that reveals much about the definition of skill, the sexual division of labor, and the meaning of power and inequality at work. Second to the physician in the medical chain of command, they reign over the rest of the hospital hierarchy. Paid far less than doctors, and less than men with comparable education and experience, nurses still enjoy higher wages and more job security than most women workers. Disadvantaged by gender, they are largely privileged by race—most nurses are white, the supervisors of women of color below them in the hierarchy. They hold an intermediate class position, drawn from working-class and middle-class families. Associated with "dirty" work in a host of popular images from cartoons to pornography, nurses also share the aura of prestige and awe that surrounds the layperson's view of esoteric medicine. The truism rings true: nursing is a good job—for a woman.

Nursing has always been a woman's job, and the structural relationship between doctors and nurses has persisted over decades of dramatic change in the setting and practice of health care. By law and custom, nurses are subordinate to physicians: in this sense they have been and still are "the physician's hand." In the new scholarship that accompanied the revitalized women's movement of the late sixties, feminists often took nursing as emblematic of the persistence of patriarchal relations: paid work, far from liberating women, might only reflect and confirm their subordination. Like other women's paid work, the argument went, nursing reproduces the social relations of domestic life: at

BARBARA MELOSH is Assistant Professor of English and American Studies at George Mason University, Fairfax, Virginia, and Curator in the Division of Medical Sciences at the National Museum of American History, Smithsonian Institution, Washington, D.C.

home, women defer to husbands and fathers and care for helpless children; at work, nurses obey doctors and do what is best for their patients.

But if this structural continuity illuminates the bonds of patriarchy, it also obscures the richness and diversity of women's experience within its confines. Over the twentieth century, the content and cultural meaning of nursing have altered as medical science and practice have developed, and as nurses themselves have pressed at the limitations of "women's" work. Nurses' experiences in three different work organizations reveal the shifting possibilities of their work. In private duty, the most common employment for nurses until 1940, nurses were individual entrepreneurs, hired to care for a single patient at home or in the hospital. In the 1920s and 1930s, a few nurses assumed influential positions in the growing public health movement, claiming a measure of autonomy through their positions in agencies that operated largely outside medical control. And after 1940, hospital employment claimed most nurses, who exchanged the precarious existence of free-lance employment for the new security—and new frustrations—of ward work. In each setting, nurses actively struggled to assert their own definitions of good work, belying the notions of subordination and passivity embedded in the phrase "the physician's hand."

Until World War II, more nurses worked in private duty than in any other arrangement, finding their cases through local doctors or through registries, employment bureaus which matched nurses seeking work with patients' requests. Nurses themselves viewed hospital staff employment as beneath the dignity of a fully trained or so-called graduate nurse; it was seen as students' work. And indeed, in the one out of four hospitals with nursing schools, students ran the wards; other hospitals functioned by hiring women without formal credentials to learn on the job under the supervision of a few nurses with hospital diplomas. Once students completed the three years of training that comprised the nursing course, they left the hospitals that had been school and work place to them as apprentices. Some graduated to supervisory positions, replacing their own teachers. A few found jobs in the prestigious public health field. But most made their way in the free-lance market of private duty nursing.[1]

On the face of it, the arrangements of private duty facilitated independence and control of work. As free-lance workers, nurses could schedule cases to suit their own needs and preferences. They could take time off to rest after a tiring stint, or take themselves off the registrar's list temporarily if sick friends or relatives needed their help. Free-lance arrangements also gave nurses the opportunity to evade unappealing work situations, a prerogative they exercised freely. Doctors, nursing leaders, and registrars complained bitterly about the practice of "case picking." One survey indicated that 61 percent of nurses routinely refused certain kinds of cases. Contagious, obstetrical, and mental cases were the most unpopular; smaller numbers of nurses refused night cases, twenty-four-hour duty, home cases, or male patients. Undoubtedly even more "case picking" occurred on an informal basis, for a nurse could declare herself off duty if confronted with a displeasing prospect.[2]

Less often, private duty nurses could manage their relationships with doctors and patients so as to enhance their control at work. Some nurses formed informal partnerships with friendly doctors, and enjoyed the security of a steady clientele and a congenial working relationship. Nurses could also avoid doctors whom they found troublesome. One nurse reported indignantly that an independent colleague had registered against seven different doctors, "because *she* does not approve of their methods." A well-established nurse enjoyed a special status in her commuinity, and could set her own terms with patients who found "their" nurse an indispensable aid in illness or childbirth.[3]

On the job, private duty gave nurses considerable autonomy in their work habits. In principle, of course, the same rules of discipline governed all nurses. In home cases, the nurse was subject to the authority of the patient's doctor; in hospitals, private duty nurses also fell under the purview of the

superintendent, who was formally responsible for all the nursing care in her institution. In practice, though, private duty nurses worked with little supervision. Doctors visited their home patients, but did not stay to oversee the nurse. Hospital nursing services sometimes had rules about the conduct and responsibilities of "special nurses" who cared for private patients. But in the actual work situation, busy head nurses rarely interfered with the bedside care that free-lancers provided. Outside the rigid hierarchy of the hospital, they escaped the discipline and demands of institutional work. As one nurse declared with satisfaction, "I am my own boss."[4]

But the exercise of this autonomy was a highly individualistic and uncertain affair even under the best of circumstances. To support themselves as free-lancers, private duty nurses had to establish a steady clientele. Dependent on hospital or private registries for their referrals, nurses had to contend with the intense loyalties of alumnae networks and cater to the demands of local doctors and patients. Hospital registries favored alumnae of their own schools, placing "outside" nurses at the bottom of their lists. Complaints of such "favoritism" filled the nursing literature. Nursing superintendents exercised considerable control over hiring special duty nurses for hospital patients, requesting their own graduates and taking special care to send work to their "pets" among the alumnae. Informal referral practices like these could help a nurse with ties to the community or the hospital, but they could also become the vehicles for a petty and arbitrary exclusivity.[5]

Although private duty nurses had limited contact with doctors on the job, their medical colleagues could exert powerful leverage over their careers. A doctor who disliked a nurse's methods, her suggestions, her personality, or even her appearance could dismiss her, might refuse to call her again, and could get her informally blacklisted in the community. Such conditions severely constrained nurses' performance and initiative on the job. Nurses who found themselves working with unethical or incompetent doctors could intervene only at considerable risk to their own futures. Whether in the isolated situation of home duty or behind closed doors in a private hospital room, the nurse could not easily appeal to outside arbitrators in conflicts with doctors. Under such circumstances, nurses' claims to expertise could have little weight against established medical authority.[6]

Hired by her patient and attending only one person at a time, the private nurse also had to shape her practice to lay standards. Wealthy and middle-class patients especially threatened the nurse's skill and craft pride. Such patients were unlikely to appreciate the fine points of a nurse's technique, or the skill involved in scrupulous observation. They often slighted the nurse's technical and scientific abilities to emphasize her personal characteristics and social demeanor. In letters to nursing journals, patients complained about their nurses' table manners, reading voices, appearances, or conversational facility. Prescriptive literature tacitly acknowledged the burden of such extraneous standards; one manual admitted, "The personality of the individual woman . . . not infrequently goes for more than skill and devotion in the nursing itself."[7]

Some patients treated their nurses like domestic servants, asking them to mend, iron, cook, scrub, do laundry, and attend children in any free moment. As one private duty nurse complained, "Many patients seem to think that they are 'getting their money's worth' only if they keep the nurse running all the time, regardless of the fact that she is removed from her patient when doing these chores." Every private duty manual offered guidance on this difficult issue, and nurses on the job developed a variety of ingenious ways to resist household tasks and to draw clearer boundaries to define nurses' special skills. Still, they had only limited resources in a market where "untrained" nurses would happily replace them, and in a situation where old-fashioned physicians sometimes sided with their patients, seeing housework as part of a nurse's duties. As one manual advised bluntly, "To succeed in nursing one must give some satisfaction to the family regardless of their unreasonableness."[8]

The loneliness of private duty haunted many nurses. One memoir summed up the work in a stark chapter titled "Isolation." She recalled the sad transition from school life to free-lancing: "I felt like a lost sheep, not to return to the hospital after each case." A nurse resuming private duty after military service during World War I exclaimed, "How one misses the comradeship of life over there," and manuals acknowledged the deprivation of the nurse working without the support and company of colleagues. The unpredictable hours of private duty disrupted sociability outside work as well. One nurse wrote plaintively, "People are too busy to bother to keep up friendship with a person who is never able to say her time is her own."[9]

Finally, free-lance work could be devastatingly insecure. Private duty was seasonal, with work abundant in the winter months and less available in the healthier seasons of summer and fall. Nurses chafed at the imposed idleness between cases and the anxious hours spent waiting for the registrar's call. Like other women workers, nurses needed their incomes: even before the depression, 53 percent of private duty nurses were responsible for partial or full support of one or more dependents. In slack seasons, or if the nurse herself became ill, she was thrown on her own limited resources.[10]

By the 1920s, the disadvantages of private duty loomed large for most free-lance nurses. They had no control over the market conditions that determined their employment, and those conditions worsened dramatically after World War I. First, nurses suffered a crisis of oversupply, the product of the historical development of American hospital-based nursing schools. Hospital managers saw student nurses as a convenient and loyal work force. As the number of hospitals multiplied between 1890 and 1920, many administrators added nursing programs to staff their floors. But, loath to hire their own finished products, hospitals turned the graduate nurses out to a rapidly swelling private duty market, recruiting new crops of students to do the ward work. Despite strenuous efforts, nursing leaders had been unable to check this expansion. The continuing stream of graduates quickly saturated the private duty market. Between 1920 and 1930, the total number of nurses doubled, while the United States' population increased only 16 percent. Private duty nurses' rising wages put their services out of the reach of many middle-class patients, and those who still hired a nurse often economized by using her for just a few days rather than retaining her through a leisurely convalescence. Caught between an oversupply of nurses and a shrinking demand, private duty nurses struggled desperately for work.[11]

Yet despite the growing constraints of free-lance work, many private duty nurses fought to retain their entrepreneurial status, and to shape their work lives according to their own conceptions of nursing's legitimate authority and proper skills. While nursing leaders pressed hospitals to hire graduate nurses for their ward work, many nurses themselves refused institutional employment, preferring to hold out for private duty. Although private duty nurses probably earned less than either public health or hospital nurses, nurses themselves widely believed that free-lancers had higher incomes than their hospital-based counterparts. In a few years, the greatly expanded and technologically complex hospital would become a desirable working environment. But in the 1920s and 1930s, nurses associated hospital work with the rigid schedules and social discipline of their student years; and indeed, most hospitals treated their fully trained workers much like students. For many resolute free-lancers, the growing risks and insecurities of private duty were still preferable to the strict paternalism of hospital employers.[12]

Free-lancers also asserted a new independence in relation to their clients. The narrowing market of private duty widened the class differences between nurses and patients. After 1920, the average private duty patient was more likely to be from the upper-middle or upper classes, that species of client most threatening to the private nurse's self-respect and autonomy at work. Earlier autobiographies, from the late nineteenth and early twentieth centuries, describe a variety of private duty work places. One nurse slept on the floor where she cared for two diphtheria patients in a shack with no running water; nursed three prostitutes through the measles in a quarantine brothel; attended a typhoid case on an isolated ranch; and then stayed with a rich woman convalescing in an elegant home. By the 1920s, similar accounts in journals and manuals depict wealthy patients almost exclusively: the diverse clientele of private duty had apparently disappeared. Available surveys confirm this impression. One survey found that growing numbers of patients felt they could not afford private nursing services. At the end of the 1930s, an American Medical Association survey found that families with annual incomes under $1,500, or 60 percent of the population, rarely used private nursing services. Most patients came from only 10 percent of the population, those families that earned over $3,000 a year. In the homes of their class superiors, nurses were most vulnerable to demands for personal service and hard put to defend their own sense of skill.[13]

Even in the harsh unemployment of the 1920s, many nurses defended their skills and their private lives by refusing to nurse home cases. Although only a few nurses admitted to registering against home cases in one survey, 40 percent of the registrars declared that they could not find nurses for home patients. As one complained, "Our nurses are most independent and want to choose their cases. They all want to nurse in the hospital." In another city, the registrar reported that favored alumnae or local nurses almost invariably refused home calls and waited for hospital special duty; only the more marginal "outside" nurses would work in patients' homes. Registrars commiserated over "this very trying and embarrassing condition" to no avail.[14]

The hospital environment tacitly enforced nurses' legitimacy as skilled workers. The visible apparatus of nursing and medicine underscored nurses' status as experts to the layperson. In contrast to their uneasy patients, nurses were insiders, initiates into the esoteric technical and institutional workings of the hospital. In the specialized workplace of the hospital, nurses gained a new social control which partially offset their patients' class prerogatives. While the nurse at home had to claim a precarious niche for herself in the established routines and social relations of the household, the hospital special worked in an environment tailored to medical and nursing routines. At home, patients commanded their own range of resources to supplement or contravene the nurse's authority. Their cooks and laundresses knew their preferences; family members and friends were at hand to run errands, to entertain them, even to support them in rebellions against medical and nursing orders. Isolated in hospitals, patients relied on their nurses for access to institutional resources and to the outside world. The nurse alone brought meals and clean linen, took messages, screened visitors, and mediated medical directives. The private patient in the hospital still retained the final prerogative of an employer, and could dismiss an unsatisfactory nurse. But short of this last recourse, the hospital patient lost much of his or her former power to define the content and practice of the nurse's work.

By insisting on hospital special duty, young nurses

struggled to preserve their old advantages as free-lance workers and to assert a new independence on the job. In the specialized work place of the hospital, they escaped many of the constraints of personal service and enjoyed better working conditions. In the end, they could not halt the broad-scale changes that were moving nursing from entrepreneurial to hospital-based practice. Still, the experience and memory of private duty influenced the first generation of nurses working in the newly dominant hospital. General duty nurses of the late 1930s and 1940s would invoke the ideal of the free-lancer's autonomy to demand better working conditions, and would appeal to traditional conceptions of the nurse's individual relationship to her patient to resist scientific management in the hospital. Although free-lancers would no longer occupy the center stage of nursing, still, their new demands on the job signaled an emerging conception of nurses as skilled workers, entitled to respect and a greater measure of authority.

As private duty nurses faced the steady decline of their work, public health nurses were building a place for themselves in the setting of the expanding public health movement. Trudging down city streets or jolting over country roads in their Fords, public health nurses brought bedside nursing services to people who could not afford private duty, and solicited patients for the new services of preventive medicine. Like private duty nurses, they often traveled to their patients, and most worked alone. But the organization of public health services and their relative independence from mainstream medicine gave public health nurses an unprecedented autonomy at work. Even as the skills and status of private duty eroded, public health nurses claimed special expertise in the developing field of preventive medicine and established themselves as an elite corps within nursing.

Coined in 1912, the term "public health nursing" reflected a growing sense of common identity among nurses working outside the usual contexts of private duty or hospital jobs. The ideal of "positive health" linked nurses in visiting nurses' associations and settlement houses, child welfare and antivenereal disease associations, factory dispensaries and department store clinics. Astute nurses working in such settings seized the chance to assert

their special expertise in the uncharted and unclaimed territory of preventive medicine. In 1912 they founded the National Organization for Public Health Nursing (NOPHN), implicitly declaring their legitimate authority to direct and organize the nursing activities related to public health.[15]

The history of public health nursing offers a glimpse of the possibilities available to nurses in a setting somewhat removed from the controlling influence of physicians. Allied with reformers, they set themselves apart from their medical colleagues and from other nurses. Located on the fringes of mainstream medicine, public health nurses worked in institutions that operated beyond the lengthening reach of the hospital and largely outside the control of the medical profession. On the job, they expanded the scope of nursing duties and responsibilities. More than either private duty or hospital nurses, public health nurses shook off their role as the physician's hand, to set out and act on their own sense of nursing's sphere and mission.

Public health nurses published a number of manuals, didactic novels, and histories that both reflected and fostered the development of a distinctive nursing specialty. This literature reinterpreted nurses' province and responsibilities in the altered context of preventive care. Manuals emphasized health education as the special contribution of the public health nurse, minimizing the traditional tasks of bedside nursing: "The nurse who tends the sick only, and teaches nothing and prevents nothing, is abortive in her work." Expert in the newly revealed "laws of health," public health nurses moved beyond the traditional service relationships of nursing to claim special expertise as teachers, "the indispensable carriers of the findings of the scientists and the laboratories to the people themselves."[16]

The work settings of public health removed nurses from direct medical control. Public health nursing associations (PHNAs) were directed by nurses who worked with lay boards. Their funding came primarily from private sources; they were also called voluntary or nonofficial agencies. The PHNAs covered the widest variety of work, active in both traditional and preventive fields. They cared for sick patients in their homes, a service in constant demand. Working to promote preventive care, they also mounted maternity and infant care programs, vaccination campaigns, case-finding and follow-up efforts. In state or municipal health departments, public health nurses worked under nursing directors or health officers, who might be either laypersons or salaried doctors. These nurses usually did little or no bedside care, concentrating on contagious disease control, screening, and "health education," a label that could cover a multitude of services. Local boards of education often hired their own school nurses. Finally, a few factories and stores employed nurses to head their dispensaries, where they administered first aid, kept records, and sometimes made safety recommendations.

Under these novel conditions, nurses' authority was extended beyond the traditional bounds set by medical prerogatives. While public health nurses formally worked under doctors' orders, physicians often supervised them from afar. Many nurses obtained standing orders, drawing up general protocols for treatment and getting the local medical society to approve them. Such orders gave nurses the license to work without direct supervision while remaining within the law that governed medical and nursing practice. Industrial nurses applied first aid and performed minor treatments without doctors. In the PHNAs, bedside nursing could be covered by standing orders for one or two visits.[17]

Nurses' new roles in case finding and health supervision eluded the existing definitions of medical and nursing prerogatives, and doctors were slow to assert an active control over preventive medicine. In situations that called for "health education," the nurse enjoyed considerable freedom, offering advice on diet, home hygiene, and child care. Maternity and infant care programs, important activities of public health agencies in the 1920s and 1930s, were almost exclusively supervised by nurses. By 1930, some public health nurses were measuring blood pressure and doing urinalyses for pregnant women, referring them to doctors if something was amiss. Although the discreet nurse would merely report her data and not diagnose overtly, the whole screening arrangement tacitly relegated a diagnostic function to the nurse.

Often public health organizations had only sporadic contact with local doctors, reinforcing the autonomy that individual nurses claimed on the job. NOPHN surveys, done in 1924 and 1934, documented the distant relationships of physicians and public health nurses. Doctors were represented on only about half of the boards that directed public health nursing agencies. By 1934, three-quarters of the agencies had separate medical advisory boards, but these physicians appeared to take little active role in the affairs of the agencies; the survey reported that most advisory boards did not meet regularly. Although most of the nursing agencies claimed that their relationships with local doctors were "friendly," the same organizations also admitted that most physicians did not send them referrals or use their services.[18]

Doctors' absence from public health created opportunities for nurses to step into the gap as the ranking experts. Conscious of the expanded scope of nursing in public health, some set forth an explicit rationale to defend their autonomy. A manual on school nursing openly challenged doctors' traditional control. "The physician, because of his medical proficiency, is nominally in charge of the situation, but is he really? The nurse . . . knows the principal, the teachers, the families of her children. The physician does not. Practically, then, the nurse really is in the best position to 'run the show.'" More often, nurses struggled to maintain their authority by bolstering their positions in the organizational structure of public health. The manuals strongly recommended nurse-controlled agencies. As one declared, "It is through the supervision of public-health nurses by public-health nurses that efficient . . . nursing services will be developed."[19]

Faced with an unreliable medical profession, nurses and reformers recognized that the survival of their work depended on their ability to mobilize lay support. Their mission was to spread the "gospel of health," to educate and inspire laypersons to demand the benefits of preventive medicine. "When the desire cometh, it is a tree of life," the NOPHN motto counseled, and public health nurses worked hard to plant and cultivate it.

Nurses' efforts to promote a new view of health revealed the dual potential of the movement itself. On the one hand, public health work expressed a genuinely democratic impulse: nurses sought to bring the benefits of scientific medicine to people who were largely neglected by private practitioners. Highly conscious of the intimidating aura of medicine, they worked to win their clients' trust and to speak in a language that laypersons could understand. Often they encouraged traditions of self-help and mutual aid. At its best, public health embodied a commitment to make medicine both accessible and accountable.

On the other hand, the broader definition of health also led to a kind of medical imperialism. By bringing virtually every aspect of human activity under the rubric of health, public health ideology provided a justification for greatly expanded medical intervention: these new experts defined health to encompass "the individual's needs, his welfare, efficiency, and happiness." Welded to the elitism underlying Progressive reform and to the public health nurse's exalted self-image, this diffuse definition of health could become the instrument for the imposition of dominant values. The goal of "right living" gave free rein to class, ethnic, and racial prejudices. Good health could become a code for middle-class standards and practices, and, like other types of reform, public health could become a vehicle for social control.[20]

In their relationships with patients, public health nurses were undoubtedly influenced by the nativism of the 1920s and the ingrained prejudices of their class. Still, in the 1920s and 1930s, these attitudes were held in check by the precarious position of public health. Traditional medical and nursing practice operated with the advantages of well-established networks of referrals and in the context of a clear lay demand for services. Operating without strong medical support, public health nurses had to work actively to win the loyalty and patronage of laypersons. Under these circumstances, nurses were forced to temper elite standards with openness to other paths toward healthful living. Repeatedly, prescriptive literature stressed personal, respectful relationships with patients as the key to successful public health work.[21]

The emphasis on an individual approach to laypersons was more than rhetorical. By the mid-1920s, nurses had restructured public health organizations to reduce the division of labor within and among agencies. Rather than visiting all the patients with tuberculosis in her city, or supervising all the young children, each nurse would care for the varied needs of the people in her assigned district. This arrangement gave variety and interest to the work, allowed considerable scope for nursing intervention, and strengthened the personal bonds between one nurse and "her" families. By 1934, all the nursing agencies in the NOPHN survey had rejected the specialization of the 1920s to embrace the generalized service. Declared Lillian Wald, "The public health nurse is the family health worker."[22]

Exchanging wealthy patients for a clientele in more modest circumstances, public health nurses could recover some of the intimacy of private duty without relinquishing their control as workers. In the 1920s, 88 percent of public health nurses had worked in private duty, and some left their wealthy patients with open relief. As one wrote, "There is greater satisfaction in doing for these poor unfortunates than in catering to patients who have lived lives of pampered luxury." Another nurse noted, "You meet a class of people who need your care and advice. . . . One is more appreciated."[23]

By the 1930s, public health had scored resounding successes. While the conservative American Medical Association remained unconvinced, many other physicians and lay observers were fervent converts to the "gospel of health." During the Depression, relief programs recognized the medical needs of the indigent. The Social Security Act of 1935 provided a long-term basis for offering tax support to the blind, the disabled, and the elderly. World War II, like World War I, led to centralization of medical services in support of the military, and this time, servicemen's families shared in benefits that included a broad program of maternity and infant care.[24]

But as public health services reorganized and expanded, nurses lost their autonomy and their distinctive identity along with their marginality. Changing patterns of funding displaced the agencies that nurses had administered and controlled. Increasing specialization among agencies disrupted the old ideal of the generalized service. And within agencies, a new division of labor further revised the individual nurse-patient relationship of the early years.

Government funding reinforced health departments and boards of education, placing the so-called nonofficial or voluntary agencies at a marked disadvantage. Hit hard by the decline in private contributions and the dwindling numbers of paying patients, many of the voluntary agencies, or PHNAs, sought affiliations with the better-funded official agencies. Administered by nurses and lay boards, the voluntary agencies had offered the most favorable environment of all the public health settings, fostering nursing initiative in the 1920s and 1930s. Public health nurses in these programs had the authority to design and direct their own work. Most of the staples of public health work—tuberculosis case finding and home care, prenatal and infant care, and school nursing—had been established through the experiments of private agencies. To many nurses, the work of the PHNAs represented the reform spirit of those years; one article pleaded for new methods of funding to preserve "the gadfly of the official agency." But even as public health expanded, these agencies faltered. Between 1933 and 1948, the private agencies lost 23 percent of their nurses. During the same period, the staffs of health departments doubled, and boards of education hired 50 percent more school nurses.[25]

The growing dominance of hospitals in the war and postwar years further altered the character of public health nursing. During the 1940s, hospital outpatient clinics or social service departments assumed much of the work formerly done in the agencies. In this institutional setting, new functions encroached on the nurse's relationship with her patient. Delivering outpatient services, instructing hospital nurses about community social services and referring patients to them, public health nurses functioned mostly as administrators; as "liaison nurses," they had little direct contact with their patients. In clinics, nurses saw many patients a day, but tight schedules and uncongenial atmosphere constrained the old intimacy of home visiting. Working in hospitals, nurses lost some of the independence of public health work to return to the traditional role of assisting doctors.[26]

As public health gained acceptance, the medical profession asserted its control, barely ruffled by public health nurses' former independence. At the same time, hospitals stripped public health nursing of much of its innovative character, replacing home visiting and individual approach with rationalized care. As the institutions and practitioners of mainstream medicine embraced the public health message, the nurse's special role was undercut. Newly converted to the "gospel of health," doctors and hospitals overlooked its elite ministers to proclaim, in the words of a popular postwar slogan, "Every nurse a public health nurse." Once proudly autonomous, the NOPHN began to negotiate for a

merger with the other professional associations in nursing. In 1953, the organization dissolved, a poignant symbol for the decline of public health nursing's separate identity.[27]

In the 1930s, graduate nurses began to move from free-lance private duty to hospital staff jobs. Nursing practice took its modern form as hospitals hired increasing numbers of graduates for general ward duty. Once run by students or attendants supervised by a single graduate nurse, hospital wards rapidly became the province of graduates. The transition took place within the space of fifteen years. In 1927, nearly three-quarters of hospitals with training schools relied exclusively on students for ward nursing services; a decade later, most reported that they had begun to employ some graduate staff nurses. By 1940, nearly half of all nurses were employed in hospitals, and by the end of World War II, a decisive majority of all active nurses held hospital jobs.[28]

The move to graduate staffing was one phase in a larger transformation in hospital management and in the organization of medical care. At bottom, a work force of dispersed free-lancers and student apprentices was increasingly inadequate to the demands of the industry. Private duty nurses' harsh experiences during the 1920s had already pointed to the underlying weakness of this organization. The Depression brought the lesson home to hospital managers as the demand for hospital care and staff nursing services sharply increased. Many middle-class patients could no longer afford the services of a special nurse at home or in the hospital, nor could they pay for hospital services. Small private hospitals closed down as their supply of paying patients dwindled, while voluntary hospitals staggered under heavy demands for their charity services. As administrators reexamined the cost of maintaining hospital nursing schools, many concluded that student staffs were no longer a real economy.[29]

Meanwhile, the demand for hospital nursing service continued to increase. Hospitals moved to a more solid economic base as insurance and federal funding grew, and the hospital industry entered a new period of consolidation and expansion. The total number of hospitals dropped as smaller institutions failed. Existing plants grew bigger, and overall the number of hospital beds increased by the thousands. Responding to this reorganization and expansion, more administrators called on graduate nurses to staff hospital wards.[30]

Before 1940, hospital employment probably gave nurses little more security than private duty. Some evidence suggests that managers used graduates as a kind of reserve labor supply, exploiting the flexibility afforded by a large pool of unemployed nurses. Few hospitals even offered written contracts. Unprotected by labor unions and vulnerable in the severe unemployment of the Depression, graduates sometimes found themselves summarily fired. As one nurse reported bitterly, the hospitals "expect you to take care of six or eight patients and as soon as they can get along without you, you are dropped." Mandatory unpaid "vacations" or indefinite layoffs were common hospital expedients for economizing on nursing service in slack times. Under circumstances like these, hospital employment probably offered few inducements even for embattled private duty nurses.[31]

Through the 1930s, hospital employment also meant a return to the paternalistic regimen of training school. On the ward, superintendents tried to apply the same strict discipline to both graduates and students. Most administrators expected or required their nurses to live in the hospital's quarters: a 1936 survey showed that 84 percent of hospitals provided room, board, and laundry as part of the nurse's wages. Even where institutional policy did not require nurses to live in the hospital, few administrators would adjust the salaries of those who wished to "live out." Nurses were increasingly unwilling to accept this arrangement; as one letter notes, "The young women of today are accustomed to 'enjoy the privileges' of independent living.... Nurses ... chafe under the inevitable restraints and irritations of constant supervision."[32]

New techniques of scientific management introduced other threats to staff nurses' autonomy. Based on Frederick Winslow Taylor's methods, the movement for "efficiency" aimed to simplify production by reducing each task to its smallest components. Studying each task closely, "efficiency experts" pared away at "wasted" motions and substituted the simplest methods. The resulting standardization of work disrupted the traditional craft process in many industries, often stripping workers of their skills and their control over production. Rationalization also lent the materials and argument for an increasingly elaborate division of labor. Once analyzed into separate components, the work process could be divided among a number of workers, each assigned to a few repetitive tasks. In nursing, as in other work, the actual application of scientific management was partial and incomplete. Nevertheless, the rhetoric of efficiency brought critical changes to the pace and organization of nursing work.

Nurses on the job viewed rationalization with a skeptical eye. They learned quickly that "efficiency" was often synonymous with speed up, recording their discontents in letters to professional journals. One wrote, "It takes young legs to keep up with the pressure and speed. . . . Sometimes nurses do more 'things' in one hour, new tests, treatments, etc., than we older women used to do in six hours." Another described the frantic work pace on her ward, and concluded, "Even the younger . . . general duty nurse is breaking under the strain, and still the surveys go on with the slogan 'Greater Efficiency!'" Others explicitly criticized the use of scientific management to stretch out increased work over smaller staffs. As one nurse insisted, "The employment of more graduate nurses in our hospital to care for patients on general duty will do for us what we have not permitted efficiency experts to do."[33]

The growing division of labor in hospitals was perhaps the most important outcome of managers' use of principles of rationalization. Throughout the twentieth century, both nursing leaders and nurses on the job had struggled to limit the use of the "subnurse," the "attendant," or the "auxiliary"—workers trained on the job to assist in nursing care, for lower wages than nurses received. But the growing pressure of ward work and the acute shortages of the war and postwar years gave these workers a permanent place in the hospital work force. After World War II, their skills and contributions were acknowledged in the creation of a new occupational category, the licensed practical nurse (LPN).

The introduction of the auxiliary nurses—or rather, their formal organization, for such workers had long formed an indispensable adjunct to hospital staffs—did raise new questions about skill and authority on the ward. A wry piece of contemporary hospital lore records the common recognition of the blurred boundaries of the nursing work force:

"A practical nurse is someone who does at night what the registered nurse does during the day." Professional leaders responded with formal structures of accreditation: they sought to define distinct credentials separating their less-trained co-workers from registered nurses. On the job, other nurses sometimes vented their insecurities in petty and divisive attacks on practicals.[34]

Although nurses faced new difficulties and constraints in the changing hospital setting, nonetheless hospital employment represented a distinct improvement. After 1940, hospital nurses worked in a climate of expansion that contrasted dramatically with the decline and marginality of private duty work. With Europe at war, Americans looked anxiously to their medical and nursing resources at home; urgent calls for more nurses lent importance to the occupation and the women in it. After United States entry into World War II, national recruiting campaigns and the debate over a nurses' draft further emphasized the critical role of nurses and nursing. In the postwar years, the continuing expansion of hospitals outpaced the supply of nurses. The 1947 Hill-Burton Act provided generous funding for hospital construction, and postwar medical advances further increased the demand for skilled workers. As a result, nurses enjoyed a favorable labor market for the first time in decades. Both the hospital work place and the changing character of medical care improved nurses' positions vis-à-vis doctors and patients.

Hospital work significantly revised the conduct of nurses' relationships with doctors. Under these new conditions, the structure of medical authority remained the same: by law and custom, doctors were nurses' superiors. But in practice, doctors lost some of their economic and social control over nurses as private duty yielded to hospital work. Hospital nurses were hired by the institution, not by the patient; and their direct supervisors were other nurses, not the physician on the case. Although hospital nurses took risks if they repeatedly irritated or challenged a powerful doctor, they were no longer directly dependent on the goodwill of any one physician.

The bureaucratic structure of the hospital diffused medical authority and offered nurses a modicum of support when conflicts arose with physicians. Doctors worked under the eyes of their peers and were subject, at least nominally, to the supervision and discipline of the medical chief-of-staff. The more public character of hospital work limited the physician's absolute authority. The private duty nurse who questioned a doctor faced the consequences alone. In the hospital, a doubtful nurse could appeal to other knowledgeable participants, or invoke the impersonal authority of bureaucratic procedures and policies. Hospital nurses had the support of small work groups and the resource of a formal structure of appeal. Buttressed by her head nurse and sympathetic colleagues, a nurse might more readily confront a doctor on the floor. If informal approaches failed, she could take the conflict through official channels, and seek arbitration through the nursing director and chief physician.

Hospital nurses occupied strategic positions in the institution. The nurse commanded the domain of her ward: she knew how to negotiate the red tape of hospital rules, placate the patients, and get the work done. Learning to win the nurse's loyalty was part of an intern's initiation, and medical lore acknowledged nurses' pivotal roles. A good nurse, every physician knew, could smooth his way—or, if she chose, impose formidable obstacles while never overstepping the bounds of her formal role. Very secure nurses might risk "forgetting" or ignoring a problematic order. In a safer (and probably more common) tactic, nurses could effectively hamstring a difficult doctor by working to rule: bringing him to the hospital at all hours by refusing to take verbal orders; invoking esoteric rules and procedures; inciting rebellion among his patients. Some obdurate doctors might persist in their claims to absolute control, but most found it simpler to concede some turf to ward nurses.[35]

Finally, the new content of medical care made nursing and medical work more interdependent. Nowhere was this more apparent than in the mushrooming special care units, where nurses assumed many functions and responsibilities formerly reserved for physicians, and assumed a new authority by virtue of their expertise. The pace and character of intensive care left no room for the old formulas of nursing deference to medical judgment. No critical care nurse would call a doctor to report meekly, "Mr. Brown's pulse appears to have ceased." She would yell for emergency equipment, pound the patient's chest, inflate his lungs, initiate closed-chest cardiac massage, perhaps even begin to administer the drugs used in resuscitation. In turn, doctors recognized and depended on the skills and judgment of these nurses.[36]

Hospital employment also dramatically increased nurses' authority with patients. In managing the tasks and relationships of patient care, nurses had long recognized the advantages of the hospital as a workplace. Free-lancers shunned hospital staff jobs, but they preferred to nurse their private cases in the hospital. Convenient facilities made the work easier, and a specialized work place supported nurses' claims to skill and control over work. The private patient lost many old prerogatives, for in the hospital nursing and medical considerations decisively outweighed lay preferences.

General duty nurses slipped altogether beyond the reach of the private duty patient's dwindling authority, for they were employed by the hospital, not by the patient. Institutional nursing released nurses from the vestiges of personal service that clung to private duty. As one former free-lancer commented, "I don't have to entertain the patient and help trim last year's hat!"[37] Responsible for more than one patient, the nurse could limit the demands of any one person. She could excuse herself from one room to answer a real or imaginary summons from another quarter, or seek a brief refuge from the entire floor by retreating to the nurses' station or the nurses' lounge. Working together, nurses also developed and enforced a shared prescription for the "good" patient. By disciplining patients to their proper roles, nurses avoided many of the disadvantages of private duty and could negotiate some respite from the quickening pace of hospital work.

Bitter at the constraints of hospital jobs, nurses themselves might object to this portrayal of the advantages of an institutional workplace. Yet in historical context, hospital work did give nurses a stronger position in the labor market and on the job. They could and did exercise considerable control as individuals, picking and choosing their shifts and workplaces in a market desperate for their skills. On the ward, they claimed middle-management positions, becoming the undisputed heads of the nursing hierarchy. In relationships with doctors and patients, they pressed the advantages of their new locations. These improvements did not constitute real control at work, and, in successive waves of postwar protest, nurses have outlined the

many limitations of institutional jobs. But a historical perspective suggests that their continuing dissatisfaction reflects more than the undeniable difficulties of hospital work. Rather, hospital jobs have supported rising expectations and facilitated collective action. Relocated from the fringes to the center of medical care, nurses have gained new responsibilities; they are demanding concomitant authority.

Nursing history illustrates the complex social meaning and expression of skill. Even the most casual observation of hospital ward work shows us that it is more than the distribution of tasks: no simple functional definition can capture the intricacy of the medical division of labor. Tasks are constantly redistributed up and down the hierarchy. In the nineteenth century, for example, most birth assistants were informally trained women; today, the male obstetrician claims a place of recognized expertise in the birthing room. In the 1920s, administration of anesthesia was "women's work," scorned by most physicians and controlled instead by nurses. Other tasks moved from physicians to nurses to LPNs to technicians or laypersons. Venipuncture, once strictly a medical prerogative, became part of the nurse's province in the 1940s; among physicians, only the lowly intern or resident now performs this task, relegated to the "scut work" of medical initiation. Blood pressure measurement passed from physician to nurse in the 1930s; today it is done by laypersons, or even by coin-operated machines set in public places. In more recent years, specialized care like respiratory therapy or dialysis has passed from physician to nurse to more narrowly trained technicians.

Faced with a notoriously flexible division of labor, some nurses have sought to use credentials to secure their own positions and to establish a claim to legitimate authority in the hospital hierarchy. The history of professionalization in nursing is largely the story of leaders' efforts to restrict access to nursing practice through state licensure and registration, to control accreditation of nursing education, and to regulate nursing practice. Perhaps the most successful occupational strategy, credentialing also reveals the ironies and ambiguities of our social definitions of skill. Of course, credentials are never wholly arbitrary: faced with the choice, most of us would want to have an inflamed appendix removed by a surgeon rather than a historian. Nonetheless, such credentials never rest *solely* on technical skill and knowledge; they are also sorting mechanisms that reflect and reproduce existing hierarchies of class, sex, and race. Moreover, they are ironic testimony to the elusive quality of skill itself: nurses and others retreat to the tautology of defining their legitimate sphere of expertise by saying it is whatever persons with their credentials say it should be. But perhaps this is no tautology at all, for credentialing is successful precisely to the degree that it confers authority to define the division of labor.

For nurses, neither technical expertise nor credentials are sufficient to explain the possibilities and limitations of work. Rather, skill is constantly renegotiated in the social world of the workplace. Confronted with threats to their own sense of skill and authority, nurses on the job worked to make and remake their experience with the resources and within the boundaries of the medical division of labor. Their history reveals the various outcomes of their efforts and suggests some of the conditions that support informal claims to skill.

The history of private duty nursing decisively undercuts the common association of free-lance status with independence and autonomy at work. Self-employment has often represented independence to Americans, whether in the celebrated autonomy of eighteenth- and nineteenth-century craft workers, in the classic American dream of owning a small business, or in the fee-for-service ideal still cherished by those physicians identified with the American Medical Association. Private duty nurses themselves apparently shared that ideal. Yet in practice, their free-lance status meant increasing vulnerability—under- and unemployment in a failing market, difficulty in asserting claims of expertise over laypersons' expectations for personal service, and isolation from the new techniques and knowledge that were enhancing the prestige and efficacy of medical care.

Public health nurses, the most independent of all nurses, offer an instructive case history that further articulates the meaning and experience of control at work. Privileged by their marginality, public health nurses were able to build and operate their own institutions; within the boundaries set by their limited influence in the larger world of medical care, they succeeded in claiming a sphere of

legitimate expertise. But when their larger goal was won—gaining the patronage of laypersons and physicians for their case—they lost the leadership of the field that they had enjoyed in the early years. On the scale of security, prestige, and authority, private duty and public health nurses were far apart. But in the end, their problem was the same: their claims to authority were increasingly hedged in by the growing dominance of hospital-based care. Private duty nurses were pressed to the fringes of medical care, isolated from the dynamic center of the hospital; public health nurses, pulled in from the fringes, were crushed in the embrace of mainstream medicine.

If self-employment stands for independence in American ideology of work, then wage work in bureaucratic institutions represents the loss of autonomy: the constraints and irritations of such institutions are one of the recurring images of twentieth-century fiction and intellectual life. Yet for hospital nurses, bureaucratic organization opened a new space for the exercise of authority and the defense of skill. For those at the top, bureaucracy did impose new restrictions: physicians suffered a relative decline in their individual authority and autonomy at work, though as a group they benefited from the new resources and prestige of advanced technology. But that shift created new opportunities for nurses, possibilities that nurses were quick to perceive and develop.

Rhetoric and wishful thinking notwithstanding, nurses are not autonomous professionals; indeed, in the large-scale and complex world of modern health care, "autonomy" is perhaps no longer an appropriate term or even a useful goal.[38] Physicians always had more leverage than nurses in that world. But they never entirely controlled it, and through the twentieth century, their own autonomy was diluted even as nurses' authority was enhanced. Patients, too, had a role in shaping the definition and experience of nursing skills. The class, race, and ethnic differences between nurses and patients created relationships of power and inequality that often outweighed mere credentials in defining skill. Confronted with an imperious wealthy patient, the private duty nurse sometimes had to defer even within her sphere of expertise; conversely, surrounded by the poorer clients of public health, nurses were able to claim more control than their credentials would justify. And finally, the workplace itself had important implications. Nurses had more control as middle managers in the central social institution of the hospital than they could gain as free-lancers or in the isolated domain of public health.

Fraught with connotations of passivity, subordination, and self-abnegation, the label of "the physician's hand" is anathema to today's nurses. Repudiating its sentimentality and paternalism, nurses are demanding recognition of their unique contributions to the work of health care. In recent years, the growth of white-collar unions and the resurgence of the women's movement have offered new ideological and organizational support. These resources have extended nurses' challenges to hospital employers, and done much to bolster their sense of entitlement to respect, higher wages, and better work lives. But nurses who look to their own history will discover that much of the impetus for the current struggle lies in long-standing occupational traditions. Whether in the declining market of private duty, the fragile institutions of public health, or the familiar setting of hospital wards, nurses have always been more than "the physician's hand."

NOTES

This article is based on material in the author's *"The Physician's Hand": Work Culture and Conflict in American Nursing* (Philadelphia: Temple University Press, 1982) and is used by permission of Temple University Press.

1 May Ayres Burgess, *Nurses, Patients, and Pocketbooks; Report of a Study of the Economics of Nursing* (New York: Committee on the Grading of Nursing Schools 1928), 197–202, 340. A rich and detailed study of nursing based on extensive questionnaire and interview data, this is an invaluable source for historians of nursing. *American Journal of Nursing* 27 (July 1927): 518.

2 Burgess, *Nurses, Patients,* 77, 98.

3 Genevieve E. Kidd, "Professional obligations of private duty nurses," *American Journal of Nursing* 20 (Jan. 1920): 290.

4 Quoted in Burgess, *Nurses, Patients,* 320.

5 Ibid., 98, 102, 104, 105, 326, 338, 362; *Trained Nurse and Hospital Review* 73 (Nov. 1924): 444; letter from M. E., Washington, *American Journal of Nursing* 28 (Aug. 1928): 831; letter from "A married nurse," ibid. 28 (Oct. 1928): 1046.

6 Manuals discussed the special problems of "professional etiquette" in the isolated situation of private duty. See, for example, Isabel Hampton Robb, *Nursing Ethics for Hospital and Private Use* (Cleveland: Koeckert, 1928; first published in 1900), 251, 257; Sara E. Parsons, *Nursing Problems and Obligations* (Boston: Whitcomb and Barrows, 1916), 58; and Mary Louise Habel and Hazel Doris Milton, *The Graduate Nurse in the Home* (Philadelphia: Lippincott, 1939), 37, 122–23.

7 For examples of patients' complaints, see "Oh wad the power gie us to see ourselves as ithers see us," *Trained Nurse and Hospital Review* 79 (Aug. 1927): 147–50 and letter from E. S.M., "Why one family was glad when the nurse left," *American Journal of Nursing* 23 (Feb. 1923): 418–19. Quotation from Robb, *Nursing Ethics,* 197.

8 Letter from R. N., Chicago, Ill., *RN: A Journal for Nurses* 2(Dec. 1938): 4; Mary E. Gladwin, *Ethics—Talks to Nurses* (Philadelphia: W. B. Saunders, 1930), 103.

9 Ida May Hadden, *First and Second Chronicles* (New York: Fleming H. Revell, 1937), 73; Lara Hartwell, "The returned nurse," *American Journal of Nursing* 20 (Jan. 1920): 294–96; quoted in Burgess, *Nurses, Patients,* 326. See also Brunettie Burrow, *Angels in White* (San Antonio, Tex.: Naylor, 1959), 11–19, 23.

10 On seasonality of private duty work, see Josephine Goldmark, *Nursing and Nursing Education in the United States: A Report of the Committee for the Study of Nursing Education* (New York: Macmillan, 1923), 168. For detailed information on private duty nurses' incomes and financial obligations, see Burgess, *Nurses, Patients,* 291–92.

11 Burgess, "More census figures—the whole United States," *American Journal of Nursing* 32 (May 1932): 516; Burgess, *Nurses, Patients,* 84–85; letter from St. Petersburg, Fla., *American Journal of Nursing* 28 (Nov. 1928): 1148; "Too many nurses—where?" ibid. 29 (March 1929): 291–300.

12 For data on annual incomes and nurses' perceptions of earnings in each field, see Burgess, *Nurses, Patients,* 353. For evidence of private duty nurses' resistance to hospital staff work, see "Official registries and professional progress," *American Journal of Nursing* 26 (Feb. 1926): 93; Adda Eldredge, "Some vocational problems," ibid. 37 (July 1937): 725; Carrie May Dokken, "The general staff nurse," ibid. 38 (Feb. 1938): 143–46; Sister M. Bernice Beck, "General staff nursing," ibid. 37 (Jan. 1937): 57–63; Elizabeth M. Jamieson, "The general duty nurse,"

ibid. 29 (July 1929): 834–37; letter from a director of nursing, *Trained Nurse and Hospital Review* 108 (Jan. 1942): 61.

13 For early memoirs of private duty nursing, see Lora Wood Hughes, *No Time for Tears* (Boston: Houghton Mifflin, 1946); Belinda Jelliffe, *For Dear Life* (New York: Charles Scribner's Sons, 1936); and Corinne Johnson Kern, *I Go Nursing* (New York: E. P. Dutton, 1933). For surveys indicating the narrowing clientele of private duty, see Burgess, *Nurses, Patients,* 148, and Margaret C. Klem, "Who purchases private duty nursing services?" *American Journal of Nursing 39 (Oct. 1939):* 1069–77.

14 Burgess, *Nurses, Patients,* 76, 98; "The registry looks at the private duty nurse," *American Journal of Nursing* 29 (Dec. 1929): 1465; "Our mutual obligation to nursing," ibid. 38 (Feb. 1938): 193; and see also Habel and Milton, *The Graduate Nurse in the Home,* vii. This manual was written in 1939, in response to the "problem" of the private duty nurse in the home. The authors noted case picking with disapproval, and indicated that nurses were somewhat less able to avoid home duty during the Depression.

15 For a detailed history and interpretation of the organization, see M. Louise Fitzpatrick, *The National Organization for Public Health Nursing, 1912–1952: Development of a Practice Field* (New York: National League for Nursing, 1975).

16 Mary Breckinridge, *Wide Neighborhoods: A Story of the Frontier Nursing Service* (New York: Harper and Brothers, 1952), 242; Mary Sewall Gardner, *Public Health Nursing,* 2d ed. (New York: Macmillan, 1933; first published 1916), 43. See also Mary Beard, *The Nurse in Public Health* (New York: Harper and Brothers, 1929), 3.

17 Manuals and articles in *Public Health Nursing* (the National Organization for Public Health Nursing journal) outlined the procedures for obtaining standing orders and stressed their importance. See Florence Swift Wright, *Industrial Nursing: For Industrial, Public Health and Pupil Nurses, and for Employers of Labor* (New York: Macmillan, 1919), 26; "Standing orders for health education," *Public Health Nursing* 22 (March 1930): 138; Violet H. Hodgson, *Public Health Nursing in Industry* (New York: Macmillan, 1933), 32; National Organization for Public Health Nursing, *Manual of Public Health Nursing* (New York: Macmillan, 1939), 10–13, 140; Bethel J. McGrath, *Nursing in Commerce and Industry* (New York: Commonwealth Fund, 1946), 51.

18 National Organization for Public Health Nursing, *Committee to Study Visiting Nursing* (New York, 1924), 22, and *Survey of Public Health Nursing: Administration and Practice* (New York: Commonwealth Fund, 1934), 127, 130; "Medical relationships in non-of-

ficial PHNAs," *Public Health Nursing* 26 (Nov. 1934): 574.

19 Dorothy Bird Nyswander, *Solving School Health Problems* (New York: Commonwealth Fund, 1942), 88–89; Beard, *The Nurse in Public Health,* 48. See also Gardner, *Public Health Nursing,* 153.

20 Quotation on scope of public health from Michael M. Davis, Jr., *Immigrant Health and the Community* (New York: Harper and Brothers, 1921), 3. For an extended analysis and critique of medicine as social control, see Ivan Illich, *Medical Nemesis: The Expropriation of Health* (New York: Pantheon, 1976).

21 For didactic short stories illustrating the ideal public health nurse's method, see Paul Stevens, "Tonsils and tact," *Hygeia* 13, no. 3 (March 1935): 356–58, and Pattie R. Saunders, "Neblett's Landing," *Public Health Nursing* 29 (June 1937): 387–88. For characteristic advice in manuals, see Ruth Gilbert, *The Public Health Nurse and Her Patient* (New York: Commonwealth Fund, 1940), 162, and Marguerite Wales, *The Public Health Nurse in Action* (New York: Macmillan, 1941), 93.

22 Annie M. Brainard, *Organization of Public Health Nursing* (New York: Macmillan, 1919), 31; Beard, *The Nurse in Public Health,* 52–59; Lillian D. Wald, *Windows on Henry Street* (Boston: Little, Brown, 1934), 91–92.

23 Quoted in Burgess, *Nurses, Patients,* 257, 269–70. See also Glee L. Hastings, "Some emotional problems of public health nurses," *Public Health Nursing* 24 (Dec. 1932): 659–60.

24 Committee on the Costs of Medical Care, *Medical Care for the American People* (Chicago: University of Chicago Press, 1932), 42; Julius B. Richmond, *Currents in American Medicine* (Cambridge, Mass.: Harvard University Press, 1969), 11–20; Lloyd C. Taylor, Jr., *The Medical Profession and Social Reform, 1885–1945* (New York: St. Martin's Press, 1974), 121–27.

25 " . . . gadfly of the official agency" in Linn Brandenberg, "Financing voluntary public health nursing agencies," *Public Health Nursing* 40 (Aug. 1948): 394; data on changing shape of funding in the 1930s and 1940s in "Public health nursing under the Social Security Act," ibid. 28 (Sept. 1936): 583; Anna L. Tittman, "New jobs for old," ibid. 30 (Jan. 1938): 11; "Better care for mothers and babies," ibid. 30 (Feb. 1938): 71–73; Mabel Reid, "1938 Census of public health nurses," ibid. 30 (Nov. 1938): 632–35; "Official agency support," ibid. 40 (Feb. 1948): 60.

26 For descriptions, mostly critical, of public health nursing in hospitals and clinics, see "Public health nursing service in clincs," *Public Health Nursing* 36 (May 1944): 210; John H. Stokes, "Public health and social hygiene," ibid. 26 (Oct. 1934): 535; Charlotte M. Inglesby, "A teaching clinic for syphilis and gon-

orrhea," ibid. 28 (Feb. 1936): 104; Karen E. Munch, "Nurse interview in the tuberculosis clinic," ibid. 38 (Feb. 1946): 73–76.

27 The slogan "every nurse a public health nurse" was quoted (and refuted) in Mary Ella Chayer, "Shall we teach them all to fly?" *Public Health Nursing* 41 (July 1949): 369–72. For examples of the vigorous debate over the merger, see Elizabeth G. Fox, "I vote no," ibid. 40 (Aug. 1948): 416–27; "Report," ibid. 40 (Nov. 1948): 534; "Non-nurse agencies in the NLA," ibid. 44 (Feb. 1952): 71–75; Editorial, ibid. 44 (June 1952): 307–8.

28 "More general staff nurses," *American Journal of Nursing* 38 (Feb. 1938): 186–90; "Did you ever see a nurse nursing?" ibid. 38 (April 1938): 30 (S); Beulah Amidon, *Better Nursing for America*, Public Affairs Pamphlets no. 60 (New York: Public Affairs Committee, 1941), 13–14; Everett C. Hughes, Helen MacGill Hughes, and Irwin Deutscher, *Twenty Thousand Nurses Tell Their Story* (Philadelphia: Lippincott, 1958), 258.

29 For recent work on the history of hospitals, see David Rosner, *A Once-Charitable Enterprise: Health Care in Brooklyn and New York, 1855–1919* (Cambridge, Eng.: Cambridge University Press, 1983), and Morris Vogel, *The Invention of the Modern Hospital: Boston, 1870–1930* (Chicago: University of Chicago Press, 1980). For discussion of nursing in the hospital workplace, see Susan Reverby, "The search for the hospital yardstick: nursing and the rationalization of hospital work," in *Health Care in America*, eds. Reverby and Rosner, (Philadelphia: Temple University Press, 1979), 117–31, and Barbara Melosh, *"The Physician's Hand": Work Culture and Conflict in American Nursing* (Philadelphia: Temple University Press, 1982), 159–205.

30 In 1932 alone, hospitals added 239,157 beds and increased their capacity by 26 percent; see "In 1932," *American Journal of Nursing* 33 (Jan. 1933): 3; Philip A. Kalisch and Beatrice J. Kalisch, *The Advance of American Nursing* (Boston: Little, Brown, 1978), 418–23, 438–41. Another useful source is Arthur C. Bachmeyer and Gerhard Hartman, eds., *The Hospital in Modern Society* (New York: Commonwealth Fund, 1943).

31 "Graduate staff nursing," *American Journal of Nursing* 36 (June 1936): 591–96; letter, ibid. 36 (Aug. 1936): 851; letter and editorial note, ibid. 39 (April 1939): 435.

32 "Graduate staff nursing," *American Journal of Nursing* 36 (June 1936): 591–96; letter from "Private Duty," *Trained Nurse and Hospital Review* 100 (Feb. 1938): 167.

33 J. M. G[eister], "An open letter on staff nursing," *Trained Nurse and Hospital Review* 106 (April 1941): 362; letter, *American Journal of Nursing* 41 (Dec. 1941): 1448; letter from "Illinois nurse," ibid. 27 (May 1927): 391; A. Faith Ankeny, "The standpoint of a nurse," *Trained Nurse and Hospital Review* 81 (Nov. 1928): 558.

34 For a more detailed discussion of the debate within nursing and the growing use of auxiliary workers, see Melosh, *"The Physician's Hand,"* 177–82.

35 See, for example, Doctor X, *Intern* (New York: Harper and Row, 1965); Elizabeth Morgan, *The Making of a Woman Surgeon* (New York: G. P. Putnam, 1980); the 1955 film *Not as a Stranger*, based on the Morton Thompson novel of the same name ("Make friends with the nurses," a senior doctor counsels his intern; "They run the hospital."). For a humorous and perceptive analysis of the informal negotiations that mediate this relationship, see Leonard I. Stein, "The doctor-nurse game," *Archives of General Psychiatry* 16 (June 1967): 699–703.

36 See, for example, Jon Franklin and Alan Doelp, *Shocktrauma* (New York: St. Martin's Press, 1980), and B. D. Colen, *Born at Risk* (New York: St. Martin's Press, 1981).

37 Quoted in Elizabeth Maury Dean, "One hundred who were private duty nurses," *American Journal of Nursing* 44 (June 1944): 560; article also provides other favorable assessments of hospital general duty compared with private duty.

38 For a discussion of the impact of state intervention and increasing corporate control of health care, see Paul Starr, *The Social Transformation of American Medicine* (New York: Basic, 1982).

35

Mabel K. Staupers
and the Integration of Black Nurses
into the Armed Forces

DARLENE CLARK HINE

World War II was a watershed in black history. Many blacks, both men and women, resolved to take advantage of the war emergency and to push for the full realization of their rights as American citizens and as human beings. Scholars have justifiably dubbed this period as "the forgotten years of the Negro Revolution." Black leaders such as A. Philip Randolph of the Brotherhood of Sleeping Car Porters and organizer of the March on Washington Movement; Walter White of the National Association for the Advancement of Colored People; Lester Granger of the National Urban League; Claude Barnett of the Associated Negro Press; James Farmer and Bayard Rustin of the Committee (later Congress) of Racial Equality employed a variety of tactics and struggled to dismantle the entire edifice of white supremacy and racial proscription.

To the dismay of black Americans, the federal government proved slow in responding to their attacks and charges of discrimination. Blacks already situated on the bottom rung of the socioeconomic ladder had suffered to a remarkable degree during the great depression. Much of the New Deal relief legislation designed to ameliorate the deprivation and suffering of impoverished Americans actually preserved Jim Crow practices. To be sure, blacks received significant amounts of work, housing, and federal relief, but this was certainly not

DARLENE CLARK HINE is Vice Provost and Associate Professor of History at Purdue University, West Lafayette, Indiana.

Reprinted with permission from *Black Leaders of the Twentieth Century*, edited by John Hope Franklin and August Meier (Champaign, Ill.: University of Illinois Press, 1982). © 1982 by the Board of Trustees of the University of Illinois.

sufficient to solve the basic problems arising from white prejudice and discrimination.

The resurgence of economic activity at the outset of World War II registered only imperceptible changes in the black condition. Private industries with and without government defense contracts continued to discriminate against blacks in hiring, wages, and promotion. While many white unions excluded blacks, the U.S. Employment Service, a federal agency, continued to fill "white only" requests from employers of defense labor. The Fair Employment Practices Commitee (FEPC) appointed by President Franklin Delano Roosevelt to implement Executive Order 8802 banning employment discrimination in government defense industries lacked enforcement powers and proved to be of only limited effectiveness. Yet, stimulated by the limited reforms of the New Deal and the democratic ideology stressed by U.S. anti-Nazi propaganda, blacks became much more militant in attacks on the racial status quo. Thus the vigilance with which black editors observed and reported accounts of racial segregation, discrimination, and civil inequalities surpassed all previous coverage.

One black leader, Mabel Keaton Staupers, heretofore unheralded and virtually ignored as executive secretary of the National Association of Colored Graduate Nurses (NACGN), successfully challenged the highly racist top echelons of the U.S. Army and Navy and forced them to accept black women nurses into the military nurses corps during World War II. This essay focuses on her leadership in the campaign to win long-denied rights for black women nurses.

Within the federal government, the Army and Navy displayed the strongest adherence to and defense of the ideology and practice of racial discrimination and segregation. Military leaders saw nothing amiss in sending a segregated Army and Navy to obliterate the forces of Fascism and Nazism to make the world safe for democracy. These contradictions were not lost upon black Americans. Walter White wrote at the time, "World War II has immeasurably magnified the Negro's awareness of the disparity between the American profession and practice of democracy."

As the country mobilized for the impending conflict, government authorities informed the major nursing organizations of the increased need for nurses. Staupers and the members of the NACGN heeded the alert. The NACGN had been founded in 1908 to champion the interests and promote the professional development of black women nurses. The leading nurses organizations, the American Nurses Association (ANA) and the National League of Nursing Education (NLNE), refused to accept individual membership from black nurses residing in seventeen, primarily southern, states. Every southern state association barred black women, thereby making the majority of black women nurses professional outcasts.

Handicapped by lack of a permanent headquarters, low membership, and insufficient funds with which to pay a salaried executive, the NACGN accomplished little during its first two decades. Thus, as late as 1930 black nurses had not obtained membership in the ANA, were excluded from the vast majority of nurse training schools, and suffered employment discrimination. One black nurse succinctly described the NACGN's plight, "There was a great need for a program which would bring into clear focus the fact that Negro nurses not only needed better educational and employment opportunities, but that these needs were aggravated by racial bias."

In 1934 the NACGN secured grants from the Julius Rosenwald Fund and the General Education Board of the Rockefeller Foundation. The money enabled the organization to move into permanent headquarters at Rockefeller Center, where all the major national nursing organizations resided. More significantly, the grant enabled the NACGN to employ an executive secretary. The time was never more propitious. The reorganization brought together Staupers and Estelle Massey Riddle, two exceptionally talented black nurses who immediately

contacted the white nursing leaders of the ANA and the NLNE and who lobbied for the removal of discriminatory policies that denied black nurses membership in state professional organizations. Staupers served as the first executive secretary from 1934 to 1946, and Riddle reigned as president of the NACGN from 1934 to 1938. Riddle, a native of Palestine, Texas, had attended the Homer G. Phillips Hospital and Nurses Training School in St. Louis, Missouri. She moved to New York in 1927 and entered Teachers College, Columbia University, becoming the first black recipient of a Rosenwald Fund Fellowship for nurses and the first black woman nurse to earn an M.A. degree.

Staupers, born in Barbados, West Indies, in 1890, had migrated with her parents to New York in 1903. After graduating from Freedmen's Hospital School of Nursing in Washington, D.C., in 1917, Staupers began her professional career as a private duty nurse in New York City. She was instrumental in organizing the Booker T. Washington Sanatorium, the first facility in the Harlem area where black doctors could treat their patients. Later Staupers served for twelve years as the executive secretary of the Harlem Committee of the New York Tuberculosis and Health Association. When the opportunity came, she unhesitatingly embraced the challenge of rebuilding and leading the NACGN. An ardent integrationist and feminist, Staupers set as her prime objective the full integration of black women nurses into the mainstream of American nursing. It would take years before her dream became a reality.

The long and arduous struggle for the professional recognition and integration of black nurses into American nursing acquired new momentum and a heightened sense of urgency with the outbreak of World War II. Between 1934 and 1940 Staupers's efforts to win for black women nurses unfettered membership in the major professional associations, particularly on the state level, had been unsuccessful. Staupers resolved therefore to seize the opportunity created by the war emergency and the increased demand for nurses to project the plight of the black nurse into the national limelight. Fully cognizant of the discrimination and exclusion black nurses suffered in World War I, Staupers vowed that history would not be repeated. In a long letter to William H. Hastie, the black civilian aide to the secretary of war, Staupers laid bare the strategy of mobilizing both blacks and whites that she would pursue in the campaign to force the complete integration of black nurses into the total war effort. Staupers viewed the acceptance of black nurses into the Army and Navy Nurse Corps as critical to the achievement of her major objective, that is, the full integration of black women into American nursing. Fortunately, the NACGN was in a much stronger position to coordinate the struggle for inclusion than it had been during the previous world conflict. She confided to Hastie: "Although we know that pressure from Negro groups will mean something, nevertheless I am spending all of my time contacting white groups, especially nursing groups. I have a feeling that if enough white nursing organizations can register a protest and enough white organizations of influence other than nurses do the same, it will create in the minds of the people in the War Department the feeling that white people do not need protection in order to save themselves from being cared for by Negro personnel."

Staupers adopted this particular strategy in order to address simultaneously two interrelated concerns. She was fully cognizant that the white American public's appreciation for nurses and the status of the nursing profession as a whole increased sharply whenever the country was involved in a war. This had been especially true during World War I. Therefore, to improve the economic, social, and educational opportunities of black nurses and their relationship with the professional nursing establishment, Staupers had to make sure that the larger white society recognized and valued the contributions of black women nurses in the Army and Navy Nurse Corps because these agencies possessed high public visibility. If the white public, especially the armed forces nurse corps, approved of and accepted black women as competent and desirable nurses, then surely the white professional nursing groups would follow suit. Her strategy was further complicated by the fact that any struggle to win public support mandated that she also attract the allegiance of sympathetic white nurses within the nursing profession.

By the time of the Japanese attack on Pearl Harbor in December 1941, Staupers had already developed a sharp sense of political timing and possessed a finely tuned facility for strategic maneuvering. She had skillfully cultivated close interaction with white nursing leaders, and as a con-

sequence the NACGN's interests were well represented by its former president, Riddle, on the National Defense Council, which was renamed in 1942 the National Nursing Council for War Service. Staupers would continue to nurture her earlier long-term friendship with Congresswoman Frances Payne Bolton of Ohio, and before long she would make contact with First Lady Eleanor Roosevelt to solicit her assistance in the integration campaign. Also, as of 1940 Staupers had purposefully arranged for officers of the major civil rights organizations to be placed on the NACGN National Advisory Committee. Finally, Staupers appreciated the value of the black press and remained in constant communication with several black editors, sending them a constant stream of NACGN press releases.

Grants from various philanthropic foundations provided the money used for her continuous travel and feminist networking activities. Staupers logged thousands of miles, spoke with hundreds of black nurses, and wielded the NACGN into a powerful instrument for social change. She urged black nurses in major urban areas to form cells of local citizens, so that they could more effectively implement the programs and strategies designed at NACGN headquarters. The NACGN organized and sponsored regional institutes to which it invited key nursing figures, white and black, to discuss openly plans for further action. They particularly emphasized the need to arouse public support against the discrimination and segregation of black women nurses.

Plans to effect the complete integration of black women into the U.S. armed forces unfolded gradually as the war progressed. During the first year of peacetime mobilization, 1940–41, Staupers concentrated on preventing the exclusion of black women from the Army and Navy Nurse Corps; once the war began she fought to have abolished the quotas that had been established by the Army. Throughout 1943 and 1944 she challenged the Army's practice of assigning black nurses only to care for German prisoners of war and not to white American soldiers. In addition Staupers cooperated with other groups to ensure that legislative measures proposed in Congress concerning nurses and hospitals contained antidiscrimination clauses. In spite of the continuous NACGN pressure, the U.S. Navy proved to be unalterably opposed to the induction of black women into the Navy Nurse Corps.

The American Red Cross Nursing Service under the leadership of Mary Beard in 1939 was, as in World War I, designated the official agency for the procurement of nursing personnel for the armed services. In the summer of that year Virginia Dunbar, Beard's assistant director, contacted Staupers to formulate the requirements for black nurses who desired to serve in the armed forces nurse corps. As most black nurses residing in southern states were barred from membership in state nurses associations, Staupers and Dunbar agreed to consider membership in the NACGN an acceptable substitute. Dunbar expressed concern that large numbers of black women would decide not to enroll, the likelihood of which was great, considering the continued hostility many blacks harbored toward the American Red Cross. For example, Hastie and Granger both questioned the desirability of designating the Red Cross as the chief procurement agency for nursing personnel in the armed forces. They cited the Red Cross's policy of separating blood donated by blacks from that given by whites as an indication of the organization's racial bias. In spite of these reservations Staupers nevertheless urged Dunbar to send letters and application forms to all black nurses training schools, nurse superintendents, and hospitals. She appealed to Barnett to publicize the fact that black nurses should enroll in the Red Cross in order to enter Army service. She asserted with determination that "we will not be left out" this time.

In addition to membership in a professional nurses association, armed forces nurses were required to be between the ages of eighteen and thirty-five. Nurses were expected to be single, divorced, or widowed. Another set of stipulations required that the potential nurse corps recruit provide references of her good moral character. Nurses in the Army and Navy Corps received a lower initial salary than any other nurse in government employ.

In spite of these deterrents, and the fact that there was so much reluctance about recruiting them, black women responded well to the call. Approximately 350 black women enrolled in the Red Cross Nursing Service, anticipating appointment in the Army Nursing Corps. As it turned out, only 117 were judged eligible for the First Reserve. Many were eliminated because of marriage and age. Several other black enrollees saw their hopes of being inducted dashed against the wall of racial exclusion. In mid-1940 they received letters informing them that the Army did not have a program that would permit the utilization of the services of black nurses. A few of the black nurses angrily forwarded copies of the rejection letters to Staupers at NACGN headquarters. An incensed Staupers wrote Beard and railed against the hypocrisy of urging black women to join up and serve their country and then callously rejecting their applications. She exploded, "We fail to understand how America can say to the World that in this country we are ready to defend democracy when its Army and Navy is committed to a policy of discrimination." The die was cast. Clearly then, the next move was up to the Army.

On October 25, 1940, on the same day Secretary of War Henry Stimson appointed Hastie, then dean of the Howard University Law School, as his Civilian Aide on Negro Affairs, James C. Magee, surgeon general of the U.S. Army, had announced the War Department's "plan for the use of colored personnel." According to the policy statement separate black wards were to be designated in station hospitals where the number of black troops was sufficient to warrant separate facilities. In the South and Southwest, where the overwhelming percentage of black troops was located, several exclusively black hospitals were to be established: Camp Livingston in Louisiana, Fort Bragg in North Carolina, and Fort Huachuca in Arizona. The black wards and hospitals were to be manned entirely by black doctors, dentists, nurses, and attendants. In a later official clarification, Magee stated, "Where only a few of that race are to be hospitalized in any given hospital . . . it would . . . be poor economy to set aside separate wards for the segregation of such cases."

The black press, nursing organizations, and black physicians immediately rallied to protest the War Department's segregation policy. In defense of his position, Magee asserted that he "would not place white soldiers in the position where they would have to accept service from Negro professionals." The War Department from the very beginning disclaimed to be an "appropriate medium for effecting social adjustments." One War Department officer would later explain to Staupers that the racial segregation supported and practiced by the U.S. Army derived from the conviction that "men who are fulfilling the same obligations, suffering the same dislocation of their private lives, and wearing the identical uniform should, within the confines of the military establishment, have the same privileges for rest and relaxation" that they enjoyed at home.

Staupers and a group of black nurses requested a meeting with Julia O. Flikke, head of the Army Nurse Corps. A few weeks following the October announcement black nurses met with Flikke, Major General George F. Lull, the deputy surgeon general for the War Department, and Colonel Love. Both Love and Lull simply reiterated the official policy: black nurses in limited numbers would be called upon to serve black troops in segregated wards and in separate military hospitals. Staupers and the NACGN committee found themselves in a dilemma. They had envisioned a broader use of black women, and what had been offered fell far short of their desires. Yet it was better than total rejection. Consequently, the NACGN decided to accept, for the time being, the half-opened door. They reasoned that once a handful of black nurses penetrated, then they could intensify agitation for more complete integration. The group refused, however, to compromise on the second proposal. Love had asked if the NACGN would be willing to assume responsibility for the recruitment of black nurses for the Army Nurse Corps as the need arose. Staupers adamantly rejected the suggestion, reminding the colonel that such tasks were the responsibility of the American Red Cross Nursing Service of which black nurses were members.

Although the meeting resulted in very little change in official Army and War Department policy, nevertheless the NACGN's militant stance initiated later changes. Magee announced in January 1941 the Army's decision to recruit fifty-six black nurses who would be assigned to the black installations at Camp Livingston and Fort Bragg. Staupers, desiring to strengthen the NACGN and to present a semblance of advancement to her followers, quickly sought to capitalize upon the announced quota. She confided to Marion B. Seymour, the chairman of the NACGN's National Defense Committee, "I hope this story will get to

the newspapers as coming from this organization before [Walter White] gets a chance to claim credit for it after all the work we have done." She quickly sent press releases to the editors of the leading black newspapers: *Chicago Defender, Amsterdam News, New York Age, Pittsburgh Courier,* and the *Norfolk Journal and Guide.*

Although she desired to obtain credit for the NACGN for the announcement of the induction of black women nurses into the Army Nurse Corps, Staupers realized that the quota of fifty-six was a slap in the face. As she pointed out, the quota implied that black nurses were inferior to the other nurses. Quotas were both floors and ceilings. The important question, simply put, now became how could she secure the foundation yet raise the roof. Like many other black leaders, Staupers found herself in a double bind, being pulled in two directions: the first toward the elimination of segregation and discrimination, while in the second attempting to exploit to the fullest the possibilities for the use of black nurses within a segregated system. For the time being, however, she turned her attention to another matter and informed a nurse colleague, "Our next job is to see that our nurses are not segregated in those states where segregation is not approved by law."

Opportunity to fight for this objective came a few months later. In March 1941 members of the subcommittee on Negro health of the Health and Medical Committee of the National Defense Council met with Magee, all of the assistant surgeon generals, Brigadier General Fairbanks, Colonel Love, and civilian aide Hastie. The subcommittee on Negro health was composed of the black Chicago physician M. O. Bousfield, chair and director of Negro health of the Julius Rosenwald Fund; Russel Dixon, dean of the Howard University School of Dentistry; A. N. Vaughn, president of the black National Medical Association; Albert W. Dent, Dillard University president and superintendent of the black Flint-Goodridge Hospital in New Orleans, and Staupers. The subcommittee at Staupers's insistence strongly urged that the plan for segregated wards for black troops not be extended to areas outside the South. Staupers pointed out that blacks had made very substantial progress in civilian life in the integration of black patients and professionals into general hospitals. The subcommittee argued that "the extension of the segregated ward plan to many areas of the country would represent an unfortunate reversal of current trends."

The members spent much time discussing the quotas which called for, in addition to the 56 nurses, only 120 doctors and 44 dentists. They unanimously objected to the quotas as being disproportionately small even for the service of black troops stationed in the South. They implored Magee to use his influence in favor of an increase. Magee adamantly supported the official policy of "segregation without discrimination." The black press castigated the obdurate Magee. The *Philadelphia Tribune* editor observed, "It has become apparent to onlookers in Washington, that at least some of the difficulties which have been experienced by black professionals in the medical branches of the armed forces have their origin in the office of one man. He is Major General James C. Magee." Most members of the military bureaucracy staunchly adhered to the quota system. Magee was, of course, reflecting the views of his superiors in the War Department, which proved unyielding in its position. Robert P. Patterson, the under secretary of war, declared that in establishing separate units the War Department could not be judged guilty of any discrimination against black nurses or physicians. He maintained that "the Medical Department has not discriminated in any sense against the Negro medical professions, nurses, or enlisted men. It has assigned Negro personnel in keeping with War Department policy and provided field and service units in support of Negro troops with Negro Personnel." Patterson continued, smugly noting that for the first time in the history of the Army opportunity had been furnished the black medical profession and ancillary services "to exercise full professional talent through the establishment of separate departments at two of our large cantonment hospitals for the care of Negro soldiers."

Thus, as far as War Department officials were concerned, segregation, implying only separation, was nondiscriminatory if equal facilities were provided. Blacks, on the other hand, considered the concept of enforced segregation discriminatory. From their perspective separation prevented freedom of movement and produced inequalities of facilities and opportunities. Traditionally minority groups possessed few means of enforcing equality guarantees. Staupers, arguing from a black perspective, contended, "My position is that, as long as either one of the Services reject Negro nurses they are discriminated against and as long as either Services continue to assign them to duty as separate Units they are segregated."

Hastie in his function as civilian aide to the secretary of war tried valiantly to convince the War Department of the unfairness of quotas and segregation. He urged that these flaws be rectified or abolished before they became too entrenched. His carefully drafted recommendations for the desegregation of the Army were summarily rejected. According to one student of the era, the general staff took the point of view that Hastie wished the Army "to carry out a complete social revolution against the will of the nation." Days before the Japanese bombed Pearl Harbor Hastie and the Army's high command had reached an impasse. General George C. Marshall wrote in response to Hastie's desegregation memorandum, "The War Department cannot ignore the social relationships between negroes and whites which have been established by the American people through custom and habit." Marshall added that "either through lack of opportunity or other causes the level of intelligence and occupational skill of the negro population is considerably below that of the white." He predicted that were the Army to engage in social experiments only "danger to efficiency, discipline, and morale" would result. Finally, he observed that the Army had attained maximum strength by properly placing its personnel in accordance with individual capabilities. This racist response coupled with several other examples of blatant disregard for him and his recommendations left Hastie no alternative than to resign as civilian aide to the secretary of war. This he did on January 31, 1943.

However, compared to the position adopted by the U.S. Navy, the Army was a model of racial enlightenment. The Navy found unnecessary the establishment of quotas, for it held black women simply ineligible and undesirable for service in the Navy Nurse Corps. According to Lt. Commander Sue S. Dauser, superintendent of the Navy Nurse Corps, Navy nurses were special nurses. They combined the responsibilities and roles of teacher, counselor, dietist, laboratory technician, X-ray operator, bookkeeper, and confidante of the sick. The Navy nurse was required to instruct hospital corpsmen in modern nursing methods. In turn the men so taught would be responsible for the welfare of the patients in the sick bays of battleships, cruisers, destroyers, and other combat vessels to which members of the Nurse Corps were not assigned. While the Army nurse engaged in some teaching activity, this was considered incidental when compared to ward or bedside duties. In sum, a Navy nurse had to be a "tactful, clearminded administrator and teacher." Presumably black women were devoid of such qualities. Furthermore, there were very few black sailors in the Navy.

Yet midway through the war both the Army and Navy moved hesitatingly toward greater integration. Staupers received notice in 1943 that the Navy had decided, at last, to place the matter of inducting black nurses "under consideration." The Army, on the other hand, had raised its quota of black nurses to 160: 30 of them were assigned to foreign duty and another 31 were deployed to form a new separate unit at Fort Clark, Texas. These actions did not appease Staupers.

Frustrated by her inability to persuade the Navy and War Department to abolish quotas completely and to institute plans for the immediate and full integration of black nurses, Staupers resolved to present the case of the black nurses to America's First Lady. Shortly after she made contact with Eleanor Roosevelt, the First Lady sent discreet inquiries to Secretary of War Stimson and to Beard. She wrote, "I have several protests lately that due to the shortage of nurses, the colored nurses be allowed to serve where there is not serious objection to it." While Stimson's response was essentially defensive and noncommittal, Beard confessed that the American Red Cross Nursing Service had been "greatly concerned with the unequal treatment of qualified Negro nurses as compared with the white nurses" servicing in the armed forces. She reassured the First Lady that the National Nursing Council for War Service was attempting quietly to influence the assignment policy of the Army and Navy Nurse Corps. Elmira B. Wickenden, executive secretary of the National Council, offered similar reassurances. Indeed, the National Nursing council in late 1943 had sent the following resolution to the surgeons general of the Army and Navy

Medical Corps: "Be it resolved that Negro graduate registered nurses be appointed to the Army (or Navy) Nurse Corps on the same basis as any other American nurses who meet the professional requirements, as was done in the last war."

Staupers's patience had grown thin; she wanted results, not promises or resolutions. Propitiously, 1944 was a presidential election year. Staupers let it be known in the appropriate political circles that she was an avowed Roosevelt supporter and did not wish to make a fuss or "give any publicity to the present situation during this pre-election period." A friend, Anna Arnold Hedgeman, the executive secretary of A. Philip Randolph's National Council for a Permanent Fair Employment Practice Committee, interceded and suggested to Eleanor Roosevelt that she invite Staupers to meet with her.

Staupers and Roosevelt met in November 1944, whereupon the NACGN executive secretary described in detail the black nurses' relationship with the armed forces. She informed the First Lady that eighty-two black nurses were serving 150 patients at the Station Hospital at Fort Huachuca at a time when the Army was complaining of a dire nursing shortage. Staupers expounded at length on the practice of using black women to take care of German prisoners of war. She asked, rhetorically, if this was to be the special role of the black nurse in the war. Staupers elaborated, "When our women hear of the great need for nurses in the Army and when they enter the Service it is with the high hopes that they will be used to nurse sick and wounded soldiers who are fighting our country's enemies and not primarily to care for these enemies." Roosevelt, apparently moved by the discussion, applied her own subtle pressure to Norman T. Kirk, surgeon general of the U.S. Army, Secretary Stimson, and the Navy's Rear Admiral W. J. C. Agnew.

As 1944 faded into 1945, events on the black nursing front took a sudden upswing. In early January 1945, Kirk announced to a crowd of three hundred nurses, politicians, and private citizens assembled at the Hotel Pierre in New York City that in order for the Army to be adequately supplied with nurses it might be advisable to institute a draft. Staupers immediately rose to her feet and pointedly asked the surgeon general, "If nurses are needed so desperately, why isn't the Army using colored nurses?" She continued, "Of 9,000 registered Negro nurses the Army has taken 247, the Navy takes none." Kirk, visibly uncomfortable according to press reports, replied, "There are 7,000 Negro nurses in comparison to a 200,000 total in the United States. I believe that the average share of colored nurses in the army is equal to the total number of Negro troops." News of the exchange received nationwide coverage and made the headlines of virtually every black newspaper in the country. The *Boston Guardian* declared, "It is difficult to find calm words to describe the folly which color prejudice assumes in the desperate shortage of nurses." The editor anticipated the kind of future action that occurred when he predicted that "the Commander-in-chief will be backed up in this instance by the great majority of the people if he orders a cessation of the outrageous ban on nurses because of skin color and thus helps to modernize the armed forces by ridding them of the fogyism which is the greatest barrier to national growth."

Compounding the tension surrounding the Kirk-Staupers incident, on January 6, 1945, in a radio-transmitted address to the U.S. Congress, President Roosevelt announced his strong desire for the enactment of legislation amending the Selective Service Act of 1940 to provide for the induction of nurses into the Army. He justified the need for such legislation on the grounds that volunteering had not produced the number of nurses required. Roosevelt adopted this position over the objections of Chief of Staff Marshall and Major General Stephen G. Henry, both of whom advised that the proposed legislation would be "most discriminatory in that it singles out a small group of especially trained women for induction under the Selective Service Act." As if on cue, however, Representative Andrew J. May (Democrat, Kentucky) introduced the Draft Nurse Bill, H. R. 1284 79th Congress, on January 9, 1945, and it was immediately referred to the Committee on Military Affairs.

An ensuing public outcry quickly forthcoming and totally unexpected jarred the military brass. Roosevelt apparently had not the slightest appreciation for the depth of public dissatisfaction with the restrictive quotas for black nurses. Staupers with alacrity sought to harness, direct, and channel the wave of public anger and sympathy. She urged black nurses, women's groups, and sympathetic

white allies across the country to send telegrams directly to Roosevelt and May, protesting the exclusion, discrimination, and segregation of black nurses. Staupers in numerous press releases pleaded, "We stress again for the Negro nurses all over the country that they rally now as never before to the support of the NACGN." And rally they did. The sheer hypocrisy of calling for a draft of nurses while excluding large numbers of black nurses willing to serve was too much for many Americans to swallow. Telegrams poured into the White House from the NAACP, the Catholic Interracial Council, National Nursing Council for War Services, Congress of Industrial Organizations, American Federation of Labor, National YWCA Board, the Alpha Kappa Alpha Sorority, the Philadelphia Fellowship Commission, the New York Citizens' Committee of the Upper West Side, the National Negro Congress, National Council of Negro Women, the United Council of Church Women, and the American Civil Liberties Union. From Cleveland, Jane Edna Hunter, president of the Ohio State Federation of Colored Women's Club and former nurse, in a telegram to the president declared: "If the proposal to draft nurses must be resorted to, then we urge that all inductees be given consideration on bases of training and fitness and allowed to serve in all branches of the Army and Navy and not restricted to Negro soldiers alone."

Buried beneath the avalanche of telegrams and seared by the heat of an inflamed public, Kirk, Agnew, and the War Department declared an end to quotas and exclusion. On January 20, 1945, Kirk stated that nurses would be accepted into the Army Nurse Corps without regard to race. On January 25, 1945, Admiral Agnew announced that the Navy Nurse Corps was now open to black women, and a few weeks later Phyllis Dailey became the first black woman to break the color barrier and receive induction into the Navy Nurse Corps. There was no outcry against the accepting of black nurses into the armed forces nurse corps.

Eventually the War Department decided to stop the entire scheme to enact a draft of nurses. Staupers's carefully orchestrated telegram campaign and tedious years of continuous effort had culminated in the breaking of at least this one link in the chain that oppressed, excluded, and prohibited black women from the full realization of their civil rights.

This was by no means the end of their war. It was, however, a welcome victory in what had been a long struggle overwhelmingly characterized by defeat, setbacks, humiliation, and frustration. The proposed nurse draft legislation and ensuing congressional debate had been the catalytic component to which Staupers and black nurses had joined their struggle for full integration into the armed forces. Presidential and congressional speeches bemoaning the shortage of nurses had only fed the fire that Staupers's public protests had generated. While Staupers and black nurses may have supported in principle the nurse draft legislation, they nevertheless used it to draw attention to the fact that they had been excluded, segregated, and discriminated against. She displayed a flawless sense of timing and political maneuvering.

The battle to integrate black women nurses into the Army and Navy Nurse Corps had been an exhaustive and draining one. In 1946 Staupers relinquished her position as executive secretary to take a much-needed and well-earned rest. This was to be of short duration, however, for Staupers considered her work incomplete. She had not accomplished her major objective, the integration of black women into the ANA. Beginning in 1934, Staupers and Riddle had appeared before the House of Delegates at the biennial meeting of the ANA. After ten years of fruitless persistence, Staupers wrote Congresswoman Bolton, "Each year although we have not gained our ultimate objective we have gained friends and are in a stronger position than ever before." After the 1944 meeting Staupers confided to Bolton her hope that "integration may be an accomplished fact before 1945."

General integration into the ANA did not come in 1945. It came three years later. In 1948 the ANA House of Delegates opened the gates to black membership, appointed a black woman nurse as assistant executive secretary in its national headquarters, and witnessed the election of Riddle to the board of directors.

For Staupers, the breakdown of the exclusion barriers was a triumphant vindication of her leadership role. In 1950 Staupers, now president of the NACGN, convinced black nurses that the purpose for which the organization had been established had now been achieved and that it was time to dissolve the NACGN. Staupers wrote in a press release dated January 26, 1951, that as far as was known the NACGN was the first major black national organization to terminate its work "because it feels that its program of activities is no longer necessary." She continued, "The doors have been opened," and the black nurse "has been given a seat in the top councils." Staupers later exulted, "We are now a part of the great organization of nurses, the American Nurses' Association."

Staupers received many accolades for her leadership in the integration fight and in the dissolution of the NACGN. By far the crowning acknowledgment and recognition of Staupers's role and contribution in the quest of black nurses for civil rights and human dignity came from a rather unexpected source. The Spingarn Award Committee of the NACGN chose Staupers to be the recipient of the Spingarn Medal for 1951. Channing H. Tobias, director of the Phelps-Stokes Fund, confided to Staupers, "I know the committee was especially appreciative of the fact that you were willing to sacrifice organization to ideals when you advocated and succeeded in realizing the full integration of Negro nurses into the organized ranks of the nursing profession of this country."

Mabel Keaton Staupers was one of the truly outstanding black women leaders in this century. The key identifying characteristic of her leadership style was the establishment of close working relationships with leading white women, black male heads of organizations, and fellow black women nurses. She secured her base first, that is, the NACGN, by maintaining continuous communication and contact with the membership. Staupers furthermore manipulated the press extremely well by releasing statements at the most strategic moment. Her public remarks unfailingly emphasized the cause for which she was fighting. In so doing she constantly reminded the country of the plight of black women nurses, of the racism and sexism that robbed them of the opportunities to develop their full human potential. Small of frame, energetic, and fast talking, Staupers knew when to accept a half-loaf of advancement and when to press on for total victory. It is unlikely that the successful integration of black women into American nursing on all levels could have been accomplished during the 1940s without Staupers at the helm of the NACGN.

SOURCES

I wish to thank Professors Leonora Woodman and Harold D. Woodman of Purdue University and William C. Hine of South Carolina State College for their thoughtful comments and thorough reading of earlier drafts of this essay. I also thank the Rockefeller Foundation, the Eleanor Roosevelt Institute, and the Rockefeller Foundation Archive Center for research grants.

UNPUBLISHED SOURCES

American Red Cross Manuscript Collection. National Archives, Washington, D.C.

Claude Barnett Papers. Chicago Historical Society, Chicago, Ill.

Frances Payne Bolton Papers. Western Reserve Historical Society, Cleveland, Ohio.

National Association of Colored Graduate Nurses Collection. New York Public Library, Schomburg Afro-American History Collection, New York, N.Y.

Eleanor Roosevelt Papers. Franklin Delano Roosevelt Library, Hyde Park, N.Y.

Rosenwald Fund Papers. Fisk University Library, Nashville, Tenn.

Mabel Keaton Staupers Papers. Amistad Research Center, New Orleans, La.

Mabel Keaton Staupers Papers. Moorland-Spingarn Research Center, Howard University, Washington, D.C.

Records of the Surgeon General's Office of the U.S. Army. National Archives Research Center, Suitland, Md.

Records of the War Department, General and Special Staff. National Archives Reseach Center, Suitland, Md.

PUBLISHED SOURCES

Staupers, Mabel Keaton, *No Time for Prejudice: A Story of the Integration of Negroes in Nursing in the United States.* New York: Macmillan Co., 1961.

Thoms, Adah B. *Pathfinders: A History of Progress of Colored Graduate Nurses.* New York: McKay, 1929.

Bibliography
Index

BIBLIOGRAPHY

GENERAL

Cott, Nancy F. *The Bonds of Womanhood: "Woman's Sphere" in New England, 1780–1835.* New Haven: Yale University Press, 1977.

Cutright, Phillips, and Shorter, Edward. "The effects of health on the completed fertility of nonwhite and white U.S. women." *Journal of Social History,* 1979, *13:* 191–217.

Degler, Carl. *At Odds: Women and the Family in America from the Revolution to the Present.* New York: Oxford University Press, 1980.

Ehrenreich, Barbara, and English, Deirdre. *Complaints and Disorders: The Sexual Politics of Sickness.* Old Westbury, N.Y.: Feminist Press, 1973.

Ehrenreich, Barbara, and English, Deirdre. *For Her Own Good: 150 Years of the Experts' Advice to Women.* New York: Anchor Press/Doubleday, 1978.

Fee, Elizabeth. "Nineteenth-century craniology: the study of the female skull." *Bulletin of the History of Medicine,* 1979, *53:* 415–33.

Hartman, Mary, and Banner, Lois, eds. *Clio's Consciousness Raised: New Perspectives on the History of Women.* New York: Harper & Row, 1974.

Kern, Stephan. *Anatomy and Destiny: A Cultural History of the Human Body.* Indianapolis: Bobbs-Merrill, 1975.

Leavitt, Judith Walzer, and Numbers, Ronald L. *Sickness and Health in America: Readings in the History of Medicine and Public Health.* Madison: University of Wisconsin Press, 1978.

Reverby, Susan, and Rosner, David, eds. *Health Care in America: Essays in Social History.* Philadelphia: Temple University Press, 1979.

Rothman, Sheila M. *Woman's Proper Place: A History of Changing Ideals and Practices, 1870 to the Present.* New York: Basic Books, 1978.

Shorter, Edward. *A History of Women's Bodies.* New York: Basic Books, 1982.

Verbrugge, Martha H. "Women and medicine in nineteenth-century America." *Signs,* 1976, *1:* 957–72.

SEXUALITY

Barker-Benfield, G. J. *The Horrors of the Half-Known Life: Male Attitudes Toward Women and Sexuality in 19th Century America.* New York: Harper, 1976.

Bullough, Vern L. *Sexual Variance in Society and History.* Chicago: University of Chicago Press, 1981.

Bullough, Vern L. "Technology and female sexuality and physiology: some implications." *Journal of Sex Research,* 1980, *16:* 59–71.

Bullough, Vern, and Bullough, Bonnie. "Lesbianism in the 1920s and 1930s: a newfound study." *Signs,* 1977, *2:* 895–904.

Bullough, Vern L., and Bullough, Bonnie. *Sin, Sickness, and Sanity: A History of Sexual Attitudes.* New York: New American Library, 1977.

Bullough, Vern L., and Voght, Martha. "Homosexuality and its confusion with the secret sin in pre-Freudian America." *Journal of the History of Medicine and Allied Sciences* 28 (April 1973).

Burnham, John C. "American historians and the subject of sex." *Societas* 2 (Aug. 1972): 307–16.

Cook, Blanche Wiesen. "Female support networks and political activism: Lillian Wald, Crystal Eastman and Emma Goldman." *Chrysalis,* 1977, no. 3: 43–61.

Ditzion, Sidney. *Marriage, Morals, and Sex in America: A History of Ideas.* New York: W. W. Norton, 1953, 1969.

Dubois, Ellen Carol, and Gordon, Linda. "Seeking ecstasy on the battlefield: danger and pleasure in nineteenth-century feminist sexual thought." *Feminist Studies*, 1983, *9:* 7–25.

Engelhardt, H. Tristram, Jr. "The disease of masturbation: values and the concept of disease." *Bulletin of the History of Medicine*, 1974, *48:* 234–48.

Faderman, Lillian. *Surpassing the Love of Men: Romantic Friendship and Love between Women from the Renaissance to the Present.* New York: William Morrow, 1981.

Foster, Lawrence. *Religion and Sexuality: Three American Communal Experiments of the Nineteenth Century.* New York: Oxford University Press, 1981.

Haller, John, and Haller, Robin. *The Physician and Sexuality in Victorian America.* Urbana: University of Illinois Press, 1974.

Hollander, Mark. "The medical profession and sex in 1900." *American Journal of Obstetrics*, 1970, *108:* 139–48.

Kern, Louis J. "Ideology and reality: sexuality and woman's status in the Oneida Community." *Radical History Review*, 1979, *20:* 180–205.

Kern, Louis J. *An Ordered Love: Sex Roles and Sexuality in Victorian Utopias—The Shakers, the Mormons, and the Oneida Community.* Chapel Hill: University of North Carolina Press, 1981.

Kushner, Howard I. "Nineteenth-century sexuality and the 'Sexual Revolution' of the Progressive Era." *Canadian Review of American Studies* 9 (Spring 1978): 34–49.

Leach, William. *True Love and Perfect Union: The Feminist Reform of Sex and Society.* New York: Basic Books, 1980.

Morgan, Edmund S. "The Puritans and sex." *New England Quarterly*, 1942, *15:* 591–607.

Muncy, Raymond Lee. *Sex and Marriage in Utopian Communities: Nineteenth-Century America.* Bloomington: Indiana University Press, 1973.

Perry, Lewis. "'Progress, not pleasure, is our aim': the sexual advice of an antebellum radical." *Journal of Social History*, 1979: *12:* 354–66.

Pivar, David J. *Purity Crusade: Sexual Morality and Social Control 1868–1900.* Westport, Conn.: Greenwood Press, 1973.

Rosenberg, Charles E. "Sexuality, Class and Role in 19th-Century America." *American Quarterly*, 1973, *25:* 131–53.

Ryan, Mary P. "The power of women's networks: a case study of female moral reform in antebellum America." *Feminist Studies*, 1979, *5:* 66–85.

Sahli, Nancy. "Sexuality in 19th- and 20th-century America: the sources and their problems." *Radical History Review*, 1979, *20:* 89–96.

Sahli, Nancy. "Smashing: women's relationships before the Fall." *Chrysalis* 8 (Summer 1979): 17–28.

Sears, Hal D. *The Sex Radicals: Free Love in High Victorian America.* Lawrence: Regents Press of Kansas, 1977.

Shade, William G. "'A mental passion': female sexuality in Victorian America," *International Journal of Women's Studies* 1 (Jan.–Feb. 1978).

Tyor, Peter L. "'Denied the power to choose the good': sexuality and mental defect in American medical practice, 1850–1920." *Journal of Social History* 10 (June 1977): 473–75.

Walters, Ronald G., ed. *Primers for Prudery: Sexual Advice to Victorian America.* Englewood Cliffs, N.J.: Prentice-Hall, 1974.

Walters, Ronald G. "Sexual matters as historical problems: a framework of analysis." *Societas* 6 (Summer 1976): 157–75.

BIRTH CONTROL

Acevedo, Zoila. "Abortion in early America." *Women and Health*, 1979, *4:* 159–67.

Brooks, Carol Flora. "The early history of the anti-contraceptive laws in Massachusetts and Connecticut." *American Quarterly*, 1966, *18:* 4–23.

Gordon, Linda. "The long struggle for reproductive rights." *Radical America*, 1981, *15:* 75–88.

Gordon, Linda. *Woman's Body, Woman's Right: A Social History of Birth Control in America.* New York: Grossman, 1976.

Himes, Norman E. *Medical History of Contraception.* Baltimore: Williams & Wilkins, 1936. Reprinted by Schocken Books, 1970.

Hoffer, Peter C., and Hall, N. E. H. *Murdering Mothers: Infanticide in England and New England, 1558–1803.* New York: New York University Press, 1981.

Katz, Michael B., and Stern, Mark J. "Fertility, class, and industrial capitalism: Erie County, New York, 1855–1915." *American Quarterly* 33 (Spring 1981): 63–70.

Kennedy, David. *Birth Control in America: The Career of Margaret Sanger.* New Haven: Yale University Press, 1970.

Mohr, James C. *Abortion in America: The Origins and Evolution of National Policy, 1800–1900.* New York: Oxford University Press, 1978.

Reed, James. *From Private Vice to Public Virtue: The Birth Control Movement and American Society since 1830.* New York: Basic Books, 1978. Reprinted under the title *The Birth Control Movement and American Society* by Princeton University Press, 1983.

Sauer, R. "Attitudes to abortion in America, 1800–1973." *Population Studies,* 1974, *28:* 53–67.

Smith, Daniel Scott, and Hindus, Michael S. "Premarital pregnancy in America, 1640–1971: an overview and interpretation." *Journal of Interdisciplinary History* 5 (Spring 1975): 537–70.

Vecoli, Rudolph J. "Sterilization: progressive measure?" *Wisconsin Magazine of History,* 1960, *43:* 190–202.

Weiner, Nella Fermi. "Of feminism and birth control propaganda (1790–1840)." *International Journal of Women's Studies* 3 (Sept./Oct. 1980): 411–30.

Williams, Donne, and Williams, Greer. *Every Child a Wanted Child: Clarence James Gamble, MD, and His Work in the Birth Control Movement.* Boston: Distributed by Harvard University Press, for the Francis A. Countway Library of Medicine, 1978.

Yates, Wilson. "Birth control literature and the medical profession in nineteenth-century America." *Journal of the History of Medicine and Allied Sciences* 31 (Jan. 1976), 42–54.

CHILDBIRTH

Antler, Joyce, and Fox, Daniel M. "The movement toward a safe maternity: physician accountability in New York City, 1915–1940." *Bulletin of the History of Medicine,* 1976, *50:* 569–95.

Bogdan, Janet. "Care or cure? childbirth practices in 19th-century America." *Feminist Studies,* 1978, *4:* 92–99.

Devitt, Neal. "The statistical case for elimination of the midwife: fact versus prejudice, 1890–1935." *Women and Health,* 1979, *4:* 81–96, 169–86.

Devitt, Neal. "The transition from home to hospital birth in the United States, 1930–1960." *Birth and the Family Journal* 4 (Summer 1977): 47–58.

Duffy, John. "Anglo-American reaction to obstetrical anesthesia." *Bulletin of the History of Medicine,* 1964, *38:* 32–44.

Dye, Nancy Schrom. "Review essay: history of childbirth in America." *Signs,* 1980, *6:* 97–108.

Eshleman, Michael. "Diet during pregnancy in the sixteenth and seventeenth centuries." *Journal of the History of Medicine,* 1975, *30, no. 1:* 23–29.

Leavitt, Judith Walzer. "'Science' enters the birthing room: obstetrics in America since the eighteenth century." *Journal of American History,* 70 (September 1983): 281–304.

Longo, Lawrence D. "Obstetrics and gynecology," in *The Education of American Physicians: Historical Essays,* ed. Ronald L. Numbers. Berkeley: University of California Press, 1980. Pp. 205–25.

Longo, Lawrence D., and Thomson, Christina M. "Prenatal care and its evolution in America," in *Childbirth: The Beginning of Motherhood, Proceedings of the Second Motherhood Symposium,* ed. Sophie Colleau. Madison: Women's Studies Research Center, 1982. Pp. 29–70.

Miller, Lawrence G. "Pain, parturition, and the profession: twilight sleep in America," in *Health Care in America: Essays in Social History,* ed. Susan Reverby and David Rosner. Philadelphia: Temple University Press, 1979.

Moseley, Caroline. "Nineteenth-century songs of childbirth, childhood and motherhood," in *Childbirth: The Beginning of Motherhood, Proceedings of the Second Motherhood Symposium,* ed. Sophie Colleau. Madison: Women's Studies Research Center, 1982. Pp. 173–92.

Rich, Adrienne. *Of Woman Born: Motherhood as Experience and Institution.* New York: W.W. Norton, 1976.

Romalis, Shelly, ed. *Childbirth: Alternatives to Medical Control.* Austin: University of Texas Press, 1981.

Siddall, A. Clair. "Bloodletting in American obstetric practice, 1800–1945." *Bulletin of the History of Medicine,* 1980, *54:* 101–10.

Wertz, Richard W., and Wertz, Dorothy C. *Lying-*

In: A History of Childbirth in America. New York: Free Press, 1977.

DISEASES AND TREATMENTS

Burnham, John C. "Medical inspection of prostitutes in America in the nineteenth century: the St. Louis experiment and its sequel." *Bulletin of the History of Medicine,* 1971, *45, no. 3:* 203–18.

Curtis, Joy, and Curtis, Bruce. "Illness and the Victorian lady: the case of Jeannie Sumner." *International Journal of Women's Studies,* 1981, *4:* 527–**43.**

Duffy, John. "Masturbation and clitoridectomy." *Journal of the American Medical Association* 186 (Oct. 19, 1963): 166–68.

Figlio, Karl. "Chlorosis and chronic disease in nineteenth-century Britain: the social constitution of somatic illness in a capitalist society." *Social History,* 1978, *3:* 167–97. See a revised version of this paper in *International Journal of Health Services,* 1978, *8:* 589–617.

Freedman, Estelle B. *Their Sisters' Keepers: Women's Prison Reform in America, 1830–1930.* Ann Arbor: University of Michigan Press, 1981.

Hudson, Robert. "The biography of disease: lessons from chlorosis." *Bulletin of the History of Medicine,* 1977, *51:* 448–63.

Sicherman, Barbara. "The uses of a diagnosis: doctors, patients and neurasthenia." *Journal of the History of Medicine and Allied Sciences,* 1977, *32:* 33–54.

Siddall, A. Clair. "Chlorosis—etiology reconsidered." *Bulletin of the History of Medicine,* 1982, *56:* 254–60.

Smith-Rosenberg, Carroll. "From puberty to menopause: the cycle of femininity in nineteenth-century America," in *Clio's Consciousness Raised,* ed. Mary Hartman and Lois Banner. New York: Harper & Row, 1974.

Smith-Rosenberg, Carroll. "The hysterical woman: sex roles and role conflict in 19th-century America." *Social Research,* 1972, *39:* 652–78.

Stage, Sarah. *Female Complaints: Lydia Pinkham and the Business of Women's Medicine.* New York: W. W. Norton, 1979.

MIDWIVES

Donegan, Jane B. *Women and Men Midwives: Medicine, Morality, and Misogyny in Early America.* Westport, Conn.: Greenwood Press, 1978.

Ehrenreich, Barbara, and English, Deirdre. *Witches, Midwives, and Nurses: A History of Women Healers.* Old Westbury, N.Y.: Feminist Press, 1973.

Ferguson, James H. "Mississippi midwives." *Journal of the History of Medicine,* 1950, *5:* 85–95.

Forbes, Thomas R. "Midwifery and witchcraft." *Journal of the History of Medicine,* 1962, *17:* 264–83.

Litoff, Judy Barrett. *American Midwives 1860 to the Present.* Westport, Conn.: Greenwood Press, 1978.

HEALTH REFORMERS

Carter, Richard. *The Gentle Legions.* New York: Doubleday, 1961.

Fellman, Anita Clair, and Fellman, Michael. *Making Sense of Self: Medical Advice Literature in Late-Nineteenth-Century America.* Philadelphia: University of Pennsylvania Press, 1981.

Himelhoch, Myra Samuels, with Arthur H. Shaffer. "Elizabeth Packard: nineteenth-century crusader for the rights of mental patients." *Journal of American Studies,* 1979, *13:* 343–75.

Hoy, Suellen M. "'Municipal housekeeping': the role of women in improving urban sanitation practices, 1880–1917," in *Pollution and Reform in American Cities,* ed. Martin Melosi. Austin: University of Texas Press, 1980. Pp. 173–98.

Johnson, James. "The role of women in the founding of the U.S. Children's Bureau," in *"Remember the Ladies": New Perspectives on Women in American History,* ed. Carol V. R. George. Syracuse: Syracuse University Press, 1975. Pp. 179–96.

Marshall, Helen E. *Dorothea Dix: Forgotten Samaritan.* Chapel Hill: University of North Carolina Press, 1973.

McCarthy, Kathleen D. *Noblesse Oblige: Charity and Cultural Philanthropy in Chicago, 1849–1929.* Chicago: University of Chicago Press, 1982.

Numbers, Ronald L. *Prophetess of Health: A Study of Ellen G. White.* New York: Harper & Row, 1976.

Sklar, Kathryn Kish. *Catharine Beecher: A Study in American Domesticity.* New Haven: Yale University Press, 1973.

Verbrugge, Martha H. "The social meaning of personal health: the Ladies' Physiological Institute of Boston and Vicinity in the 1850s," in

Health Care in America: Essays in Social History, ed. Susan Reverby and David Rosner. Philadelphia: Temple University Press, 1979. Pp. 45–66.

Vertinsky, Patricia. "Sexual equality and the legacy of Catharine Beecher." *Journal of Sport History* 6 (Spring 1979): 38–49.

Whorton, James. *Crusaders for Fitness: The History of American Health Reformers.* Princeton: Princeton University Press, 1982.

PHYSICIANS

Blake, John B. "Women and medicine in antebellum America." *Bulletin of the History of Medicine,* 1965, *39:* 99–123.

Chaff, Sandra L.; Haimbach, Ruth; Fenichel, Carol; and Woodside, Nina B., eds. *Women in Medicine: A Bibliography of the Literature on Women Physicians.* Metuchen, N.J.: Scarecrow Press, 1977.

Drachman, Virginia. "Female solidarity and professional success: the dilemma of women doctors in late-nineteenth-century America." *Journal of Social History* 15 (Summer 1982): 607–19.

Harris, Barbara. *Beyond Her Sphere: Women and the Professions in American History.* Westport, Conn.: Greenwood Press, 1978.

Kaufman, Martin. "The admission of women to nineteenth-century American medical societies." *Bulletin of the History of Medicine,* 1976, *50:* 251–60.

King, John W., and King, Caroline R. "Early women physicians in Vermont." *Bulletin of the History of Medicine,* 1951, *25:* 429–41.

Morantz, Regina Markell. "The 'connecting link': the case for the woman doctor in 19th-century America," in *Sickness and Health in America: Readings in the History of Medicine and Public Health,* ed. Judith Walzer Leavitt and Ronald L. Numbers. Madison: University of Wisconsin Press, 1978. Pp. 117–28.

Morantz, Regina Markell. "Morality vs. science: the views of Elizabeth Blackwell and Mary Putnam Jacobi." *American Quarterly,* forthcoming.

Morantz, Regina Markell; Pomerleau, Cynthia Stodola; and Fenichel, Carol Hansen, eds. *In Her Own Words: Oral Histories of Women Physicians.* Westport, Conn.: Greenwood Press, 1982.

Shryock, Richard Harrison. "Women in American Medicine." *Journal of the American Medical Women's Association* 5 (Sept. 1950): 371–79.

Walsh, Mary Roth. *"Doctors Wanted: No Women Need Apply": Sexual Barriers in the Medical Profession.* New Haven: Yale University Press, 1978.

NURSES

Ashley, JoAnn. *Hospitals, Paternalism, and the Role of the Nurse.* New York: Teachers College Press, 1976.

Bullough, Vern, and Bullough, Bonnie. *The Care of the Sick: The Emergence of Modern Nursing.* London: Croom Helm, 1979.

Bullough, Vern L.; Bullough, Bonnie; and Elcano, Barrett. *Nursing: A Historical Bibliography.* New York: Garland, 1981.

Davies, C., ed. *Rewriting Nursing History.* London: Croom Helm; Totowa, N.J.: Barnes & Noble, 1980.

James, Janet Wilson. "Isabel Hampton and the professionalization of nursing in the 1890s," in *The Therapeutic Revolution: Essays in the Social History of American Medicine,* ed. Morris Vogel and Charles Rosenberg. Philadelphia: University of Pennsylvania Press, 1979. Pp. 201–44.

Kalish, Phillip, and Kalish, Beatrice. *The Advance of American Nursing.* Boston: Little, Brown, 1978.

Lagemann, Ellen Condliffe, ed. *Nursing History: New Perspectives, New Possibilities.* New York: Teachers College Press, 1983.

Marshall, Helen E. *Mary Adelaide Nutting: Pioneer of Modern Nursing.* Baltimore: Johns Hopkins University Press, 1972.

Melosh, Barbara. *"The Physician's Hand": Work Culture and Conflict in American Nursing.* Philadelphia: Temple University Press, 1982.

Mottus, Jane E. *New York Nightingales: The Emergence of the Nursing Profession at Bellevue and New York Hospital, 1850–1920.* Ann Arbor, Mich.: UMI Research Press, 1980.

Reverby, Susan. *One Strong Voice . . . A Brief History of Women Health Workers and Their Changing Role.* Bread and Roses Project, District 1199, National Union of Hospital and Health Care Employees/RWDSU/AFL-CIO.

Reverby, Susan. "The search for the hospital yardstick: nursing and the rationalization of hospital work," in *Health Care in America: Essays in Social History,* ed. Susan Reverby and David Rosner. Philadelphia: Temple University Press, 1979. Pp. 206–225.

Safier, Gwendolyn. *Contemporary American Leaders in Nursing: An Oral History.* New York: McGraw-Hill, 1977.

Sanes, Samuel. "Elizabeth Blackwell: her first medical publication." *Bulletin of the History of Medicine,* 1944, *16:* 83–88.

Santos, Elvin H., and Stainbrook, Edward. "A history of psychiatric nursing in the nineteenth century." *Journal of the History of Medicine,* 1949, *4:* 48–74.

Shryock, Richard Harrison. "Nursing emerges as a profession: the American experience." *Clio Medica,* 1968, *3:* 131–147.

INDEX

Prepared by Lisa MacPherson

COMPOSED BY GRAPHIC COMPOSITION, INC.
ATHENS, GEORGIA
MANUFACTURED BY FAIRFIELD GRAPHICS
FAIRFIELD, PENNSYLVANIA
TEXT AND DISPLAY LINES ARE SET IN BASKERVILLE

Library of Congress Cataloging in Publication Data
Main entry under title:

Women and health in America.

Bibliography: pp. 509–514.
Includes index.
1. Women—Health and hygiene—United States—History
Addresses, essays, lectures. 2. Women—United States—
Sexual behavior—History—Addresses, essays, lectures.
3. Women—Diseases—United States—History—Addresses,
essays, lectures. 4. Women in medicine—United States—
History—Addresses, essays, lectures. I. Leavitt,
Judith Walzer. [DNLM: 1. History of medicine, Modern—
United States. 2. Women—History—United States.
3. Gynecology—History—United States. 4. Obstetrics—
History—United States. 5. Health occupations—History
—United States. 6. Family planning—History—United
States. WZ 70 AA1 W8]
RA778.W744 1984   362.1′088042   83-40267
ISBN 0-299-09640-8
ISBN 0-299-09644-0 (pbk.)